general urology

general urology

8th
EDITION

DONALD R. SMITH, MD

Professor of Urology and
Chairman of the Division of Urology
University of California School of Medicine
San Francisco

Consulting Urologist, San Francisco General Hospital
Consulting Surgeon (Urology)
Veterans Administration Hospital, San Francisco

Los Altos, California   **LANGE Medical Publications**

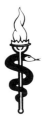

A Concise Medical Library for Practitioner and Student

General Urology, 8th ed. $11.00

Current Medical Diagnosis & Treatment 1975 (annual revision). Edited by M.A. Krupp and M.J. Chatton. 1044 pp.	1975
Current Pediatric Diagnosis & Treatment, 3rd ed. Edited by C.H. Kempe, H.K. Silver, and D. O'Brien. 1020 pp, *illus.*	1974
Current Surgical Diagnosis & Treatment, 2nd ed. Edited by J.E. Dunphy and L.W. Way. 1123 pp, *illus.*	1975
Review of Physiological Chemistry, 15th ed. H.A. Harper. 570 pp, *illus.*	1975
Review of Medical Physiology, 7th ed. W.F. Ganong. 587 pp, *illus.*	1975
Review of Medical Microbiology, 11th ed. E. Jawetz, J.L. Melnick, and E.A. Adelberg. 528 pp, *illus.*	1974
Review of Medical Pharmacology, 4th ed. F.H. Meyers, E. Jawetz, and A. Goldfien. 721 pp, *illus.*	1974
General Ophthalmology, 7th ed. D. Vaughan and T. Asbury. 334 pp, *illus.*	1974
Correlative Neuroanatomy & Functional Neurology, 15th ed. J.G. Chusid. 429 pp, *illus.*	1973
Principles of Clinical Electrocardiography, 8th ed. M.J. Goldman. 400 pp, *illus.*	1973
Handbook of Psychiatry, 3rd ed. Edited by P. Solomon and V.D. Patch. 706 pp.	1974
Handbook of Surgery, 5th ed. Edited by J.L. Wilson. 877 pp, *illus.*	1973
Handbook of Obstetrics & Gynecology, 5th ed. R.C. Benson. 770 pp, *illus.*	1974
Physician's Handbook, 17th ed. M.A. Krupp, N.J. Sweet, E. Jawetz, E.G. Biglieri, and R.L. Roe. 728 pp, *illus.*	1973
Handbook of Medical Treatment, 14th ed. Edited by M.J. Chatton. 640 pp.	1974
Handbook of Pediatrics, 11th ed. H.K. Silver, C.H. Kempe, and H.B. Bruyn. 710 pp, *illus.*	1975
Handbook of Poisoning: Diagnosis & Treatment, 8th ed. R.H. Dreisbach. 517 pp.	1974

Table of Contents

Preface

This book was originally written with the medical student in mind, but as new editions appeared it became evident that urologic residents as well as urologists and physicians in other fields were finding it useful.

The thesis of the book is that, although many urologic disorders produce few or no symptoms, the clues to their presence lie in careful history taking and physical examination and, above all, a personally performed study of the fresh, stained urinary sediment and utilization of the PSP renal function test, which also permits estimation of the amount of residual urine. In addition to excretory urograms, the need for voiding cystourethrograms has become increasingly apparent for demonstrating posterior urethral valves, congenital urethral stenosis in girls, and vesicoureteral reflux (the most common cause of acute and chronic pyelonephritis).

I am particularly pleased with this edition because of the opportunities that have arisen to include new subject areas and revised concepts of established urologic entities with the aid of the eminent men whose names now adorn the new table of contents. Ultrasonography has gained an important place in urologic diagnosis, and Dr Granville C. Coggs has prepared a chapter explaining the clinically important aspects of this subject to our readers. Drs Malcolm R. Powell and Jerome M. Weiss have considerably revised their chapter on radioisotopic kidney studies because of the many new and useful radiopharmaceutical preparations that have recently appeared. Dr Felix O. Kolb, an endocrinologist with a special interest in the metabolism of stone formation, has collaborated with me on the chapter on urinary stones with reference to etiology, diagnosis, and prevention. He has also revised the section on nephrocalcinosis. Drs J. Vivian Wells and H. Hugh Fudenberg have contributed an important chapter on the immunology of genitourinary tumors.

Dr Peter H. Forsham has completely rewritten the chapter on disorders of the adrenal glands. The chapter covering diagnosis of medical renal diseases has been expanded by Dr Marcus A. Krupp. Dr William J.C. Amend Jr, a nephrologist, has collaborated with Drs Oscar Salvatierra Jr and Folkert O. Belzer to write a new chapter on chronic renal failure, dialysis, and renal transplantation. Finally, my chapter on intersex has been replaced with one prepared by Drs Felix A. Conte, Edward O. Reiter, and Melvin M. Grumbach entitled Abnormalities of Sexual Differentiation.

The extensive bibliographies, which have received much favorable comment, have been brought up to date.

It is a pleasure to note that the Spanish edition of this book published by El Manual Moderno of Mexico City, the German translation under the imprint of Urban & Schwarzenberg in Munich, and the French translation prepared by Flammarion Médecine-Sciences of Paris continue to receive wide acceptance. Since the publication of the last American edition, both a Polish and a Portuguese translation have appeared. The publication of a Japanese edition is imminent.

Donald R. Smith, MD

San Francisco, California
August, 1975

1...

Anatomy of the Genitourinary Tract

Urology deals with diseases and disorders of the genitourinary tract in the male and of the urinary tract in the female. Surgical diseases of the adrenal gland are also included. These systems are illustrated in Figs 1−1 and 1−2.

ADRENALS

Gross Appearance

A. Anatomy: Each kidney is capped by an adrenal gland, and both organs are enclosed within Gerota's (perirenal) fascia. Each adrenal weighs about 5 g. The right adrenal is triangular in shape; the left is more rounded and crescentic. Each gland is composed of a cortex, chiefly influenced by the pituitary gland, and a medulla derived from chromaffin tissue.

B. Relations: Fig 1−3 shows the relation of the adrenals to other organs. The right adrenal lies between the liver and the vena cava. The left gland lies close to the aorta and is covered on its lower surface by the pancreas; superiorly and laterally, it is related to the spleen.

Histology

The adrenal cortex is composed of 3 distinct layers: the outer zona glomerulosa, the middle zona fasciculata, and the inner zona reticularis. The medulla lies centrally and is made up of polyhedral cells containing eosinophilic granular cytoplasm. These chromaffin cells are accompanied by ganglion and small round cells.

Blood Supply

A. Arterial: Each adrenal receives 3 arteries: one from the inferior phrenic artery, one from the aorta, and one from the renal artery.

B. Venous: The right adrenal blood is drained by a very short vein which empties into the vena cava; the left adrenal vein terminates in the left renal vein.

Lymphatics

The lymphatic vessels accompany the suprarenal vein and drain into the lumbar lymph nodes.

KIDNEYS

Gross Appearance

A. Anatomy: The kidneys lie along the borders of the psoas muscles and are therefore obliquely placed. The position of the liver causes the right kidney to be lower than the left (Figs 1−3 and 1−4). The adult kidney weighs about 150 g.

The kidneys are supported by the perirenal fat (which is enclosed in the perirenal fascia), the renal vascular pedicle, abdominal muscle tone, and the general bulk of the abdominal viscera. Variations in these factors permit variations in the degree of renal mobility. The average descent on inspiration or on assuming the upright position is 4−5 cm. Lack of mobility suggests abnormal fixation (eg, perinephritis), but extreme mobility is not necessarily pathologic.

On longitudinal section (Fig 1−5), the kidney is seen to be made up of an outer cortex, a central medulla, and the internal calyces and pelvis. The cortex is homogeneous in appearance. Portions of it project toward the pelvis between the papillae and fornices and are called the columns of Bertin. The medulla consists of numerous pyramids formed by the converging collecting renal tubules, which drain into the minor calyces.

B. Relations: Figs 1−3 and 1−4 show the relations of the kidneys to adjacent organs and structures. Their intimacy with intraperitoneal organs explains, in part, some of the gastrointestinal symptoms which accompany genitourinary disease.

Histology

A. Nephron: The functioning unit of the kidney is the nephron, which is composed of a tubule which has both secretory and excretory functions (Fig 1−5). The secretory portion is contained largely within the cortex and consists of a renal corpuscle and the secretory part of the renal tubule. The excretory portion of this duct lies in the medulla. The renal corpuscle is composed of the vascular glomerulus, which projects into Bowman's capsule, which, in turn, is continuous with the epithelium of the proximal convoluted tubule. The secretory portion of the renal tubule is made up of the proximal convoluted tubule, the loop of Henle, and the distal convoluted tubule.

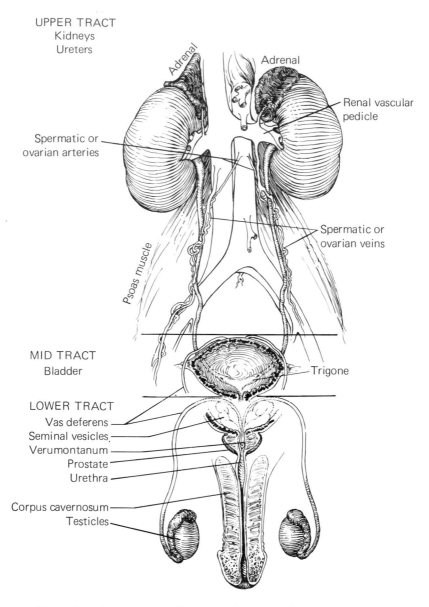

Figure 1—1. Anatomy of the male genitourinary tract. The upper and mid tracts have urologic function only. The lower tract has both genital and urinary functions.

The excretory portion of the nephron is the collecting tubule, which is continuous with the distal end of the ascending limb of the convoluted tubule. It empties its contents through the tip (papilla) of a pyramid into a minor calyx.

B. Supporting Tissue: The renal stroma is composed of loose connective tissue and contains blood vessels, capillaries, nerves, and lymphatics.

Blood Supply (Figs 1–3 and 1–5)

A. Arterial: Usually there is one renal artery, a branch of the aorta, which enters the hilum of the kidney between the pelvis, which normally lies posteriorly, and the renal vein. It may branch before it reaches the kidney, and 2 or more separate arteries may be noted. In duplication of the pelvis and ureter, it is usual for each renal segment to have its own arterial supply.

This artery further divides into the interlobular arteries, which ascend in the columns of Bertin (between the pyramids) and then arch along the base of the pyramids (arcuate arteries). From these vessels smaller (afferent) branches pass to the glomeruli. From the glomerular tuft, efferent arterioles pass to the tubules in the stroma.

B. Venous: The renal veins are paired with the arteries, but any of them will drain the entire kidney if the others are tied off.

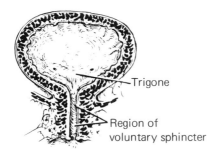

Figure 1—2. Anatomy of the mid and lower tracts in the female.

Although the renal artery and vein are usually the sole blood vessels of the kidney, accessory renal vessels are common and may be of clinical importance if they are so placed as to compress the ureter, in which case hydronephrosis may result.

Lymphatics

The lymphatics of the kidney drain into the lumbar lymph nodes (Figs 18—1 and 18—2).

CALYCES, RENAL PELVIS, & URETER

Gross Appearance

 A. Anatomy:

 1. Calyces—The tips of the minor calyces (4—12 in number) are indented by the projecting pyramids (Fig 1—5). These calyces unite to form 2 or 3 major calyces, which join the renal pelvis.

 2. Renal pelvis—The pelvis may be entirely intrarenal or partly intrarenal and partly extrarenal. Inferomedially, it tapers to form the ureter.

 3. Ureter—The adult ureter is about 30 cm long, varying in direct relation to the height of the individual. It follows a rather smooth S curve. Areas of constriction are found (1) at the ureteropelvic junction, (2) where the ureter crosses over the iliac vessels, and (3) where it courses through the bladder wall.

 B. Relations:

 1. Calyces—The calyces are intrarenal and are intimately related to the renal parenchyma.

 2. Renal pelvis—If the pelvis is partly extrarenal, it lies along the lateral border of the psoas muscle and

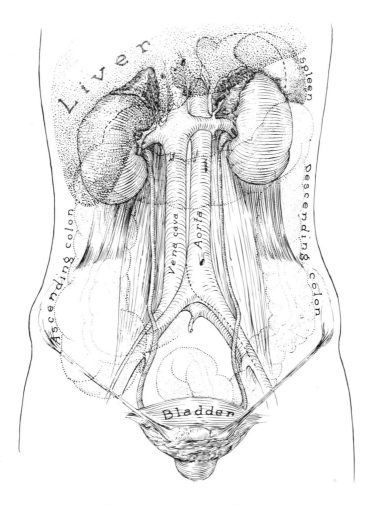

Figure 1—3. Relations of kidney, ureters, and bladder (anterior aspect).

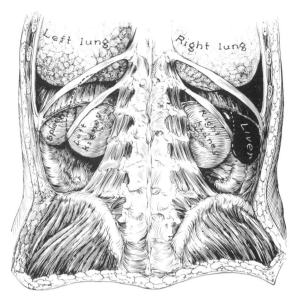

Figure 1–4. Relations of kidneys (posterior aspect).

on the quadratus lumborum muscle; the renal vascular pedicle is placed just anterior to it. The left renal pelvis lies at the level of the first or second lumbar vertebra; the right pelvis is a little lower.

3. Ureter—As followed from above downward, the ureters lie on the psoas muscles, pass medially to the sacroiliac joints, and then swing laterally near the ischial spines before passing medially to penetrate the base of the bladder (Fig 1–3). The uterine arteries are closely related to the juxtavesical portion of the ureters. The ureters are covered by the posterior peritoneum; their lowermost portions are closely attached to it, while the juxtavesical portions are embedded in vascular retroperitoneal fat.

As the vasa deferentia leave the prostate, they lie just medial to the ureters; just above the trigonal area, the vasa pass anteriorly to the ureters on their way to the internal inguinal rings (Fig 1–6).

Histology (Fig 1–5)

The walls of the calyces, pelvis, and ureters are composed of transitional cell epithelium under which lies loose connective and elastic tissue (lamina propria). External to these are a mixture of spiral and longitudinal smooth muscle fibers. They are not arranged in definite layers. The outermost adventitial coat is composed of fibrous connective tissue.

Blood Supply

A. Arterial: The renal calyces, pelvis, and upper ureters derive their blood supply from the renal arteries; the mid ureter is fed by the internal spermatic (or ovarian) arteries. The lowermost portion of the ureter is served by branches from the common iliac, hypogastric, and vesical arteries.

B. Venous: The veins of the renal calyces, pelvis, and ureters are paired with the arteries.

Lymphatics

The lymphatics of the upper portions of the ureters as well as those from the pelvis and calyces enter the lumbar lymph nodes. The lymphatics of the mid ureter pass to the hypogastric and common iliac lymph nodes; the lower ureteral lymphatics empty into the vesical and hypogastric lymph nodes (Figs 18–1 and 18–2).

BLADDER

Gross Appearance

The bladder is a hollow muscular organ which serves as a reservoir for urine. In women, its posterior wall and dome are invaginated by the uterus. The adult bladder has a capacity of 350–450 ml.

A. Anatomy: When empty, the adult bladder lies behind the symphysis pubis and is largely a pelvic organ. In infants and children, it is situated higher. When it is full, it rises well above the symphysis and can readily be palpated or percussed. When overdistended, as in acute or chronic urinary retention, it may cause the lower abdomen to bulge visibly.

Extending from the dome of the bladder to the umbilicus is a fibrous cord, the medial umbilical ligament, which represents the obliterated urachus. The ureters enter the bladder posteroinferiorly in an oblique manner and at these points are placed about 2.5 cm apart (Fig 1–6). The orifices are situated at the extremities of the crescent-shaped interureteric ridge which forms the proximal border of the trigone. The trigone occupies the area between the ridge and the bladder neck.

The internal sphincter, or bladder neck, is not a true circular sphincter but a thickening formed by interlaced and converging muscle fibers of the detrusor as they pass distally to become the smooth musculature of the urethra.

B. Relations: In the male, the bladder is related posteriorly to the seminal vesicles, vasa deferentia, ureters, and rectum (Figs 1–8 and 1–9). In the female, the uterus and vagina are interposed between the bladder and rectum (Fig 1–10). The dome and posterior surfaces are covered by peritoneum; hence, in this area the bladder is closely related to the small intestine and sigmoid colon. In both male and female, the bladder is related to the posterior surface of the symphysis pubis, and, when distended, it is in contact with the lower abdominal wall.

Histology (Fig 1–7)

The mucosa of the bladder is composed of transitional epithelium. Beneath it is a well-developed submucosal layer formed largely of connective and elastic tissues. External to the submucosa is the detrusor muscle, made up of a mixture of smooth muscle fibers which are arranged at random in a longitudinal, circular, and spiral manner.

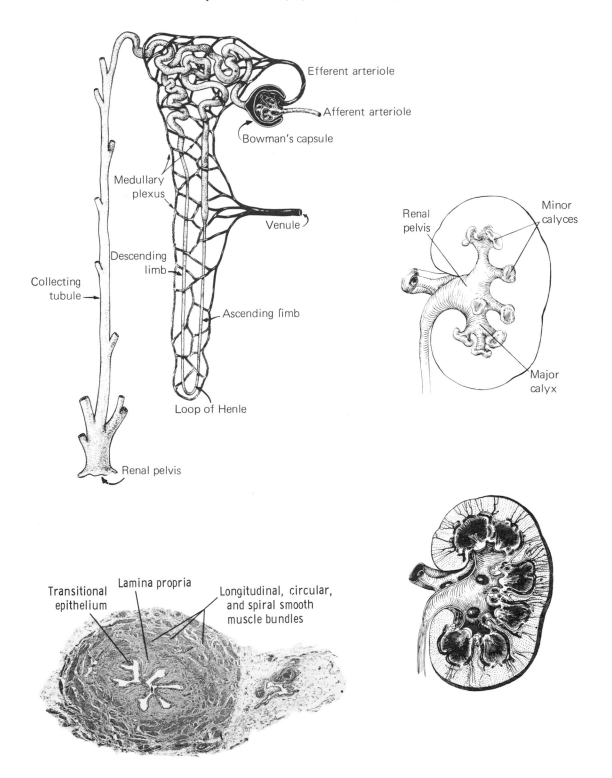

Figure 1–5. Anatomy and histology of the kidney and ureter. *Above left:* Diagram of the nephron and its blood supply. (Courtesy of Merck Sharp & Dohme: Seminar:9[3], 1947.) *Above right:* Renal calyces, pelvis, and ureter (posterior aspect). *Below left:* Histology of the ureter. The smooth muscle bundles are arranged in both a spiral and longitudinal manner. *Below right:* Longitudinal section of kidney showing calyces, pelvis, ureter, and renal blood supply (posterior aspect).

Blood Supply

A. Arterial: The arterial supply to the bladder comes from the superior, middle, and inferior vesical arteries, which arise from the anterior trunk of the hypogastric artery. Smaller branches from the obturator and inferior gluteal arteries also reach this organ. In the female, the uterine and vaginal arteries also send branches to the bladder.

B. Venous: Surrounding the bladder is a rich plexus of veins which ultimately empties into the hypogastric veins.

Lymphatics

The lymphatics of the bladder drain into the vesical, external iliac, hypogastric, and common iliac lymph nodes (Figs 18–1 and 18–2).

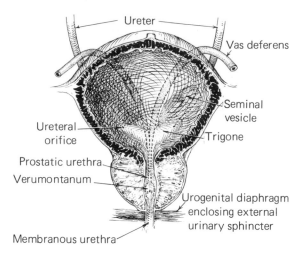

Figure 1–6. Anatomy and relations of the ureters, bladder, prostate, seminal vesicles, and vasa deferentia (anterior view).

PROSTATE GLAND

Gross Appearance

A. Anatomy: The prostate is a fibromuscular and glandular organ lying just inferior to the bladder (Figs 1–6 and 1–8). The normal prostate weighs about 20 g and contains the posterior urethra, which is about 2.5 cm in length. It is supported anteriorly by the puboprostatic ligaments and inferiorly by the urogenital diaphragm (Fig 1–6). The prostate is perforated posteriorly by the ejaculatory ducts, which pass obliquely to empty through the verumontanum on the floor of the prostatic urethra just proximal to the striated external urinary sphincter.

According to the classification of Lowsley (Hutch & Rambo), the prostate consists of 6 lobes: anterior, posterior, median, subcervical, and right and left lateral. The latter 3 lie between the inner longitudinal layer of smooth muscle (which is continuous with the similar layer of the vesical wall) and the outer circular smooth muscle layer of the urethra (which is an extension of the outer layer of the bladder). These circular fibers represent the true involuntary sphincter of the posterior urethra. These 3 lobes tend to undergo hypertrophy with advancing age.

The other 3 lobes lie outside of the urethral lumen and are therefore not involved in the reaction of hyperplasia. The posterior lobe, however, is prone to cancerous degeneration.

B. Relations: The prostate gland lies behind the symphysis pubis. Closely applied to its posterosuperior surface are the vasa deferentia and seminal vesicles (Fig 1–8). Posteriorly, it is separated from the rectum by the 2 layers of Denonvilliers' fascia, serosal rudiments of the pouch of Douglas which once extended to the urogenital diaphragm (Fig 1–9).

Histology (Fig 1–7)

The prostate consists of a thin fibrous capsule under which are circularly oriented smooth muscle fibers and collagenous tissue that surrounds the urethra (involuntary sphincter). Deep to this layer lies the prostatic stroma, composed of connective and elastic tissues and smooth muscle fibers in which are embedded the epithelial glands. These glands drain into the major excretory ducts (about 25 in number) which open chiefly on the floor of the urethra between the verumontanum and the vesical neck. Just beneath the transitional epithelium of the prostatic urethra lie the periurethral glands.

Blood Supply

A. Arterial: The arterial supply to the prostate is derived from the inferior vesical, internal pudendal, and middle hemorrhoidal arteries.

B. Venous: The veins from the prostate drain into the periprostatic plexus, which has connections with the deep dorsal vein of the penis and the hypogastric veins.

Lymphatics

The lymphatics from the prostate drain into the hypogastric, sacral, vesical, and external iliac lymph nodes (Figs 18–1 and 18–2).

SEMINAL VESICLES

Gross Appearance

The seminal vesicles lie just cephalad to the prostate under the base of the bladder (Figs 1–8 and 1–9). They are about 6 cm long and quite soft. Each vesicle joins its corresponding vas deferens to form the ejaculatory duct. The ureters lie medial to each, and the rectum is contiguous with their posterior surfaces.

Histology

The mucous membrane is pseudostratified. The

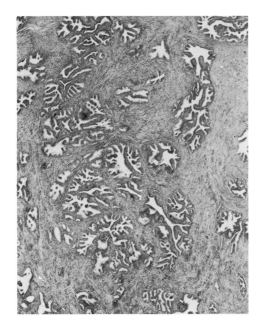 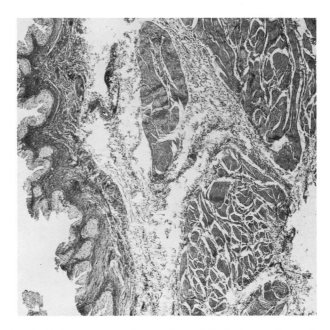

Figure 1—7. *Left:* Histology of the prostate. Epithelial glands embedded in a mixture of connective and elastic tissue and smooth muscle. *Right:* Histology of the bladder. The mucosa is transitional cell in type and lies upon a well-developed submucosal layer of connective tissue. The detrusor muscle is composed of interlacing longitudinal, circular, and spiral smooth muscle bundles.

submucosa consists of dense connective tissue covered by a thin layer of muscle which in turn is encapsulated by connective tissue.

Blood Supply

The blood supply is similar to that of the prostate gland.

Lymphatics

The lymphatics of the seminal vesicles are those that serve the prostate (Figs 18—1 and 18—2).

SPERMATIC CORD

Gross Appearance

The 2 spermatic cords extend from the internal inguinal rings through the inguinal canals to the testicles (Fig 1—8). Each cord contains the vas deferens, the internal and external spermatic arteries, the artery of the vas, the venous pampiniform plexus (which forms the spermatic vein superiorly), lymph vessels, and nerves. All of the above are enclosed in investing layers of thin fascia. A few fibers of the cremaster muscle insert on the cords in the inguinal canal.

Histology

The fascia covering the cord is formed of loose connective tissue which supports arteries, veins, and lymphatics. The vas deferens is a small, thick-walled tube consisting of an internal mucosa and submucosa surrounded by 3 well-defined layers of smooth muscle encased in a covering of fibrous tissue. Above the testes, this tube is straight. Its proximal 4 cm tend to be convoluted.

Blood Supply

A. Arterial: The external spermatic artery, a branch of the inferior epigastric, supplies the fascial coverings of the cord. The internal spermatic artery passes through the cord on its way to the testis. The deferential artery is close to the vas.

B. Venous: The veins from the testis and the coverings of the spermatic cord form the pampiniform plexus, which, at the internal inguinal ring, unites to form the spermatic vein.

Lymphatics

The lymphatics from the spermatic cord empty into the external iliac lymph nodes (Figs 18—1 and 18—2).

EPIDIDYMIS

Gross Appearance

A. Anatomy: The upper portion of the epididymis (globus major) is connected to the testis by numerous efferent ducts from the testis (Fig 1—8). The epididymis consists of a markedly coiled duct which,

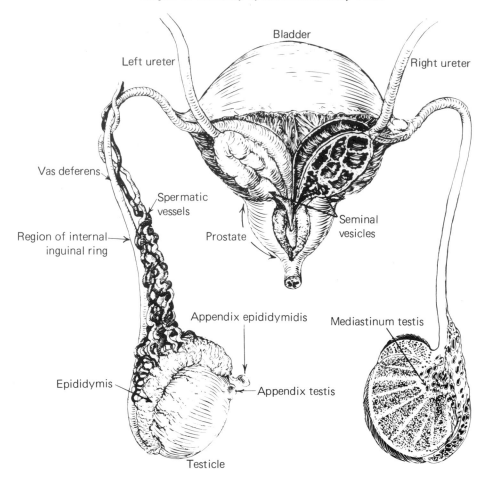

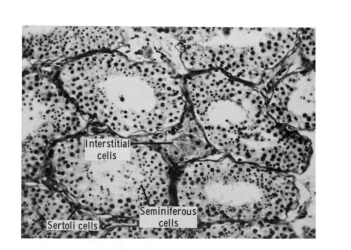

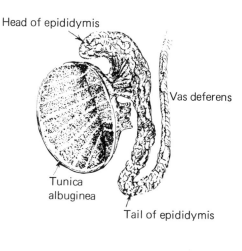

Figure 1—8. *Above:* Gross anatomy and relations of ureters, bladder, prostate, seminal vesicles, vasa deferentia, testes, and epididymides. *Below left:* Histology of the testis. Seminiferous tubules lined by supporting basement membrane for the Sertoli and spermatogenic cells. The latter are in various stages of development. *Below right:* Cross section of testis showing fibrous septa dividing organ into lobules.

at its lower pole (globus minor), is continuous with the vas deferens. An appendix of the epididymis is often seen on its upper pole; this is a cystic body which sometimes is pedunculated but at other times is sessile.

B. Relations: The epididymis lies posterolateral to the testis and is nearest to the testis at its upper pole. Its lower pole is connected to the testis by fibrous tissue. The vas lies posteromedial to the epididymis.

Histology

The epididymis is covered by serosa. The ductus epididymidis is lined by pseudostratified columnar epithelium throughout its length.

Blood Supply

A. Arterial: The arterial supply to the epididymis comes from the internal spermatic artery and the artery of the vas (deferential artery).

B. Venous: The venous blood drains into the pampiniform plexus, which becomes the spermatic vein.

Lymphatics

The lymphatics drain into the external iliac and hypogastric lymph nodes (Figs 18–1 and 18–2).

TESTIS

Gross Appearance

A. Anatomy: The average testicle measures about 4 × 3 × 2.5 cm (Fig 1–8). It has a dense fascial covering called the tunica albuginea testis, which, posteriorly, is invaginated somewhat into the body of the testis to form the mediastinum testis. This fibrous mediastinum sends fibrous septa into the testis, thus separating it into about 250 lobules.

The testis is covered anteriorly and laterally by the visceral layer of the serous tunica vaginalis, which is continuous with the parietal layer that separates the testis from the scrotal wall.

At the upper pole of the testis is the appendix testis, a small pedunculated or sessile body which is similar in appearance to the appendix of the epididymis.

B. Relations: The testis is closely attached posterolaterally to the epididymis, particularly at its upper and lower poles.

Histology (Fig 1–8)

Each lobule contains 1–4 markedly convoluted seminiferous tubules each of which is about 60 cm long. These ducts converge at the mediastinum testis, where they connect with the efferent ducts which drain into the epididymis.

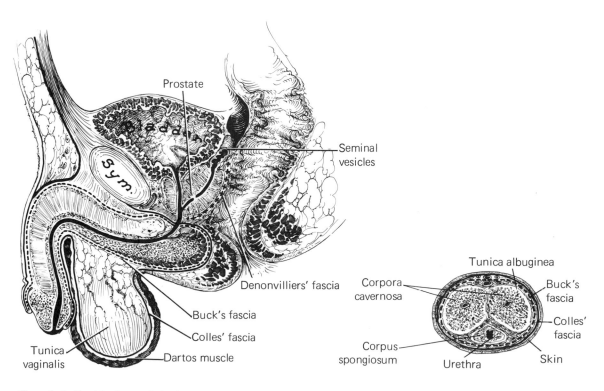

Figure 1–9. Fascial planes of the lower genitourinary tract. (After Wesson.) *Left:* Relations of the bladder, prostate, seminal vesicles, penis, urethra, and scrotal contents. *Right:* Transverse section through the penis. The paired upper structures are the corpora cavernosa. The single lower body surrounding the urethra is the corpus spongiosum.

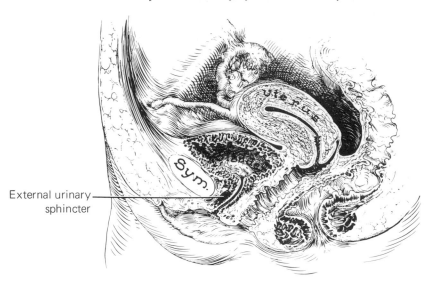

Figure 1—10. Anatomy and relations of the bladder, urethra, uterus and ovary, vagina, and rectum.

External urinary sphincter

The seminiferous tubule has a basement membrane containing connective and elastic tissue. This supports the seminiferous cells, which are of 2 types: (1) Sertoli (supporting) cells and (2) spermatogenic cells. The stroma between the seminiferous tubules contains connective tissue in which the interstitial Leydig cells are located.

Blood Supply

The blood supply to the testes is closely associated with that to the kidneys because of the common embryologic origin of the 2 organs.

A. Arterial: The arteries to the testes (internal spermatics) arise from the aorta just below the renal arteries and course through the spermatic cords to the testes, where they anastomose with the arteries of the vasa which branch off from the hypogastric artery.

B. Venous: The blood from the testis returns in the pampiniform plexus of the spermatic cord. At the internal inguinal ring, the pampiniform plexus forms the spermatic vein.

The right spermatic vein enters the vena cava just below the right renal vein; the left spermatic vein empties into the left renal vein.

Lymphatics

The lymphatic vessels from the testes pass to the lumbar lymph nodes, which, in turn, are connected to the mediastinal nodes (Figs 18—1 and 18—2).

SCROTUM

Gross Appearance

Beneath the corrugated skin of the scrotum lies the dartos muscle. Deep to this are the 3 fascial layers derived from the abdominal wall at the time of testicular descent. Beneath these is the parietal layer of the tunica vaginalis.

The scrotum is divided into 2 sacs by a septum of connective tissue. The scrotum not only supports the testes but, by relaxation or contraction of its muscular layer, helps to regulate their environmental temperature.

Histology

The dartos muscle, under the skin of the scrotum, is unstriated. The deeper layer is made up of connective tissue.

Blood Supply

A. Arterial: The arteries to the scrotum arise from the femoral, internal pudendal, and inferior epigastric arteries.

B. Venous: The veins are paired with the arteries.

Lymphatics

The lymphatics drain into the superficial inguinal and subinguinal lymph nodes (Figs 18—1 and 18—2).

PENIS & MALE URETHRA

Gross Appearance

The penis is composed of 2 corpora cavernosa and the corpus spongiosum, which contains the urethra, whose diameter is 8—9 mm. These corpora are capped distally by the glans. Each corpus is enclosed in a fascial sheath (tunica albuginea), and all are surrounded by a thick fibrous envelope known as Buck's fascia. A covering of skin, devoid of fat, is loosely applied about these bodies. The prepuce forms a hood over the glans.

Beneath the skin of the penis (and scrotum) and extending from the base of the glans to the urogenital diaphragm is Colles' fascia, which is continuous with Scarpa's fascia of the lower abdominal wall (Fig 1–9).

The proximal ends of the corpora cavernosa are attached to the pelvic bones just anterior to the ischial tuberosities. Occupying a depression on their ventral surface in the midline is the corpus spongiosum, which is connected proximally to the undersurface of the urogenital diaphragm through which emerges the membranous urethra. This portion of the corpus spongiosum is surrounded by the bulbocavernosus muscle. Its distal end expands to form the glans penis.

The suspensory ligament of the penis arises from the linea alba and symphysis pubis and inserts into the fascial covering of the corpora cavernosa.

Histology

A. Corpora and Glans Penis: The corpora cavernosa, the corpus spongiosum, and the glans penis are composed of septa of smooth muscle and erectile tissue which enclose vascular cavities.

B. Urethra: The urethral mucosa which traverses the glans penis is formed of squamous epithelium. Proximal to this, the mucosa is transitional in type. Underneath the mucosa is the submucosa, which contains connective and elastic tissue and smooth muscle. In the submucosa are the numerous glands of Littré, whose ducts connect with the urethral lumen.

The urethra is surrounded by the vascular corpus spongiosum and the glans penis.

Blood Supply

A. Arterial: The penis and urethra are supplied by the internal pudendal arteries. Each artery divides into a profunda artery of the penis (which supplies the corpora cavernosa), a dorsal artery of the penis, and the bulbourethral artery. These latter branches supply the corpus spongiosum, the glans penis, and the urethra.

B. Venous: The superficial dorsal vein lies external to Buck's fascia. The deep dorsal vein is placed beneath Buck's fascia and lies between the dorsal arteries. These veins connect with the pudendal plexus, which drains into the internal pudendal vein.

Lymphatics

Lymphatic drainage from the skin of the penis is to the superficial inguinal and subinguinal lymph nodes. The lymphatics from the glans penis pass to the subinguinal and external iliac nodes. The lymphatics from the deep urethra drain into the hypogastric and common iliac lymph nodes (Figs 18–1 and 18–2).

FEMALE URETHRA

The adult female urethra is about 3.5–4 cm long and 8 mm in diameter. It is slightly curved and lies beneath the symphysis pubis just anterior to the vagina.

The epithelial lining of the female urethra is squamous in its distal portion and pseudostratified or transitional in the remainder. The submucosa is made up of connective and elastic tissues and spongy venous spaces. Embedded in it are many periurethral glands, which are most numerous distally; the largest of these are the periurethral glands of Skene, which open on the floor of the urethra just inside the meatus.

External to the submucosa is a longitudinal layer of smooth muscle which is continuous with the inner longitudinal layer of the bladder wall. Surrounding this is a heavy layer of circular smooth muscle fibers which extend from the external vesical muscular layer. They constitute the true involuntary urethral sphincter. External to this is the circular striated (voluntary) sphincter surrounding the middle third of the urethra. It is part of the pelvic floor and levator muscles.

The arterial supply to the female urethra is derived from the inferior vesical, vaginal, and internal pudendal arteries. Blood from the urethra drains into the internal pudendal veins.

Lymphatic drainage from the external portion of the urethra is to the inguinal and subinguinal lymph nodes. Drainage from the deep urethra is into the hypogastric lymph nodes (Figs 18–1 and 18–2).

Nerve Supply to the Genitourinary Organs

See Figs 3–1, 3–2, and 19–1.

•   •   •

References

Adrenals

Ivemark B, Ekström T, Lagergren C: The vasculature of the developing and mature human adrenal gland. Acta paediat scandinav 56:601, 1967.

Johnstone FRC: The surgical anatomy of the adrenal glands with particular reference to the suprarenal vein. S Clin North America 44:1315, 1964.

Kidneys

Barger AC, Herd JA: The renal circulation. New England J Med 284:482, 1971.

Fetterman GH & others: The growth and maturation of human glomeruli and proximal convolutions from term to adulthood. Pediatrics 35:601, 1965.

Graves FT: The arterial anatomy of the congenitally abnormal kidney. Brit J Surg 56:533, 1969.

Hegedüs V: Arterial anatomy of the kidney: A three-dimensional angiographic investigation. Acta radiol (diag) 12:604, 1972.

Hodson J: The lobar structure of the kidney. Brit J Urol 44:246, 1972.

Layton JM: The structure of the kidney from the gross to the molecular. J Urol 90:502, 1963.

Mayerson HS: The lymphatic system with particular reference to the kidney. Surg Gynec Obst 116:259, 1963.

Potter EL: Development of the human glomerulus. Arch Path 80:241, 1965.

Roddie IC: Modern views of physiology. 20. The kidney. Practitioner 205:242, 1970.

Zamboni L, DeMartino C: Embryogenesis of the human renal glomerulus. 1. A histologic study. Arch Path 86:279, 1968.

Calyces, Renal Pelvis, & Ureters

Cussen LJ: The structure of the normal human ureter in infancy and childhood. Invest Urol 5:179, 1967.

Elbadawi A, Amaku EO, Frank IN: Trilaminar musculature of submucosal ureter: Anatomy and functional implications. Urology 2:409, 1973.

Osathanondh V, Potter EL: Development of human kidney shown by microdissection. 2. Renal pelvis, calyces, and papillae. 3. Formation and interrelationships of collecting tubules and nephrons. 4. Formation of tubular portions of nephrons. 5. Development of vascular pattern of glomerulus. Arch Path 76:277, 290, 1963; 82:391, 403, 1966.

Sykes D: The morphology of renal lobulations and calyces, and their relationship to partial nephrectomy. Brit J Surg 51:294, 1964.

Bladder

Elbadawi A, Schenk EA: A new theory of the innervation of bladder musculature. 4. Innervation of the vesicourethral function and external urethral sphincter. J Urol 111:613, 1974.

Hodges CV: Surgical anatomy of the urinary bladder and pelvic ureter. S Clin North America 44:1327, 1964.

Hutch JA: The internal urinary sphincter: A double loop system. J Urol 105:375, 1971.

Hutch JA: *Anatomy and Physiology of the Bladder, Trigone and Urethra.* Appleton-Century-Crofts, 1972.

Tanagho EA, Miller ER: Functional considerations of urethral sphincteric dynamics. J Urol 109:273, 1973.

Tanagho EA, Smith DR: The anatomy and function of the bladder neck. Brit J Urol 38:54, 1966.

Tanagho EA & others: Observations in the dynamics of the bladder neck. Brit J Urol 38:72, 1966.

Prostate Gland

Hutch JA, Rambo ON Jr: A study of the anatomy of the prostate, prostatic urethra and the urinary sphincter system. J Urol 104:443, 1970.

McNeal JE: The prostate and prostatic urethra: A morphologic study. J Urol 107:1008, 1972.

Spermatic Cord

Ahlberg NE, Bartley O, Chidekel N: Right and left gonadal veins: An anatomical and statistical study. Acta radiol (diag) 4:593, 1966.

Bergman LL: The regional anatomy of the inguinal canal. GP 26:114, Oct 1962.

Testis

Busch FM, Sayegh ES: Roentgenographic visualization of human testicular lymphatics: A preliminary report. J Urol 89:106, 1963.

Female Urethra

Lindner HH, Feldman SE: Surgical anatomy of the perineum. S Clin North America 42:877, 1962.

Zacharin RF: The anatomic supports of the female urethra. Obst Gynec 32:754, 1968.

2...

Embryology of the Genitourinary System

Emil A. Tanagho, MD

At birth, the genital and urinary systems are related only in the sense that they share certain common passages. Embryologically, however, they are intimately related. Because of the complex interrelationships of the embryonic phases of the 2 systems, they will be discussed here as 5 subdivisions: the nephric system, the vesicourethral unit, the gonads, the genital duct system, and the external genitalia.

THE NEPHRIC SYSTEM

The nephric system develops progressively as 3 distinct entities: pronephros, mesonephros, and metanephros.

Pronephros

This is the earliest nephric stage in man, and it corresponds to the mature structure of the most primitive vertebrate. It extends from the fourth to the fourteenth somites and consists of 6–10 pairs of tubules. These open into a pair of primary ducts that are also formed at that same level, extend caudally, and eventually reach and open into the cloaca. The pronephros is a vestigial structure that disappears completely by the fourth week of embryonic life (Fig 2–1).

Mesonephros

The mature excretory organ of the higher fish and amphibians corresponds to the embryonic mesonephros. It is the principal excretory organ during early embryonic life (4–8 weeks). It, too, gradually degenerates, although parts of its duct system become associated with the male reproductive organs. The mesonephric tubules develop from the intermediate mesoderm caudad to the pronephros shortly before pronephric degeneration. The mesonephric tubules differ from those of the pronephros in that they develop a cuplike outgrowth into which a knot of capillaries is pushed. This is called Bowman's capsule, and the tuft

Emil A. Tanagho is Professor of Urology, University of California School of Medicine, San Francisco.

of capillaries is called a glomerulus. In their growth, the mesonephric tubules extend toward and establish a connection with the nearby primary nephric duct as it grows caudally to join the cloaca (Fig 2–1). This primary nephric duct is now called the mesonephric duct. After establishing their connection with the nephric duct, the primordial tubules elongate and become S-shaped. As the tubules elongate, a series of secondary branchings increases their surface exposure, thereby enhancing their capacity for interchanging material with the blood in adjacent capillaries. Leaving the glomerulus, the blood is carried by one or more efferent vessels that soon break up into a rich capillary plexus closely related to the mesonephric tubules. This is physiologically important. The mesonephros, which forms early in the fourth week, reaches its maximum size by the end of the second month.

Metanephros

The final phase of the development of the nephric system originates from both the intermediate mesoderm and the mesonephric duct. Development begins in the 5–6 mm embryo with a budlike outgrowth from the mesonephric duct as it bends to join the cloaca. This ureteral bud grows cephalad and collects mesoderm from the nephrogenic cord of the intermediate mesoderm around its tip. This mesoderm with the metanephric cap moves, with the growing ureteral bud, more and more cephalad from its point of origin. During this cephalad migration, the metanephric cap becomes progressively larger, and rapid internal differentiation takes place. Meanwhile, the cephalad end of the ureteral bud expands within the growing mass of metanephrogenic tissue to form the renal pelvis (Fig 2–1). Numerous outgrowths from the renal pelvic dilatation push radially into this growing mass and form into hollow ducts that branch and rebranch as they push their way toward the periphery. These form the primary collecting ducts of the kidney. Mesodermal cells become arranged in small vesicular masses that lie in close proximity to the blind end of the collecting ducts. Each of these vesicular masses will form a uriniferous tubule draining into the duct nearest to its point of origin. As the kidney grows, increasing numbers of tubules are formed in its peripheral zone. These vesicular masses develop a central cavity and become S-shaped. One end of the S coalesces with the terminal

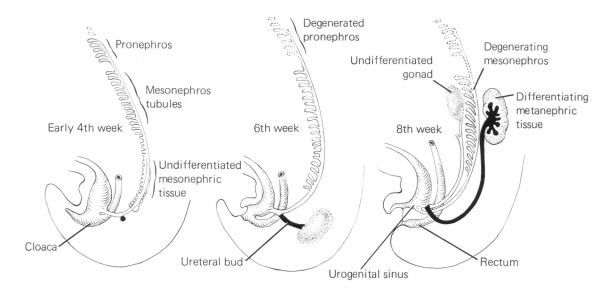

Figure 2—1. Schematic representation of the development of the nephric system. Only a few of the tubules of the pronephros are seen early in the fourth week, while the mesonephric tissue differentiates into mesonephric tubules that progressively join the mesonephric duct. The first sign of the ureteral bud from the mesonephric duct is seen. At 6 weeks, the pronephros has completely degenerated and the mesonephric tubules start to do so. The ureteral bud grows dorsocranially and has met the metanephrogenic cap. At the eighth week, there is cranial migration of the differentiating metanephros. The cranial end of the ureteric bud expands and starts to show multiple successive outgrowths. (Adapted from several sources.)

portion of the collecting tubules, resulting in a continuous canal. The proximal portion develops into the distal and proximal convoluted tubules and into Henle's loop; the distal end becomes the glomerulus and Bowman's capsule. At this stage, the undifferentiated mesoderm and the immature glomeruli are readily visible on microscopic examination (Fig 2—2). The glomeruli are fully developed by the thirty-sixth week or when the fetus weighs 2500 g (Potter). The metanephros arises opposite the twenty-eighth somite (fourth lumbar segment). At term, it has ascended to the level of the first lumbar or even the twelfth thoracic vertebra. This ascent of the kidney is due not only to actual cephalad migration but to differential growth in the caudal part of the body as well. During the early period of ascent (seventh to ninth weeks), the kidney slides up above the arterial bifurcation and rotates 90 degrees. Its convex border is now directed laterally instead of dorsally. Further ascent proceeds more slowly until the kidney reaches its final position.

Certain features of these 3 phases of development must be emphasized: (1) The 3 successive units of the system develop from the intermediate mesoderm. (2) The tubules at all levels appear as independent primordia and only secondarily unite with the duct system. (3) The nephric duct is laid down as the duct of the pronephros and develops from the union of the ends of the anterior pronephric tubules. (4) This pronephric duct serves subsequently as the mesonephric duct and as such gives rise to the ureter. (5) The nephric duct reaches the cloaca by independent caudal growth. (6) The embryonic ureter is an outgrowth of the nephric duct, yet the kidney tubules differentiate from adjacent metanephric blastema.

ANOMALIES OF THE NEPHRIC SYSTEM

Failure of the metanephros to ascend leads to **ectopic kidney.** An ectopic kidney may be on the proper side but low (simple ectopy) or on the opposite side (crossed ectopy) with or without fusion. Failure to rotate during ascent causes a **malrotated kidney.**

Fusion of the paired metanephric masses leads to various anomalies—most commonly **horseshoe kidney.**

The ureteral bud from the mesonephric duct may bifurcate, causing a **bifid ureter** at varying levels depending on the time of the bud's subdivision. An accessory ureteral bud may develop from the mesonephric duct, thereby forming a **duplicated ureter,** usually meeting the same metanephric mass. Rarely, each bud has a separate metanephric mass, resulting in **supernumerary kidneys.**

If the double ureteral buds are close together on the mesonephric duct, they will open near each other in the bladder. In this case, the main ureteral bud, which is the first to appear and the most caudal on the mesonephric ducts, will reach the bladder first. It will then start to move upward and laterally and will be followed later by the second accessory bud as it

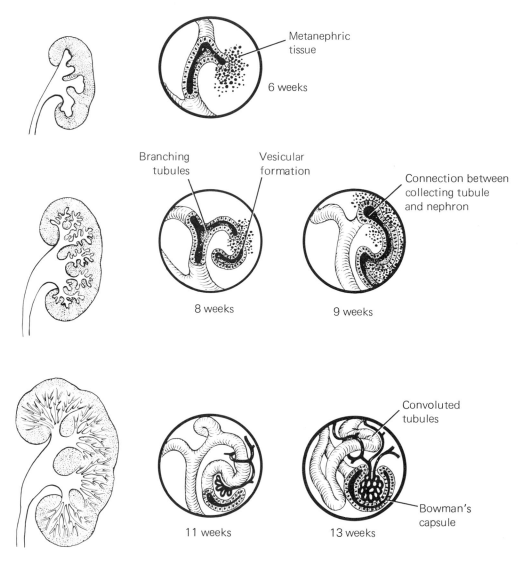

Figure 2—2. Progressive stages in the differentiation of the nephrons and their linkage with the branching collecting tubules. A small lump of metanephric tissue is associated with each terminal collecting tubule. These are then arranged in vesicular masses which later differentiate into a uriniferous tubule draining into the duct near which it arises. At one end, Bowman's capsule and the glomerulus differentiate; the other end establishes communication with the nearby collecting tubules.

reaches the urogenital sinus. The main ureteral bud (now more cranial on the urogenital sinus) will drain the lower portion of the kidney. The 2 ureteral buds have reversed their relationship as they moved from the mesonephric duct to the urogenital sinus. This is why double ureters usually cross (Weigert-Meyer law). If the 2 ureteral buds are widely separated on the mesonephric duct, the accessory bud appears more proximal at the duct and will end in the bladder with an ectopic orifice lower than the normal one. This ectopic orifice could still be in the bladder close to its outlet, in the urethra, or even in the genital duct system (Fig 2—3). A single ureteral bud that arises higher than normal on the mesonephric duct can also end in a similar ectopic location.

Lack of development of a ureteral bud will result in a **solitary kidney** and a hemitrigone.

THE VESICOURETHRAL UNIT

The blind end of the hindgut caudad to the point of origin of the allantois expands to form the cloaca, which is separated from the outside by an ectodermal depression under the root of the tail. This depression is called the proctodeum, and a thin plate of tissue

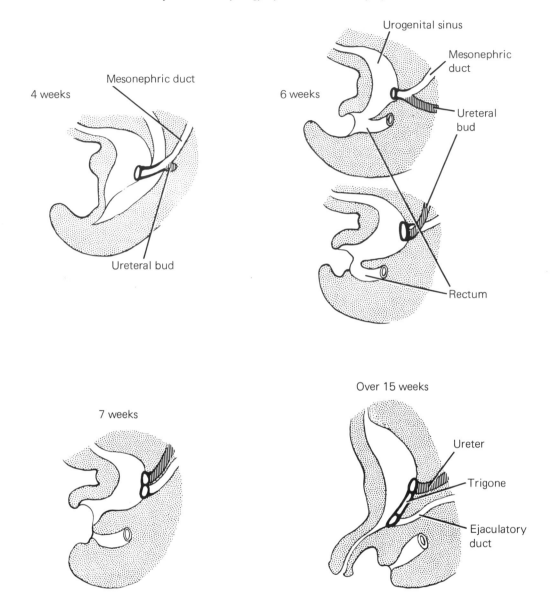

Figure 2–3. The development of the ureteral bud from the mesonephric duct and their relationship to the urogenital sinus. The ureteral bud appears at the fourth week. The mesonephric duct distal to this ureteral bud will be gradually absorbed into the urogenital sinus, resulting in separate endings for the ureter and the mesonephric duct. The mesonephric tissue that is incorporated into the urogenital sinus will expand and form the trigonal tissue.

closing the hindgut is the cloacal membrane. At the 4 mm stage, starting at the cephalad portion of the cloaca where the allantois and gut meet, the cloaca progressively divides into 2 compartments by the caudad growth of a crescentic fold, the urorectal fold. The 2 limbs of the fold bulge into the lumen of the cloaca from either side, eventually meeting and fusing. The division of the cloaca into ventral (urogenital sinus) and dorsal (rectum) is completed during the seventh week. During the development of the urorectal septum, the cloacal membrane undergoes a reverse rotation so that the ectodermal surface is no longer directed toward the developing anterior abdominal wall but gradually faces caudally and slightly posteriorly. This growth change facilitates the subdivision of the cloaca and is brought about mainly by the development of the infraumbilical portion of the anterior abdominal wall and by regression of the tail. The mesoderm that passes around the cloacal membrane to the caudal attachment of the umbilical cord proliferates and grows, forming a surface elevation, the genital tubercle. The further growth of this part of the abdominal wall progressively separates the umbilical cord from the genital tubercle. The division of the cloaca is completed before the cloacal membrane ruptures, and its 2 parts therefore open separately. The ventral part is the primitive urogenital sinus, which has the shape of an elongated cylinder and is continuous cranially with the allantois.

The urogenital sinus receives the mesonephric ducts. The caudad end of the mesonephric duct distal to the ureteral bud is progressively absorbed into the urogenital sinus. By the seventh week, both mesonephric duct and ureteral bud have independent opening sites. This will introduce an island of mesodermal tissue amid the surrounding endoderm of the urogenital sinus. As development progresses, the opening of the mesonephric duct (which will become the ejaculatory duct) migrates downward and medially. The opening of the ureteral bud (which will become the ureteral orifice) migrates upward and laterally. The absorbed mesoderm of the mesonephric duct expands with this migration to occupy the area limited by the final position of these tubes (Fig 2–3). This will later

be differentiated as the trigonal structure, which is the only mesodermal inclusion in the endodermal vesicourethral unit.

The urogenital sinus can be divided into 2 main segments; the dividing line is the junction of the combined Müllerian ducts with the urogenital sinus (Müller's tubercle), which is the most fixed reference point in the whole structure and which will be discussed below. The segments are as follows:

(1) The ventral and pelvic portion will form the bladder, part of the urethra in the male, and the whole urethra in the female. This portion receives the ureter.

(2) The urethral or phallic portion receives the mesonephric and the fused Müllerian ducts. This will be part of the urethra in the male and forms the lower fifth of the vagina and the vaginal vestibule in the female.

During the third month, the ventral part of the urogenital sinus starts to expand and forms an epithe-

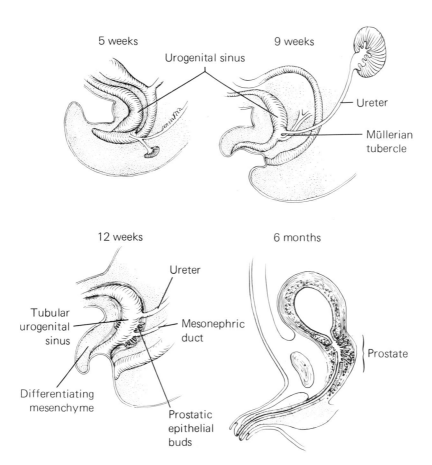

Figure 2–4. Differentiation of the urogenital sinus in the male. At the fifth week, the progressively growing urorectal septum is separating the urogenital sinus from the rectum. The former receives the mesonephric duct and the ureteral bud. It retains its tubular structure until the twelfth week, when the surrounding mesenchyme starts to differentiate into muscle fibers around the whole structure. The prostatic gland develops as multiple epithelial outgrowths just above and below the mesonephric duct. During the third month the ventral part expands to form the bladder proper while the pelvic part remains narrow and tubular, forming part of the urethra. (Reproduced, with permission, from Tanagho & Smith: Mechanisms of urinary continence. 1. Embryologic, anatomic, and pathologic considerations. J Urol 100:640, 1969.)

lial sac whose apex tapers into an elongated, narrowed urachus. The pelvic portion remains narrow and tubular, and this will form the whole urethra in the female and the supramontanal portion of the prostatic urethra in the male. The splanchnic mesoderm surrounding the ventral and pelvic portion of the urogenital sinus begins to differentiate into interlacing bands of smooth muscle fibers and an outer fibrous connective tissue coat. By the twelfth week, the layers characteristic of the adult urethra and bladder are recognizable (Fig 2–4).

The part of the urogenital sinus caudad to the opening of the Müllerian duct will form the vaginal vestibule and contribute to the lower fifth of the vagina in the female (Fig 2–5). In the male, it forms the inframontanal part of the prostatic urethra and the membranous urethra. The penile urethra is formed by the fusion of the urethral folds on the ventral surface of the genital tubercle. In the female, the urethral folds remain separate and form the labia minora. The glandular urethra in the male is formed by the canalization of the urethral plate. The bladder originally extends up to the umbilicus, where it is connected to the allantois that extends into the umbilical cord. The allantois usually is obliterated at the level of the umbilicus by the fifteenth week. The bladder then starts to descend by the eighteenth week. As it descends, its apex becomes stretched and narrowed and it pulls on the already obliterated allantois, now called the urachus. By the twentieth week, the bladder is well

separated from the umbilicus and the stretched urachus will become the middle umbilical ligament.

THE PROSTATE

The prostate develops as multiple solid outgrowths of the urethral epithelium both above and below the entrance of the mesonephric duct. These simple, tubular outgrowths begin to develop in 5 distinct groups at the end of the eleventh week and are complete by the sixteenth week (112 mm). They branch and rebranch, ending in a complex ductal system that encounters the differentiating mesenchymal cells around this segment of the urogenital sinus. These mesenchymal cells start to develop around the tubules by the sixteenth week and become denser at the periphery to form the prostatic capsule. By the twenty-second week, the muscular stroma is considerably developed and continues to progressively increase until birth.

From the 5 groups of epithelial buds, 5 lobes are eventually formed: anterior, posterior, median, and 2 lateral. Initially, these lobes are widely separated, but later they meet, with no definite septa dividing them. Tubules of each lobe do not intermingle with each other but simply lie side by side.

The anterior lobe tubules begin to develop simul-

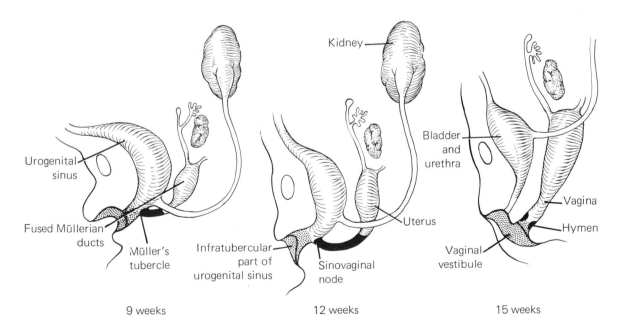

9 weeks   12 weeks   15 weeks

Figure 2–5. Differentiation of the urogenital sinus and the Müllerian ducts in the female embryo. At 9 weeks, the urogenital sinus receives the fused Müllerian ducts at Müller's tubercle (sinovaginal node), which is solidly packed with cells. As the urogenital sinus distal to Müller's tubercle becomes wider and shallower (15 weeks), the urethra and fused Müllerian duct will have separate openings. The distal part of the urogenital sinus will form the vaginal vestibule and the lower fifth of the vagina (shaded area), and that part above Müller's tubercle will form the urinary bladder and the entire female urethra. The fused Müllerian ducts will form the uterus and the upper four-fifths of the vagina. The hymen is formed at the junction of the sinovaginal node and the urogenital sinus.

taneously with those of the other lobes. Although in the early stages the anterior lobe tubules are large and show multiple branches, gradually they contract and lose most of these branches. They continue to shrink so that at birth they show no lumen and appear as small, solid embryonic epithelial outgrowths. In contrast, the tubules of the posterior lobe are fewer in number yet relatively larger, with extensive branching. These tubules, as they grow, extend posterior to the developing median and lateral lobes and form the posterior aspect of the gland, which may be felt rectally.

ANOMALIES OF THE VESICOURETHRAL UNIT

Failure of the cloaca to subdivide is rare and results in a **persistent cloaca.** Incomplete subdivision is more frequent, ending with **rectovesical, rectourethral,** or **rectovestibular fistulas** (usually with **imperforate anus** or **anal atresia**).

Failure of descent or incomplete descent of the bladder leads to a **urinary umbilical fistula (urethral fistula), urachal cyst,** or **urachal diverticulum** depending on the stage and degree of maldescent.

Development of the genital primordia in an area more caudal than normal can result in formation of the corpora cavernosa just caudad to the urogenital sinus outlet, with the urethral groove on its dorsal surface. This defect results in complete or incomplete **epispadias** depending on its degree. A more extensive defect results in **vesical exstrophy.** Failure of fusion of urethral folds leads to various grades of **hypospadias.** This defect, because of its mechanism, never extends proximal to the bulbous urethra. This is in contrast to epispadias, which usually involves the entire urethra up to the internal meatus.

THE GONADS

Most of the structures which make up the embryonic genital system have been taken over from other systems, and their readaptation to genital function is a secondary and relatively late phase in their development. The early differentiation of such structures is therefore independent of sexuality. Furthermore, each embryo is at first morphologically bisexual, possessing all the necessary structures for either sex. The development of one set of sex primordia and the gradual involution of the other is determined by the sex type of the gonad.

The sexually undifferentiated gonad is a composite structure. Male and female potentials are repre-

sented by specific histologic elements (medulla and cortex) which have alternative roles in gonadogenesis. Normal differentiation involves the gradual predominance of one component.

The primitive sex glands make their appearance during the fifth and sixth weeks within a localized region of the thickening known as the urogenital ridge (this contains both the nephric and genital primordia). At the sixth week, the gonad consists of a superficial germinal epithelium and an internal blastema. The blastemal mass is derived mainly from proliferative ingrowth from the superficial epithelium that comes loose from its basement membrane.

During the seventh week, the gonad begins to assume the characteristics of a testis or ovary. Differentiation of the ovary usually occurs somewhat later than that of the testis.

If the gonad develops into a testis, the gland increases in size and shortens into a more compact organ while achieving a more caudal location. Its broad attachment to the mesonephros is converted into a gonadal mesentery known as the mesorchium. The cells of the germinal epithelium grow into the underlying mesenchyme and form cordlike masses. These are radially arranged and converge toward the mesorchium, where a dense portion of the blastemal mass is also emerging as the primordium of the rete testis. A network of strands soon forms which is continuous with the testis cords. The latter also split into 3–4 daughter cords. These eventually become differentiated into the seminiferous tubules by which the spermatozoa are produced. The rete testis unites with the mesonephric components that will form the male genital ducts, as discussed below (Fig 2–6).

If the gonad develops into an ovary, it (like the testis) gains a mesentery (mesovarium) and settles in a more caudal position. The internal blastema differentiates in the ninth week into a primary cortex beneath the germinal epithelium and a loose primary medulla. A compact cellular mass bulges from the medulla into the mesovarium and establishes the primitive rete ovarii. At 3–4 months of age, the internal cell mass becomes young ova. A new definitive cortex is formed from the germinal epithelium as well as from the blastema in the form of distinct cellular cords (Pflüger's tubes), and a permanent medulla is formed. The cortex differentiates into ovarian follicles containing ova.

Descent of the Gonads

A. The Testis: In addition to its early caudal migration, the testis later leaves the abdominal cavity and descends into the scrotum. By the third month of fetal life, the testis is located retroperitoneally in the false pelvis. A fibromuscular band (the gubernaculum) extends from the lower pole of the testis through the developing muscular layers of the anterior abdominal wall to terminate in the subcutaneous tissue of the scrotal swelling. The gubernaculum also has several other subsidiary strands that extend to adjacent regions. Just below the lower pole of the testis, the

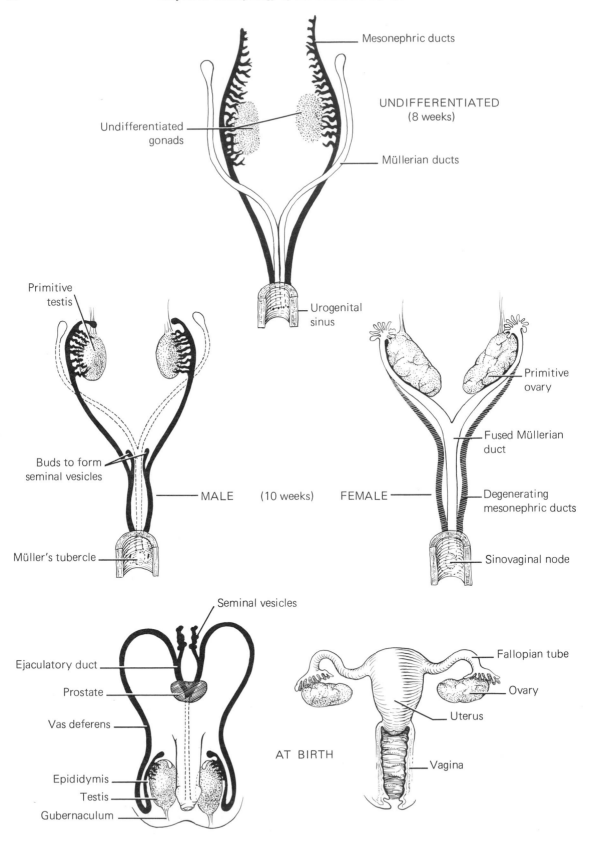

Figure 2—6. Transformation of the undifferentiated genital system into the definitive male and female systems.

peritoneum herniates as a diverticulum along the anterior aspect of the gubernaculum, eventually reaching the scrotal sac through the anterior abdominal muscles (the processus vaginalis). The testis remains at the abdominal end of the inguinal canal until the seventh month. It then passes through the inguinal canal behind (but invaginating) the processus vaginalis (Fig 2–6). Normally, it reaches the scrotal sac by the end of the eighth month.

B. The Ovary: In addition to an early internal descent, the ovary becomes attached through the gubernaculum to the tissues of the genital fold and then attaches itself to the developing uterovaginal canal at its junction with the uterine tubes. This part of the gubernaculum between the ovary and uterus becomes the round ligament of the ovary; the part between the uterus and the labia majora becomes the round ligament of the uterus. This prevents extra-abdominal descent, and the ovary enters the true pelvis. It eventually lies posterior to the uterine tubes on the superior surface of the urogenital mesentery, which has descended with the ovary and now forms the broad ligament. A small processus vaginalis forms and passes toward the labial swelling, but it is usually obliterated at full term.

GONADAL ANOMALIES

Lack of development of the gonads leads to **gonadal agenesis.** Incomplete development with arrest at a certain phase leads to **hypogenesis. Supernumerary gonads** are rare. The commonest anomaly involves descent of the gonads, especially the testis. Retention of the testis in the abdomen or arrest of its descent at any point along its natural pathway leads to **cryptorchism,** which may be either unilateral or bilateral. If the testis does not follow the main gubernaculum structure but follows one of its subsidiary strands, it will end in an abnormal position, resulting in **ectopic testis.**

Failure of union between the rete testis and mesonephros results in a testis separate from the male genital ducts (the epididymis).

THE GENITAL DUCT SYSTEM

Alongside the indifferent gonads, there are, early in embryonic life, 2 different yet closely related ducts. One is primarily a nephric duct (Wolffian duct), yet it will also serve as a genital duct if the embryo develops into a male. The other (Müllerian duct) is primarily a genital structure from the start.

Both ducts grow caudally to join the primitive urogenital sinus. The Wolffian duct (known as the pronephric duct at the 4 mm stage) joins the ventral part of the cloaca, which will be the urogenital sinus. This duct gives rise to the ureteral bud close to its caudal end. The ureteral bud will grow cranially and meet metanephrogenic tissue. That part of each mesonephric duct caudad to the origin of the ureteric bud becomes absorbed into the wall of the primitive urogenital sinus so that the mesonephric duct and ureter open independently. This is achieved at the 15 mm stage (seventh week). During this period, starting at the 10 mm stage, the Müllerian ducts start to develop. They reach the urogenital sinus relatively late—at the 30 mm embryonic stage (ninth week). This is the most constant and reliable point of reference in the whole system.

If the embryo develops into a male and the gonad starts to develop into a testis (17 mm, seventh week), the Wolffian duct will start to differentiate into the male duct system, forming the epididymis, vas deferens, seminal vesicles, and ejaculatory ducts. At this time, the Müllerian duct proceeds toward its junction with the urogenital sinus and immediately starts to degenerate. It will only remain as a rudimentary structure.

If the embryo develops into a female and the gonad starts to differentiate into an ovary (22 mm, eighth week), the Müllerian duct system forms the uterine (Fallopian) tubes, uterus, and most of the vagina. The Wolffian ducts, aside from their contribution to the urogenital sinus, remain rudimentary.

THE MALE DUCT SYSTEM

The Epididymis

Because of the proximity of the differentiating gonads and the nephric duct, some of the mesonephric tubules are retained as the efferent ductules and their lumens become continuous with those of the rete testis. These tubules, together with that part of the mesonephric duct into which they empty, will form the epididymis. Each coiled ductule makes a conical mass known as the lobule of the epididymis. The cranial end of the mesonephric duct becomes highly convoluted, completing the formation of the epididymis. This is an example of direct inclusion of a nephric structure into the genital system. Additional mesonephric tubules, both cephalad and caudad to those that were included in the formation of the epididymis, will remain as rudimentary structures, ie, the appendix of the epididymis and the paradidymis.

Vas Deferens, Seminal Vesicles, & Ejaculatory Ducts

The mesonephric duct caudad to that portion forming the epididymis will form the vas deferens. Shortly before this duct joins the urethra (urogenital sinus), a localized dilatation (ampulla) develops and the saccular convoluted structure that will form the seminal vesicle is evaginated from its wall. The mesonephric duct between the origin of the seminal vesicle and the urethra will form the ejaculatory duct. The whole mesonephric duct now achieves its characteristic thick investment of smooth muscle with a narrow lumen along most of its length.

Both above and below the point of entrance of the mesonephric duct into the urethra, multiple outgrowths of urethral epithelium mark the beginning of the development of the prostate. As these epithelial buds grow, they meet the developing muscular fibers around the urogenital sinus, and some of these fibers become entangled in the branching tubules of the growing prostate and become incorporated into it, forming its muscular stroma (Fig 2–6).

THE FEMALE DUCT SYSTEM

The Müllerian ducts, which are a paired system, are seen alongside the mesonephric duct. It is not known whether they arise directly from the mesonephric ducts or separately as an invagination of the celomic epithelium into the parenchyma lateral to the cranial extremity of the mesonephric duct, but the latter theory is favored. The Müllerian duct develops and runs lateral to the mesonephric duct. Its opening with the celomic cavity persists as the peritoneal ostium of the uterine tube (later it develops fimbriae). The other end grows caudally as a solid tip and then crosses in front of the mesonephric duct at the caudad extremity of the mesonephros. It continues its growth in a caudomedial direction until it meets and fuses with the Müllerian duct of the opposite side. The fusion is partial at first, so there is a temporary septum between the 2 lumens. This later disappears, leaving one cavity that will form the uterovaginal canal. The potential lumen of the vaginal canal is completely packed with cells. The solid tip of this cord pushes the epithelium of the urogenital sinus outward, where it becomes Müller's tubercle (33 mm stage, ninth week). They actually fuse at the 63 mm stage (thirteenth week), forming the sinovaginal node, which receives a limited contribution from the urogenital sinus. (This contribution will form the lower fifth of the vagina.)

The urogenital sinus distal to Müller's tubercle, originally narrow and deep, shortens, widens, and opens to form the floor of the pudendal or vulval cleft. This results in separate openings for the vagina and urethra and also brings the vaginal orifice to its final position nearer the surface. At the same time, the vaginal segment increases appreciably in length. The vaginal vestibule is derived from the infratubercular segment of the urogenital sinus (in the male, the same segment will form the inframontanal part of the

Table 2–1. Male and female homologous structures.

Embryonic Structure	Male	Female
Mesonephric duct	Epididymis Vas deferens and seminal vesicles Ejaculatory ducts Appendix epididymidis Ureter, renal pelvis, etc Trigonal structure	Duct of epoophoron Gartner's duct Vesicular appendage Ureter, renal pelvis, etc Trigonal structure
Müllerian duct	Appendix testis Prostatic utricle	Fallopian tubes Uterus Vagina (upper four-fifths)
Müller's tubercle	Verumontanum	Hymen (site of)
Sinovaginal bulb from urogenital sinus	Part of prostatic utricle	Lower one-fifth of vagina
Junction of sinovaginal bulb and urogenital sinus	Disappears normally (remnants probably form prostatic valves)	Hymen
Urogenital sinus Ventral and pelvic part	Urinary bladder (except the trigone) Supramontanal part of prostatic urethra	Urinary bladder (except the trigone) Whole urethra
Phallic or urethral portion	Inframontanal part of prostatic urethra Membranous urethra	Vaginal vestibule
Genital tubercle	Penis	Clitoris
Urethral folds	Penile urethra	Labia minora
Genital swellings	Scrotum	Labia majora
Gubernaculum	Gubernaculum testis	Ligament of ovary Round ligament of uterus
Genital glands	Testis	Ovary
Germinal cords	Seminiferous tubules	Pflüger's tube

prostatic urethra and the membranous urethra). The labia minora are formed from the urethral folds (in the male they will form the pendulous urethra). The hymen is the remnant of the Müllerian tubercle. The lower fifth of the vagina is derived from the contribution of the urogenital sinus with the sinovaginal node. The remainder of the vagina and the uterus are formed from the lower fused third of the Müllerian ducts. The Fallopian tubes are the cephalad two-thirds of the Müllerian ducts (Fig 2–6).

ANOMALIES OF THE GONADAL DUCT SYSTEM

Nonunion of the rete testis and the efferent ductules can occur and, if bilateral, lead to **azoospermia and sterility**. Failure of the Müllerian ducts to approximate or incomplete fusion can lead to various degrees of **duplication** in the genital ducts. **Congenital absence** of one or both uterine tubes or of the uterus or vagina occurs rarely.

Arrested development of the infratubercular segment of the urogenital sinus leads to its persistence, with the urethra and vagina having a common duct to the outside (**urogenital sinus**).

THE EXTERNAL GENITALIA

During the eighth week, external sex differentiation begins to occur. Not until 3 months, however, do the progressively developing external genitalia attain characteristics that can be recognized as distinctively male or female. During the indifferent stage of sexual development, 3 small protuberances appear on the external aspect of the cloacal membrane. In front is the genital tubercle, and on either side of the membrane are the genital swellings.

By the breakdown of the urogenital membrane (17 mm, seventh week), the primitive urogenital sinus achieves a separate opening on the undersurface of the genital tubercle.

MALE EXTERNAL GENITALIA

The urogenital sinus opening extends on the ventral aspect of the genital tubercle as the urethral groove. The primitive urogenital orifice and the urethral groove are bounded on either side by the urethral folds. The genital tubercle becomes elongated to form the phallus. The corpora cavernosa are indicated in the seventh week as paired mesenchymal columns within the shaft of the penis. By the tenth week, the urethral folds start to fuse from the urogenital sinus orifice

toward the tip of the phallus. At the fourteenth week, the fusion is complete and results in the formation of the penile urethra. The corpus spongiosum results from the differentiation of the mesenchymal masses around the formed penile urethra.

The glans penis becomes defined by the development of a circular coronary sulcus around the distal part of the phallus. The urethral groove and the fusing folds do not extend beyond the coronary sulcus. The glandular urethra develops as a result of canalization of an ectodermal epithelial cord that has grown through the glans. This canalization reaches and communicates with the distal end of the previously formed penile urethra. During the third month, a fold of skin at the base of the glans begins growing distally and, 2 months later, surrounds the glans. This forms the prepuce. Meanwhile, the genital swellings shift caudally and are recognizable as scrotal swellings. They meet and fuse, resulting in the formation of the scrotum, with 2 compartments partially separated by a median septum and a median raphe, indicating their line of fusion.

FEMALE EXTERNAL GENITALIA

Until the eighth week, the appearance of the female external genitalia closely resembles that of the male except that the urethral groove is shorter. The genital tubercle, which becomes bent caudally and lags in development, becomes the clitoris. As in the male (though on a minor scale), mesenchymal columns differentiate into corpora cavernosa and a coronary sulcus identifies the glans clitoridis. The most caudal part of the urogenital sinus shortens and widens, forming the vaginal vestibule. The urethral folds do not fuse but remain separate as the labia minora. The genital swellings meet in front of the anus, forming the posterior commissure, while the swellings as a whole enlarge and remain separated on either side of the vestibule and form the labia majora.

ANOMALIES OF THE EXTERNAL GENITALIA

Absence or duplication of the penis or clitoris is very rare. More commonly, the penis remains rudimentary or the clitoris may show hypertrophy. These may be seen alone or, more frequently, in association with **pseudohermaphroditism**. Concealed penis and transposition of penis and scrotum are relatively rare anomalies.

Failure or incomplete fusion of the urethral folds results in **hypospadias** (see above). Penile development is also anomalous in cases of **epispadias** and **exstrophy** (see above).

• • •

References

General

Allan FD: *Essentials of Human Embryology*. Oxford Univ Press, 1960.

Arey LB: *Developmental Anatomy: A Textbook and Laboratory Manual of Embryology,* 6th ed. Saunders, 1954.

Blechschmidt E: *The Stages of Human Development Before Birth; An Introduction to Human Embryology.* Saunders, 1961.

Frazer JES, Baxter JS: *Manual of Embryology. The Development of the Human Body,* 3rd ed. Williams & Wilkins, 1953.

Keith A: *Human Embryology and Morphology,* 6th ed. Williams & Wilkins, 1948.

Kjellberg SR, Ericsson NO, Rudhe U: *The Lower Urinary Tract in Childhood: Some Correlated Clinical and Roentgenologic Observations.* Year Book, 1957.

Patten BM: *Human Embryology,* 2nd ed. Blakiston, 1953.

Anomalies of the Nephric System

Ashley DJB, Mostofi FK: Renal agenesis and dysgenesis. J Urol 83:211, 1960.

Cowinn JL, Landry BW: Cystic diseases of the kidney in infants and children. Radiol Clin North America 6:191, 1968.

Murphy WK, Palubinskas AJ, Smith DR: Sponge kidney: Report of 7 cases. J Urol 85:866, 1961.

Osathanondh V, Potter EL: Pathogenesis of polycystic kidneys: Survey of results of microdissection. Arch Path 77:510, 1964.

Osathanondh V, Potter EL: Pathogenesis of polycystic kidneys: Type 4 due to urethral obstruction. Arch Path 77:502, 1964.

Persky L, Izant R, Bolande R: Renal dysplasia. J Urol 98:431, 1967.

Traut HF: The structural unit of the human kidney. Contribution to Embryology, No. 76, Carnegie Inst Pub No. 332, 15:103, 1923.

The Vesicourethral Unit

Begg RC: The urachus, its anatomy, histology and development. J Anat 64:170, 1930.

Browne D: Some congenital deformities of the rectum, anus, vagina and urethra. (Hunterian Lecture). Ann Roy Coll Surg England 8:173, 1951.

Cullen TS: *Embryology, Anatomy and Diseases of the Umbilicus Together With Diseases of the Urachus.* Saunders, 1916.

Dant RV, Emmett JL, Kennedy RLJ: Congenital absence of abdominal muscles with urologic complications; report on a patient successfully treated. Proc Staff Mayo Clin 22:8, 1947.

Eagle JR Jr, Barrett GS: Congenital deficiency of abdominal musculature with associated genitourinary abnormalities: A syndrome. Report of nine cases. Pediatrics 6:721, 1950.

Hinman F Jr: Surgical disorders of the bladder and umbilicus of urachal origin. Surg Gynec Obst 113:605, 1961.

Lattimer JK: Congenital deficiency of the abdominal musculature and associated genitourinary anomalies: A report of 22 cases. J Urol 79:343, 1958.

Lowsley OO: Persistent cloaca in the female: Report of two cases corrected by operation. J Urol 59:692, 1948.

Lowsley OS: Congenital malformation of the posterior urethra. Ann Surg 60:733, 1914.

Ney C, Friedenberg RM: Radiographic findings in anomalies of the urachus. J Urol 99:288, 1968.

Stephens FD: The female anus, perineum and vestibule: Embryogenesis and deformities. J Obstet Gynaec Brit Common 8:55, 1968.

Stephens FD: *Congenital Malformations of the Rectum, Anus and Genitourinary Tracts.* Livingstone, 1963.

Wainstein ML, Persky L: Superior vesical fistula: An unusual form of exstrophy of the urinary bladder. Am J Surg 115:397, 1968.

Anomalies of the Vesicourethral Unit

Amar AD, Hutch JA: Anomalies of the ureter. Page 98 in: *Encyclopedia of Urology.* Vol 7: *Malformations.* Springer, 1968.

Chwalle R: The process of formation of cystic dilatations of the vesical end of the ureter and of diverticula at the ureteral ostium. Urol Cutan Rev 31:499, 1927.

Ericsson NO: Ectopic ureterocele in infants and children: A clinical study. Acta chir scandinav Suppl 197, 1954.

Lenaghan D: Bifid ureters in children: An anatomical, physiological and clinical study. J Urol 87:808, 1962.

Meyer R: Normal and abnormal development of the ureter in the human embryo: A mechanistic consideration. Anat Rec 96:355, 1946.

Randall A, Campbell EW: Anomalous relationship of the right ureter to the vena cava. J Urol 34:565, 1935.

Wershub LP, Kirwin TJ: Ureterocele, its etiology, pathogenesis and diagnosis. Am J Surg 88:317, 1954.

Gonadal Anomalies

Burns RK: Hormones and the differentiation of sex. In: *Survey of Biological Progress,* Vol 1. Academic Press, 1949.

Grossman H, Ririe SDG: The incidence of urinary tract anomalies in cryptorchid boys. Am J Roentgenol 103:210, 1968.

Gruenwald P: The relation of the growing Müllerian duct to the Wolffian duct and its importance for the genesis of malformations. Anat Rec 81:1, 1949.

Sugrue D: Male urogenital hypoplasia. Am J Surg 115:390, 1968.

3...

Symptoms of Disorders of the Genitourinary Tract

In the work-up of any patient, the history is of paramount importance; this is particularly true in urology. It will be necessary to discuss here only those urologic symptoms which are apt to be brought to the physician's attention by the patient. It is important not only to know whether the disease is acute or chronic but also whether it is recurrent, since recurring symptoms may represent acute exacerbations of chronic disease.

SYSTEMIC MANIFESTATIONS

Symptoms of fever, weight loss, and malaise should be sought. The presence of fever associated with other symptoms of urinary tract infection may be helpful in evaluating the site of the infection. Simple acute cystitis is essentially an afebrile disease. Acute pyelonephritis or prostatitis is apt to cause high temperatures (to 40 °C [104 °F]), often accompanied by violent chills. Infants and children suffering from acute pyelonephritis may have high temperatures without other localizing symptoms or signs. Such a clinical picture, therefore, *invariably* requires bacteriologic study of the urine.

A history of unexplained attacks of fever occurring even years before may have been due to an otherwise asymptomatic pyelonephritis. Renal carcinoma sometimes causes fever which may reach 39 °C (102.2 °F) or more. The absence of fever does not by any means rule out renal infection, for it is the rule that chronic pyelonephritis does not cause fever.

Weight loss is to be expected in the advanced stages of cancer, but it may also be noticed when renal insufficiency due to obstruction or infection supervenes.

General malaise may be noted with neoplasm, chronic pyelonephritis, or renal failure.

LOCAL & REFERRED PAIN

Two types of pain have their origins in the genitourinary organs: local and referred. The latter is unusually common.

Local pain is felt in or near the involved organ. Thus, the pain from a diseased kidney (T10–12, L1) is felt in the costovertebral angle and in the flank in the region of and below the twelfth rib. Pain from an inflamed testicle is felt in the gonad itself.

Referred pain originates in a diseased organ but is felt at some distance from that organ. The ureteral colic (Fig 3–3) caused by a stone in the upper ureter may be associated with severe pain in the ipsilateral testicle; this is explained by the common innervation of these 2 structures (T11–12). A stone in the lower ureter may cause pain referred to the scrotal wall; in this instance, the testis itself is not hyperesthetic. The burning pain with voiding which accompanies acute cystitis is felt in the distal urethra in the female or in the glandular urethra in the male (S2–3).

Abnormalities of a urologic organ can also cause pain in any other organ (eg, gastrointestinal, gynecologic) that has a sensory nerve supply common to both (Fig 3–2).

Kidney Pain (Fig 3–3)

Typical renal pain is usually felt as a dull and constant ache in the costovertebral angle just lateral to the sacrospinalis muscle and just below the twelfth rib. This pain often spreads along the subcostal area toward the umbilicus. It may be expected in those renal diseases which cause sudden distention of the renal capsule. Acute pyelonephritis (with its sudden edema) and acute ureteral obstruction (with its sudden renal back pressure) both cause this typical pain. It should be pointed out, however, that many urologic renal diseases are painless because their progression is so slow that sudden capsular distention does not occur. Such diseases include cancer, chronic pyelonephritis, staghorn calculus, tuberculosis, and hydronephrosis due to mild ureteral obstruction. Radiculitis commonly mimics renal pain.

Ureteral Pain (Fig 3–3)

Ureteral pain is typically stimulated by acute ob-

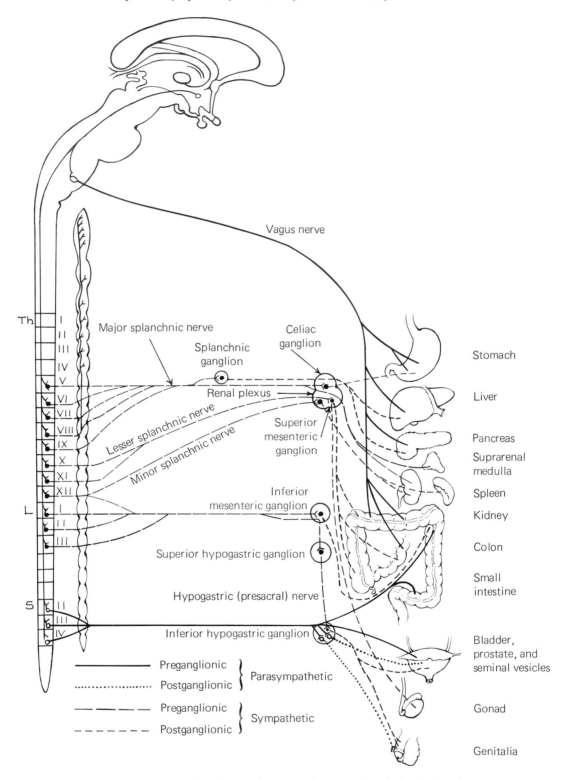

Figure 3–1. Diagrammatic representation of autonomic nerve supply to gastrointestinal and genitourinary tracts.

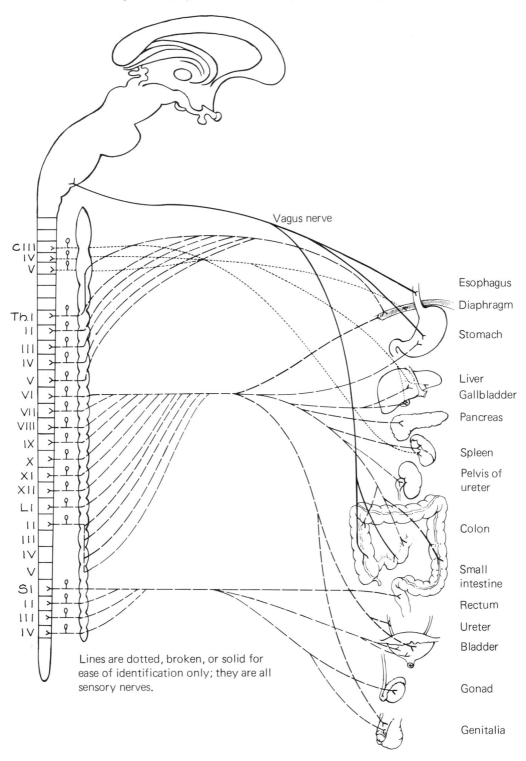

Figure 3–2. Diagrammatic representation of the sensory nerves of the gastrointestinal and genitourinary tracts.

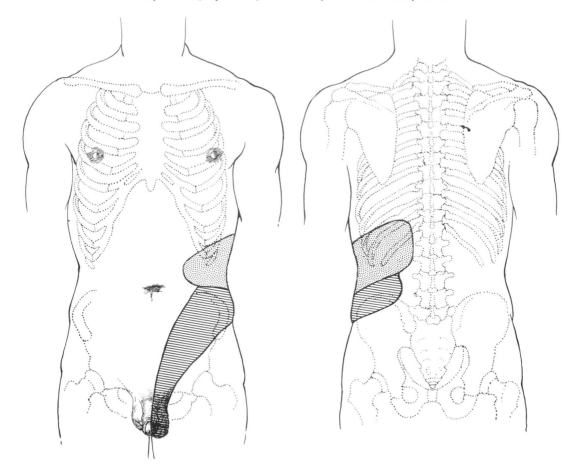

Figure 3—3. Referred pain from kidney (dotted areas) and ureter (shaded areas).

struction (passage of a stone or a blood clot). In this instance, there is back pain from capsular distention combined with severe colicky pain (due to renal pelvic and ureteral muscle spasm) that radiates from the costovertebral angle down toward the lower anterior abdominal quadrant, along the course of the ureter. In men it may also be felt in the bladder, scrotum, or testicle. In women it may radiate into the vulva. The severity and colicky nature of this pain are caused by the hyperperistalsis and spasm of this smooth muscle organ as it attempts to rid itself of a foreign body or to overcome obstruction.

The physician may be able to judge the position of a ureteral stone by the history of pain and the site of referral. If the stone is lodged in the upper ureter, the pain radiates to the testicle, since the nerve supply of this organ is similar to that of the kidney and upper ureter (T11—12). With stones in the mid portion of the ureter on the right side, the pain is referred to McBurney's point and may therefore simulate appendicitis; on the left side, it may resemble diverticulitis or other diseases of the descending or sigmoid colon (T12, L1). As the stone approaches the bladder, inflammation and edema of the ureteral orifice ensue and symptoms of vesical irritability may occur. It is

important to realize, however, that in mild ureteral obstruction, as seen in the congenital stenoses, there is usually no pain, either renal or ureteral.

Vesical Pain

The overdistended bladder of the patient in acute urinary retention will cause agonizing pain in the suprapubic area. Other than this, however, constant suprapubic pain not related to the act of urination is usually not of urologic origin. The relatively uncommon interstitial cystitis and vesical ulceration caused by tuberculosis may cause suprapubic discomfort when the bladder becomes full, but this discomfort is usually relieved by urination.

The patient in chronic urinary retention due to bladder neck obstruction or to a neurogenic bladder may experience little or no suprapubic discomfort even though the bladder reaches the umbilicus.

The common cause of bladder pain is infection; the pain is usually not felt over the bladder but is referred to the distal urethra and is related to the act of urination. Terminal dysuria may be severe.

Prostatic Pain

Direct pain from the prostate gland is not common. Occasionally, when the prostate is inflamed, the patient may feel a vague discomfort or fullness in the perineal or rectal area (S2–4). Lumbosacral backache is occasionally experienced as a referred pain from the prostate, but is not a common symptom of prostatitis. Inflammation of the gland may cause symptoms of cystitis.

Testicular Pain

Testicular pain due to trauma or infection is very severe and is felt locally, although there may be some radiation of the discomfort along the spermatic cord into the lower abdomen. It may involve the costovertebral area as well. Uninfected hydrocele and tumor of the testes do not commonly cause pain. A varicocele may cause a dull ache in the testicle that is increased after heavy exercise. At times the first symptom of an early indirect inguinal hernia may be testicular pain (referred). Pain from a stone in the upper ureter may be referred to the testicle.

Epididymal Pain

Acute infection of the epididymis is the only painful disease of this organ and is quite common. Some degree of neighborhood inflammatory reaction involves the adjacent testis as well, further aggravating the discomfort. In the early stages of epididymitis, pain may first be felt in the groin or lower abdominal quadrant. (If on the right side, it may simulate appendicitis.) This may be a referred type of pain but can be secondary to associated inflammation of the vas deferens. The discomfort associated with epididymitis may reach the costal angle and may mimic ureteral stone.

Back & Leg Pain

Pain low in the back and radiating down one or both legs, especially when associated with symptoms of vesical neck obstruction, suggests metastases to the pelvic bones from cancer of the prostate.

GASTROINTESTINAL SYMPTOMS OF UROLOGIC DISEASES

Whether renal or ureteral disease is painful or not, gastrointestinal symptoms are often present. The patient with acute pyelonephritis will suffer not only from localized back pain, symptoms of vesical irritability, chills, and fever but also from generalized abdominal pain and distention. The patient who is passing a stone down the ureter will have typical renal and ureteral colic and, usually, hematuria, and may experience severe nausea and vomiting as well as abdominal distention. However, the urinary symptoms so far overshadow the gastrointestinal symptoms that the latter are usually ignored. Inadvertent overdistention of the renal pelvis (eg, with opaque material in order to obtain adequate retrograde urograms) may cause the pa-

tient to become nauseated, to vomit, and to complain of cramplike pain in the abdomen. This clinical experiment demonstrates the renointestinal reflex, which may lead to confusing symptomatology. In the very common "silent" urologic diseases, some degree of gastrointestinal symptomatology may be present which could mislead the clinician into seeking the diagnosis in the intraperitoneal zone.

Cause of the Mimicry

A. Renointestinal Reflexes: These account for most of the confusion. They arise because of the common autonomic and sensory innervations of the 2 systems (Figs 3–1 and 3–2). Afferent stimuli from the renal capsule or musculature of the pelvis may, by reflex action, cause pylorospasm (symptoms of peptic ulcer) or other changes in tone of the smooth muscles of the enteric tract and its adnexa.

B. Organ Relationships: The right kidney is closely related to the hepatic flexure of the colon, the duodenum, the head of the pancreas, the common bile duct, the liver, and the gallbladder (Fig 1–3). The left kidney lies just behind the splenic flexure of the colon and is closely related to the stomach, pancreas, and spleen. Inflammations or tumors in the retroperitoneum thus may extend into or displace intraperitoneal organs, causing them to produce symptoms.

C. Peritoneal Irritation: The anterior surfaces of the kidneys are covered by peritoneum. Renal inflammation, therefore, will cause peritoneal irritation, which leads to muscle rigidity and rebound tenderness.

The symptoms arising from chronic renal disease (eg, uninfected hydronephrosis, staghorn calculus, cancer, chronic pyelonephritis) may be entirely gastrointestinal and may simulate in every way the syndromes of peptic ulcer, gallbladder disease, appendicitis, or other less specific gastrointestinal complaints. If a thorough survey of the gastrointestinal tract fails to demonstrate suspected disease processes, the physician should give every consideration to study of the urinary tract.

SYMPTOMS RELATED TO THE ACT OF URINATION

Many conditions cause symptoms of "cystitis." These include infections of the bladder, vesical inflammation due to chemical or x-ray radiation reactions, interstitial cystitis, prostatitis, senile urethritis, psychoneurosis, torsion or rupture of an ovarian cyst, and foreign bodies in the bladder. Often, however, the patient with chronic cystitis notices no symptoms of vesical irritability. In children who have taken bubble baths, symptoms resembling cystitis may be noted secondary to the resulting urethritis.

Frequency, Nocturia, & Urgency

The normal capacity of the bladder is about 400

ml. Frequency may be caused by residual urine which decreases the functional capacity of the organ. When the mucosa, submucosa, and even the muscularis become inflamed (eg, infection, foreign body, stones, tumor), the capacity of the bladder decreases sharply. This decrease is due to 2 factors: the pain which results from even mild stretching of the bladder and the loss of bladder elasticity which results from inflammatory edema. When the bladder is normal, urination can be delayed if circumstances require it, but this is not so in acute cystitis. Once the diminished bladder capacity is reached, any further distention may be agonizing, and the patient may actually urinate involuntarily if he does not void immediately. During very severe acute infections, the desire to urinate may be constant, and each voiding may produce only a few milliliters of urine. Day frequency without nocturia and acute or chronic frequency lasting only a few hours suggest nervous tension (see Chapter 34).

Diseases that cause fibrosis of the bladder are accompanied by frequency of urination. Examples of such diseases are tuberculosis, interstitial cystitis, and bilharziasis. The presence of stones or foreign bodies causes vesical irritability, but secondary infection is almost always present.

Nocturia is often a symptom of renal disease related to a decrease in the functioning renal parenchyma with loss of concentrating power. Nocturia may occur in the absence of disease by persons who drink excessive amounts of fluids in the late evening. Coffee and alcoholic beverages, because of their specific diuretic effect, often produce nocturia if consumed just before bedtime. In older people, when ambulatory, some fluid retention may develop secondary to mild heart failure or varicose veins. With recumbency at night, this fluid is mobilized, leading to nocturia.

A very low or very high urine pH can irritate the bladder and cause frequency of urination. In chronic obstructive pulmonary disease, the $P_{a_{CO_2}}$ is elevated. Compensation requires increased urinary excretion of chloride, leading to a low pH (Farcon & Morales, 1972). With hyperventilation, the urine becomes strongly alkaline.

Burning Upon Urination

This is common in acute cystitis and prostatitis. In men, it is usually felt in the distal urethra just proximal to or in the glans. In women, it is ordinarily referred to the urethra. It is important to remember that it is rarely felt in the suprapubic area. This burning sensation occurs in association with the act of urination, although it may be more marked at the beginning of, during, at the end of, or occasionally after urination. It may be very severe. Vague pain in the urethra not associated with the act of voiding is usually not caused by urinary system disease. In men, it is apt to be a psychosexual symptom; in women, however, it may occasionally be caused by chronic urethritis.

Enuresis

Strictly speaking, enuresis means bedwetting at night. It is physiologic during the first 2 or 3 years of life but becomes troublesome, particularly to parents, after that age. It may be functional or secondary to delayed neuromuscular maturation of the urethrovesical component, but it may present as a symptom of organic disease (eg, infection, distal urethral stenosis in girls, posterior urethral valves in boys, neurogenic bladder). If, however, wetting occurs also during the daytime or if there are other urinary symptoms—or if the enuresis persists beyond the age of 6 or 7 years— urologic investigation is essential. In adult life, enuresis may be replaced by nocturia for which no organic basis can be found.

Symptoms of Prostatic Obstruction

(See also Chapters 10 and 18.)

A. Hesitancy and Straining: Hesitancy in initiating the urinary stream is one of the early symptoms of enlarged prostate. As the degree of obstruction increases, hesitancy is prolonged; the patient may have to strain in order to initiate urination.

B. Loss of Force and Decrease of Caliber of the Stream: Progressive loss of force and caliber of the urinary stream is noted as urethral resistance increases despite the generation of increased intravesical pressure.

C. Terminal Dribbling: This becomes more and more noticeable as obstruction progresses and is a most distressing symptom.

D. Acute Urinary Retention: Sudden inability to urinate may supervene. The patient experiences increasingly agonizing suprapubic pain associated with severe urgency. He may dribble only small amounts of urine.

E. Chronic Urinary Retention: This may cause little discomfort to the patient even though there is great hesitancy in starting the stream and marked reduction of its force and caliber. Constant dribbling of urine (paradoxical incontinence) may be experienced. It may be likened to water pouring over a dam.

F. Interruption of the Urinary Stream: Interruption may be abrupt and accompanied by severe pain radiating down the urethra. This type of reaction strongly suggests the complication of vesical calculus.

G. Sense of Residual Urine: The patient often feels he still has urine in his bladder when he has finished urinating.

H. Cystitis: Recurring episodes of acute cystitis suggest the presence of residual urine.

Symptoms of Urethral Obstruction

In the male, the combination of a slow and bifurcated stream suggests urethral stricture. A slow, weak stream in the male infant or little boy is compatible with posterior urethral valves or congenital urethral stricture.

Little girls with or without urinary infection may have a slow, hesitant, or interrupted stream. This should suggest involuntary spasm of the periurethral striated musculature secondary to distal urethral stenosis (see Chapter 28). Some women complain of constant impairment of urinary flow, in which case the possibility of urethral stricture should be investigated. Often, however, careful questioning will reveal that some voidings are slow while others are quite free. This is compatible with periodic periurethral muscle spasm on a psychogenic basis, or with urethritis.

Incontinence

There are many reasons for incontinence. The history often gives a clue to its cause.

A. True Incontinence: The patient may lose urine without warning; this may be a constant or periodic symptom. The more obvious causes include exstrophy of the bladder, epispadias, vesicovaginal fistula, and ectopic ureteral orifice. Injury to the urethral smooth muscle sphincters may occur during prostatectomy or childbirth. Congenital or acquired neurogenic diseases may lead to dysfunction of the bladder and incontinence.

B. Stress Incontinence: When slight weakness of the sphincteric mechanisms is present, urine may be lost in association with physical strain (eg, coughing, laughing, rising from a chair). This is common with vesical neurogenic disease. The patient stays dry while lying in bed.

C. Urgency Incontinence: This type of urgency may be so precipitate and severe that there is involuntary loss of urine. Urgency incontinence not infrequently occurs with acute cystitis, particularly in women, since they seem to have relatively poor anatomic sphincters. Urgency incontinence is a common symptom of an upper motor neuron lesion. It is often seen also in tense, anxious women even in the absence of infection.

D. Paradoxical (Overflow or False) Incontinence: This is loss of urine due to chronic urinary retention or secondary to a flaccid bladder. The intravesical pressure finally equals the urethral resistance; urine then constantly dribbles forth.

Oliguria & Anuria

Oliguria and anuria may be caused by acute renal failure (due to shock or dehydration), fluid-ion imbalance, or bilateral ureteral obstruction.

Pneumaturia

The passage of gas in the urine almost always means that there is a fistula between the urinary tract and the bowel. This occurs most commonly in the bladder or urethra but may be seen also in the ureter or renal pelvis. Carcinoma of the sigmoid colon, diverticulitis with abscess formation, regional enteritis, and trauma cause most vesical fistulas. Congenital anomalies account for most urethral fistulas. Certain bacteria, by the process of fermentation, may rarely liberate gas.

Cloudy Urine

Patients often complain of cloudy urine, but it is most often cloudy merely because it is alkaline; this causes the precipitation of phosphate. Chyluria is a rare cause of cloudy urine. A properly performed urinalysis will reveal the cause of cloudiness.

Bloody Urine

Hematuria is a danger signal that cannot be ignored. It is important to know whether urination is painful or not, whether the hematuria is associated with symptoms of vesical irritability, and whether blood is seen in all or only a portion of the urinary stream. Some individuals will pass red urine after eating beets (particularly if they are anemic) or taking laxatives containing phenolphthalein, in which case the urine is translucent rather than opaque and contains no red cells. Because of the wide use of rhodamine B as a coloring agent in cookies, cakes, cold drinks, and fruit juices, children commonly pass red urine after the ingestion of these foods. This is the so-called Monday morning disorder. The hemoglobinuria that occurs as a feature of the hemolytic syndromes may also cause the urine to be red.

A. Bloody Urine in Relation to Symptoms and Diseases: Hematuria associated with renal colic suggests ureteral stone, although a clot from a bleeding renal tumor can cause the same type of pain.

Hematuria is not uncommonly associated with nonspecific or tuberculous infection of the bladder. The bleeding is often terminal (bladder neck or prostate), although it may be present throughout urination (vesical or upper tract). Stone in the bladder often causes hematuria, but infection is usually present and there are symptoms of bladder neck obstruction, neurogenic bladder, or cystocele. When a tumor of the bladder ulcerates, it is often complicated by infection and bleeding. Thus, symptoms of cystitis and hematuria are also compatible with neoplasm.

Dilated veins may develop at the bladder neck secondary to enlargement of the prostate. These may rupture when the patient strains to urinate.

Hematuria without other symptoms ("silent") must be regarded as a symptom of tumor of the bladder or kidney until proved otherwise. It is usually intermittent; bleeding may not recur for months. Complacency because the bleeding stops spontaneously must be condemned. Less common causes of silent hematuria are staghorn calculus, polycystic kidneys, solitary renal cyst, sickle cell disease, and hydronephrosis. Painless bleeding is common with acute glomerulonephritis. Recurrent bleeding is occasionally seen in children suffering from focal glomerulitis.

B. Time of Hematuria: Learning whether the hematuria is partial (initial, terminal) or total (present throughout urination) is often of help in placing the site of the bleeding. Initial hematuria suggests an anterior urethral lesion (eg, urethritis, stricture, meatal stenosis in young boys). Terminal hematuria usually arises from the posterior urethra, bladder neck, or trigone. Among the common causes are posterior urethritis and polyps and tumors of the vesical neck.

Total hematuria has its source at or above the level of the bladder (eg, stone, tumor, tuberculosis, nephritis).

Unusual Consequences of Micturition

Postmicturition syncope has been observed occasionally in men. Orthostatic hypotension and cardiac standstill have been observed in one patient. Psychomotor epilepsy and angina pectoris may be triggered by voiding.

MANIFESTATIONS RELATED TO SEXUAL ORGANS

Symptoms

Many people suffer from genitourinary complaints on a purely psychologic or emotional basis. In others, organic symptoms may be increased in severity because of tension states. It is therefore important to seek clues which might give evidence of emotional stress.

In women, the relationship of the menses to ureteral pain or vesical complaints should be determined, although menstruation may exacerbate both organic and functional vesical and renal difficulties.

Many patients, particularly women, recognize that the state of their "nerves" has a direct effect on their symptoms. They often realize that their "cystitis" develops following a tension-producing or anxiety-producing episode in their personal or occupational environment.

A. Sex Difficulties in the Male: Men may complain directly of sexual difficulty. However, they are often so ashamed of loss of sexual power that they cannot admit it even to a physician. In such cases they come to him asking for "prostate treatment," hoping that the physician will understand that they have sexual complaints and that they will be treated accordingly. The main sexual symptoms include impaired quality of erection, premature loss of erection, absence of ejaculate with orgasm, premature ejaculation, and even loss of desire. Since these symptoms are usually psychologic in origin, this area must therefore be explored.

B. Sex Difficulties in the Female: Women suffering from the psychosomatic cystitis syndrome almost always admit to an unhappy sex life. They notice that frequency or vaginal-urethral pain often occurs on the day following the incomplete sexual act. Many of them recognize the inadequacy of their sexual experiences as one of the underlying causes of their urologic complaints; too frequently, however, the doctor either does not ask them pertinent questions or, if the patient volunteers this information, he ignores it.

In treating sex difficulties of suspected psychosomatic origin, the physician should explore pertinent facts concerning childhood, adolescence (sex education and experiences), marriage problems, and relationships with relatives, business associates, etc. Even if psychosomatic disease is strongly suspected before the history-taking has been completed, a thorough examination and laboratory survey must be done. Both psyche and soma may be involved, and the patient requires assurance that he is not suffering from serious organic disease. Although sexual interest and activity decline with advancing years, physically healthy men may continue to be sexually active into their eighth or ninth decades.

Objective Manifestations

(See also Infertility, Chapter 33.)

On occasion, a patient may have objective signs. The most common include urethral discharge, lesions of the skin, and scrotal, perineal, or abdominal masses.

Another symptom referable to the sex organs is bloody ejaculation. This is often associated with prostatitis, prostatic congestion, or hypertrophy of the mucosa of the seminal vesicles.

•   •   •

References

Local & Referred Pain

Dowd JB: Flank pain in nonurologic disease. M Clin North America 47:437, 1963.

Gastrointestinal Symptoms of Urologic Diseases

Takacs FJ: The interrelationships of gastrointestinal and renal diseases. M Clin North America 50:507, 1966.

Symptoms Related to the Act of Urination

Bennett MA, Heslop RW, Meynell MJ: Massive haematuria associated with sickle-cell trait. Brit MJ 1:677, 1967.

Davidson AIG, Matheson NA: Ovarian cysts and urinary symptoms. Brit J Surg 51:908, 1964.

Farcon EM, Morales PA: The association of chronic obstructive pulmonary disease (COPD) and lower urinary tract symptoms. J Urol 108:619, 1972.

Fiala M & others: Role of adenovirus type II in hemorrhagic cystitis secondary to immunosuppression. J Urol 112:595, 1974.

Glasgow EF, Moncrieff MW, White RHR: Symptomless haematuria in childhood. Brit MJ 2:687, 1970.

Hoffman RB, Zucker MO: A new technique in the treatment of renal bleeding: Epinephrine infusion in a patient with sickle cell trait. California Med 118:49, June 1973.

Levin S: Red urine: The Monday morning disorder of children. Pediatrics 36:134, 1965.

Low AI, Matz LR: Haematuria and renal fornical lesions. Brit J Urol 44:681, 1972.

Marshall S: The effect of bubble bath on the urinary tract. J Urol 93:112, 1965.

Morris JJ, McIntosh HD: Angina of micturition. Circulation 27:85, 1963.

Redman JF, Mobley JE: Sickle cell disease: Renal colic and microscopic hematuria. J Urol 100:594, 1968.

Schoenberg BS, Kuglitsch JF, Varnes WE: Micturition syncope: Not a single entity. JAMA 229:1631, 1974.

Spear GS & others: Idiopathic hematuria of childhood: Pathologic findings in the kidney in six patients. Human Path 4:349, 1973.

Tresidder GC: "Prostatism." Practitioner 212:208, 1974.

Wiggelinkhuizen J, Landman C, Greenberg E: Chyluria. Am J Dis Child 124:99, 1972.

Zivin I, Rowley W: Psychomotor epilepsy with micturition. Arch Int Med 113:8, 1964.

4...

Physical Examination of the Genitourinary Tract

The history will suggest whether a complete or partial examination is indicated. The symptom of urethral discharge probably does not require a thorough physical examination; on the other hand, painless hematuria would certainly require a careful examination of the genitourinary tract. In this chapter are discussed the urologic aspects of the physical examination of the patient.

EXAMINATION OF THE KIDNEYS

Inspection

On occasion, a mass may be visible in the upper abdominal area which, if soft (eg, as in hydronephrosis), may be difficult to palpate. Fullness in the costovertebral angle may be consistent with malignancy (eg, neuroblastoma in children) or perinephric infection. The presence and persistence of indentations in the skin from lying on wrinkled sheets suggest edema of the skin secondary to perinephric abscess. If this disease is suspected, have the patient lie on a rough towel and observe for indentations.

Palpation of the Kidneys

The kidneys lie rather high under the diaphragm and lower ribs and are therefore well protected from injury. Because of the position of the liver, the right kidney is lower than the left. The kidneys are difficult to palpate in men because of the resistance of abdominal muscle tone and because the kidneys in men are more fixed than those of women and move only slightly with change of posture or respiration. The lower part of the right kidney can sometimes be felt, but the left kidney cannot usually be felt unless it is grossly enlarged or displaced.

The most successful method of renal palpation is carried out with the patient lying supine on a hard surface (Fig 4–1). The kidney is lifted by one hand in the costovertebral angle. On deep inspiration, the kidney moves downward, and when it is lowest the other hand is pushed firmly and deeply beneath the costal margin in an effort to trap the kidney below that point. If this is successful, the anterior hand can palpate the size, shape, and consistency of the organ as it slips back into its normal position.

The kidney can sometimes best be palpated with the patient sitting and the examiner standing behind him. At other times, if the patient is lying on his side, the uppermost kidney drops downward and medially, thereby making it more accessible to palpation.

An enlarged renal mass suggests compensatory hypertrophy (if the other kidney is absent or atrophic), hydronephrosis, tumor, cyst, or polycystic disease. A mass in this area, however, may be a retroperitoneal tumor, the spleen, a lesion of the bowel (eg, tumor, abscess), a lesion of the gallbladder, or a pancreatic cyst. Tumors may have the consistency of normal tissue; they may also be nodular. Hydronephroses may be firm or soft. Polycystic kidneys are usually nodular.

An acutely infected kidney is tender, but this is difficult to elicit since marked muscle spasm is usually present. Since normal kidneys are often tender also, this sign is not always helpful.

Although renal pain may be diffusely felt in the back, tenderness is usually well localized just lateral to the sacrospinalis muscle and just below the twelfth rib. This may be brought out by palpation or, more sharply, by fist percussion over that area.

Percussion of the Kidneys

At times a greatly enlarged kidney cannot be felt on palpation, particularly if it is soft. This can be true of hydronephrosis. Such masses, however, may be readily outlined by percussion, both anteriorly and posteriorly; this part of the examination should never be omitted. Percussion is of particular value in outlining an enlarging mass in the flank following renal trauma (progressive hemorrhage), where tenderness and muscle spasm prevent proper palpation.

Transillumination

This maneuver may prove quite helpful in the child under 1 year of age who presents with a suprapubic or flank mass. A 2- or 3-cell flashlight with an opaque flange protruding beyond the lens is an adequate instrument. The flashlight is applied at right angles to the abdomen. The fiberoptic light cord, used to illuminate various optical instruments, is an excellent source of cold light. A dark room is required. A distended bladder or cystic mass will transilluminate; a solid mass will not. Flank masses may also be tested by applying the light posteriorly.

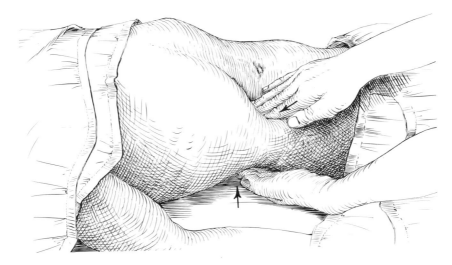

Figure 4–1. Method of palpation of the kidney. The posterior hand lifts the kidney upward. The anterior hand feels for the kidney. The patient then takes a deep breath; this causes the kidney to descend. As the patient inhales, the fingers of the anterior hand are plunged inward at the costal margin. If the kidney is mobile or enlarged, it can be felt between the 2 hands.

Differentiation of Renal & Radicular Pain

Radicular pain is commonly felt in the costovertebral and subcostal areas. It may spread along the course of the ureter as well and is the most common cause of so-called "kidney" pain. Every patient who complains of flank pain should be examined for evidence of nerve root irritation. The cause is often poor posture, arthritis, or intervertebral disk disease. Radicular pain may be noted as an aftermath of a flank incision wherein a rib may become dislocated, causing the costal nerve to impinge on the edge of a ligament. Pain experienced during the preeruptive phase of herpes zoster involving any of the segments between T11 and L2 may also simulate pain of renal origin.

Radiculitis usually causes hyperesthesia of the area of skin served by the irritated peripheral nerve. This hypersensitivity can be elicited by means of the pinwheel or by grasping and pinching both skin and fat of the abdomen and flanks. Pressure exerted by the thumb over the costovertebral joints will reveal local tenderness at the point of emergence of the involved peripheral nerve.

Auscultation

Auscultation of the costovertebral areas and upper abdominal quadrants may reveal a systolic bruit which is often associated with stenosis or aneurysm of the renal artery. Bruits over the femoral arteries may be found in association with the Leriche syndrome, which may be a cause of impotence.

EXAMINATION OF THE BLADDER

The bladder cannot be felt unless it is moderately distended. In the adult, if it is percussible, it contains at least 150 ml of urine. In acute or (more commonly) in chronic urinary retention, the bladder may reach or even rise above the umbilicus, in which case its outline may be seen and usually felt. (In chronic retention, where the bladder wall is flabby, the bladder may be difficult to palpate. In this instance, percussion is of great value.)

In the male infant or little boy, palpation of a hard mass deep in the center of the pelvis is compatible with a thickened hypertrophied bladder secondary to obstruction caused by posterior urethral valves.

A few instances have been reported wherein marked edema of the legs has developed secondary to compression of the iliac vessels by a distended bladder. Bimanual (abdominorectal or abdominovaginal) palpation may reveal the extent of a vesical neoplasm. To be successful, it must be done under anesthesia.

EXAMINATION OF THE EXTERNAL MALE GENITALIA

PENIS

Inspection

If the patient has not been circumcised, the foreskin should be retracted. This may reveal tumor or balanitis as the cause of a foul discharge. If retraction is not possible (ie, phimosis), surgical correction (dorsal slit or circumcision) is indicated.

The observation of a poor urinary stream is significant. In the newborn, neurogenic bladder or the presence of posterior urethral valves should be considered.

In men, such a finding suggests urethral stricture or prostatic obstruction.

The scars of healed syphilis may be an important clue. An active ulcer requires bacteriologic or pathologic study (eg, syphilitic chancre, epithelioma). Superficial ulcers or vesicles are compatible with herpes simplex; they are often interpreted by the patient as a serious venereal disease, possibly syphilis.

Meatal stenosis is a common cause of bloody spotting in the male infant. On rare occasions, it may be of such degree as to cause advanced bilateral hydronephrosis. It is easily corrected by meatotomy.

The position of the meatus should be noted. It may be located proximal to the tip of the glans on either the dorsum (epispadias) or the ventral surface (hypospadias). In either instance, there is apt to be abnormal curvature of the penis—dorsally with epispadias, ventrally with hypospadias. The urethral orifice is often stenotic.

Palpation

Palpation of the shaft may reveal a fibrous plaque involving the fascial covering of the corpora cavernosa. This is typical of Peyronie's disease. Tender areas of induration felt along the urethra may signify periurethritis secondary to urethral stricture.

Urethral Discharge

Urethral discharge is the most common complaint referable to the male sex organ. Gonococcal pus is usually profuse, thick, and yellow or gray-brown. Nonspecific discharges may be similar in appearance but are often thin, mucoid, and scanty. Although gonorrhea must be ruled out as the cause of a urethral discharge, a high percentage of such cases will be found to be nonspecific. Patients with urethral discharge should also be examined for other venereal diseases; double infection is not uncommon.

Bloody discharge should suggest the possibility of a foreign body in the urethra (male or female), urethral stricture, or neoplasm.

Urethral discharge must always be sought before the patient is asked to void.

SCROTUM

Infections and inflammations of the skin of the scrotum are not common. Small sebaceous cysts are occasionally seen. Malignant tumors are rare. The scrotum is bifid when midscrotal or perineal hypospadias is present.

Elephantiasis of the scrotum is caused by obstruction to lymphatic drainage. It is endemic in the tropics and is due to filariasis. Elephantiasis may result from radical resection of the lymph nodes of the inguinal and femoral areas, in which case the skin of the penis is also involved. Small hemangiomas of the skin are common and may bleed spontaneously.

TESTIS

The testes should be carefully palpated with the fingers of both hands. A hard area in the testis proper must be regarded as a malignant tumor until proved otherwise. Transillumination of all scrotal masses should be a routine procedure. With the patient in a dark room, a strong flashlight is placed against the scrotal sac posteriorly. A hydrocele will cause the intrascrotal mass to glow red. Light will not be transmitted through a solid tumor. Tumors are often smooth but may be nodular. They seem abnormally heavy. A testis replaced by tumor or damaged by gumma is insensitive to pressure, and the usual sickening sensation is absent. About 10% of tumors are associated with a secondary hydrocele which may have to be aspirated before definitive palpation can be done.

The testis may be absent from the scrotum. This may represent transient (physiologic retractile testis) or true cryptorchism. Palpation of the groins may reveal the presence of the organ.

The atrophic testis (following postoperative orchiopexy, mumps orchitis, or torsion of the spermatic cord) is usually flabby and at times hypersensitive. Although spermatogenesis may be lost, androgen function is usually intact.

EPIDIDYMIS

The epididymis is sometimes rather closely attached to the posterior surface of the testis, and at other times it is quite free of it. The epididymis should be carefully palpated for size and induration. Induration means infection (primary tumors are exceedingly rare).

In the acute stage of epididymitis, the testis and epididymis are indistinguishable by palpation; the testicle and epididymis may be adherent to the scrotum, which is usually quite red. Tenderness is exquisite.

Chronic painless induration should suggest tuberculosis, although nonspecific chronic epididymitis is also a possibility. Other signs of tuberculosis of the genitourinary tract usually present include "sterile" pyuria, a thickened seminal vesicle, a nodular prostate, and "beading" of the vas deferens.

SPERMATIC CORD & VAS DEFERENS

A swelling in the spermatic cord may be cystic (eg, hydrocele or hernia) or solid (eg, connective tissue tumor). The latter is rare. Lipoma in the investing fascia of the cord may simulate hernia. Diffuse swelling and induration of the cord are seen with filarial funiculitis.

Careful palpation of the vas deferens may reveal thickening (eg, chronic infection), fusiform enlargements (the "beading" caused by tuberculosis), or even its absence. The latter finding is of importance in the infertile male; it is rare.

TESTICULAR TUNICS & ADNEXA

Hydroceles are usually cystic but on occasion are so tense that they simulate solid tumors. Transillumination makes the differential diagnosis. They may develop secondary to nonspecific acute or tuberculous epididymitis, trauma, or tumor of the testis. The latter is a distinct possibility if hydrocele appears "spontaneously" between the ages of 18–35. It should be aspirated to permit careful palpation of underlying structures.

Hydrocele usually surrounds the testis completely. Cystic masses that are separate from but in the region of the upper pole of the testis are probably spermatoceles. Aspiration reveals the typical thin, milky fluid, which contains sperms.

VAGINAL EXAMINATION

Diseases of the female genital tract may secondarily involve the urinary organs, thereby making a thorough gynecologic examination essential. Commonly associated are urethrocystitis secondary to urethral diverticulitis or cervicitis, pyelonephritis during pregnancy, and ureteral obstruction from metastatic nodes or direct extension in cancer of the cervix.

Inspection

The urinary meatus may reveal a reddened, tender, friable lesion (urethral caruncle) or a reddened, everted posterior lip which is often seen with senile urethritis and vaginitis. Biopsy is indicated if a malignant tumor cannot be ruled out. Smears of discharges should be made. The diagnosis of senile vaginitis (and urethritis) is established by staining a smear of the vaginal epithelium with Lugol's solution. It should be examined immediately after rinsing because the brown dye in the cells quickly fades. Cells lacking glycogen (hypoestrogenism) do not take up the stain, whereas normal cells do.

Evidence of skenitis and bartholinitis may reveal the source of persistent urethritis or cystitis. The condition of the vaginal wall should be observed. Bacteriologic study of the secretions may be helpful. Urethrocele and cystocele may cause residual urine and lead to persistent infection of the bladder. They are often found in association with stress incontinence. A bulge in the anterior vaginal wall might represent a urethral diverticulum. The cervix should be visualized in order to note the presence of malignancy or infection. Taking biopsy specimens or making Papanicolaou preparations may be indicated.

Palpation

At times the urethra, the base of the bladder, and the lower ureters may be tender on palpation, but little can be deduced from this. Induration of the urethra or trigonal area or a mass involving either may be a clue to an existing neoplasm. A soft mass found in this area could be a urethral diverticulum. Pressure on such a lesion may cause pus to extrude from the urethra. A stone in the lower ureter may be palpable. Evidence of enlargement of the uterus (eg, pregnancy, myomas) or diseases or inflammations of the colon or adnexa may afford a clue to the cause of urinary symptoms (eg, compression of a ureter by a malignant ovarian tumor, endometriosis, or diverticulitis of sigmoid colon adherent to the bladder).

Carcinoma of the cervix may invade the base of the bladder, causing vesical irritability or hematuria; or its metastases to iliac lymph nodes may compress the ureters.

Rectal examination may afford further information and is the obvious route of examination in children and virgins.

RECTAL EXAMINATION OF THE MALE

SPHINCTER & LOWER RECTUM

The estimation of sphincter tone is of great importance. Laxity of the muscle strongly suggests similar changes in the urinary sphincters and detrusor and may be a clue to the diagnosis of neurogenic disease. In addition to the digital prostatic examination, the examiner should palpate the entire lower rectum and rule out stenosis, internal hemorrhoids, cryptitis, rectal fistulas, mucosal polyps, and rectal malignancies.

PROSTATE

Before the rectal examination is made, a specimen of urine for routine analysis should be collected. This is of the utmost importance, since prostatic massage (or even palpation at times) will force prostatic secretion into the posterior urethra. If this secretion contains pus, a specimen of urine voided after the rectal examination will be contaminated by it.

Size

The average prostate is about 4 cm in length and width. It is widest superiorly at the bladder neck. As the gland enlarges, the lateral sulci become relatively deeper and the median furrow becomes obliterated. The prostate may also elongate. It is necessary to realize that the clinical importance of prostatic hyperplasia is measured by the severity of symptoms and the amount of residual urine and not by the size of the gland. On rectal examination, the prostate may be of normal size and consistency in a patient with acute urinary retention.

Consistency

Normally, the consistency of the gland is similar to that of the contracted thenar eminence of the thumb (with the thumb completely opposed to the little finger). It is rather rubbery. It may be mushy if congested (due to lack of intercourse or to chronic infection with impaired drainage), indurated (due to chronic infection with or without calculi), or stony hard (due to advanced carcinoma).

The difficulty lies in differentiating firm areas in the prostate: fibrosis from nonspecific infection, granulomatous prostatitis, nodulation from tuberculosis, firm areas due to prostatic calculi or early cancer. Generally speaking, nodules caused by infection are raised above the surface of the gland. At their edges, the induration gradually fades to the normal softness of surrounding tissue. In cancer, conversely, the suspicious lesion is usually not raised; it is hard and has a sharp edge, ie, there is an abrupt change in consistency on the same plane. It tends to arise in the lateral sulcus (Fig 4–2).

Even the most experienced clinicians sometimes have trouble making this differentiation. In the absence of other signs of tuberculosis and in the absence of pus in the prostatic secretion, cancer is likely, particularly if an x-ray fails to show prostatic calculi (which are seen just behind or above the symphysis).

Serum acid phosphatase determinations and radiographs of bones are of no help in diagnosing early carcinoma of the prostate.

Mobility

The mobility of the gland varies. Occasionally it has great mobility; at other times, very little. In advanced neoplasm it is fixed because of local extension through the capsule. The prostate should be routinely massaged in the adult and its secretion examined microscopically. It should not be massaged, however, in the presence of an acute urethral discharge, acute prostatitis, acute prostatocystitis, in men near the stage of complete urinary retention (because it may precipitate complete retention), or in men suffering from obvious cancer of the gland. Even in the absence of symptoms, massage is necessary, for prostatitis is commonly asymptomatic. Diagnosis and treatment of such silent disease is important in preventing cystitis and epididymitis.

Technic of Massage

The patient should lean over the examining table so that his body is horizontal. His legs should be straight and his feet somewhat apart.

Methods of massage vary, but the basic maneuver is to press the gland substance firmly with the pad of the index finger in order to express secretion into the prostatic urethra. Start laterally and superiorly and massage toward the midline. A rolling motion of the finger is less traumatic to the rectal mucosa and prostate gland and is better tolerated by the patient. Finally, the seminal vesicles should be stripped from above downward and medially (Fig 4–3).

Copious amounts of secretion may be obtained from some prostate glands and little or none from others. This of course depends to some extent upon the vigor with which the massage is carried out. If no secretion is obtained, have the patient void even a few drops of urine; this will contain adequate secretion for

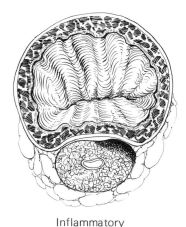
Inflammatory

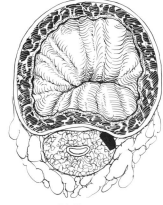
Malignant

Figure 4–2. Differential diagnosis of prostatic nodules. *Left:* Inflammatory area is raised above the surface of the gland; induration decreases gradually at its periphery. *Right:* Cancerous nodule is not raised; there is an abrupt change in consistency at its edges.

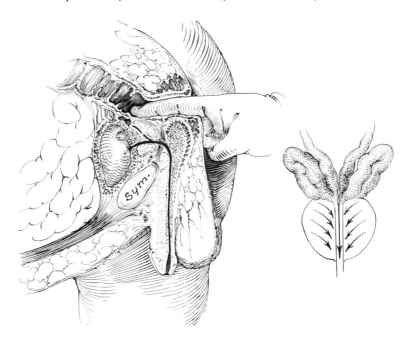

Figure 4—3. Technic of prostatic massage. The glandular substance is compressed from its lateral edges to the urethra, which lies in the center. (Drawing at right shows direction of pressure.) The seminal vesicles are then stripped from above downward.

examination. Microscopic examination of the secretion is done under low-power magnification. Normal secretion contains numerous lecithin bodies, which are refractile, like red cells, but much smaller than red cells. Only an occasional white cell is present. A few epithelial cells and, rarely, corpora amylacea are seen. Sperms may be present, but the absence of sperms is of no significance.

The presence of large numbers of pus cells is pathologic and makes the diagnosis of prostatitis. Stained smears are usually impractical. It is difficult to fix this material on the slide, and even when this is successful pyogenic bacteria are usually not found. Acid-fast organisms can often be found by appropriate staining methods.

On occasion it may be necessary to obtain cultures of prostatic secretion in order to demonstrate nonspecific organisms or *Mycobacterium tuberculosis.* After thorough cleansing of the glans and emptying of the bladder (to mechanically cleanse the urethra), massage is done. Drops of secretion are collected in a sterile tube of culture medium. Bacteriologic diagnosis is usually not helpful because antibiotic therapy is of little value in the treatment of chronic prostatitis.

SEMINAL VESICLES

Palpation of the seminal vesicles should be attempted. The vesicles are situated under the base of the bladder and diverge from below upward (Fig 1–8).

Normal seminal vesicles are usually not palpable, but when they are overdistended they may feel quite cystic. In the presence of chronic infection (particularly tuberculosis) or in association with advanced carcinoma of the prostate, they may be markedly indurated. Stripping of the seminal vesicles should be done in association with prostatic massage, for the vesicles are usually infected when prostatitis is present. Primary tumors of the vesicles are very rare.

EXAMINATION OF LYMPH NODES
(Figs 18–1 and 18–2)

Inguinal & Subinguinal Lymph Nodes

With inflammatory lesions of the skin of the penis and scrotum or vulva, the inguinal and subinguinal lymph nodes may be involved. Such diseases include chancroid, syphilitic chancre, lymphogranuloma venereum, and, on occasion, gonorrhea.

Malignancies (squamous cell carcinoma) involving the penis, glans, scrotal skin, or distal urethra in women metastasize to the inguinal and subinguinal nodes. Testicular tumors do not spread to these nodes unless they have invaded the scrotal skin or have been subjected to previous orchiopexy.

Other Lymph Nodes

Tumors of the testis and prostate may involve the left supraclavicular nodes. Tumors of the bladder and prostate typically metastasize to the hypogastric, external iliac, and preaortic nodes, although only occasionally are they so large as to be palpable. Masses near the midline in the upper abdomen in a young man should suggest metastases from cancer of the testis; the primary growth may be minute and completely hidden in the substance of what appears to be a normal testicle.

NEUROLOGIC EXAMINATION

A careful neurologic survey may uncover sensory or motor impairment which will account for residual urine (neurogenic bladder) or incontinence. Since the bladder and its sphincter are innervated by the second to fourth sacral segments, much information can be gained by testing anal sphincter tone and the sensation of the perianal skin and by eliciting the Achilles tendon and bulbocavernosus reflexes. The bulbocavernosus reflex is normal if, with a finger in the rectum, the external anal sphincter and bulbocavernosus muscle can be felt to contract when the glans penis or clitoris is squeezed or an indwelling Foley catheter is jerked. If no contraction occurs, interruption of the sacral reflex arc (lower motor neuron lesion) is present.

•   •   •

References

Examination of the Kidneys

Bearn JG, Pilkington TRE: Organs palpable in the normal adult abdomen. Lancet 2:212, 1959.

Hand M: Radicular pain simulating urologic disease. J Urol 85:668, 1961.

Koop CE: Abdominal mass in the newborn infant. New England J Med 289:569, 1973.

Marshall S, Lapp M, Schulte JW: Lesions of the pancreas mimicking renal disease. J Urol 93:41, 1965.

Mofenson HC, Greensher J: Transillumination of the abdomen in infants. Am J Dis Child 115:428, 1968.

Moser RJ, Caldwell JR: Abdominal murmurs: An aid in the diagnosis of renal artery disease in hypertension. Ann Int Med 56:471, 1962.

Museles M, Gaudry CL Jr, Bason WM: Renal anomalies in the newborn found by deep palpation. Pediatrics 47:97, 1971.

Pieretti R, Gilday D, Jeffs R: Differential kidney scan in pediatric urology. Urology 4:665, 1974.

Examination of the Bladder

Boyarsky S, Goldenberg J: Detection of bladder distention by suprapubic percussion. New York J Med 62:1804, 1962.

Carlsson E, Garsten P: Compression of the common iliac vessels by dilatation of the bladder. Acta radiol 53:449, 1960.

Patil UB: Estimation of residual urine in bladder: Use of vesical "thrill" test. Urology 4:737, 1974.

Stoutz HL: Massive edema of lower extremities associated with overdistention of bladder. J Urol 86:503, 1961.

Neurologic Examination

Bors E, Blenn KA: Bulbocavernosus reflex. J Urol 82:128, 1959.

5 . . .
Urologic Laboratory Examination

BLOOD COUNT

Hypochromic anemia may occur in association with chronic pyelonephritis, uremia, and carcinoma. Most infections will be accompanied by an increased white cell count with a shift to the left.

Erythrocytosis has been noted in association with 3–4% of urologic renal diseases, including carcinoma, hydronephrosis, and simple cyst. A number of instances have also been seen in association with uterine myomas and hepatoma. The erythropoietin level in the plasma is increased. Following definitive surgery, the erythropoietin level and the increased red cell count return to normal. If metastases develop later, erythrocytosis returns. (*Note:* Platelets, leukocytes, and other blood elements are usually not increased; the term polycythemia as applied to red blood cell count elevation in these disorders is a misnomer.)

EXAMINATION OF URETHRAL DISCHARGE IN THE MALE

A specimen of the discharge should be obtained before the patient voids. If discharge is absent at the time of examination, the urethra should be "milked" or the first portion of the voided urine can be collected and centrifuged. This sediment is similar to gross discharge.

The sediment or the actual discharge should be examined while wet. Trichomonads are seen as motile round bodies which are a little larger than pus cells. They may be cultured in a liquid liver or other suitable medium. The presence of lecithin bodies suggests that the discharge may be of prostatic origin. Pus and epithelial cells should be noted. If many epithelial cells are seen, chronic infection is probably present.

These secretions should also be stained. Methylene blue preparations permit clear observation of bacterial morphology. If cocci are present, Gram's stain (for gonococci) must be done.

EXAMINATION OF THE URINE

Urinalysis is without doubt the most important and most fruitful of all laboratory screening tests, yet it is the most poorly performed laboratory test in all medicine. There are 3 reasons for the inadequacy of so many urinalyses: (1) the urine is too often improperly collected, (2) it is not examined when fresh, and (3) examination of the sediment is frequently incomplete.

It is essential that the urine specimen be collected before the rectal examination is made. This guarantees that the urine will not be contaminated by infected prostatic secretion which may drain into the posterior urethra following this manipulation.

Proper Collection of Urine

In both men and women, the urethra harbors bacteria and a few pus cells. Any urine specimen voided into a single container will for this reason be contaminated by the normal urethral flora. This immediately clouds the interpretation of microscopic findings and often leads to the diagnosis of cystitis when the bladder urine actually contains no pus cells or bacteria. This applies particularly to women, in whom voiding causes urine to flow over the vulva and, at times, into the vagina.

A. Collecting Specimens From Men: The simplest method of collecting urine from a man is to give him a clean glass and instruct him to start his stream into the toilet bowl or urinal. He should be instructed to retract a redundant foreskin. After the stream has thoroughly cleansed the urethra, it should be directed into the glass (without interrupting the act of urination); before voiding has been completed, the glass should be removed. This affords a "midstream" (second glass) specimen which is as clean as that obtained by catheter.

A "2-glass" test affords the most information. The patient is instructed to begin voiding in one glass. After 10–15 ml have been passed, the stream should be directed into the second glass. If the patient complains of a scant discharge but none can be expressed at the time of examination, the first glass will contain the elements of the discharge. It should be centrifuged and examined as discharge. Pus in the first glass without white cells in the second suggests prostatitis if the patient denies the presence of discharge.

B. Collecting Specimens From Women: Women should be placed in the lithotomy position. The labia are held apart. After the vulva has been cleansed—and with the labia still separated—the patient is instructed to start voiding into a bowl held close to the vulva. The midportion of the stream should be collected in a sterile container. It is almost impossible for a woman to accomplish this without help.

Catheterization is also satisfactory and should not be avoided because of the fear of introducing infection with the catheter; the advantages of obtaining a "sterile" specimen far overshadow this slight risk, which may be further diminished by thorough irrigation of the bladder and the instillation of 30—60 ml of 1:5000 aqueous chlorhexidine solution or 0.5% neomycin. The passage of a catheter of moderate size (22F) in women also permits exploration of the urethra and may reveal stenosis, which may be the predisposing cause of the urinary infection.

C. Collecting Specimens From Children: If the boy or girl is old enough to cooperate, a midstream specimen can be collected as described above for men and women. The use of a plastic bag (after thorough antiseptic cleansing) for collection of urine in the neonate and infant is unsatisfactory from the bacteriologic standpoint. Kelalis & others (1973) have shown that when little girls void in the supine position more than half of them reflux urine into the vagina. Boehm & Haynes (1966), utilizing a technic which they term "midstream catch," report minimal bacterial contamination. After feeding, and before the infant voids, the genital area is thoroughly cleansed with hexachlorophene detergent. The child is then held in the prone position (Fig 5—1). The spinal reflex of Perez is then elicited by stroking the back along the paravertebral muscles. Spontaneous voiding usually occurs within 5 minutes. The stream is directed into a sterile container.

One should not hesitate to catheterize little girls if other methods of urine collection fail. In similar circumstances, suprapubic aspiration may be considered in the male.

Examination While Fresh

The "morning urine" is not an adequate urine specimen for routine examination of the urinary sediment. Even though the specific gravity of such a specimen is acceptable as a fairly dependable renal function test, the urinary sediment is abnormally altered after standing a few hours. Red cells break up and casts disintegrate as the urine becomes alkaline; bacteria, if not present in the fresh urine, enter the container and multiply rapidly. This can lead to the erroneous diagnosis of "urinary tract infection." Whether the physician is interested in the presence of red cells, casts, pus cells, or bacteria, a specimen that is not fresh is of little value. If urinalysis is to be dependable, the specimen must be collected properly and examined immediately.

Microscopic Examination of Sediment After Centrifuging

The stained smear of urinary sediment, examined

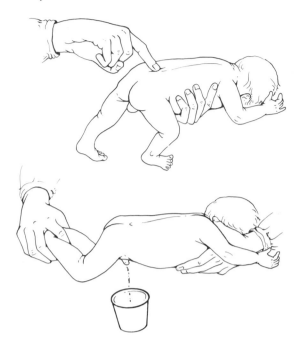

Figure 5—1. "Midstream catch" urine by the method of Boehm and Haynes. (Redrawn from Boehm JJ, Hyanes JL: Bacteriology of "midstream catch" urines: Studies in newborn infants. Am J Dis Child 111:366, 1966.)

personally, is of the greatest importance as a screening test for the presence of bacteriuria. On occasion, although bacteria are seen on a stained smear, the cultures are returned as "negative." Since finding bacteria on a stained smear means that there are at least 10,000 organisms per ml, such a finding is pathognomonic of infection, and a negative culture in this instance should be ignored. A stained smear gives quick information so that immediate treatment can be instituted; a culture takes many hours to complete with loss of valuable time. Studies show that the correlation of stained smears with cultures is good. If the patient has symptoms compatible with cystitis but pyuria and bacteriuria are absent, a culture should be obtained. This may negate the few errors encountered with the stained smear.

A. Wet Smear: This should be examined under low and medium power. White cells, red cells, crystals, and casts should be searched for, and the types of casts present should be noted (Fig 5—2). Squamous epithelial cells from the urethra and bladder neck are to be expected in the urine of the female; they are absent in men except in patients who are receiving estrogen therapy for cancer of the prostate. Trichomonads and yeast cells may also be seen.

B. Staining of the Sediment: Whether the wet smear reveals abnormalities or not, a stained smear must be examined. If pus cells appear to be present in a wet smear, staining of the sediment will aid in differentiating leukocytes and epithelial cells. The finding of transitional (mononuclear) epithelial cells, singly or in

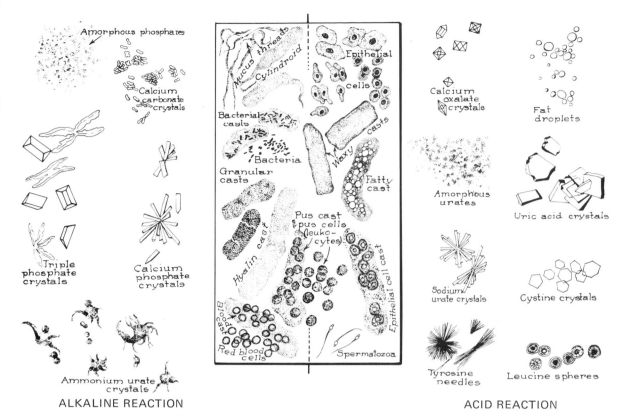

ALKALINE REACTION   ACID REACTION

Figure 5—2. Microscopic examination of urine sediment. (Redrawn after Todd & Sanford.)

clumps, strongly suggests vesical neoplasm (Fig 5 -3). The stained smear will also tentatively identify the bacteria. This will allow the physician to select an antibiotic or chemotherapeutic agent immediately and on the basis of objective clinical information. Staining the urine when pus is present may also reveal that no bacteria can be seen. Such a "sterile" pyuria strongly suggests tuberculosis of the urinary tract. Death from renal tuberculosis may occur if the diagnosis is delayed, and late diagnosis is usually due to improperly performed urinalyses.

If no pus is found on the wet preparation, the sediment must still be stained, since about 30% of patients with chronic urinary tract infection or urinary stasis have apyuric bacteriuria. One should not wait for the presence of pyuria or symptoms suggesting urinary tract diseases before considering such a possibility. This means that routine urinalysis in all patients, no matter what their symptoms, requires staining of the urinary sediment; until this has been done, urinary tract infection has not been ruled out.

1. For pyogenic organisms—

a. Triple-strength methylene blue is the stain of choice:

Methylene blue	1.5
Alcohol	30.0
0.1 N potassium hydroxide	2.0
Distilled water, qs ad	120.0

Fix the sediment on the slide with heat. Take care to only *warm* the slide, since too much heat will distort the stained cells. Flood the slide with the dye for 10—20 seconds, then rinse and dry with mild heat. Do not blot since this is apt to remove the sediment. It is helpful to mark the slide through the area containing the stained sediment with a red wax pencil before the immersion oil is applied. This allows the microscopist to find the plane of the sediment with ease when the oil immersion lens is used. A cover slip is not necessary.

b. Gram's stain is of limited value in the study of urinary sediment. If rods are found, they are usually gram-negative; if cocci are found, they are usually gram-positive. Gram's stain has the disadvantage of repeated staining and washing, which may cause the sediment to be washed from the slide. It is useful in the identification of the gonococcus.

(1) Fix smear by heat.

(2) Cover with crystal violet for 1 minute.

(3) Wash with water. Do not blot.

(4) Cover with Gram's iodine for 1 minute.

(5) Wash with water. Do not blot.

(6) Decolorize for 10—30 seconds with gentle agitation in acetone (30 ml) and alcohol (70 ml).

(7) Wash with water. Do not blot.

(8) Cover for 10—30 seconds with safranin (2.5% solution in 95% alcohol).

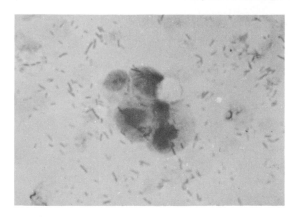

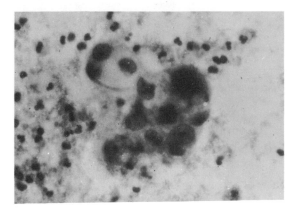

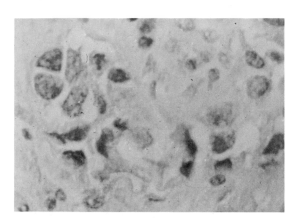

Figure 5–3. Urinary cytology. *Above left:* Triple-strength methylene blue stain of urinary sediment showing clumps of transitional cells with irregular and relatively large nuclei. Note presence of bacteria. *Above right:* Papanicolaou stain from same urinary sediment. Note similarity to methylene blue stain. *Left:* Biopsy of papillary vesical neoplasm from same patient. Clump of transitional cells in upper left hand corner is similar to those seen in urinary sediment.

(9) Wash with water and let dry.

2. Acid-fast (Ziehl-Neelsen) stains—Acid-fast staining should be done if a "sterile pyuria" is found or if urinary tuberculosis is suspected. The centrifuged sediment from 15 ml of urine discloses tubercle bacilli in half of such cases. If a 24-hour urine specimen is centrifuged, it will reveal tubercle bacilli in about 70–80%. The technic for Ziehl-Neelsen staining is as follows:

a. Stain heat-fixed smear with steaming Ziehl's carbolfuchsin for 5 minutes, or leave in cold stain for 24 hours. Cold Kinyoun carbolfuchsin acid-fast stain may be applied for 5 minutes.

b. Wash in tap water.

c. Decolorize with acid-alcohol until only a slight pink tinge remains.

d. Wash in tap water.

e. Counterstain with triple-strength methylene blue for 10–20 seconds.

f. Wash in tap water and dry with heat.

Cultures for Bacteria

A. Quantitative Cultures: Some type of quantitative estimation of the number of bacteria must be made. It is essential that the colony count be judged in the light of the specific gravity of the specimen. A count of 1000 organisms per ml in urine with a specific gravity of 1.002 is significant. A similar count in 1.030 urine might be compatible with urethral contamina-

tion. If urine which is not too dilute has been collected properly and plated immediately, a count of fewer than 1000 organisms per ml is compatible with urethral contamination. Only counts above 1000 organisms per ml should be considered significant. The acceptance of the popular concept that 100,000 organisms per ml is the "breaking point" between contamination and true infection causes many urinary tract infections to be missed. This high count was chosen to allow for errors in collection of the urine and delays in transport to the laboratory. Quantitative cultures are also useful for preparing antibiotic sensitivity tests, which are helpful in the definitive treatment of infections.

Many authors* have described and evaluated simplified methods of quantitative urine culture applicable to office practice. The advantages of such office procedures are absolute control of the method of collection of urine by the physician and the opportunity for immediate plating. Few hospitals can compete with these technics, which make available a quantitative culture within hours. With such a method, a colony count of 1000 per ml is significant. Drug sensitivity disks can be placed on another plate, thus affording quick guidance in the choice of antibiotic.

---

*Stamey, 1967; McLin & Tavel, 1971; Kunin & Bergeron, 1972; Jackaman, Darrell, & Shackman, 1973; and Narins & Whitehead, 1972.

B. Cultures for Tubercle Bacilli: If stained smears are negative for tubercle bacilli, cultures should be made. Even if the smears reveal acid-fast organisms, cultures should be done, since the finding of the bacteria in the stained sediment, although it is strong presumptive evidence, is not definitive proof of the presence of tuberculosis.

Other Tests of the Urine

A. Urinary pH: Normal kidneys contribute to the control of body pH by excreting urine in the pH ranges of 4.5 to about 7.5. The former figure is typical of diabetic acidosis. Readings above 7.5 mean that urea-splitting organisms are present. Despite a low blood pH, the urinary pH in renal tubular acidosis varies between 6.0 and 7.0.

B. Cytologic Examination: (Fig 5–3.) Transitional cells shed from tumors of the urinary tract may be demonstrated either by the Papanicolaou technic or by methylene blue stain. The latter is as efficient as the former. Men do not shed epithelial cells unless they are taking estrogens, in which case squamous cells are seen. Women commonly shed squamous cells from the bladder neck and urethra. Both may pass small round transitional cells, however, if acute cystitis is present.

These stains correlate well with the presence of transitional cell neoplasms of the renal pelvis, ureter, or bladder but have not been too helpful in suggesting the presence of adenocarcinoma of the kidney.

C. Hormone Tests: In the presence of a testicular tumor, estimates of the amount of chorionic gonadotropin are of great importance in calculating the prognosis and may help to evaluate the presence or absence of metastases after the primary tumor has been removed. Determination of the amounts of plasma testosterone, pituitary gonadotropins, corticosteroids, and estrogens in the urine may be helpful in certain endocrine disorders, including infertility in the male.

D. Sulkowitch Test: The Sulkowitch test affords a rough estimate of the amount of calcium excreted in the urine. The patient should be instructed to refrain from drinking milk or eating cheese 3–4 days before the test is done. The Sulkowitch test is useful in uncovering hyperparathyroidism as a cause of urinary calculus formation. Sulkowitch reagent is made up according to the following formula:

Oxalic acid	2.5
Ammonium oxalate	2.5
Glacial acetic acid	5.0
Distilled water, qs ad	150.0

To 5 ml of urine, add 2 ml of Sulkowitch reagent. The amount of calcium is estimated by the speed of precipitation and the intensity of the cloud; it is graded from 0–4+.

Lack of reaction is compatible with hypoparathyroidism (it may be negative in acute pancreatitis), whereas a strongly positive test means hypercalciuria and suggests the presence of hypercalcemia. This test is indispensable in the study and management of patients

Table 5–1. Urinary levels of LDH and alkaline phosphatases in disease states.

Diseases	Urinary Levels Of	
	LDH	Alkaline Phosphatase
Cancer of bladder Chronic pyelonephritis Sclerosing glomerulonephritis Malignant hypertension	↑	Normal

Cancer of kidney, prostate
Adrenocortical adenoma and
    cancer
Acute and chronic glomerulone-
    phritis (various types)
Acute tubular necrosis
	↑	↑

suffering from urinary stone; it must, however, be correlated with the specific gravity of the urine.

E. Lactic Acid Dehydrogenase (LDH): This enzyme has been found to be significantly elevated in most potentially fatal medical renal diseases and chronic pyelonephritis. Increased levels are also observed in patients with cancer of the kidney, bladder, and prostate.

Amador, Dorfman, & Wacker (1965) have studied the urinary levels of LDH and alkaline phosphatase activities in the differential diagnosis of renal and other diseases (Table 5–1). The levels of both enzymes are normal in renal cyst, adrenocortical hyperplasia, benign prostatic hyperplasia, benign essential hypertension, and acute cystitis and pyelonephritis. Since the LDH test is rather nonspecific and since 75% of patients with an elevated level of the enzyme prove to have urinary infection, the simple test of urinalysis is usually definitive. Gault and Geggie have found this a poor diagnostic step.

F. Vanilmandelic Acid (VMA): Vanilmandelic acid is the urinary metabolite of the catecholamines, including dopa, dopamine, norepinephrine, normetanephrine, and metanephrine. VMA levels are elevated in patients with pheochromocytoma, neuroblastoma, and ganglioneuroma. VMA determination is, therefore, a simple yet efficient screening test for these conditions. Estimation of the various catecholamines probably affords somewhat better diagnostic accuracy.

Summary

The stained smear of the sediment from a properly collected urine is all that is needed to diagnose most cases of urinary tract infection. Bacteriologic cultures and sensitivity tests are required in patients who are acutely ill or in those who suffer from chronic or recurrent disease.

RENAL FUNCTION TESTS

The kidneys have 3 primary functions: (1) the regulation of sodium chloride, potassium, and water (fluid and ion) balance, (2) the regulation of body pH, and (3) the excretion of the end products of metabolism.

Proteinuria

The presence of proteinuria as measured by sulfosalicylic acid or indicator papers must be explained, although random tests may be misleading. Proteinuria must be correlated with the specific gravity of the specimen. A mere trace of protein in urine with a specific gravity of 1.004–1.010 is compatible with a significant 24-hour loss of protein in a patient with marked impairment of renal function, even uremia. Amounts of protein up to 100 mg per 24 hours are normal.

Sulfosalicylic acid (but not Albustix) gives a positive test for proteinuria in the presence of some radiopaque chemicals used in excretory urography.

Heavy proteinuria is seen in nephrosis and, at times, glomerulonephritis; but the clinical picture and other findings in the urinary sediment usually lead to the proper diagnosis. The heaviest proteinuria may be noted in children with high fever and severe dehydration and in orthostatic proteinuria. Proteinuria is not, therefore, necessarily pathognomonic of intrinsic renal disease.

Urine Specific Gravity

The specific gravity of the urine is a simple and significant test of renal function, although determination of osmolality may be more accurate. Normal kidneys in young persons can concentrate to 1.040; at age 40, to 1.036; at age 50, to 1.030. Thus, a specific gravity of 1.030 in a man 70 years old implies not only excellent renal function but also intense dehydration. With marked hydration, the specific gravity may fall to 1.000. Urine densities above 1.040 suggest that the specimen contains radiopaque fluid.

In the presence of diminishing renal function, there is progressive loss of concentrating power until 1.006–1.010 is reached. The power of dilution, however, tends to be maintained until renal damage is extreme. Even in uremia, although the concentrating power is limited to 1.010, dilution in the range of 1.002–1.004 may still be found. Therefore, a specific gravity of 1.004 in a random urine specimen does not guarantee adequate renal function. Oddly, the fixation point of specific gravity with advanced hydronephrosis is closer to 1.006, and even in this circumstance dilution may reach 1.002.

Urinary specific gravity rises as the radiopaque medium used in excretory urography is excreted. Total renal function may be estimated by subtracting the specific gravity of the preinjection specimen from the specific gravity of the urine voided any time up to 2 hours after the infusion. An increase of 0.025 units or more indicates good total renal function. Less than this implies impaired function. In the uremic patient, little change is observed.

The PSP (Phenol Red) Test

(Also a measure of residual urine.)

The patient is instructed to void. Exactly 1 ml of phenosulfonphthalein (containing 6 mg of the dye) is then given intravenously with a tuberculin syringe (the ampule contains 1.2 ml). The patient should drink no more than 200 ml of water during each of the 2 subsequent half-hour periods. (Do not force fluids before or during the test, since excretion of PSP is not dependent upon urine flow. Furthermore, rapid vesical filling causes an obstructed bladder to lose tone, and the amount of residual urine is thereby increased.) Collect urine specimens one-half hour and, if excretion is less than 50%, 1 hour after the injection. Alkalinize with 5–10 ml of 10% NaOH to bring out the red color. Dilute the specimen with water to a volume of 1000 ml if the dye appears in good concentration. If the specimen is pale, dilute with only 250 ml or 500 ml, in which case the resulting percentage should be divided by 4 or 2, respectively. The percentage of dye recovered is measured by means of colorimetry. Collections beyond the first hour are of no value.

At times the urine may have a brownish hue; this usually occurs in "stagnant" (residual) urine. The azo dyes (eg, Pyridium, Azo Gantrisin) and Bromsulphalein interfere with accurate estimation of PSP excretion. Probenecid (Benemid) depresses PSP excretion by 67% because it interferes with the transport of the dye.

If a catheter is in the bladder, it is necessary to irrigate it at the time of collection of each specimen because an indwelling catheter does not completely empty the bladder. The PSP excretion may be low if the test is done shortly after excretory urography, for both the radiopaque fluid and PSP compete for transport on protein molecules.

The average amount of dye normally recovered in the first half-hour specimen is 50–60%; the second specimen contains 10–15%. The normal total, then, for 1 hour is 60–75%. The normal PSP in children (infants excepted) is 5–10% higher than in the adult. An unusually high PSP in an adult is compatible with surgical or congenital absence of one kidney with compensatory hypertrophy of its mate.

A "diaper" PSP test can be done on infants, even the newborn. The dye is given intramuscularly and the diaper is removed after 3 hours. It is placed in a graduate which is filled to the 1000 ml mark. The normal PSP in infants is 50% or more in 3 hours. Even at the age of 3 days, at least 30% will be excreted in 3 hours. In the presence of vesical outlet obstruction, bilateral renal damage, or vesicoureteral reflux, little of the dye may be recovered. Such a finding requires explanation.

The PSP test is a test of renal blood flow and tubular function. Since urologic renal diseases primarily affect the tubules, the test has obvious value as an index of the presence and extent of urologic renal damage. The test has the advantage of being simple,

Table 5—2. Examples of PSP excretion.

	I		II		III	
½ hour	25 ml	15%	30 ml	35%	25 ml	25%
1 hour	55 ml	25%	40 ml	25%	50 ml	25%
Totals	80 ml	40%	70 ml	60%	75 ml	50%

From such excretion curves the approximate amounts of residual urine can be estimated:

$$\frac{Vol^1\ (50\ or\ 60\ -\ PSP^1)}{PSP^1} = \text{Approximate amount of residual urine (in ml)}$$

Vol^1 = the volume of the first specimen.
PSP^1 = the percentage of PSP recovered in the first specimen.
"50 or 60" = the expected normal PSP excretion after ½ hour.
(The second half-hour does not enter into this calculation.)

The amount of residual urine in each of the above examples can therefore be calculated as follows:

$$\text{I} \quad \frac{25\ (60\ -\ 15)}{15} = \frac{1125}{15} = \text{About 75 ml residual urine}$$

$$\text{II} \quad \frac{30\ (60\ -\ 35)}{35} = \frac{750}{35} = \text{About 21 ml residual urine}$$

$$\text{III} \quad \frac{25\ (60\ -\ 25)}{25} = \frac{875}{25} = \text{About 35 ml residual urine}$$

and in most cases it also affords a fairly accurate estimate of residual urine. If the urine specimen collected half an hour after the intravenous injection contains 50% or more of the dye, renal function is good and, if the urine volume is small (eg, 25–50 ml), there can be no significant residual urine. The test can therefore be stopped at that point, for nothing further can be learned from a second specimen. If the first specimen does not contain the normal amount of dye, a second specimen should be collected at the end of the second half-hour.

The presence of residual urine (vesical or bilateral ureterorenal) is suggested if a "flat" or "uphill" curve is obtained in association with (1) a fairly good total PSP in 1 hour, (2) a morning specific gravity of 1.024 or better, or (3) a normal serum creatinine. With increasing degrees of renal damage and in the absence of residual urine, the following PSP curves are to be expected in 1 hour: 40%–15%, 30%–10%, and 20%–10%. Even poorly functioning kidneys do not produce an "uphill" curve since 70% of the dye is cleared the first time around. When damage is severe, the total PSP is low and the curve "flat" (10%–10%, 5%–5%, Trace–Trace).

The examples of PSP excretion in Table 5–2 therefore imply the presence of residual urine, for the curves are "flat" or nearly so, or "uphill."

When PSP curves are flat and their totals are low (eg, 20%–15%, 10%–10%, or 5%–5%), a serum creatinine should be obtained. If normal, a PSP of 50%–60% in the first half-hour can be assumed and the calculation of the amount of residual urine made. The same would be true if the specific gravity of the urine were 1.024 or higher. If there is doubt in the physician's mind, immediate catheterization should be performed and the PSP content of the retained urine added to that obtained during the test. This maneuver will show total PSP excretion and give an estimation of residual urine.

The use of the PSP test for estimation of total renal function and of residual urine, if present, makes it one of the most valuable routine office diagnostic procedures. It is a more useful test of renal function than measurement of nitrogen retention. It is inexpensive and affords real information in one-half hour, and it estimates degrees of renal damage before the uremic stage is reached. This test should be a routine laboratory procedure like the complete blood count and urinalysis. Since so many serious renal diseases are silent, the PSP test may occasionally pick up such a case. Many patients in uremia both feel and look well. A PSP of better than 30% in the first half-hour rules out uremia due to renal failure; only when it is 30% or less should tests for nitrogen retention be done.

In unilateral renal disease (eg, hydronephrosis), the specific gravity or concentration tests may show impairment because of the mixing of the urine from the good kidney with that from the diseased. The PSP, however, will usually be normal, because of the compensatory hypertrophy of the good kidney. In this instance, then, the PSP is a more dependable test of total renal function than concentrating power.

The same is true when residual urine is present in the bladder. A dilute urine retained in the bladder will lower the specific gravity of the concentrated fluid which is produced by dehydration, and the inference of renal impairment may be made. The PSP, however, will give a "flat" curve with a fairly normal total (eg, 25%–20%: total, 45%), which suggests the presence of residual urine.

For these reasons, concentration tests should be performed in conjunction with the PSP. This will help to prevent errors which might occur in the interpretation of the concentration test in certain urologic disorders.

Gault and others have described the 60-minute plasma PSP concentration as a test of renal function. One mg of PSP/kg body weight is given IV. The residual plasma level at 1 hour is estimated by colorimetry. The normal value is in the range of 110 μg. A high level implies impaired renal function. This method is of value if the urine is bloody, but in other circumstances the routine PSP test or determination of the blood urea nitrogen and creatinine levels seems simpler.

Endogenous Creatinine Clearance

Although creatinine is filtered through the glomerulus and PSP is excreted by the tubules, these tests tend to parallel each other because most renal diseases involve both renal elements (Table 5–3). Thus, the creatinine clearance is roughly equal to twice the excretion of PSP in the first half-hour. The clearance of endogenous creatinine approximates the glomerular filtration rate (GFR) as measured by inulin. The normal values vary between 72–140 ml/minute.

Blood Nitrogen Levels

In the face of bilateral ureteral or bladder neck obstruction, bilateral vesicoureteral reflux, shock, or heart failure, the flow of urine down the tubules is slowed. This allows overreabsorption of urea nitrogen; creatinine is not so affected. Such a phenomenon is compatible with the countercurrent theory of renal function. When the urinary tract is normal and unobstructed, the plasma urea:creatinine ratio is 10:1. When there is significant bilateral urinary stasis or diminished renal blood flow, the urea:creatinine ratio rises to 20–30:1. A similar pattern is seen when there is extravasation of urine into the peritoneal cavity. Thus, the combination of both blood urea nitrogen and creatinine determinations is of considerable diagnostic importance as a screening test.

In the adult, the upper limits of normal are creatinine, 1.4 mg/100 ml, and blood urea nitrogen, 20 mg/100 ml. Up to age 5, the normal creatinine is 0.6 mg/100 ml and the blood urea nitrogen 8 mg/100 ml.

Young children with advanced bilateral hydronephrosis may have a fixed specific gravity of 1.006 with

Table 5–3. Correlation of PSP test, serum creatinine, and creatinine clearance (no residual urine).

Half-Hour PSP	Specific Gravity	Serum Creatinine (mg/100 ml)	Creatinine Clearance (ml/min)
50 and higher	1.015–1.040	to 1.4 (normal)	100 and higher
30	1.010	1.7	60
20	1.010	2.0	40
10	1.010	2.4	20
5	1.010	3.4	10
0	1.010	4.0 and higher	5 or less

a trace of protein and yet have a serum creatinine level within the normal range. A "diaper" PSP test will reveal the renal damage or suggest residual urine.

Serum Electrolytes

(See Inside Back Cover.)

The estimation of the concentration of serum electrolytes is important in patients with suspected fluid-ion imbalance or oliguria, hyperparathyroidism, hyperaldosteronism, and chronic renal failure.

Urine Chloride Concentration
(Bedside Test of Scribner)

One of the prime functions of the kidneys is the regulation of body sodium chloride in relation to body water. In the face of sodium chloride excess, the kidneys can excrete up to 375 mEq/liter of salt. With sodium chloride deprivation, normal kidneys can so efficiently withhold salt that its concentration in the urine falls to zero. As renal function fails, the specific gravity becomes fixed at 1.006–1.010 (stage of uremia); with further damage, the PSP excretion finally falls to a trace. The last measurable function that the kidneys lose is sodium chloride regulation. In lower nephron nephrosis (acute tubular necrosis), the chloride concentration becomes fixed at 30–40 mEq/liter. The only exception to this rule is the relatively rare incomplete tubular lesion in which the chloride concentration may be fixed at a point between 20–100 mEq/liter.

It is obvious, then, that estimation of the urine chloride is helpful in the treatment of fluid and electrolyte derangements and in the estimate of renal function. A urine chloride of 250 mEq/liter implies good renal tubular function and sodium chloride excess. Similarly, a chloride concentration of 1–2 mEq/liter also implies adequate tubular function but sodium chloride depletion or retention (eg, heart failure).

When specific gravity becomes fixed, those mechanisms having to do with ammonia and bicarbonate substitution are sharply limited. Under these circumstances, the urine sodium concentration tends to equal the level of chloride in the urine unless the patient is receiving excess base (sodium lactate or bicarbonate).

•　　•　　•

References

Examination of the Urine

Amador E, Dorfman LE, Wacker WEC: Urinary alkaline phosphatase and LDH activities in the differential diagnosis of renal disease. Ann Int Med 62:30, 1965.

Aronson AS, Gustafson B, Svenningsen NW: Combined suprapubic aspiration and clean-voided urine examination in infants and children. Acta paediat scandinav 62:396, 1973.

Boehm JJ, Haynes JL: Bacteriology of "midstream catch" urines: Studies in newborn infants. Am J Dis Child 111:366, 1966.

Bower BF, Gordan GS: Hormonal effects of nonendocrine tumors. Ann Rev Med 16:83, 1965.

Brody LH, Salladay JR, Armbruster K: Urinalysis and the urinary sediment. M Clin North America 55:243, 1971.

Cohen SN, Kass EH: A simple method for quantitative urine culture. New England J Med 277:176, 1967.

Emanuel B, Aronson N: Neonatal hematuria. Am J Dis Child 128:204, 1974.

Friedman SA, Gladstone JL: The effects of hydration and bladder incubation time on urine colony counts. J Urol 105:428, 1971.

Gault MH, Geggie PHS: Clinical significance of urinary LDH, alkaline phosphatase and other enzymes. Canad MAJ 101:208, 1969.

Gavan TL: In vitro antimicrobial susceptibility testing: Clinical implications and limitations. M Clin North America 58:493, 1974.

Hakulinen A: Urinary excretion of vanilmandelic acid of children in normal and certain pathological conditions. Acta paediat scandinav (Suppl 212), 1971.

Hendler ED, Kashgarian M, Hayslett JP: Clinicopathological correlations of primary haematuria. Lancet 1:458, 1972.

Jackaman FR, Darrell JH, Shackman R: The dip-slide in urology. Brit MJ 1:207, 1973.

Jonsson K: Renal angiography in patients with hematuria. Am J Roentgenol 116:758, 1972.

Kelalis PP & others: Urinary vaginal reflux in children. Pediatrics 51:941, 1973.

Kunin CM, Bergeron JA: A simple quantitative urine culture method using an internally coated plastic pipette. Am J Clin Path 58:271, 1972.

Labovitz ED & others: "Benign" hematuria with focal glomerulitis in adults. Ann Int Med 77:723, 1972.

Lawson JS, Hewstone AS: Microscopic appearance of urine in the neonatal period. Arch Dis Childhood 39:287, 1964.

McLin P, Tavel FR: Urine culture and direct sensitivity testing: A rapid simple method for use in the office. Clin Med 78:16, 1971.

Narins DJ, Whitehead ED: Simplified office bacteriology: A method of urine culture and sensitivity testing. J Urol 108:780, 1972.

Park C-H & others: Reliability of positive exfoliative cytology study of the urine in urinary tract malignancy. J Urol 102:91, 1969.

Pryles CV, Lustik B: Laboratory diagnosis of urinary tract infection. P Clin North America 18:233, 1971.

Ritter S, Spencer H, Smachson J: The Sulkowitch and quantitative urine calcium excretion. J Lab Clin Med 56:314, 1960.

Rubin MI, Baliah T: Urinalysis and its clinical interpretation. P Clin North America 18:245, 1971.

Schulte JW & others: A simple technic for recognizing abnormal epithelial cells in the urine. J Urol 89:615, 1963.

Stamey TA: Office bacteriology. J Urol 97:926, 1967.

Tunnessen WW, Smith C, Oski FA: Beeturia: A sign of iron deficiency. Am J Dis Child 117:424, 1969.

Renal Function Tests

Barsocchini LM, Smith DR: Diaper phenolsulfonphthalein test in the newborn infant. J Urol 91:195, 1964.

Berliner RW, Bennett CM: Concentration of urine in the mammalian kidney. Am J Med 42:777, 1967.

Dossetor JB: Creatininemia versus uremia: The relative significance of blood urea nitrogen and serum creatinine concentrations in azotemia. Ann Int Med 65:1287, 1966.

Galambos JT, Herndon EG Jr, Reynolds GH: Specific-gravity determination: Fact or fancy. New England J Med 270:506, 1964.

Gault MH, Fox I: The sixty-minute plasma phenolsulfonphthalein concentration as a test of renal function. Am J Clin Path 52:345, 1969.

Griner PF, Liptzin B: Use of the laboratory in a teaching hospital: Implications for patient care, education and hospital costs. Ann Int Med 75:157, 1971.

Harrow BR, Sloane JA, Salhanick L: Clinical evaluation of renal function tests. J Urol 87:527, 1962.

Harrow BR, Sloane JA: Value of concentration test in determining renal function. Postgrad Med 37:A48, Jan 1965.

Jensen H, Henriksen K: Proteinuria in non-renal infectious disease. Acta med scandinav 196:75, 1974.

Laboratory tests: Misuse and abuse. (Editorial.) JAMA 218:90, 1971.

Lindeman RD, Van Buren HC, Raisz LG: Osmolar renal concentrating ability in healthy young men and hospitalized patients without renal disease. New England J Med 262:1306, 1960.

Lyon RP: Hypogravic urine with uremia and normotension. J Urol 82:558, 1959.

Lyon RP: Measurement of urine chloride as a test of renal function. J Urol 85:884, 1961.

Marshall S: A test of renal function: Excretion of contrast medium as measured by urinary specific gravity. Brit J Urol 36:519, 1964.

Newcombe DS, Cohen AS: Uricosuric agents and phenolsulfonphthalein excretion. Arch Int Med 112:738, 1963.

Richardson JA, Philbin PE: The one-hour creatinine clearance rate in healthy men. JAMA 216:987, 1971.

Scribner BH: Bedside determination of chloride. Proc Staff Meet Mayo Clin 25:209, 1950.

Smith DR: Estimation of the amount of residual urine by means of the phenolsulfonphathalein test. J Urol 83:188, 1960.

Tjan HL & others: Creatinine clearance in clinical medicine. California Med 98:121, 1963.

Young JD Jr, de Mendonca PP, Bendhack D: A comparison of phenolsulfonphthalein excretion with the renal clearance of creatinine and PAH. Ann Surg 169:724, 1969.

6...
Roentgenographic Examination of the Urinary Tract

PLAIN FILM OF ABDOMEN

A plain film of the abdomen, also called a KUB (kidney, ureter, and bladder), is a helpful step in the presumptive diagnosis of genitourinary disease (Figs 6–1 and 6–2). Since gastrointestinal and urologic diseases tend to mimic each other, it may be helpful in differential diagnosis as well.

Renal Shadows

A. Kidney Size: A plain film of the abdomen will usually show the renal outlines. They may be obscured, however, by bowel content, lack of perinephric fat, or a perinephric hematoma or abscess, which typically obliterates the renal shadow. This difficulty, however, may be overcome by tomography. Congenital absence or possible ectopy of a kidney may be suggested. If both kidneys are unusually large, polycystic kidney disease, multiple myeloma, lymphoma, amyloid disease, or hydronephrosis may be present. If both are small, the end stage of glomerulonephritis or bilateral atrophic pyelonephritis must be considered. Unilateral enlargement should suggest renal tumor, cyst, or hydronephrosis, whereas a small kidney on one side is compatible with congenital hypoplasia, atrophic pyelonephritis, or an ischemic kidney. Normally, the left kidney is 0.5 cm longer than its mate. Discrepancy in the relative size of one kidney may imply renal ischemia.

The normal kidney extends from the top of the first to the bottom of the third to fourth lumbar vertebra.

B. Position: In 90% of cases, the right kidney is lower than the left, because of displacement by the liver. If a kidney appears to be abnormally displaced, a retroperitoneal tumor should be suspected (eg, adrenal tumor, pancreatic pseudocyst).

The axes of the kidneys are oblique to the spine; their lower poles are farther apart than their upper poles because they lie along the borders of the psoas muscles. If their axes are parallel to the spine (which means that the lower ends of the kidneys are lying on the psoas muscles), the possibility of "horseshoe" kidney should be considered.

C. Shape: The shape of the kidney should be studied. A lobulated edge might suggest polycystic kidney disease. An expansion of one pole of a kidney is compatible with tumor, cyst, or carbuncle. Indentations on the lateral border of a small kidney suggest scarring from previous attacks of pyelonephritis.

Calcification

Because a plain film of the abdomen is 2-dimensional, it is practically impossible to make a positive diagnosis of stone in the urinary tract except in the instance of a staghorn calculus, which forms a perfect cast of the pelvis and calyces, thereby simulating a urogram. All one can usually say from study of a plain film is that there are opaque bodies in the region of the adrenal, kidney, ureter, bladder, or prostate. Oblique and lateral films, as well as visualization of the urinary tract with radiopaque fluids, are necessary in order to actually determine the position of the calcification in the respective organs.

Punctate calcification in the adrenals suggests tuberculous involvement (Fig 13–2) or neuroblastoma (Fig 20–3). Adrenal calcification follows spontaneous hemorrhage into the gland (Fig 6–14). Numerous small calcific bodies in the parenchyma of a kidney may suggest tuberculosis (Fig 6–2) or medullary sponge kidney (Fig 21–9), although nephrocalcinosis (Fig 15–12) caused by primary or secondary hyperparathyroidism or hypercalciuria should be considered. About 7% of malignant renal tumors contain some calcification. Calcifications in the veins in the perivesical area (phleboliths) may simulate stone in the ureter, but as a rule they are perfectly round, often laminated, and contain radiolucent centers. Calcified mesenteric lymph nodes may also resemble stone. Linear calcification lying to the left of the lumbar spine is compatible with aneurysm of the abdominal aorta. An aneurysm of the right renal artery (Fig 21–11) may be confused with a gallstone. Calcifications at the junction of the hypogastric and iliac arteries are often seen just below the sacroiliac joints and may therefore be confused with ureteral stones. A stone in the appendix may occasionally be confused with stone in the ureter. Radiopaque gallstones may overlie the kidney, but an oblique or lateral film will demonstrate that the opacity is anterior to the kidney. Uterine fibroids and, occasionally, diseased ovaries may undergo pathologic calcification. Moles on the skin and swallowed pills or foreign bodies may be radi-

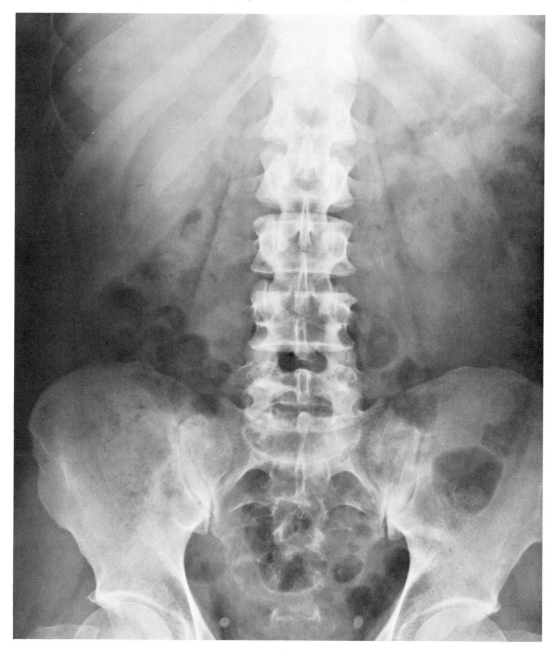

Figure 6—1. Normal plain film of abdomen. Bones are normal, psoas shadows well demarcated, renal shadows normal. The bladder contains some urine. Two phleboliths are seen in the region of the lower ureters and bladder.

opaque. The wall of an adrenal or renal cyst may contain calcium.

The use of tomography will show indistinct calcifications often missed on a plain film.

Psoas Shadows

The psoas muscles usually stand out sharply. If one is obliterated and the kidney shadow on that side is absent, and if there is scoliosis of the spine with its concavity on the side of the defect, perinephric or paranephric abscess or hematoma is a possibility.

Bone Shadows

Survey of the bones may reveal arthritic change, which may suggest that what was thought to be kidney pain is really caused by radiculitis. Gross spina bifida may be noted; the sacrum may be absent. Such findings would suggest the presence of neurogenic bladder (Fig 6—17). Metastases should also be sought. If osteoblastic, they almost certainly arise from the prostate; if osteolytic, the common primary sites are in the breast, thyroid, lung, and kidney.

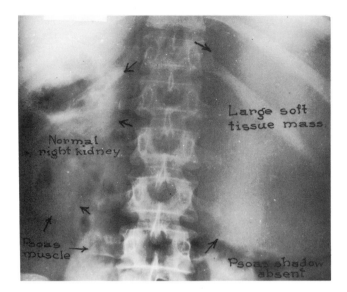

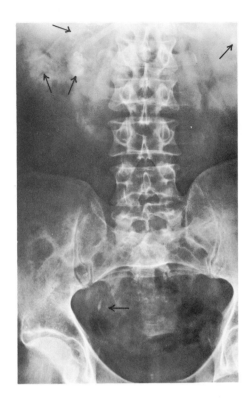

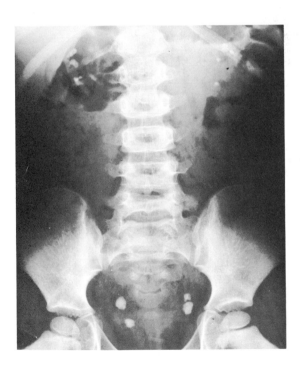

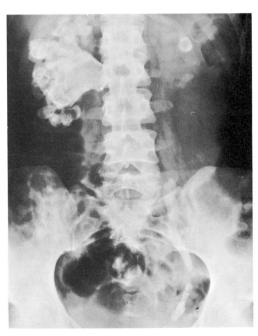

Figure 6–2. Abnormal plain films of the abdomen. *Above left:* Large soft tissue mass in left upper abdomen (simple cyst of kidney). Absence of intestinal gas (displacement of bowel) over mass (see Fig 6–17, below left and right, same patient). *Above right:* Calcification in small functionless right kidney and lower right ureter typical of advanced tuberculosis. There is a stone in the left kidney. *Below left:* Multiple renal and ureteral calcium oxalate stones in 12-year-old boy suffering from hyperoxaluria. *Below right:* Large staghorn calculus in right kidney and multiple stones in left kidney and lower half of ureter.

Gastrointestinal Shadows

A plain film, by demonstrating gas in the small bowel, may lead to the diagnosis of bowel obstruction, although the initial impression may have been disease of the urinary tract. Gas under the diaphragm with the patient in an upright posture makes the diagnosis of a ruptured viscus (eg, perforated peptic ulcer). A large renal mass may displace all intestinal gas from that area (Fig 6–2).

EXCRETORY UROGRAMS

During the past 20 years, improvements in intravenous radiographic media have been such that they now rival retrograde urograms in quality. This very efficiency has impaired their usefulness as a test of renal function. Although nausea, vomiting, and pain in the arm are occasionally experienced after intravenous injection of radiopaque material, these reactions are usually less disturbing to the patient than the sequelae of retrograde urography (nausea and vomiting, abdominal and renal pain). Rare allergic reactions (eg, urticaria, asthma, shock) following intravenous infusion of these iodized substances are apparently usually aborted by the addition of an antihistamine to the radiopaque fluid.

Excretory urograms illustrate the urinary excretory tract in the most physiologic manner. The renal pelves and calyces are not distorted by the overdistention which may be produced with retrograde filling.

The cystogram which is obtained on the later films may reveal trabeculation, diverticula, or a space-occupying lesion (Fig 18–9). A postvoiding film may demonstrate residual urine in the bladder.

Note: For 1–2 hours after injection of the radiopaque medium, the normal specific gravity of the urine is 1.040–1.060. Under these circumstances, a specific gravity of 1.020 or less indicates that renal function is severely impaired.

Indications

Excretory urograms are indicated when disease of the urinary tract is suspected. Diseases which should be investigated by this means include cysts and tumors of the kidney (space-occupying lesions), tuberculosis of the kidney (ulceration of calyces), pyelonephritis, hydronephrosis, vesicoureteral reflux, hypertension, and stone in the urinary tract.

Excretory urograms may also be of value in patients suffering from gastrointestinal complaints in whom no organic disease of the gastrointestinal tract can be demonstrated. A urologic cause for the symptoms may be shown.

Because the radiographic fluid increases the density of the kidneys to x-rays, the size of the kidneys and their outlines become clearer. This is an advantage when evidence of expansion of the renal parenchyma (eg, tumor) or change in size of the kidney is sought.

If renal injury is suspected, excretory urograms should be obtained as soon as practicable (primarily to make certain that the uninjured contralateral kidney is normal). This is invaluable information if emergency removal of the injured kidney becomes imperative as a lifesaving measure.

Excretory urograms are indispensable in infants, particularly male infants, where cystoscopy may be unduly traumatic. During the first month of life, delayed concentration and prolonged excretion of urographic contrast medium is observed. In this age group, the usual early films should be deleted and late films (1–2 hours) taken. A few months later, however, the best film may be noted 6 minutes after injection in the nondehydrated child.

Contraindications

Excretory urograms are contraindicated if there is evidence of hypersensitivity: history of allergic reactions to previous intravenous urography, iodine sensitivity, or other allergic manifestations such as hives or asthma. Although the routine addition of an antihistamine to the contrast medium may reduce the incidence of allergic reactions, it would be unwise to depend upon this precaution if the patient has manifested hypersensitivity in the past. Excretory radiopaque material may be lethal in patients with multiple myeloma. This risk is markedly lessened if the patient is well hydrated beforehand. Preliminary dehydration in patients suspected of or having primary hyperparathyroidism may precipitate irreversible hypercalcemia. Fortunately, fairly good urograms can be obtained in association with normal fluid intake, particularly if the dose of the opaque medium is increased.

A few deaths have been reported in infants due to pulmonary injury. This is thought to be caused by the hypertonicity of the contrast medium. Preliminary dehydration should therefore be condemned.

If the PSP test is less than 30% in 1 hour or if blood nitrogen retention is demonstrated, it will be necessary to administer a larger dose of radiopaque fluid (eg, double the usual dose or use a 90% concentration of the medium) or to perform infusion urography. Adequate films may thus be obtained when the blood urea nitrogen is as high as 100 mg/100 ml.

In women, urography is most safely performed during the 10 days following the onset of menses. It presents a genetic hazard during pregnancy.

Technic

A. Preparation of the Patient: No food or fluids should be taken for at lease 6 hours before the procedure is scheduled, although in infants dehydration should not be practiced. A cathartic (eg, castor oil) taken the night before will decrease the amount of gas and fecal material in the bowel, thus ensuring clearer delineation of the urinary tract. An enema is less effective. If urograms are urgently desired and the patient is hydrated, satisfactory films are still obtainable. A 3-minute film should be added to the series, since the

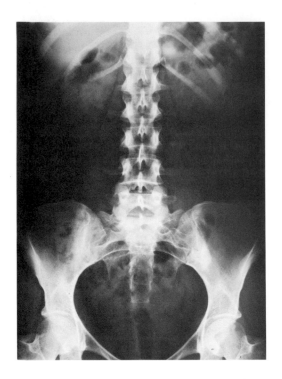
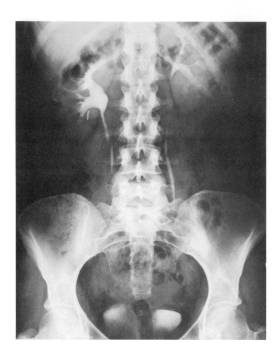
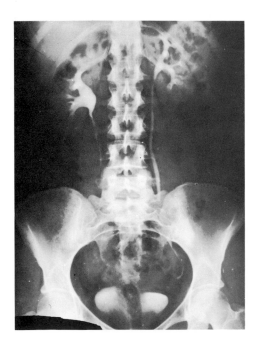
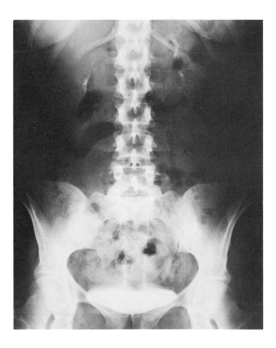

Figure 6—3. Normal excretory urogram. *Above left:* Plain abdominal film. Bones normal, renal shadows fairly well seen, psoas margins distinct. Black oblong shadow below coccyx is a vaginal menstrual tampon. *Above right:* Five minutes after injection of radiopaque material. Prompt excretion in good concentration. Lower calyces of left kidney indistinct, upper ureters well outlined. Note area of systole in both upper ureters. Some radiopaque material in bladder. *Below left:* Fifteen-minute film. Calyces of left kidney now well filled. All calyces are well cupped. Differences in ureteral diameter are caused by systolic contractions. *Below right:* Twenty-five-minute film, prone. Excellent drainage of opaque material. Each kidney drops a distance equal to height of one-half vertebra.

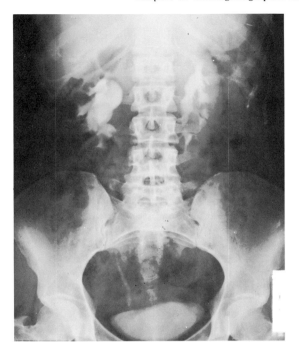
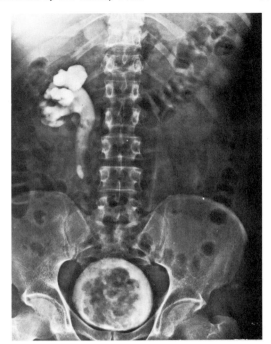
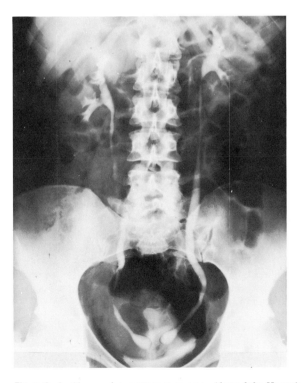
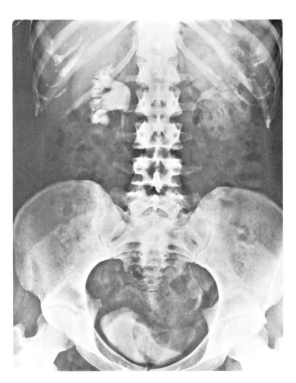

Figure 6–4. Abnormal excretory urograms. ***Above left:*** Horseshoe kidney. Axes of renal masses vertical, lower calyces on psoas muscles. ***Above right:*** Right ureteral stone causing hydronephrosis. Large irregular filling defect from unsuspected vesical neoplasm. ***Below left:*** Bilateral ureteroceles causing a minimum of obstruction. ***Below right:*** Moderate right hydronephrosis with obstruction at ureteropelvic junction due to aberrant vessel. Compression of left side of bladder from enlarged uterus.

radiopaque material under these circumstances is excreted more promptly. A double dose of the iodide will further enhance the quality of the films.

B. Procedure:

1. Preliminary plain film—This must be taken not only to check on the quality of the radiographic technic and the position of the patient but also to demonstrate urinary stones which might be obscured by the radiopaque medium.

2. Injection of the radiopaque fluid—The amount of fluid which should be injected varies with the type of fluid and the age of the patient. (Follow the manufacturer's directions.) One of the antihistamines should be added to the infusion material.

a. Intravenous injection—This is the method of choice if venipuncture is feasible. Since allergic reactions may occur and death may ensue (rarely), preliminary tests for hypersensitivity should be performed. If one or more tests are positive, this examination should not be done. Unfortunately, none of these tests guarantees complete safety, although the intravenous test is more reliable than the ocular or subcutaneous test.

(1) Tests for sensitivity—

(a) Ocular test—One drop of the contrast medium is instilled into the eye. If erythema is produced, the test is positive.

(b) Subcutaneous test—Inject 0.1 ml subcut. If induration and erythema develop promptly, the test is positive.

(c) Intravenous test—Inject 1 ml of the medium IV. If no signs of hypersensitivity (eg, urticaria, asthma) are observed, the test is negative.

(2) Manifestations of sensitivity—If symptoms and signs of hypersensitivity are manifested by the patient during the injection, it should be stopped immediately. Warning signs of allergic reaction include respiratory difficulty; sneezing, itching, or urticaria; nausea and vomiting; and fainting. Treatment consists of oxygen for anoxia, hypertensive drugs and intravenous dextrose solutions for shock, intravenous barbiturates for convulsions, and the intravenous injection of an antihistamine if allergic reactions are observed.

b. Extravascular infusion—This procedure is indicated if venipuncture is impossible (eg, in the infant). (See manufacturer's directions for dosage.) The ocular and intradermal tests should be performed first. If sensitivity is demonstrated by these tests, the infusion should be withheld. The ampule of radiopaque medium (to which an antihistamine has been added) is diluted to 100 ml with normal saline solution. Equal parts of the solution are given subcutaneously over the scapular areas. Excretion is maximal on the 30- to 60-minute films.

3. Routine urograms—The infusion should be given rapidly. Radiograms are taken at 10 seconds for the nephrogram effect, and at 5, 10, and 15 minutes with the patient in the supine position. Films taken 2 and 3 minutes after the beginning of the injection (minute sequence) should be routine in all patients who are hypertensive, for these radiograms, by revealing delayed concentration of the dye in one kidney, may suggest decreased renal function and blood flow. At 25 minutes, a film is also taken with the patient erect in order to demonstrate the mobility of the kidneys, to obtain ureterograms, and to observe the efficiency with which the renal pelves and ureters drain. All films should include the kidney, ureter, and bladder areas since subtle changes in the ureters which imply the presence of vesicoureteral reflux may otherwise be missed.

In infants and children, the films should be taken at 3, 5, 8, and 12 minutes, for their kidneys excrete the fluid more rapidly than do those of the adult. If the renal areas are obscured by bowel content, the child should be offered 150–240 ml of a carbonated beverage. The resulting gas-filled stomach displaces the bowel and thus improves visualization of the kidneys.

Ureteral compression may be helpful if the first urogram shows poor concentration of the medium. The urine is thus held in the upper urinary tracts, affording enhanced filling. Compression, however, may cause spontaneous extravasation of urine in the region of the pelvis. This is not pathologic.

4. Supplementary urograms—As soon as the routine exposures are taken and developed, they should be viewed. Oblique, lateral, or supine films may then be indicated in order to localize calcific bodies more accurately and to gain a third dimension of the urogram; this may be helpful if calyceal distortion is suspected. Taking films in the prone position, particularly in children, may lead to improved filling of some calyces and the ureter. Troublesome gas shadows may also be displaced.

If excretion of the urographic fluid is delayed, films should be taken periodically for as long as 4 hours or even 24 hours after the injection. Advanced hydronephrosis and dilated ureters may become apparent only then. It is feasible to inject additional radiopaque medium if there is impaired concentration on the initial films.

5. X-ray of the bladder region after voiding—This should be routine in all urologic patients, no matter what age or sex. At the conclusion of the urographic study, the patient should be instructed to void; a film of the bladder area should be taken immediately. This will demonstrate the presence or absence of residual urine. Partial urinary retention is common but is often not suspected. Normal and abnormal urograms are shown in Figs 6–3 and 6–4.

INFUSION UROGRAPHY

This technic of excretory urography is indicated in patients suffering from renal insufficiency (blood urea nitrogen up to 100 mg/100 ml) and when maximum detail is required. Preliminary dehydration is unnecessary. Give 25% sodium diatrizoate (Hypaque) or similar radiopaque fluid, 2–4 ml/kg in a similar volume of normal saline. This is infused through an 18-

gauge needle over a period of 5–10 minutes. Films are exposed at 10, 20, and 30 minutes, though additional films and views may be indicated. This technic lends itself well to tomography, which can be executed at the completion of the infusion.

The routine use of this type of urography, particularly in children, should be condemned. Preliminary hydration plus the marked osmotic diuresis stimulated by the larger dose of the radiopaque fluid causes the ureters to be completely full and somewhat dilated, thus simulating the changes compatible with vesicoureteral reflux.

If the patient is being studied for hypertension, exposure should be made at 2, 3, 4, and 5 minutes as well. This procedure also lends itself to the urea washout test, which can be done as the final step.

In a few instances, opacification of the uterus and even myomas may be noted.

UREA WASHOUT TEST

Since the basic phenomenon in renal ischemia is the overreabsorption of water by the renal tubules, a hyperconcentration of the radiopaque medium in this kidney should be seen on urography. This change can be accentuated by osmotic diuresis produced by urea.

After preliminary dehydration, (1) infuse 50 ml of 50% sodium diatrizoate (Hypaque)—or other opaque medium—rapidly through a 16-gauge needle; (2) expose films at 30 seconds and at 2, 3, 5, 8, 15, and 20 minutes; (3) give 40 g urea and 30 ml of sodium diatrizoate in 500 ml of normal saline in a 15-minute period; and (4) take a film every 3 minutes until one or both kidneys have "washed out" the radiopaque medium. Normally, both are washed out in 15 minutes. If one kidney retains the "dye" 6–9 minutes longer than the other kidney, the test is considered positive for renal ischemia.

ANGIONEPHROTOMOGRAMS
(Intravenous Renal Angiograms)

Nephrotomography has its greatest usefulness in the differentiation of renal cyst and tumor. Briefly, this technic involves the rapid intravenous injection of a bolus of radiopaque material which opacifies vascularized tissues in the kidney. The space occupied by a cyst or abscess fails to opacify (Fig 6–5); a malignant tumor shows normal or increased opacification because of its increased blood supply (Fig 18–4). Renal angiography is more efficient in this differential diagnosis.

Technic

(1) Preparation of the patient and tests for sensitivity to the radiographic fluid are carried out as de-

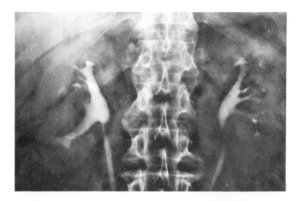

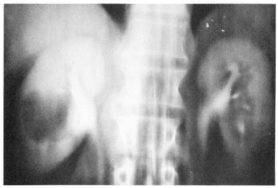

Figure 6–5. Angionephrotomogram. *Above:* Excretory urogram showing space-occupying lesion in the center of the right kidney; calyces distorted and displaced. *Below:* Nephrotomogram showing lack of opacification of the lesion which, therefore, is a simple cyst. Note the similarity of this urogram to that in Fig 18–3 (bottom right), which proved to be cancer.

scribed for excretory urograms.

(2) Take a plain film of the renal areas, and then take test tomograms to demonstrate the kidneys (usually 8–11 cm from the tabletop). Insert a No. 12 needle into one antecubital vein or one No. 16 needle into each antecubital vein. Establish the circulation time by injecting 2.5 ml of 20% sodium dehydrocholate (Decholin) in 10 ml of normal saline solution. Inject 30 ml of 50% sodium diatrizoate (Hypaque) or other opaque medium to enhance the nephrogram. Rapidly inject 50 ml of 90% sodium diatrizoate, take a plain film at the predetermined circulation time, and follow immediately with 4–6 tomograms.

RETROGRADE UROGRAMS

Only this type of radiography requires special training in urologic instrumentation. The indications, contraindications, and technic of the preliminary cystoscopy and ureteral catheterization are discussed in Chapter 9.

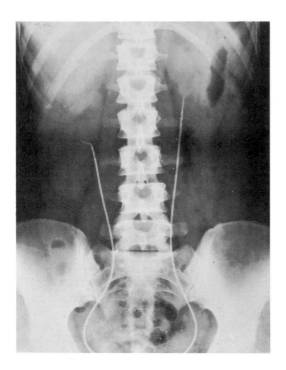
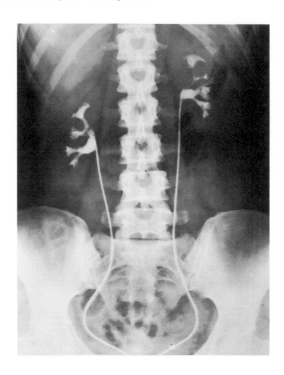
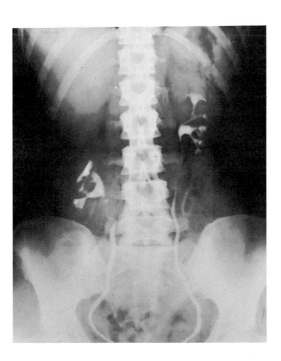
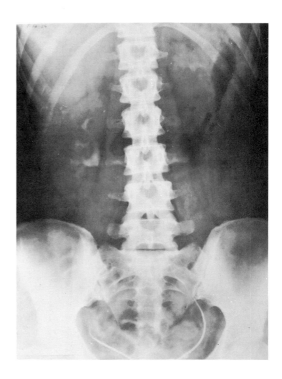

Figure 6—6. Normal retrograde urogram. *Above left:* Plain abdominal film showing radiopaque ureteral catheters in the renal pelves. *Above right:* Film taken in the supine position. Calyces are well cupped and there is no dilatation of the pelves. *Below left:* Urogram taken in the upright position with catheters drawn down into the lower ureters. The right kidney drops the height of one and one-half vertebrae, causing some redundancy of the upper ureter. The left kidney drops the height of one vertebra. *Below right:* Film taken 15 minutes later, showing almost complete drainage of both kidneys.

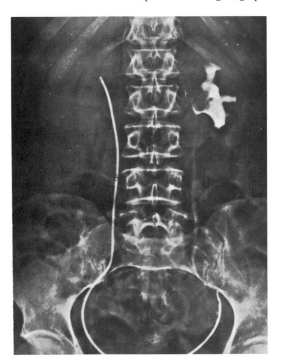
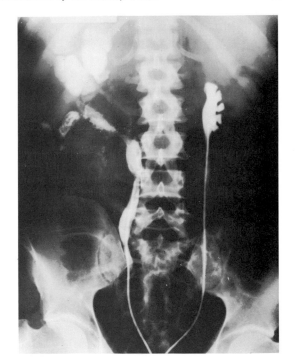
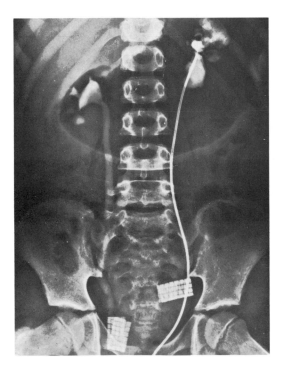
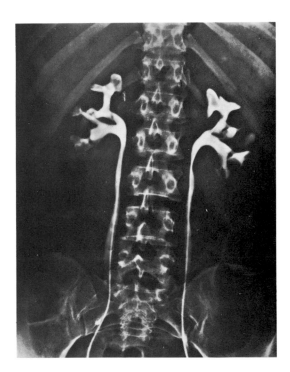

Figure 6–7. Abnormal retrograde urograms. *Above left:* Space-occupying lesion of left renal pelvis. Transitional cell carcinoma. *Above right:* Stones in right renal pelvis and upper ureter; calculus pyonephrosis. Atrophic kidney, left. *Below left:* Bilateral renal tuberculosis. Motheaten appearance of calyces of left kidney, obliteration of upper calyx, and dilated and foreshortened ureter on right. *Below right:* Bilateral papillary necrosis. All papillae have sloughed. Upper medial and lowest calyces on left show "negative" shadows representing retained papillae.

After catheters have been passed to the renal pelves, a "split" renal function test (PSP) should be performed (see Chapter 5) and urine specimens obtained for microscopic examination and culture. Undiluted radiopaque material is then allowed to flow up the catheters. The average normal renal pelvis has a capacity of 3–4 ml. Overdistention causes painful renal pelvic and ureteral spasms (colic) and capsular (costovertebral) pain. Overfilling may also distort the urogram; if the pelvis is extrarenal, a normal pelvis and calyces may appear hydronephrotic (Figs 6–6 and 6–7).

Indications

A. Infection: When upper tract abnormality is suspected and pyuria is present, catheterization of the ureters affords separate urine specimens from the kidneys for bacteriologic study, thus establishing the site of the infection. Retrograde urograms can then be done.

B. Inadequate Excretory Urograms: If excretory urograms (even the infusion type) do not adequately demonstrate ureteropelvic detail, retrograde urograms may be needed.

C. Impaired Total Renal Function: If renal function is decreased to the point where excretory urograms will prove inadequate, retrograde filling of the renal pelves will be necessary.

D. Assessment of Degree of Ureteral Obstruction: If excretory urograms portray ureteropelvic junction or ureteral obstruction, its degree may be best judged by instilling radiopaque fluid into the renal pelvis. In the absence of significant obstruction, most of the medium will have drained out in 15 minutes, whereas marked stenosis may cause retention of the iodide for hours.

E. Sensitivity to Intravenous Radiopaque Fluid: If excretory urograms are contraindicated because of allergy, retrograde urograms must be substituted.

F. Need for Oblique and Lateral Radiograms: Since the radiopaque medium given intravenously is diluted by urine, the density of the excreted fluid is less than that obtained with retrograde filling. If oblique and lateral films are desired, the density of the tissues through which the x-rays must pass is increased; retrograde instillation may prove more satisfactory in some instances.

Contraindications

Although there are contraindications to cystoscopy and ureteral catheterization, there are none to retrograde urography itself.

Technic

A. Preparation of the Patient: Fluids can be taken as tolerated unless general anesthesia is to be employed for the procedure. The bowel should first be cleansed by catharsis (eg, castor oil).

B. Procedure:

1. Cystoscopy and ureteral catheterization—These are done first.

2. Preliminary plain film of abdomen (supine)—This checks on the position of the patient and the catheters and on the radiographic technic, and demonstrates calcific densities in the urinary tract which might be obscured by the radiopaque medium.

3. Instillation of the radiopaque fluid—

a. Supine urogram—If the capacity of the renal pelvis is not known, 3–4 ml of undiluted urographic medium should be instilled by gravity under low pressure (20 cm of water). A radiogram is then taken, developed, and viewed. If filling is incomplete, another x-ray film can be exposed after more fluid is introduced.

b. Oblique or lateral radiograms—These should then be taken as indicated.

c. Upright ureteropyelogram—The patient is then placed in the semi-erect position, and, while the urographic fluid is still being introduced, the catheters are slowly withdrawn into the lower ureters and a film taken. This affords good ureterograms and shows the degree of mobility of the kidneys.

If ureteral filling is inadequate, the patient should be placed in the Trendelenburg position and more of the contrast medium instilled; an x-ray exposure is again made.

d. "Emptying" or delayed films—If the ureteropyelograms reveal evidence of obstruction, an x-ray should be taken 15 minutes after the previous one without further introduction of radiopaque medium. If some of the medium is still retained, later films should be made in order to assess the degree of obstruction.

BULB URETEROPYELOGRAM

If optimum ureteral detail is essential, a bulb ureteropyelogram should be obtained. This is accomplished by forcing a bulbous tipped catheter tightly into the ureteral orifice. Radiopaque fluid is then instilled with a syringe.

OPACIFICATION OF RENAL CYSTS

One of the most difficult problems in diagnosis is the differentiation of renal cyst and tumor. Some urologists, fearing the complications of cancer on the wall of a cyst, tend to explore all kidneys showing evidence of a space-occupying lesion as revealed by urography. Others will not resort to surgery if the diagnosis of cyst can be established. Renal angiography (particularly of the selective type) establishes the diagnosis of vascular adenocarcinomas, but what appears to be a nonvascular mass, although almost always a cyst, could be a necrotic tumor or an abscess. In this instance, renal cystography can be performed.

Under fluoroscopic control and after administration of a radiopaque fluid intravenously (although some clinicians needle blindly, using previous urograms as a guide), a 7-inch, 18-gauge needle is introduced into the presumed cyst. In most instances, clear fluid will be obtained; this should be subjected to cytologic study. Radiopaque fluid is then instilled into the cystic cavity and a film taken. If the radiopaque fluid is homogeneous, the edges of the cavity smooth, and cytology negative, the diagnosis of simple cyst is warranted, thus negating the need for surgery (Fig 21–5). The return of bloody fluid or just a little blood implies the presence of carcinoma; surgery is indicated.

ANTEGRADE UROGRAMS

If excretory or infusion urograms reveal the presence of advanced hydronephrosis or a large nonfunctioning renal mass and radiopaque fluid introduced into the lower ureter fails to reach the renal pelvis because of ureteral stenosis, antegrade urograms can be procured. A high-dose infusion urogram should first be obtained. Under fluoroscopic control, an 18-gauge needle, 15 cm long, should be passed into a dilated calyx or pelvis. Radiopaque material can then be instilled and appropriate films taken.

In order to afford temporary drainage, a small plastic catheter can be passed through the needle as a nephrostomy tube. The needle can then be removed.

CYSTOGRAMS

Cystograms are made by instilling radiopaque fluid into the bladder through a catheter. Roentgenograms then show an outline of the bladder wall. In addition, ureteropyelograms may be obtained if the ureterovesical "valves" are incompetent (see Chapter 11).

RETROGRADE CYSTOGRAMS

Indications

A. When Cystoscopy Is Not Feasible: In male infants, the small caliber of the urethra may preclude passage of the smallest cystoscope or panendoscope. If mechanical difficulties prevent passage of an optical instrument to the bladder but a catheter can be successfully passed, a cystogram may reveal a vesical tumor, vesicoureteral reflux, or protrusion of an enlarged prostate into the vesical cavity.

If a catheter cannot be introduced through the urethra, a small plastic tube can be placed in the bladder through the barrel of a needle passed suprapubically.

B. Study of the Neurogenic Bladder: Particularly in the spastic type of neurogenic bladder, ureterovesical reflux is common. Cystograms will reveal this reflux as well as the degree of damage from hydronephrosis or pyelonephritis.

C. Rupture of the Bladder: Cystography is the best method of testing for extravasation of urine (Fig 16–7).

D. Recurrent Infection: Cystography should be routine in the study of any patient suffering from recurrent infection, particularly children. Vesicoureteral reflux is one of the common causes of perpetuation of infection. This procedure may also delineate vesical fistulous communications and is of great help in the study of urinary incontinence in both males and females.

E. Lateral Cystogram: This is an important step in the evaluation of the woman with stress incontinence. (See Chapter 26.)

Contraindications

During acute attacks or exacerbations of chronic urinary infection, the instillation of radiopaque medium under pressure may increase the seriousness of the infection (eg, bacteremia), particularly if reflux exists.

Technic

(1) If vesicoureteral reflux is suspected, a KUB should be made. If vesical disease only is to be studied (eg, rupture), a film of the bladder area alone is sufficient.

(2) A catheter is passed to the bladder. The urine it contains should be drained off.

(3) Introduction of radiopaque fluid: In the adult, 250–350 ml are sufficient. In a child 1 year old, the normal vesical capacity is 75–100 ml. Any fluid used for excretory or retrograde urography diluted with 3 parts of water or normal saline solution can be used.

(4) The catheter is then clamped off and an x-ray taken with the patient supine. This may reveal trabeculation and diverticula, intravesical protrusion of an enlarged prostate, vesical tumors, or vesicoureteral reflux.

(5) Left and right oblique radiograms will visualize diverticula which lie behind the bladder or a fistulous tract into the vagina.

(6) Cystograms taken in the true lateral position are helpful in delineating the cause of urinary incontinence, particularly in women (Figs 6–9 and 26–2).

(7) The vesical fluid is then allowed to drain out and another x-ray film exposed. Diverticula or a fistulous tract into the vagina will still contain the radiopaque fluid and will be clearly defined. Intraperitoneal or extraperitoneal extravasation of the contrast medium behind the bladder will be shown. Fig 6–8 demonstrates the normal and some abnormal cystograms.

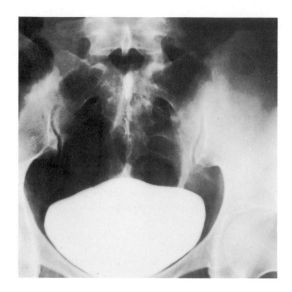
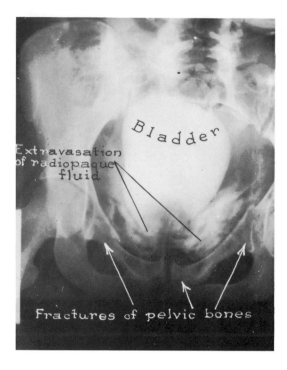
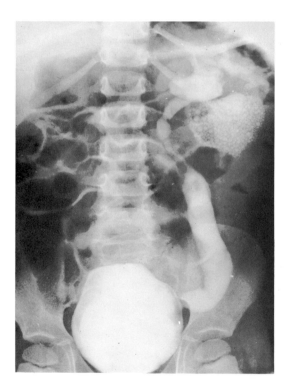
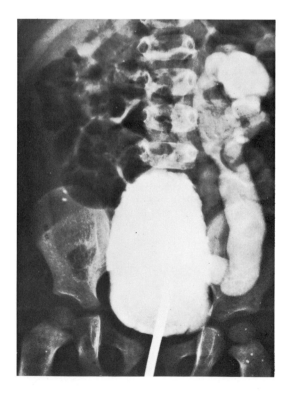

Figure 6–8. Normal and abnormal cystograms. *Above left:* Normal cystogram. *Above right:* Avulsion of prostatic urethra secondary to pelvic fracture. Extraperitoneal extravasation. *Below left:* Light iodized oil (Lipiodol) instilled into bladder to seek evidence of residual urine. Lipiodol refluxed up second left ureter to fill hydronephrotic lower pole (same patient as below right). *Below right:* Trabeculated bladder and left ureteral reflux demonstrating marked hydroureteronephrosis.

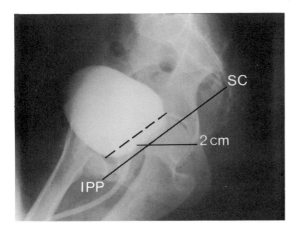 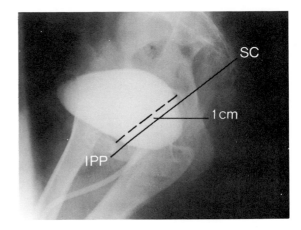

Figure 6—9. Lateral cystogram in stress incontinence. The dashed line shows the normal position of the base of the normal bladder. Line SCIPP is a reference line drawn from the sacrococcygeal (SC) joint to the inferior point of the pubic bone (IPP). *Left:* Resting cystogram in stress incontinence. The bladder base lies 2 cm below the normal position. *Right:* Cystogram taken with straining in a patient with stress incontinence. Normally, the base of the bladder should lie on the dashed line. The base of the bladder descends about 4 cm, revealing poor support of the urethrovesical junction.

DELAYED CYSTOGRAMS

Simple cystography often fails to demonstrate ureterovesical reflux, although incompetency of the vesicoureteral valves exists. Stewart (1955) has shown that "delayed" cystograms reveal this reflux more efficiently. If voiding cystourethrography is attempted but the patient cannot void, delayed cystograms should be resorted to.

Technic
(1) Preliminary film of abdomen should be made.
(2) A small catheter is passed to the bladder and the urine drained off.
(3) Radiopaque fluid is then introduced into the bladder. The amount varies from 30 ml in an infant to 120 ml for a child 8 years of age and 200—300 ml for adults. The least noxious fluid is urographic medium diluted with 3 parts of water or normal saline solution.
(4) The catheter is then removed.
(5) Serial x-ray films are then exposed every 15—30 minutes during the next 1—3 hours. Ureteral reflux may appear on one "delayed" film only to be absent on the next. One kidney may reveal reflux, whereas on the next exposure only the opposite kidney may contain the radiopaque fluid.

VOIDING CYSTOURETHROGRAMS

This technic often shows ureteral reflux when both the simple and delayed cystograms fail to do so because of the increased intravesical pressure generated at the time of voiding. The voiding cystourethrogram may also reveal the presence of posterior urethral valves (Fig 27—1) or urethral strictures (Fig 27—4). If catheterization is impossible or thought to be contraindicated, radiopaque fluid can be instilled by suprapubic vesical puncture.

Immediately following the conclusion of the series of delayed cystograms or after filling the bladder with the radiopaque medium, the patient is instructed to void. During the act of urination, one or more x-rays are taken.

CYSTOURETHROGRAMS

Cystourethrograms combine simple cystography with urethrography. Vesical and urethral abnormalities are thereby visualized.

A catheter is passed to the bladder and a plain film of the bladder area is taken. About 200—300 ml of radiopaque fluid or air are then introduced into the bladder, a plain x-ray film exposed, and oblique views made. With the patient lying at a 45-degree angle, 20 ml of radiopaque water-soluble lubricant are injected into the urethra and a radiogram made (Fig 6—9).

•   •   •

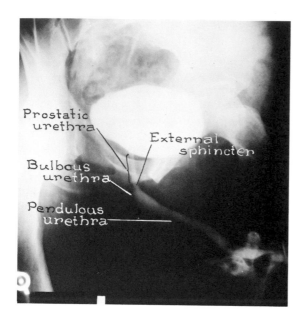

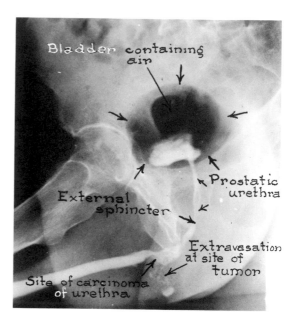

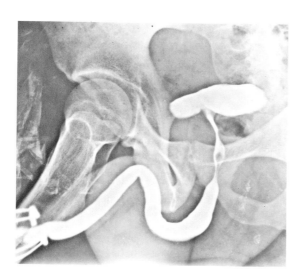

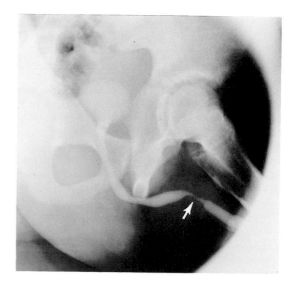

Figure 6–10. Normal and abnormal cystourethrograms and retrograde urethrograms. *Above left:* Normal cystourethrogram. *Above right:* Cystourethrogram showing carcinoma of urethra. *Below left:* Normal urethrogram. Note "negative" shadow over pubic bone representing the verumontanum. *Below right:* Oblique retrograde urethrogram showing stricture of pendulous urethra.

RETROGRADE URETHROGRAMS

Stenoses of the urethra and enlargements of the prostate and even some posterior urethral valves (Fig 27–1) can be shown on films by introducing into the urethra 20–30 ml of a water-soluble lubricant in which there is an equal amount of radiopaque fluid. Oily media (eg, iodized oil [Lipiodol]) are contraindicated since they may cause pulmonary emboli. The radiogram should be taken while the fluid is being injected. Oblique films of the area of the urethra and prostate will demonstrate narrowings, diverticula, fistulas, and other diseases of these organs (Fig 6–10).

ESTIMATION OF RESIDUAL URINE IN CHILDREN

Instill 5 ml of ascendant iodized oil (Lipiodol) into the bladder. If the child does not retain urine, a film taken 24 hours later will show no retention of the opaque material. If some urinary retention does exist, the fluid may remain in the bladder for many days. If vesicoureteral reflux is present, the iodized oil may be visualized in the kidney (Fig 6–8).

CINERADIOGRAPHY

Cineradiography, formerly only a research tool, is now of practical value in clinical diagnosis. It reveals a higher incidence and degree of reflux than cystography and the voiding cystourethrogram and affords a dynamic picture of this abnormality.

The bladder is gradually filled with radiopaque fluid. The ureters are studied for transient or persistent reflux. The efficiency of peristalsis may also be studied. Reflux may only be demonstrated during the act of voiding, when intravesical pressure is high. About half of children suffering from urinary tract infection will show vesicoureteral reflux. This phenomenon is also revealed in a significant number of adults with chronic pyelonephritis.

PRESACRAL RETROPERITONEAL PNEUMOGRAMS

The main value of retroperitoneal pneumograms is visualization of the adrenal glands and renal outlines. Excision of adrenal tumors or even total bilateral adrenalectomy has become a routine surgical procedure now that potent hormonal replacement preparations are available. Direct perirenal air insufflation

fell into disrepute 15–20 years ago because it caused a number of deaths from gas embolus. It is safe, however, if CO_2 is used. The use of angiography has reduced the indications for this procedure.

During the past 20 years, the presacral technic has been used extensively. However, a few deaths from gas embolism have been reported where air and even oxygen have been used. Because CO_2 is much more soluble than oxygen in body tissues and blood, its use has recently been recommended as a safety measure. The great disadvantage of CO_2 is the rapidity of its absorption (20–30 minutes). Tomograms, which are essential if presacral retroperitoneal pneumograms are to attain a high degree of diagnostic accuracy, are therefore more difficult to obtain. The importance of slow low-pressure insufflation cannot be overemphasized. The author has no knowledge of a death from gas embolism when oxygen has been instilled with a low-pressure apparatus as described below.

Presacral pneumograms should not be made if the proper diagnosis can be established by simpler (and possibly safer) methods (eg, plain films, tomograms, excretory urograms, angiography).

Technic

A. Preparation of the Patient: A sedative and opiate should be administered 1 hour before the procedure is to be done.

B. Procedure (Fig 6–11).

1. The patient is placed on his right side (if the physician is right-handed) with his knees drawn up on the abdomen. The skin of the sacral area is prepared with soap and water and a skin antiseptic. The area is sterilely draped.

2. A wheal of 1% procaine hydrochloride is raised on the skin just below the tip of the coccyx. The tissues deep to this point are then anesthetized.

3. A No. 18 spinal needle (stiff enough to be accurately guided) is passed to a point just below the tip of the coccyx; it is then directed upward so that its point lies just anterior to the end of the coccyx. This placement is facilitated by palpation of the area with the left index finger inserted in the rectum.

4. The needle is aspirated to be sure it has not entered a blood vessel. Ten ml of air are then introduced by syringe. It should enter with minimal resistance. If it does not, the needle should be remanipulated.

5. A pneumothorax type of machine should then be connected to the spinal needle. The upper bottle contains sterile water; the lower one is filled with oxygen. The oxygen should flow slowly when the levels of the respective bottles are about 20 cm apart. If higher pressure is required, the position of the needle should be changed. Seven ml of oxygen per kg body weight should be introduced.

If bilateral insufflation is desired, the tubing should be disconnected from the spinal needle and the patient instructed to roll slowly onto his abdomen and then onto his left side. The tubing is again connected to the needle and an equal amount of oxygen allowed

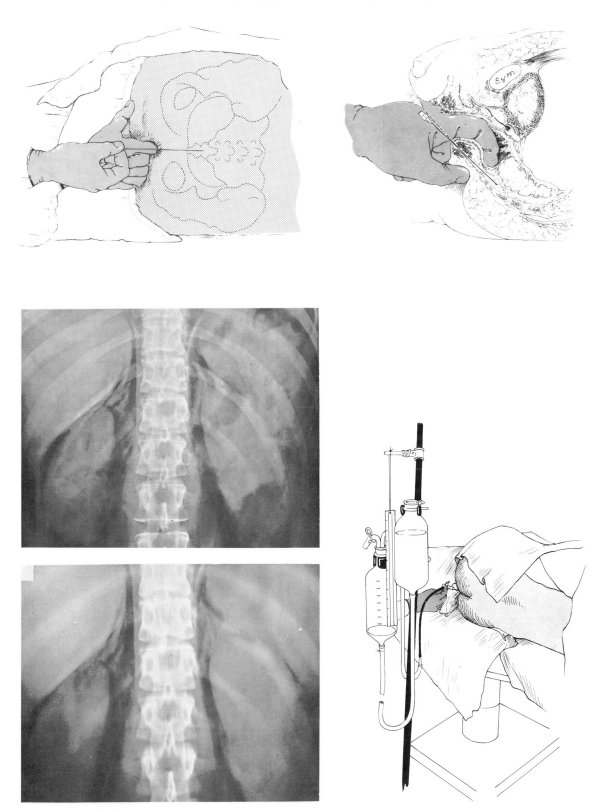

Figure 6–11. Technic of presacral retroperitoneal pneumography; normal pneumogram. *Above:* Technic of placing needle. *Below right:* Pneumothorax apparatus used for insufflation. *Center left:* Normal pneumogram showing kidneys and adrenals. *Below left:* Tomogram of same patient. Details of organs enhanced.

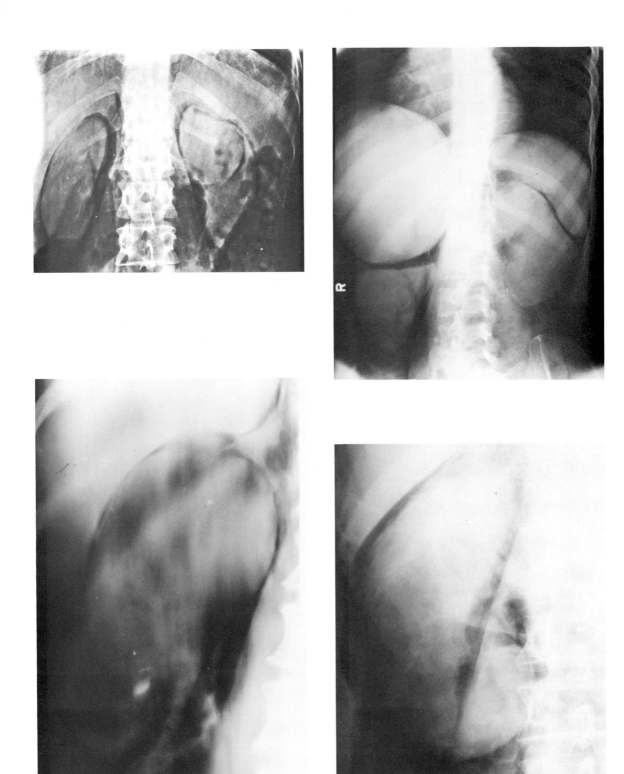

Figure 6–12. Abnormal retroperitoneal pneumograms. *Above left:* Presacral oxygen showing pheochromocytoma overlying upper half of left kidney. *Above right:* Massive androgenic tumor of right adrenal with downward displacement of right kidney. Spleen clearly shown above left kidney. *Below left:* Carcinoma of upper pole of right kidney. Note expansion of this pole; normal adrenal above it. *Below right:* Cyst of lower pole of right kidney overlying psoas muscle, which is visible through mass.

to fill the right side. By changing position for each insufflation, equal distribution of the gas is obtained.

Warning: If syncope or circulatory collapse occurs, the patient should be placed immediately on his left side. If the cause is gas embolus, this position will allow the oxygen trapped in the right ventricle to pass into the lungs; death is thereby prevented.

6. The patient is then placed prone with the head of the table or cart elevated 20 degrees; this causes the gas to rise to the perirenal area. This position should be maintained at all times except when supine x-ray films are taken.

7. Plain x-ray films of the renal area are then exposed immediately after insufflation and every 30—60 minutes thereafter until the clearest delineation of the kidney and adrenals is obtained. When visualization of the organ in question is at its maximum, tomograms should be taken. This procedure is essential since it affords optimum detail of the adrenals and kidneys (Figs 6—11 and 6—12).

8. Simultaneous excretory urography may further enhance the study.

C. Recovery of the Patient: Six hours after the insufflation, 75% of the oxygen has been absorbed as judged by radiography. During this period, the patient should be flat in bed. Ambulation causes the gas to rise to the mediastinum and neck, causing the patient some apprehension.

RENAL ANGIOGRAPHY

Although renal angiograms can be procured by direct lumbar needle puncture of the aorta, this technic has been superseded by percutaneous femoral angi-ography wherein a catheter is passed to the level of the renal arteries under fluoroscopic control. Percutaneous catheterization of the brachial or axillary artery is also feasible. Twelve to 24 ml of radiopaque fluid suitable for intravenous urography (eg, meglumine diatrizoate, 66%, and sodium diatrizoate, 10%, [Renografin-76]) are rapidly introduced into the aorta, and serial films are immediately taken (midstream technic). About 10 exposures are made over a period of 10 seconds, but 2 per second are exposed for the first 3 seconds. A second or even a third injection may be indicated for oblique views. Besides demonstrating the caliber of the great vessels, this procedure shows the renal arterial circulation (Fig 6—13). Fig 32—3 reveals stenosis of the renal artery as the cause of hypertension. A pheochromocytoma is shown in Fig 20—8.

Selective renal angiography is accomplished by passing a femoral catheter into one of the renal arteries under fluoroscopic control. About 8 ml of contrast medium are injected, and approximately 16 exposures are made during the first few seconds (Fig 6—13). The intrarenal vascular detail demonstrated by this technic is superior to the midstream method and is therefore of particular value in the differential diagnosis of renal cyst (Fig 21—5) and tumor (Fig 18—3). The space occupied by a cyst fails to opacify. Neovascularity followed by increased density on late films is typical of tumor.

In cases where the lesion is small or obscured by overlying arteries, epinephrine can first be injected into the catheter followed by instillation of radiopaque medium. This technic causes spasm of normal vessels but has no effect on arteries in tumors.

There is a good correlation between the renal angiogram and the technetium (camera) scan (see Chapter 8).

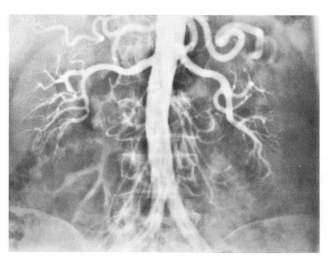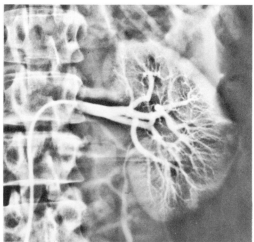

Figure 6—13. Normal percutaneous femoral renal angiograms. *Left:* Midstream technic. Renal arteries and their branches are of normal caliber and distribution. The celiac axis, splenic artery, and branches of the superior mesenteric arteries are well outlined. *Right:* Selective renal angiogram. Detail of smaller arterial branches is enhanced. They are evenly distributed throughout the kidney.

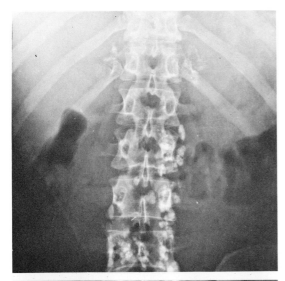

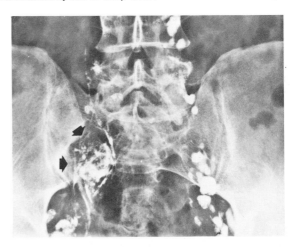

Figure 6—15. Abnormal lymphangiogram. Carcinoma of the penis with metastases to right common iliac nodes, overlying sacroiliac joint, which have blocked ascent of contrast medium.

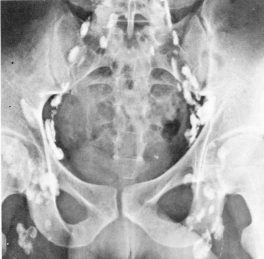

Figure 6—14. Normal lymphangiogram. (Composite of 2 films.) Note calcifications of both adrenal glands, probably secondary to spontaneous hemorrhage. Compare with Fig 6—15.

VESICAL ANGIOGRAPHY

In order to judge the size and depth of penetration of vesical neoplasms, the following technic can be employed. A Seldinger catheter is passed to the bifurcation of the aorta, and the vessels are "flooded" with 30 ml of 90% contrast material. As an alternative, each hypogastric artery is selectively catheterized and into each of them are instilled 10 ml of radiopaque fluid. Films are rapidly exposed over a period of 8 seconds. The series is repeated in the oblique position, affording a tangential view of the tumor. These roentgenograms reveal the typical pattern or "stain" of an invasive tumor (Fig 18—9), thus improving accuracy of staging of

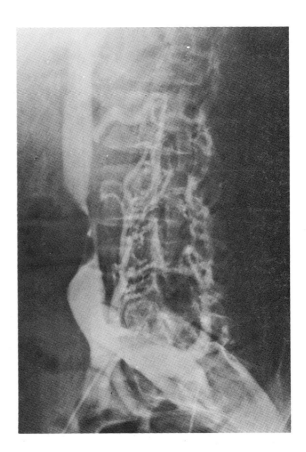

Figure 6—16. Venacavogram. Right posterior oblique exposure revealing defect caused by metastases to lumbar lymph nodes from seminoma of right testis. (See Fig 18—15 for retrograde ureterogram on same patient.)

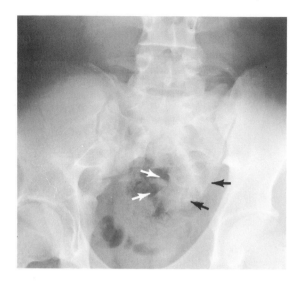

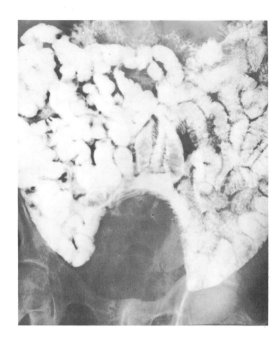

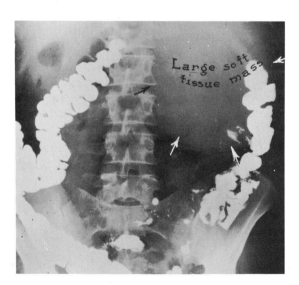

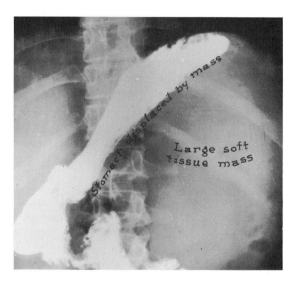

Figure 6–17. Miscellaneous x-ray studies. *Above left:* Study of bones reveals scimitar-shaped sacrum on the right side. Typical of anterior meningomyelocele. Patient had a neuorgenic bladder. *Above right:* Patient with low midline mass and cramping abdominal pain. Gastrointestinal series showing the cause of the symptoms—a distended bladder. *Below left:* Barium enema showing displacement of transverse colon by large cyst of left kidney. *Below right:* Gastrointestinal series (same patient) showing displacement of stomach by cyst of left kidney.

the lesion. The study may be enhanced if 60 ml of CO_2 are first instilled into the bladder.

LYMPHANGIOGRAPHY

Cannulation of a lymphatic vessel in the foot and injection of an oily contrast medium leads to x-ray opacification of the inguinal, pelvic, retroperitoneal, and supraclavicular lymphatic systems (Fig 6–14). The main value of this procedure is the demonstration of metastatic infiltration in regional lymph nodes (Fig 6–15). It therefore lends itself to the study of patients with cancers of the testes (Fig 18–15), penis, bladder, or prostate. It can demonstrate the lymphatic connections to the kidney in patients with chyluria.

VENACAVOGRAPHY

Retrograde catheterization of the femoral veins affords a route for the injection of radiopaque material into the vena cava (Fig 25–5). Evidence of masses in the right retroperitoneal areas are demonstrated by encroachment on the vessel. Thus, this technic is one of particular value in outlining enlarged retroperitoneal lymph nodes (eg, testicular tumor; Fig 6–16). This technic may also reveal tumor thrombus in the adrenal vein or vena cava.

SELECTIVE RENAL VENOGRAPHY

While venacavography may reveal gross extension of renal carcinoma into the vena cava, it may miss minor defects in the renal veins themselves because of the "washout" of the veins by a large volume of blood. Selective renal venography overcomes this deficiency. It is an excellent method of demonstrating renal vein thrombosis (Fig 21–12).

The washout effect can be decreased by injection of epinephrine into the renal artery 10 seconds before the venous infusion of 35–60 ml of radiopaque mate-

rial. If indicated, a blood sample from the renal vein can be subjected to analysis for renin.

SELECTIVE ADRENAL VENOGRAPHY

Transfemoral catheterization of one or both adrenal veins can be accomplished. This allows estimation of the concentration of hormones (eg, aldosterone, cortisol, 11-deoxycortisol) in the venous blood and phlebography. It is particularly useful in the endocrinologic and radiographic diagnosis of Cushing's disease, hyperaldosteronism, carcinoma, and bilateral adrenal hyperplasia.

OTHER X-RAY STUDIES

Roentgenograms of the gastrointestinal tract, chest, and bones may contribute to urologic diagnosis.

Gastrointestinal Series (Fig 6–17)
A barium enema may show displacement of the colon—a cardinal sign of retroperitoneal tumor. The stomach may also be displaced by large retroperitoneal masses (eg, kidney, spleen, pancreas).

Cholecystograms
Films of the gallbladder may show evidence of gallbladder disease. Extensive renal carcinoma may invade the common duct. Cholecystitis or cholelithiasis may be the cause of pseudorenal pain.

Chest Film
An x-ray of the chest may reveal the source of a tuberculous infection of the kidney or may show metastasis from renal, testicular, or other tumors (Fig 18–4).

Osteograms
Films of bones may reveal evidence of metastases (Figs 18–4 and 18–13), spina bifida (Fig 6–17), or changes compatible with hyperparathyroidism (Fig 15–4), or osteitis fibrosa generalisata as often seen in patients with renal tubular acidosis.

•　　•　　•

References

General

Hope JW, Borns PF: Radiologic diagnosis of primary and metastatic cancer in infants and children. Radiol Clin North America 3:353, 1965.

Lowman RM: Retroperitoneal tumors: A survey and assessment of Roentgen techniques. Radiol Clin North America 3:543, 1965.

Symposium on urinary tract (radiologic aspects). Radiol Clin North America 3:3, 1965.

Tucker AS: The Roentgen diagnosis of abdominal masses in children: Intravenous urography vs inferior venacavography. Am J Roentgenol 95:76, 1965.

Plain Film of Abdomen

Batson PG, Keats TE: The roentgenographic determination of normal adult kidney size as related to vertebral height. Am J Roentgenol 116:737, 1972.

Daniel WW Jr & others: Calcified renal masses: A review of ten years experience at the Mayo Clinic. Radiology 103:503, 1972.

Duggan HE: The radiological interpretation of the scout film in the acute abdomen. S Clin North America 40:1221, 1960.

Elkin M, Cohen G: Diagnostic value of the psoas shadow. Clin Radiol 13:210, 1962.

Jaffe R: Anterior sacral meningocele. Obst Gynec 28:684, 1966.

Madsen EH: The value of tomography for the demonstration of small intrarenal calcifications. Brit J Radiol 45:203, 1972.

McAfee JG, Donner MW: Differential diagnosis of calcifications encountered in abnormal radiographs. Am J Med Sc 243:609, 1962.

Mogg RA: Urinary tract displacements. Brit J Urol 32:472, 1960.

Olurin EO, Olurin O: Pancreatic calcification: A report of 45 cases. Brit MJ 4:534, 1969.

Shemilt P: The origin of phleboliths. Brit J Surg 59:695, 1972.

Stevenson J, MacGregor AM, Connelly P: Calcification of the adrenal glands in young children. Arch Dis Childhood 36:316, 1961.

Excretory Urograms

Allen TD: Extensive displacement of the kidney by intraperitoneal disease. J Urol 97:823, 1967.

Cerny JC, Kendall AR, Nesbit RM: Subcutaneous pyelography in infants: A reappraisal. J Urol 98:405, 1967.

Chait A & others: Vascular impressions on the ureter. Am J Roentgenol 111:729, 1971.

Daughtridge TG: Mucosal folds in the upper urinary tract. Am J Roentgenol 107:743, 1969.

Dunbar JS, Nogrady B: Excretory urography in the first year of life. Radiol Clin North America 10:365, 1972.

Esho JO, Cass AS: Medial deviation of ureters following abdominoperineal resection for carcinoma of large bowel. Urology 2:658, 1973.

Feingold M, Fine RN, Ingall D: Intravenous pyelography in infants with single umbilical artery. New England J Med 270:1178, 1964.

Filly RA & others: Urinary tract infections in children. 2.

Roentgenologic aspects. Western J Med 121:374, 1974.

Fischer HW, Doust VL: An evaluation of pretesting in the problem of serious and fatal reactions to excretory urography. Radiology 103:497, 1972.

Fischer HW, Rothfield NJH: Whither urography? J Urol 107:120, 1972.

Fletcher EWL, Lecky JW: The normal position of the upper ureter in lateral intravenous pyelography. Brit J Urol 41:554, 1969.

Ford WH Jr, Palubinskas AJ: Renal extravasation during excretory urography using abdominal compression. J Urol 97:983, 1967.

Friedenberg RM & others: Clinical significance of deviations of the lower ureter. J Urol 96:146, 1966.

Gates DF, Ceccarelli FE: Benadryl and the IVP reaction. J Urol 108:627, 1972.

Geraghty JA: An approach to the problem of intestinal gas in diagnostic radiology. Brit J Radiol 39:42, 1966.

Gilbert EF & others: Hemorrhagic renal necrosis in infancy: Relationship to radiopaque compounds. J Pediat 76:49, 1970.

Grainger RG: Renal toxicity of radiological contrast media. Brit M Bull 28:191, 1972.

Kassner EG, Elguezabal A, Pochaczevsky R: Death during intravenous urography: Overdose syndrome in young infants. New York J Med 73:1958, 1973.

Lopez FA & others: The nephrogram: A valuable indicator or renal abnormalities. Am J Roentgenol 106:614, 1969.

Myers GH Jr, Witten DM: Acute renal failure after excretory urography in multiple myeloma. (Editorial.) Am J Roentgenol 113:583, 1971.

Nebesar RA, Pollard JJ, Fraley EE: Renal vascular impressions: Incidence and clinical significance. Am J Roentgenol 101:719, 1967.

Nogrady MB, Dunbar JS: Delayed concentration and prolonged excretion of urographic contrast medium in the first month of life. Am J Roentgenol 104:289, 1968.

Olsson O: Excretion of sodium metrizoate through the liver during urography. Acta radiol diag 11:85, 1971.

Pillay VKG & others: Acute renal failure following intravenous urography in patients with long-standing diabetes mellitus and azotemia. Radiology 95:633, 1970.

Poole CA, Viamonte M Jr: Unusual renal masses in the pediatric age group. Am J Roentgenol 109:368, 1970.

Reekie D, Davidson JK: The radiation hazard in radiography of the female abdomen and pelvis. Brit J Radiol 40:849, 1967.

Riggs W Jr, Hagood JH, Andrews AE: Anatomic changes in the normal urinary tract between supine and prone urograms. Radiology 94:107, 1970.

Saldino RM, Palubinskas AJ: Medial placement of the ureter: A normal variant which may simulate retroperitoneal fibrosis. J Urol 107:582, 1972.

Swick M: Uroradiographic media. Urology 4:750, 1974.

Wilkiemeyer RM, Boyce WH, Malek RS: Validity of the intravenous pyelogram in assessment of renal function. Surg Gynec Obst 135:897, 1972.

Wilson MC & others: Improved excretory urograms by use of second injection of contrast medium. J Urol 87:1010, 1962.

Witten DM, Hirsch FD, Hartman GW: Acute reactions to urographic contrast medium: Incidence, clinical characteristics and relationship to history of hypersensitivity states. Am J Roentgenol 119:832, 1973.

Infusion Urography

Birnholz JC: Uterine opacification during excretory urography: Definition of a previously unreported sign. Radiology 105:303, 1972.

Bosniak MA: Nephrotomography: A relatively unappreciated but extremely valuable diagnostic tool. Radiology 113:313, 1974.

Duré-Smith P: Drip infusion and routine urography: A comparative trial. Brit J Radiol 39:655, 1966.

Evans AT, Knoblaugh RA: Routine drip infusion pyelography. Am J Surg 119:656, 1970.

Greene LF & others: Routine use of tomography in excretory urography. J Urol 110:714, 1973.

Taylor DA, Macken KL, Fiore AS: Mannitol pyelography: A simpliification of the drip infusion technic. Radiology 88:1115, 1967.

Urea Washout Test

Harwood-Nash DCF, Lansdown EL: Evaluation of the urea washout pyelogram and urography in the assessment of renovascular hypertension. Canad MAJ 96:245, 1967.

Schreiber MH & others: The normal pyelogram urea washout test. Am J Roentgenol 98:88, 1966.

Angionephrotomograms

Athanasoulis CA & others: Angionephrotomography and subtraction: Relative value in renal mass lesions. Am J Roentgenol 117:108, 1973.

Becker JA: The nonvisualized kidney: The value of nephrotomography. Radiology 89:676, 1967.

Peterson CC Jr, Jackson JH Jr, Moore JG: A re-evaluation of nephrotomography stressing limitations of the procedure. J Urol 98:721; 1967.

Pfister RC, Shea TE: Nephrotomography: Performance and interpretation. Radiol Clin North America 9:41, 1971.

Opacification of Renal Cysts

Buttarazzi PJ & others: Aspiration of renal cyst. J Urol 100:591, 1968.

Lalli AF: Percutaneous aspiration of renal masses. Am J Roentgenol 101:700, 1967.

Witherington R, Rinker JR: Percutaneous needle puncture in the diagnosis of renal cysts. J Urol 95:733, 1966.

Antegrade Urograms

Fletcher EWL, Gough MH: Antegrade pyelography in children. Brit J Radiol 46:191, 1973.

Navarrette RV: Repeat direct pyelography via needle nephrostomy. Acta radiol diag 11:33, 1971.

Sherwood T, Stevenson JJ: Antegrade pyelography: A further look at an old technique. Brit J Radiol 45:812, 1972.

Cystourethrograms

Bartley O, Helander CG: Double-contrast cystography in

tumors of the urinary bladder. Acta radiol 54:161, 1960.

Berson JW, Alexander RL, Mehan DJ: Cystourethrography as a teaching aid for residents. South MJ 60:943, 1967.

Currarino G: Narrowings of the male urethra caused by contractions or spasm of the bulbocavernosus muscle: Cystourethrographic observations. Am J Roentgenol 108:641, 1970.

Hutch JA, Shopfner CE: The lateral cystogram as an aid to urologic diagnosis. J Urol 99:202, 1968.

Hyman RM, Yulis GB: An improved technique for male urethrocystography. J Urol 93:62, 1965.

McAlister WH, Cacciarelli A, Shackelford GD: Complications associated with cystography in children. Radiol 111:167, 1974.

Rudhe U: Roentgenographic diagnosis of obstructive disorders of the lower urinary tract in infancy and childhood. Postgrad Med 35:29, 1964.

Shopfner CE: Cystourethrography: Methodology, normal anatomy and pathology. J Urol 103:92, 1970.

Simon G, Berdon WE: Suprapubic bladder puncture for voiding cystourethrography. J Pediat 81:555, 1972.

Stewart CM: Delayed cystography and voiding cystourethrography. J Urol 74:749, 1955.

Theander G: Roentgen appearance of prostatic channels in infancy and childhood. Acta radiol diag 11:467, 1971.

Tucker AS, Persky L: Cystography in childhood tumors and pseudotumors. Am J Roentgenol 109:390, 1970.

Verga-Pires JA, Elebute EA: Urethrocystography in the male. Brit J Urol 39:194, 1967.

Retrograde Urethrograms

McClennan BL, Becker JA, Robinson T: Venous extravasation at retrograde urethrography: Precautions. J Urol 106:412, 1971.

Morales O, Nilsson S, Romanus R: Urethrographic studies of the posterior urethra. (2 parts.) Acta radiol diag 2:81, 305, 1964.

Mukerjee MG & others: Urethrovascular reflux and its significance in urology. J Urol 112:608, 1974.

Mullin EM, Peterson LJ, Paulson DF: Retrograde urethrogram: Diagnostic aid and hazard. J Urol 110:464, 1973.

Shopfner CE, Hutch JA: The normal urethrogram. Radiol Clin North America 6:165, 1968.

Estimation of Residual Urine in Children

Young BW, Anderson WG, King GG: Radiographic estimation of residual urine in children. J Urol 75:263, 1956.

Cineradiography

Mitsuya H & others: Cinefluorography of the upper urinary tract. Urol Internat 13:236, 1962.

Tanagho EA, Hutch JA, Miller ER: Diagnostic procedures and cinefluoroscopy in vesico-ureteral reflux. Brit J Urol 38:435, 1966.

Tristan TA & others: Cinefluorographic investigation of genitourinary tract function. Am J Roentgenol 90:1, 1963.

Presacral Retroperitoneal Pneumograms

Anderson EE, Glenn JF: Carbon dioxide contrast studies

in retroperitoneal masses. J Urol 101:530, 1969.

Landes RR, Ransom CL: Presacral retroperitoneal pneumography utilizing carbon dioxide. J Urol 82:670, 1959.

Renal Angiography

Alfidi RJ, Gill WM, Klein HJ: Arteriography of adrenal neoplasms. Am J Roentgenol 106:635, 1969.

Baum S, Gillenwater JY: Renal artery impressions on the renal pelvis. J Urol 95:139, 1966.

Becker JA & others: Misleading appearances in renal angiography. Radiology 88:691, 1967.

Caine M, Kedar SS, Schwartz A: Renal angiography by the percutaneous noncatheter left brachial technique. Brit J Urol 39:571, 1967.

Casarella WJ: Magnification renal arteriography. Urology 1:501, 1973.

Crane C: Renal angiography: Lumbar approach. Am J Surg 107:74, 1964.

Goldstein HM, Reuter SR, Wallace S: Pseudotumor of the renal pelvis caused by arterial impression. J Urol 111:735, 1974.

Hegeoüs V: Three-dimensional selective angiography in the diagnosis of renal masses. Acta radiol diag 15:401, 1974.

Hotchkiss RS, Sammons BP: Selective renal angiography. J Urol 93:309, 1965.

Kahn PC, Wise HM Jr: The use of epinephrine in selective angiography of renal masses. J Urol 99:133, 1968.

Killen DA, Foster JH: Spinal cord injury as a complication of contrast angiography. Surgery 59:969, 1966.

Lang EK: Roentgenographic assessment of asymptomatic 'renal lesions: An analysis of the confidence level of diagnoses established by sequential roentgenographic investigation. Radiology 109:257, 1973.

Meaney TF: Complications of percutaneous femoral angiography. Geriatrics 29:61, 1974.

Meyers MA, Whalen JP, Evans JA: Diagnosis of perirenal and subcapsular masses: Anatomic-radiologic correlation. Am J Roentgenol 121:523, 1974.

Moes CAF, Burrington JD: The use of aortography in the diagnosis of abdominal masses in children. Radiology 98:59, 1971.

Roy P: Percutaneous catheterization via the axillary artery. Am J Roentgenol 94:1, 1965.

Vesical Angiography

Wise HW Jr, Fainsinger MH: Angiography in the evaluation of carcinoma of the bladder. JAMA 192:1027, 1965.

Lymphangiography

Chavez CM: Lymphangiography. Am J Med Sc 248:225, 1964.

Fraley EE, Clouse M, Litwin SB: The uses of lymphography, lymphadenography and color lymphadenography in urology. J Urol 93:319, 1965.

Mahaffy RG: Lymphography and the urologist. Postgrad MJ 41:452, 1965.

Oritz F, Walzak MP, Marshall VF: Chyluria: Lymphatic-urinary fistula demonstrated by lymphangiography. J Urol 91:608, 1964.

Wallace S & others: Lymphangiographic interpretation. Radiol Clin North America 3:467, 1965.

Venacavography

Berdon WE, Baker DH, Santulli TV: Factors producing spurious obstruction of the inferior vena cava in infants and children with abdominal tumor. Radiology 88:111, 1967.

Hayt DB: Upright inferior vena cavagraphy. Radiology 86:865, 1966.

Hipona FA, Crummy AB: The roentgen diagnosis of renal vein thrombosis. Am J Roentgenol 98:122, 1966.

Simon H, Moquin R, Dameshek W: The inferior venacavagram and lymphoproliferative disorders. JAMA 184:978, 1963.

Wendel RG, Evans AT, Wiot JF: A new technique for inferior venacavagraphy. J Urol 100:705, 1968.

Selective Renal Venography

Kahn PC: Selective venography in renal parenchymal disease. Radiology 92:345, 1969.

Selective Adrenal Venography

Cope C, Isard HJ, Wesolowski WE: Selective adrenal phlebography. Radiology 90:1105, 1968.

Nicolis GL & others: Percutaneous adrenal venography: A clinical study of 50 patients. Ann Int Med 76:899, 1972.

7 . . .
Ultrasonic Examination of the Urinary Tract

Granville C. Coggs, MD

PHYSICAL BACKGROUND & EXAMINATION TECHNICS

Diagnostic ultrasound utilizes high-frequency sound waves, usually 2 million cycles per second (2 MHz), to produce images of organs within the body. A transducer—a combination sound generator and sound receiver—is used to direct a narrow sound beam into the body. As the sound beam passes through tissue interfaces of differing densities, part of the sound is reflected—"echoed"—at such interfaces back to the transducer. In "A" mode ultrasound, these echoes are presented as peak deviations from a zero voltage baseline on an oscilloscope. In "B" scanning, these echoes are converted into electrical currents and transformed into dots on an oscilloscope screen corresponding to the position of the transducer on the body. "B" mode scanning is the more generally used method of ultrasound presentation for urologic tract examinations because the resultant dot pictures more closely resemble body section radiographs or tomograms. A permanent recording of the oscilloscope image may be accomplished in several ways. These include photographing the oscilloscope with a polaroid camera which produces a positive image (white dots); and electrostatic copying on 8½ × 11 inch paper, which produces a negative image (black dots). For examination of the kidney, the patient is placed in the prone position and mineral oil is applied to his back to provide sonic contact between the skin surface and the transducer face. The transducer is moved with a rocking motion (Figs 7−1 and 7−2) along the skin and a cross-sectional image of the underlying structures is produced (Figs 7−3 and 7−4). A series of transverse and longitudinal scans is usually made at 2 cm intervals over the area of interest (eg, kidney). Each scan of the series takes about 30 seconds, and the total time required for evaluation of the kidneys is about 30 minutes. For examination of the bladder, the patient is usually placed in the supine position and scans of this area (Fig 7−5) are obtained.

Diagnostic ultrasound involves no hazard because

Granville C. Coggs is Professor of Radiology, University of Texas School of Medicine, San Antonio; formerly a faculty member of the University of California School of Medicine, San Francisco.

the power level used, approximately 1 mW/sq cm, is approximately 1/1000 of that used in therapeutic ultrasound and is applied in short pulses for less than 1% of the total time that the machine is in operation. After more than 20 years of clinical use, no deleterious effects have been observed in young adults whose mothers were examined by diagnostic ultrasound during pregnancy.

DIFFERENTIAL DIAGNOSIS OF RENAL CYSTS & TUMORS

With increasing refinement of urographic technics, unsuspected renal masses are being found with increased frequency. Diagnostic ultrasound is rapidly increasing in use and is becoming the principal method in the investigation of renal masses.

Many authors now feel that renal sonography should be the next step in evaluation after demonstration of a renal mass by urography. Renal sonography should be followed by nephrotomography, arteriography, or percutaneous puncture as necessary for preoperative definitive diagnosis approaching 100% accuracy. In general, patients whose renal sonograms show a cystic pattern are further examined by nephrotomography or cyst puncture (or both), whereas patients whose sonograms show a solid pattern are further examined by arteriography.

The typical appearance of a cyst shows displacement of the calyceal echoes, an anechoic area surrounded by a sharply defined border, and increased sound transmission associated with the far wall of the anechoic mass. The center of the mass remains relatively anechoic with increasing intensity of the diagnostic sound beam.

A renal tumor also generally shows displacement of the calyceal echoes. Increasing gain produces increased number of echoes within the mass. The outline of the mass is usually irregular and does not show increased sound transmission through the far wall. Fig 7−6 shows the typical sonographic appearance of a renal cyst. Fig 7−7 is a sonographic transverse section of a woman with bilateral renal masses. The left kidney shows a large renal tumor; the right kidney shows a typical renal cyst.

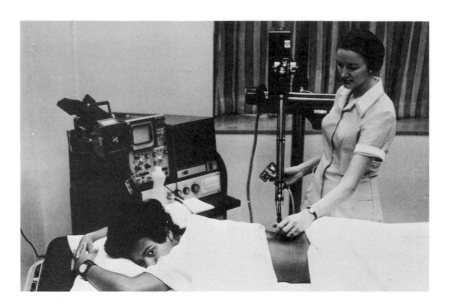

Figure 7—1. Production of a transverse B scan of the renal areas. Transverse cross sections of the kidneys pictured on the larger oscilloscope are shown in detail in Fig 7—3.

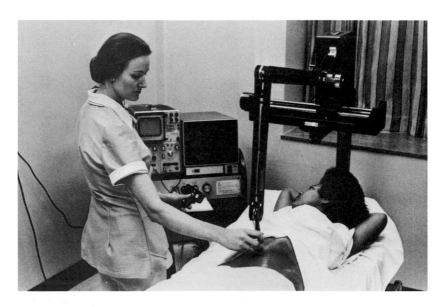

Figure 7—2. Production of a longitudinal B scan of the lower abdomen. The midline longitudinal cross section of the bladder and uterus pictured on the larger oscilloscope is shown in detail in Fig 7—5.

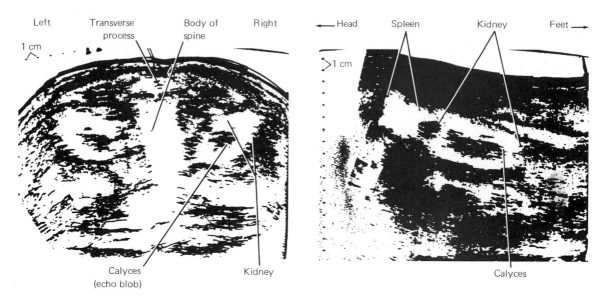

Figure 7–3. Prone transverse section at a level through the mid-section of normal kidneys.

Figure 7–4. B scan longitudinal section of the lumbar region performed 8 cm to the left of the spine, showing sections of the spleen and left kidney.

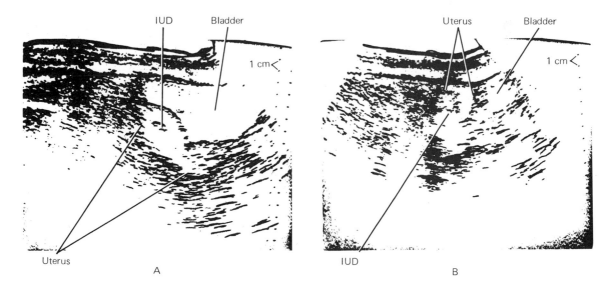

Figure 7–5. Longitudinal midline B scans of lower abdomen showing outline of normal bladder prevoiding *(A)* and postvoiding *(B).* Note IUD in normal uterus.

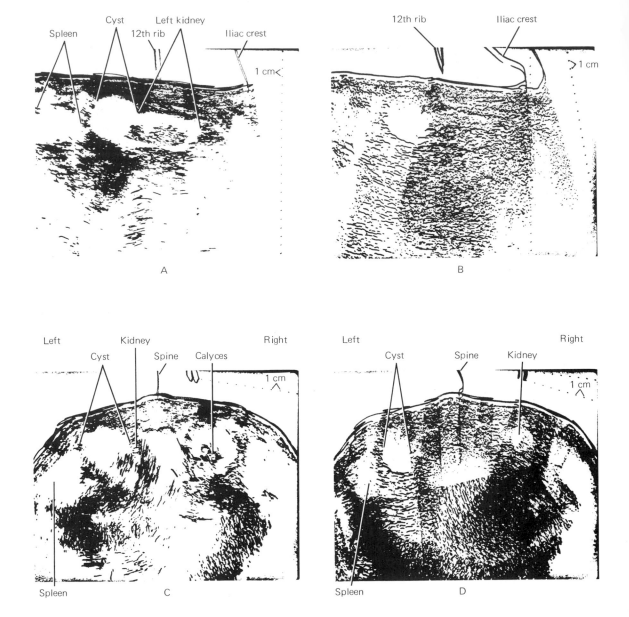

Figure 7–6. Cyst of upper pole of left kidney. Longitudinal B scans 6 cm to the left of the spine at medium gain *(A)* and at high gain *(B)*. Transverse B scans of cyst of upper pole of left kidney, sections taken 12 cm superior to iliac crests. Scans were taken at medium gain *(C)* and high gain *(D)*. Cyst proved by aspiration.

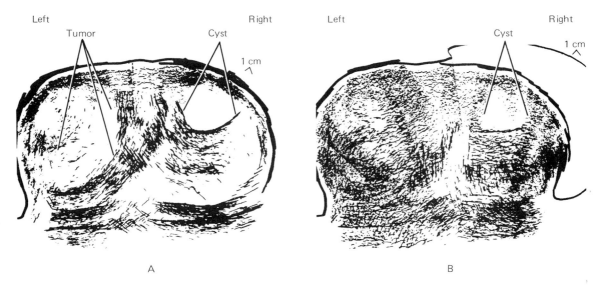

Figure 7–7. Prone transverse B scans through the kidneys at medium gain *(A)* and high gain *(B)*. The homogeneous fluid contents of the cyst do not fill in with echoes (black dots) at high gain as do the heterogeneous tissues of the "solid" tumor.

Sonography is about 95% accurate as a means of distinguishing between solid and cystic renal masses.

EVALUATION OF POLYCYSTIC KIDNEYS

Polycystic kidneys present a characteristic sonographic picture. The kidneys are irregularly enlarged to several times normal size. The various cysts are usually of differing sizes and present sonolucent patterns similar to isolated cysts.

Polycystic kidneys are often associated with polycystic liver disease. An example of combined involvement of the liver and kidneys is shown in Fig 7–8.

ASSISTANCE IN PERCUTANEOUS ASPIRATION OF RENAL CYSTS & PERCUTANEOUS RENAL BIOPSY

Kristensen and Holm in Copenhagen and Goldberg in Philadelphia were leaders in utilizing transducers with central holes to facilitate percutaneous puncture of renal cysts (Fig 7–9).

The region of the cyst is first mapped out on the patient's skin, and the depth of the center of the cyst from the skin surface is determined from the B scan. The transducer with the hole in the center is then moved over the general region of the cyst until the characteristic appearance of the cyst appears on the oscilloscope positioned beneath the transducer. The puncture needle is then passed through the center of

the transducer hole to the appropriate predetermined depth and the cyst fluid is aspirated. The tip of the needle can usually be seen advancing into the anechoic area of the cyst (Fig 7–10).

Clear cyst fluid obtained on aspiration usually indicates a benign lesion. Radiography of the cyst with a horizontal x-ray beam after instillation of radiopaque contrast media and air and demonstration of smooth, sharply defined cyst walls gives further evidence that the cyst is benign. The aspirated fluid should be sent to the laboratory for determination of cells, fat, and lactic acid dehydrogenase to further assess the character of the cyst.

Some writers feel that percutaneous aspiration of cysts should be restricted to selected cases because of the rare simultaneous occurrence of a tumor within a cyst. Von Schreeb showed in a prospective study of 150 renal tumors with subsequent nephrectomy that there were no significant differences in 5-year survival in 77 patients whose tumors were percutaneously punctured and contrast media instilled, compared to 73 patients who underwent nephrectomy without prior percutaneous puncture.

Percutaneous renal biopsy is facilitated by using the B scan as guidance in outlining on the patient's skin the relative position of the kidney underneath. Although a high degree of accuracy in locating the inferior border of the kidney can be obtained if the patient breathes quietly, greater accuracy is obtained if the lower border of the kidney is marked in the same phase of inspiration for localization as for percutaneous biopsy.

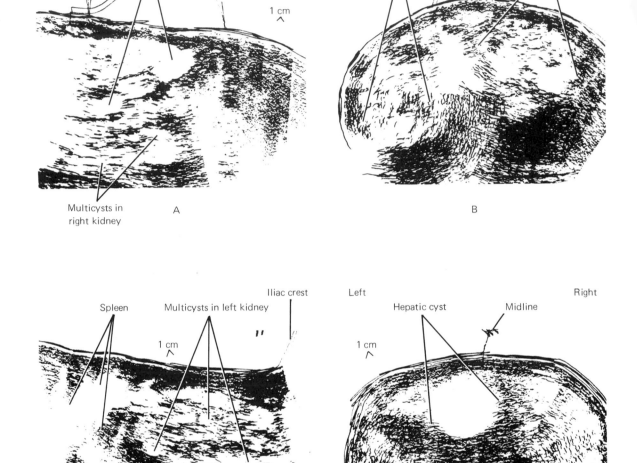

Figure 7—8. Polycystic kidneys and liver. *A:* Longitudinal supine scan 8 cm to right of midline showing polycystic right kidney and liver. *B:* Transverse prone section, level 4 cm superior to iliac crest, through midsections of polycystic kidneys. *C:* Longitudinal prone section, 8 cm to left of spine; polycystic left kidney and spleen. *D:* Transverse supine section, 16 cm superior to umbilicus, large hepatic cyst.

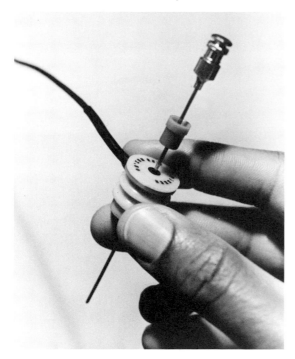

Figure 7–9. Needle aspiration transducer.

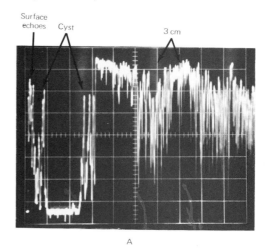

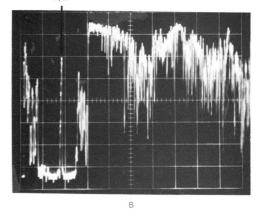

Figure 7–10. Cyst model shown before insertion of needle *(top)* and after insertion of needle tip into center of cyst *(bottom)*. Needle tip echo is indicated by arrow. Dimension of sides of small square is 3 cm.

DIAGNOSIS OF PERIRENAL ABSCESS & RETROPERITONEAL HEMORRHAGE OR MASSES

Structures or spaces which are primarily liquid in nature are fairly easily diagnosed by ultrasound. Perirenal abscesses and subcapsular renal hematomas fall into this category. A retroperitoneal hematoma secondary to rupture of an aneurysm of the splenic artery has been diagnosed by ultrasound. Retroperitoneal fluid collections or tumor masses are more easily recognized when they produce displacement of a kidney. A large adrenal tumor producing downward and anterior displacement of the left kidney is shown in Fig 7–11. Serial examinations which show progressive kidney displacement are useful in evaluating rate of tumor growth or, in cases of retroperitoneal bleeding, whether bleeding is continuing.

EVALUATION OF RENAL TRANSPLANTS

The relatively superficial position of most renal transplants makes transplant evaluation by diagnostic ultrasound relatively easy.

There is usually a slow increase in size of the transplanted kidney during the first 6 months after transplant. A sudden increase to 20% more than the initial donor kidney size occurring soon after transplant usually indicates acute rejection. Holmes states that the calyceal-pelvic "echo blob" normally occupies less than 15% of the total area of the kidney. Increase in area of the "echo blob" may suggest obstruction or intrapelvic tumor.

Fluid collections about the transplanted kidney, secondary to bleeding or lymphatic obstruction, may be well demonstrated by diagnostic ultrasound. We have observed in serial fashion the status of a renal transplant during a twin pregnancy. The appearance of this transplant during the mid trimester of pregnancy is shown in Fig 7–12.

ESTIMATION OF RESIDUAL URINE

The urine-filled bladder is readily outlined by diagnostic ultrasound. Holmes has described a procedure utilizing a planimeter whereby the volume of

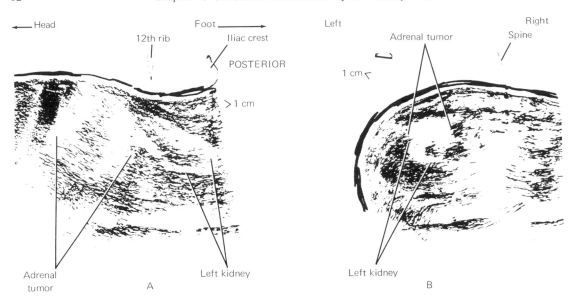

Figure 7–11. Prone longitudinal B scan 7 cm to the left of the spine *(A)* and transverse B scan through lumbar area *(B)* showing large adrenal tumor displacing the left kidney downward and anteriorly.

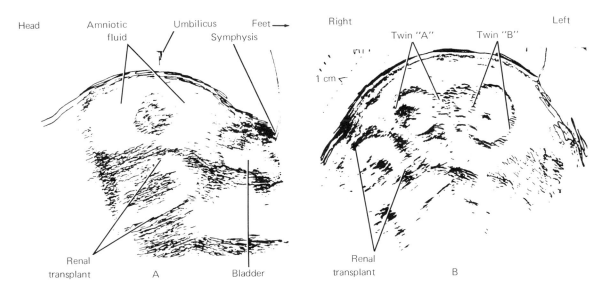

Figure 7–12. Longitudinal B scan, 12 cm to right of midline *(A)* and transverse B scan 8 cm superior to symphysis pubis *(B)*. Renal transplant and twin fetuses are shown.

urine in the bladder can be calculated to an accuracy of ± 10%. Goldberg has described the usefulness of ultrasound in determining the volume of urine in the bladder prior to suprapubic percutaneous aspiration of urine in pediatric patients. This capability is useful in older patients to determine the amount of residual urine after voiding without catheterization. Evaluation of changes of the bladder contour is useful in detecting other intrapelvic disease when it distorts the bladder contour. Congenital urachal anomalies are well demonstrated by ultrasound. An example of change in blad-

der contour in a normal woman before and after voiding is shown in Fig 7–5.

PROSTATIC EVALUATION

In recent years there has been increased interest in evaluation of the prostate by ultrasound. Earlier, Whittingham evaluated the prostate via the suprapubic approach using a commercially available B scanner.

Since that time, Watanabe and King have used the rectal approach in prostatic evaluation. More recently, Holm has described a transurethral approach for prostatic evaluation.

It seems that the transrectal and transurethral approaches more reliably determine prostatic volume and give more information regarding whether there may be hyperplasia or neoplasia involving the prostate.

Additional experience is needed for more definitive assessment of the value of ultrasound in prostatic evaluation.

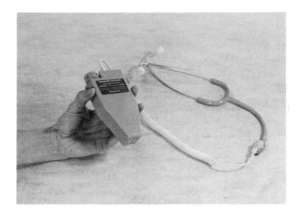

Figure 7–13. Doppler ultrasonic stethoscope.

DIAGNOSIS OF TORSION OF THE TESTIS USING DOPPLER ULTRASOUND

The distinguishing feature of torsion of the testis is loss of blood flow. Hahn and his associates have used isotope scans to demonstrate this, but the procedure is cumbersome and time-consuming. Levy and Pedersen and their associates have used the Doppler ultrasonic stethoscope to accurately distinguish acute testicular torsion from epididymitis in 8 patients.

The Doppler ultrasonic stethoscope is a pocket-sized instrument with a stethoscope headset (Fig 7–13). It operates on the Doppler shift principle. Two transducers are incorporated into the head of the stethoscope. One transducer continuously sends high-frequency sound waves into the tissues. The other transducer continuously receives high-frequency sound waves reflected back from the tissues. If the tissue is stationary, no sound will be heard. The periodic intermittent blood flow in vessels is received and heard as pulsatile sound.

The testis to be examined is supported against the scrotal skin with one hand, and the instrument is guided over the surface with the other. The testis is systematically auscultated, beginning behind the testis directly over the testicular artery as it enters the testis. The instrument is then guided anteriorly over the ventral surface, and the change in sound intensity is recorded.

Absence of pulsatile sound from the painful testis is diagnostic of testicular torsion. Examination of the noninvolved testis serves as a control. The examination requires about 5 minutes.

● ● ●

References

General References
    King DL (editor): *Diagnostic Ultrasound*. Mosby, 1974.

Physical Background & Examination Technics
    Hasch E: Ultrasound in the investigation of disease of the kidney and urinary tract in children. Acta paediat scandinav 63:42, 1974.
    Stuber JL, Templeton AW, Bishop K: Ultrasonic evaluation of the kidneys. Radiology 104:139, 1972.
    Von Micsky LI: Clinical sonography in urology. Urology 1:506, 1973.

Polycystic Kidneys
    Asher WM, Leopold GR: A streamlined diagnostic approach to renal mass lesions with renal echogram. J Urol 108:205, 1972.
    Doust DB, Maklad NF: Control of renal cyst puncture by transverse ultrasonic B scanning. Radiology 109:679, 1973.
    Goldberg BB, Capitanio MA, Kirkpatrick JA: Ultrasonic evaluation of masses in pediatric patients. Am J Roentgenol 116:677, 1972.
    Goldberg BB, Pollack HM: Ultrasonically guided renal cyst aspiration. J Urol 109:5, 1973.
    Goldberg BB, Pollack HM: Ultrasonic aspiration transducer. Radiology 102:187, 1972.
    Igawa K, Miyagishi T: The use of scintillation and ultrasonic scanning to disclose polycystic kidneys and liver. J Urol 108:685, 1972.
    Jeans WP, Perry JB, Roylance J: Renal puncture. Clin Radiol 23:298, 1972.
    King DL: Renal ultrasonography. Radiology 105:633, 1972.
    Kristensen JK & others: Ultrasonic guided percutaneous puncture of renal masses. Scandinav J Urol Nephrol (Suppl 15)6:49, 1972.
    Kristensen JK & others: Ultrasound in the demonstration of renal masses. Brit J Urol 44:517, 1972.
    Lalli AF: Percutaneous aspiration of renal masses. Am J Roentgenol 101:700, 1967.
    Leopold GR & others: Renal ultrasound: An updated approach to the diagnosis of renal cyst. Radiology 109:671, 1973.
    Lufkin EG & others: Polycystic kidney disease: Earlier diagnosis using ultrasound. Urology 4:5, 1974.
    Pederson JF: Percutaneous nephrostomy guided by ultra-

sound. J Urol 112:157, 1974.

Pollack HM & others: A systematized approach to the differential diagnosis of renal masses. Radiology 113:653, 1974.

Romeister RS, Walls WH, Valk WL: B-scan ultrasound in the evaluation of renal mass lesions. J Urol 112:8, 1974.

Silverman J, Kilhenny C: Tumor in the wall of a simple renal cyst. Radiology 93:95, 1969.

Von Schreeb T: Is there a risk of spreading tumor in diagnostic puncture? Scandinav J Urol Nephrol 1:270, 1967.

Perirenal Abscess; Retroperitoneal Hemorrhage or Masses

Holm HH & others: Indications for abdominal scanning in abdominal diagnostics. J Clin Ultrasound 1:5, 1974.

Holmes JH: Urologic ultrasonography. Pages 242–259 in: *Diagnostic Ultrasound.* King DL (editor). Mosby, 1974.

Renal Transplants

Holmes JH: Urologic ultrasonography. Pages 242–259 in: *Diagnostic Ultrasound.* King DL (editor). Mosby, 1974.

Leopold GR: Renal transplant size measured by reflected ultrasound. Radiology 95:687, 1970.

Sampson D: Ultrasonic method for detection of human renal allotransplants. Lancet 2:976, 1969.

Winterberger AR, Palma LD, Murphy GP: Ultrasonic testing in human renal allografts. JAMA 219:475, 1972.

Residual Urine

Barrett E, Morley P: Ultrasound in the investigation of space-occupying lesions of the urinary tract. Brit J Radiol 44:733, 1971.

Goldberg BB, Meyer H: Ultrasonically guided suprapubic urinary bladder aspiration. Pediatrics 51:70, 1973.

Holmes JH: Ultrasonic studies of the bladder. J Urol 97:654, 1967.

Sanders RS, Oh KS, Dorst JP: B-scan ultrasound: Positive and negative contrast material evaluation of congenital urachal anomaly. Am J Roentgenol 120:448, 1974.

Prostatic Evaluation

Holm HH, Northeved A: A transurethral ultrasonic scanner. J Urol 111:238, 1974.

King WW & others: Current status of prostatic echography. JAMA 226:444, 1973.

Watanabe H & others: Development and application of new equipment for transrectal ultrasonography. J Clin Ultrasound 2:91, 1974.

Watanabe H & others: Diagnostic application of ultrasonotomography to the prostate. Invest Urol 8:548, 1970.

Torsion of the Testis

Hahn LC & others: Testicular scanning: A new modality for the preoperative diagnosis of testicular torsion. J Urol 113:60, 1975.

Levy BJ: The diagnosis of torsion of the testicle using the Doppler ultrasonic stethoscope. J Urol 113:63, 1975.

Pedersen JF, Holm HH, Hald T: Torsion of the testis diagnosed by ultrasound. J Urol 113:66, 1975.

8...
Radioisotopic Kidney Studies

Malcolm R. Powell, MD, & Jerome M. Weiss, MD

Radioisotopic tracer procedures provide means of studying the structure and function of internal organs without disturbing their normal physiologic processes. None of the radiopharmaceuticals used in the evaluation of kidney function and disorders impose the hypertonic and chemical stress associated with the use of intravenous contrast media. The content of iodide in the iodinated renal radiopharmaceuticals is so low that there is not even an iodide hypersensitivity hazard. The presence of radiopharmaceuticals in the kidney is detected by an external instrument after peripheral intravenous injection, thus avoiding the instrumentation common to other methods of urologic evaluation. These studies can be performed with acceptable radiation exposure in all age groups, although some methods are modified for children.

The specific advantage of radioisotopes over x-rays is the ease with which radioisotope concentration can be estimated by counting radioactive disintegrations while a simultaneous image of radioisotope distribution is produced. X-ray images are not readily susceptible to numerical quantification, but they do show higher spatial resolution and in this respect are greatly superior to radioisotopic images produced by current equipment. Although roentgenographic methods provide very high resolution of renovascular structures and of calyceal and pelvic anatomy, special procedures such as nephrotomography during infusion urography may be required to provide information about renal cortical structure. Images of the kidney with radionuclides, on the other hand, provide a simpler means of evaluating the renal cortex. Many of the factors that handicap roentgenographic methods for kidney evaluation—eg, excessive bowel gas, marked obesity, and uremia—have little effect on the diagnostic usefulness of radioisotopic imaging studies.

Study of an internal organ by means of a radioactive tracer requires that the radioisotope be concentrated by the organ. The process of concentration is referred to as "labeling." The kidney concentrates a number of radioactive labels by several mechanisms

Malcolm R. Powell is Assistant Clinical Professor of Radiology and Medicine, University of California School of Medicine (San Francisco). Jerome M. Weiss is Assistant Clinical Professor of Urology, University of California School of Medicine (San Francisco).

and is therefore readily susceptible to these methods of study.

Although the exact place of radioisotopic procedures in the diagnosis of genitourinary disorders is not yet well defined, they are versatile and provide information that cannot be obtained in other ways. The information is generally of a screening nature. The relative simplicity, the low cost, and the large amount of information provided by the radioisotopic methods has led to their increasing acceptance.

Current clinical evaluation of the kidney in the nuclear medicine laboratory includes static imaging studies of radiopharmaceutical distributions within the kidney and urinary tract, function studies to image radiopharmaceutical accumulation and excretion, and blood clearance measurements.

MEANS OF RENAL EVALUATION WITH RADIOPHARMACEUTICALS

Radiopharmaceuticals

Four general types of renal radioisotopic labels are in current use. Classified according to the mechanisms of labeling, they are as follows: (1) renal cortex labels, which are retained in the renal tubular cells; (2) renal tubular function labels, which briefly label the renal cortex as they are accumulated by renal tubular cells and then are passed into the urine and cleared from the kidney; (3) intravascular compartment labels; and (4) substances cleared solely by glomerular filtration, allowing radioactive tracer determination of glomerular filtration rate. Tables 8–1A and B list the characteristics of the more useful radiopharmaceuticals in these categories, and Fig 8–1 illustrates their use.

Until about 1973, the most commonly used renal cortical labels were the radioactive mercury-labeled chlormerodrins. More recently, a number of new renal cortical labels employing ^{99m}Tc in various compounds have been introduced. These ^{99m}Tc compounds deliver a smaller radiation absorbed dose to the kidneys than do the radioactive mercury agents and improve the static kidney images by providing more radioactive events for recording the image. After peripheral intravenous injection, these tracers are accumulated in renal

Table 8—1A. Radiopharmaceuticals for urologic diagnosis: Characteristics of the commonly used radionuclide labels.

Radionuclide	Physical Half-Life	Gamma Ray Energies (keV) and Abundance	Gamma Camera Sensitivity (Dots/Min/μCi for Various Collimators)	Advantages and Disadvantages
Technetium-99m (^{99m}Tc)	6.0 hours	140 (90%)	336—1080*	Very large numbers of gamma rays (photons) for radiation absorbed dose (no beta particles). Photon energy ideal. Readily available.
Iodine-131 (^{131}I)	8.1 days	364 (82%) 637 (6.8%) 284 (5.4%) etc	101*	Easy to bind to complex molecules without significant denaturation. Radiation absorbed dose per available photon high.
Iodine-125 (^{125}I)	60.2 days	27 (K x-ray) 35 (7%)	Not useful (energy too low for resolution)	Long shelf life when used to tag complex molecules. Low energy most suitable for in vitro measurements.
Mercury-197 (^{197}Hg)	2.71 days	67 (K x-ray) 77 (18%) 191 (2%)	Marginal usefulness: low spatial resolution	Reduces kidney radiation dose by factor of 10 compared to ^{203}Hg. Low photon energy reduces resolution by gamma camera.
Mercury-203 (^{203}Hg)	46.9 days	279 (77%)	150—500*	Ideal photon energy for excellent spatial resolution by gamma camera but a low number of photons for large radiation dose.
Gallium-67 (^{67}Ga)	3.24 days	93 (68%) 184 (23%) 296 (21%) 388 (8%)	Low sensitivity (improved by dual spectrometer)	Specially ordered for each test. Cost relatively high. Best currently available tracer to detect neoplasms and abscesses.

*Data from Anger HO: Radioisotope cameras. Chapter 10 in: *Instrumentation in Nuclear Medicine.* Hine GJ (editor). Academic Press, 1967.

Table 8—1B. Radiopharmaceuticals for urologic diagnosis.

Radiopharmaceutical	Usual Dose (μCi)	Radiation Absorbed Dose (Rads) From Usual Doses — Renal	Whole Body	Usual Scintiphoto Exposure Time and Imaging Time Postdose	Use
Urologic Radiopharmaceuticals					
^{99m}Tc-Fe-ascorbate DTPA ^{99m}Tc-glucoheptonate ^{99m}Tc-methylsuccinate	2000	1.0	0.008	4 second serial photos, 0—30 second, and 2—4 minute static photos at 30 minutes.	Localized in renal cortex by deposition and retention in renal tubular cells. Uptake is proportionate to regional renal blood flow. Rapid serial photos show renal blood flow distribution.
^{197}Hg-chlormerodrin ^{203}Hg-chlormerodrin	150 100	1.8 15.0	0.02	10—15 minute photos 30 minutes after dose.	Localizes in renal cortex; allows only static imaging and with less resolution than ^{99m}Tc agents.
^{99m}Tc-Sn-DTPA	2000	0.10	0.030	1 or 2 minute serial photos 0—20 minutes or longer. Also useful to image blood flow.	Excreted solely by glomerular filtration. Useful for function imaging, but cortical definition vs background less than with other ^{99m}Tc agents.
^{125}I-iothalamate	50	Negligible	0.00015	Not useful for imaging.	Glomerular filtration rate measurement.
^{131}I-hippurate	200	0.080	0.0042 (assumes normal clearance)	2—10 minute photos (depending on renal function): 0—30 minutes for normal function to 1—2 hours for poor function.	Excreted by tubular function (like para-aminohippurate). 70—80% extraction causes rapid clearance in normal. Prolonged cortical transit time occurs in ischemic or other forms of tubular damage with increased water reabsorption. Unique in labeling damaged renal cortex.
Other Nonrenal Radiopharmaceuticals Useful in Urology					
^{99m}Tc-polyphosphate ^{99m}Tc-pyrophosphate ^{99m}Tc-diphosphonate	15,000	1.05	0.15	2—4 minutes per view at 2—4 hours (30 minutes for whole body scan).	Bone imaging to detect reactive bone formation at sites of metastases before x-rays become abnormal (prostatic, renal cell, and testicular cancer). Excreted by kidney and affords genitourinary tract information.
^{67}Ga-citrate	4000	6.0	1.0	5 minutes per view; at 4—6 hours for abscesses and 48 hours for tumors (1 hour for whole body scan).	Detects occult neoplasms and abscesses. Used to stage testicular neoplasms by detecting lymph node involvement. Requires bowel preparation before scanning.

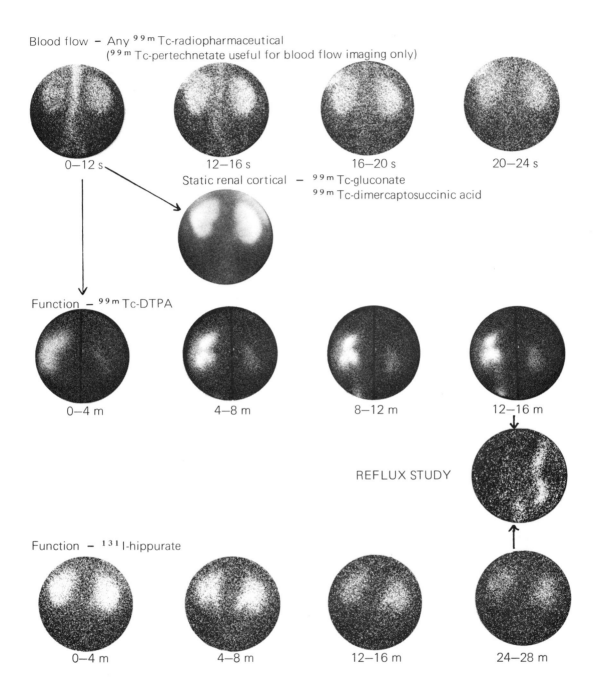

Blood flow — Any ^{99m}Tc-radiopharmaceutical
(^{99m}Tc-pertechnetate useful for blood flow imaging only)

0–12 s   12–16 s   16–20 s   20–24 s

Static renal cortical — ^{99m}Tc-gluconate
^{99m}Tc-dimercaptosuccinic acid

Function — ^{99m}Tc-DTPA

0–4 m   4–8 m   8–12 m   12–16 m

REFLUX STUDY

Function — ^{131}I-hippurate

0–4 m   4–8 m   12–16 m   24–28 m

Figure 8–1. Sequence required for nuclear medicine imaging procedures to evaluate the kidneys and urinary tract. As diagrammed by this illustration, a single radiopharmaceutical can be used for more than one purpose. Any technetium-99m-labeled agent may be used to obtain a blood flow study since all that is needed is to provide a large number of radioactive disintegrations per brief time interval used for each photograph. Some of these agents localize in the renal cortex and afford excellent static images of the kidney 20 minutes to an hour or more after injection. Typical of these agents are technetium-99m-gluconate and technetium-99m-dimercaptosuccinic acid. A function evaluation can be performed either with technetium-99m-DTPA, as it is excreted by glomerular filtration, or by I-131-hippurate, which is excreted by tubular function. Once bladder filling occurs, these agents can be used for a reflux study, either during micturition or with compression of a filled bladder. Thus, the current utilization of a "triple isotope study" is to obtain a scintiphotographic evaluation of kidney structure, blood flow, and function using usually 2 agents or sometimes only one agent. s = seconds; m = minutes.

tubular epithelium, labeling the renal cortex, while a portion of the injected dose passes into the urine. These substances are dependent upon renal blood flow for cortical labeling and, once fixed in the renal tubular cells, make it possible to record images of the renal cortex. The renal uptake of mercury has been used to estimate renal blood flow.

The intravascular compartment of the kidney may be imaged immediately after peripheral intravenous injection of 5 or preferably 10 mCi of any ^{99m}Tc-labeled radiopharmaceutical. A series of 3- to 5-second posterior view photographs of the kidneys is obtained during the first pass filling of the kidneys before the tracer is lost by active uptake or by dilution in the blood and exchange with other spaces. Since amounts of ^{99m}Tc agents can be used which provide large numbers of disintegrations per minute at quite acceptable patient radiation exposures, good definition of renal blood flow is recorded. These photographs are different from arteriograms in that they depict transit times of the tracer through various portions of the kidney rather than instantaneous intravascular distributions. In a normal renal vascular flow study, film exposure in renal cortical areas should be similar to that seen during maximal aortic filling in the same series of pictures. A renal vascular flow study can also be performed with nonrenal agents such as ^{99m}Tc pertechnetate or ^{99m}Tc-labeled human serum albumin, since this procedure is not dependent upon renal uptake of the tracer but only upon renal blood flow, which constitutes over 20% of the cardiac output. Subsequent to the blood flow study, renal static imaging may be accomplished with the same radiopharmaceutical if one of the renal cortical labeling agents such as ^{99m}Tc-glucoheptonate was used.

The long half-lives of the radiomercury-labeled chlormerodrins are sometimes useful when serial static images must be made over longer periods of time, eg, for multiple determinations of kidney position or serial reevaluation of kidney structures after trauma. None of the renal cortical agents are particularly useful in static renal imaging during uremia or for detection of poorly functioning renal tissue with normal kidney function—eg, congenital renal duplication with a poorly functioning supernumerary kidney.

Iodide-131 orthoiodohippurate is used for renal tubular function studies. It is excreted into the urine by the renal tubular epithelium and is used in radioisotope renography. A radioisotope renogram is simply a recording of the amount of radioactivity detected over each kidney from the time of injection of the labeled hippurate. After peripheral intravenous injection of hippurate, the count rate increases in a few seconds with delivery of 20% of the injected tracer to the kidneys by renal blood flow. The normal kidney rapidly accumulates hippurate as a function of effective renal plasma flow, and the amount of radioactivity detected over the kidney continues to rise until loss of radioactivity by urine drainage exceeds the rate of accumulation by the renal cortex. Beyond that point, if renal drainage is normal, the amount of radioactivity

in the kidney continues to decrease because the radiopharmaceutical was given as a single injection and the amount available in the blood for clearance has decreased throughout the period of observation. In uremia there is slower accumulation and prolonged cortical retention of hippurate, so that late scintiphotographs usually show a useful image of the kidney analogous to the image produced by renal cortical agents. The kidney may be evaluated with radiohippurate in patients with severe uremia when neither intravenous urograms nor radiochlormerodrin images can be obtained. Hippurate is also useful for detection of poorly functioning renal tissue in the absence of uremia.

Several other radiopharmaceuticals are useful to the urologist in special circumstances. Agents which are excreted solely by glomerular function may be used to determine the glomerular filtration rate. The 2 which are most commonly available are ^{99m}Tc(Sn)-DTPA, a pure chelate of technetium, and radioiodinated iothalamate. It should be noted that ^{99m}Tc-DTPA must be prepared with tin reduction of the technetium as indicated by the designation ^{99m}Tc(Sn)-DTPA or it will not be a true glomerular agent owing to lack of complete reduction. Several commercial agents have been available which were referred to as ^{99m}Tc-DTPA but which actually are complex mixtures of technetium pertechnetate, technetium DTPA, and other complexing agents such as iron ascorbate. The ^{99m}Tc(Sn)-DTPA can also be used for renal imaging, although the definition of the renal cortex is not as clear as with agents which localize within the cortex and remain there. The ^{99m}Tc(Sn)-DTPA excretion study is useful for constructing a radioisotope urogram and can be used for studies of ureteral reflux, as can be accomplished with ^{131}I hippurate. Both of these agents can be imaged during reflux from the bladder after peripheral intravenous administration of the tracer.

Other radiopharmaceuticals of urologic interest are those used for detection of primary malignancies and their metastases and for the detection of abscesses. Since most genitourinary tumors have a tendency to metastasize to bone, radionuclide bone imaging is an important part of the evaluation of patients who are suspected of having these malignancies. Bone metastases may be detected much earlier by a radionuclide bone imaging study than by conventional radiographic screening methods. Several bone imaging agents are listed in Table 8–1B.

Occult malignant tumors and abscesses can be detected by the so-called "tumor scan." For this purpose, gallium-67 citrate seems to be as useful an agent as any presently available. It is injected intravenously, and the scans are performed after a variable delay as described in Table 8–1B. Bowel preparation is necessary prior to scanning. Since uptake in purulent abscesses is usually much greater than in neoplasms, detection of an abscess is subject to less interference by normal uptake of the tracer in surrounding structures.

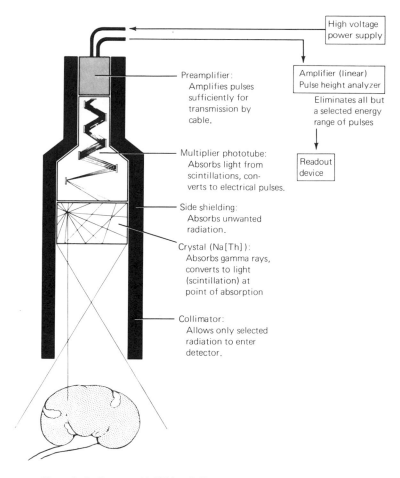

Figure 8—2. Detector. NaI(Th) = thallium-activated sodium iodide crystal.

Instrumentation

All of the radiopharmaceuticals discussed above are labeled with gamma radiation-emitting isotopes. Gamma radiation is necessary for external detection of radiation during in vivo studies. Gamma rays penetrate tissue as do x-rays; beta particles have charge and mass which cause rapid absorption with passage through tissue.

Table 8—2 illustrates in diagrammatic form the general types of gamma radiation detectors used in kidney tests. Several functions are common to all (Fig 8—2). A gamma radiation detector containing a sodium iodide crystal converts each gamma ray to a minute flash of light. When the gamma ray is absorbed in the sodium iodide crystal, an instantaneous flash of light (scintillation) is emitted at the point of absorption. The scintillations are detected and converted to electrical pulses by photomultiplier tubes with photosensitive surfaces applied to one surface of the crystal. The magnitude of each electrical pulse is proportionate to the original gamma ray energy and can be analyzed by a spectrometer set to detect only the radiation energy characteristic of the radioisotope being studied. Since each gamma-emitting radioisotope emits one or more

gamma rays with characteristic radiation energies, spectrometry allows detection of one type of radioisotope in the presence of others. This is analogous to spectrophotometry, in which transmission of a range of light of rather limited wavelength is measured to the exclusion of all other wavelengths. Once recognized as a preselected gamma ray energy, each of these gamma absorption events is recorded in one of several different ways that is appropriate to the instrument being used.

In addition to detectors and spectrometers, gamma radiation detecting instrumentation requires a means of limiting the radiation detected to that emitted from an area of interest. An area that is of interest to a clinical investigator may be the contents of a test tube, a kidney in vivo, or an even smaller region of interest in vivo. Restriction of the gamma rays absorbed by the detector crystal to gamma rays coming from a selected region of interest requires that the detector crystal be protected from all other gamma rays coming from other regions. This is accomplished by lead shielding. The shielding that protects the crystal from extraneous gamma rays is referred to as "side shielding" or "back shielding." The shielding that

Table 8–2. Differences in radiation detecting instruments.

Instrument	Well Counter	Probe Counter	Rectilinear Scanner	Gamma Camera
Function	Measures radioactivity in a test tube.	Detects radioactivity in a limited region in vivo and records quantitative changes of a radiopharmaceutical versus time.	Forms a life-sized image (planar projection) of the distribution of a radiopharmaceutical in vivo. Moving detector scans area by to and fro motion.	Forms a miniature image of radiopharmaceutical distribution in vivo; records changing distributions (stop-motion images) and numerical data.
Basic detector differences	Test tube; Well in crystal. *Note:* Detector orientation is inverted for well counting compared to Fig. 8–2.	Crystal; Cylindric collimator	Crystal; Focused collimator	37 multiplier phototubes determine where each scintillation occurred in crystal. Parallel hole collimator. Crystal one-half inch thick, 12 inches in diameter
Readout	Scaler: Reads either total counts in a preset time or total time to reach preset count.	Ratemeter and strip chart recorder record count rate as a function of time. (Radioisotope renogram) COUNTS PER MINUTE — TIME	Mechanical positioning of image formation; detector and image move as unit. (a) Tap scan produced by scaler and printer; one print for preset number of counts. (b) Photoscan produced by ratemeter linked x-ray film exposure.	Electronic positioning of imaged event by oscilloscope display of light flash ("dot") at position corresponding to the original gamma ray absorption in the crystal. Oscilloscope display is continuously photographed.

limits the field of view of the detector crystal is referred to as "collimation."

In other respects, the various gamma radiation detecting instruments used in medical diagnosis have differences which make them suitable for their specific uses.

Well counters are simple systems designed to count test tube content of radioactivity. The crystal of the detector contains a hole referred to as a well into which a test tube containing the sample is inserted for in vitro counting. In addition to the basic system, consisting of a detector with a well in the crystal and a spectrometer, the system has a "scaler" that registers either the number of counts detected in a preset time or the time required to reach a preset number of counts. These instruments are used for in vitro counting of the type required in glomerular filtration rate determination.

The probe counter is a somewhat more complicated instrument used in radioisotope renography. It has 2 or more detectors which are used to count radioactivity in each kidney, and often a third or fourth field of view such as the bladder or the cardiac blood pool. Each detector has a scintillation crystal with a cylindric collimator limiting the field of view to a cone-shaped area, as shown in Table 8–2. After gamma spectrometry, the radioactive disintegrations detected in each field of view are continuously converted to average count rates by rate meters and then are plotted as functions of time by a recorder. When these instruments are designed principally for radioisotope renography, the collimator is designed so that the field of view will encompass an entire kidney at the usual kidney depth. The probe counter, therefore, will provide a graphic and numerical recording of radiopharmaceutical content versus time in each kidney and perhaps the cardiac blood pool or bladder. The detectors provide information averaging the events in a whole kidney. This may prove misleading in some patients since the precise location of radioactivity within the kidney is not recorded.

Probe counters are used less frequently now in renal studies since scintillation cameras are generally available and will obtain radioactive counts versus time in addition to kidney images. However, the probe counter does have one virtue which assures that it will continue to be used in large centers, its sensitivity in detecting radiation. A cylindric collimator is many times as sensitive as a scintillation camera detector and allows use of very small doses of tracer with more frequently repeated tests.

Radionuclide imaging instrumentation is designed to provide an image of the distribution of gamma rays emitted from an organ or a tissue rather than to detect only the count rate of radioactivity in a region or an organ. Two general types of radionuclide imaging equipment are now in general clinical use: radionuclide scanners and stationary detector radionuclide imaging devices. Of the latter instruments, only the Anger type of scintillation camera is in general use and will be described here.

The radionuclide scanner is a moving detector instrument which makes an image of radiation distribution as it systematically scans the whole region of interest. It detects radiation from a specific focal volume at a distance from the surface of the detector. This is done by means of a lead collimator which has holes converging to a focal point several inches beyond the collimator. Only gamma rays originating from within the focus pass through the holes and into the detector, others being absorbed in the lead septa between the holes and in the side shielding of the detector. As a scanning detector is moved over a subject in a rectilinear raster pattern, a systematic point-to-point recording of radioactivity count rate is obtained. The results are printed out by a mechanical linkage, either by a "tapper" on paper or by exposure of x-ray film proportionate to the count rate detected. The resulting "scan" then shows areas of intense radioactivity as black exposure of the film, and lesser degrees of exposure are roughly proportionate to lesser amounts of radioactivity. The necessity for detector motion in a scanner limits these instruments to the imaging of fairly static distributions of radioactivity.

The Anger scintillation camera or gamma camera is the most generally used of the newer stationary detector gamma-imaging instruments. The detector of this instrument uses a half-inch-thick disk of sodium iodide 12 inches or more in diameter. The field of view is limited to a diameter approximately 2 inches less than the crystal diameter by a lead collimator which has parallel holes perpendicular to the crystal surface. These holes allow only those gamma rays that are vertically oriented to enter the detector. The scintillations produced in the crystal are detected by an array of photomultiplier tubes that allow a computer in the instrument to "take a fix" on where the event occurred in the crystal plane. This is electronically relayed to an oscilloscope that flashes a point of light in a position approximating the originally detected event. The oscilloscope display is photographed continuously to produce photographs composed of large numbers of dots. Each dot recorded came from a gamma ray traveling vertically from its point of origin in the subject; therefore, the dots accumulate to make a pattern representative of the in vivo distribution of radioactivity. The result is referred to as a "scintiphoto." Because the scintillation camera detector is stationary, continuous photographs can be made showing all the scintillations detected from both kidneys over an interval of time. The scintiphotograph produced may represent an interval as brief as a few seconds or as long as many minutes. Thus, the scintillation camera allows photography either of static or of rapidly changing distributions of radionuclide labels. Radioactivity concentration changes are imaged in rapid dynamic studies such as those showing blood flow or in slower dynamic studies such as those following concentration and excretion of a label in the urine. In addition, the information collected with a scintillation camera can be electronically processed to provide numerical information from small defined areas in the field of view. This numerical information can be subjected to computer analysis to provide quantification of regional renal function.

SCINTIPHOTOGRAPHY

Since evaluation of kidney structure and function by means of the scintillation camera combines aspects of most of the other nuclear medicine methods—and since the image sequences are an effective device for explaining the clinical uses of nuclear medicine tests—scintiphotography will be discussed first.

The scintillation camera is used to perform kidney evaluation with as many as 3 differing distributions of radiopharmaceuticals. It is possible either to image different distributions of a single radiopharmaceutical or to use 2 or 3 different radiopharmaceuticals to image the structure, function, and blood flow distributions. By comparison of images without change of patient position, studies of sequential distributions of radiopharmaceuticals provide greater information than in a single evaluation. The studies are performed rapidly and without patient discomfort. Gamma spectroscopy allows imaging of each radioactive label used without interference by previously injected labels.

The original multiple radiopharmaceutical study described was the "triple isotope study" utilizing ^{203}Hg-chlormerodrin for positioning and static imaging of renal structure, ^{131}I-hippurate for evaluation of renal function and to image poorly functioning renal tissue, and ^{99m}Tc-pertechnetate for imaging renal blood flow distribution. ^{203}Hg-chlormerodrin was used with the scintillation camera rather than ^{197}Hg-chlormerodrin because its higher energy afforded better resolution in the images with less internal absorption of photons emitted from deep structures. Because of the sensitivity of the scintillation camera, a lower dose of radioactivity could be used than for conventional scanning procedures. Although it was not necessary in every patient to use all 3 radiopharmaceuticals, triple studies were generally performed for evaluation of mass lesions, renal ischemia, and trauma. If the patient was uremic, it was customary to limit the evaluation to ^{131}I-hippurate scintiphotography plus a blood flow study if indicated. For sequential evaluation of renal function after acute tubular necrosis, transplantation, or other forms of renal damage, only the ^{131}I-hippurate study was performed.

With the availability of the newer ^{99m}Tc-labeled radiopharmaceuticals, renal evaluation can be obtained using the new cortical labeling agents both for renal structure evaluation and for blood flow imaging. ^{131}I-hippurate remains an important agent for evaluation of renal function.

Kidney scintiphotography is best obtained with the patient prone and the abdomen compressed in order to prevent renal rotation and to position the kidneys closer to the detector and to the midline of the patient with their long axes parallel to the plane of the detector. A parallel hole multichannel collimator is used. Scintiphotographs can be obtained in other positions to evaluate the dynamic effects of patient position on renal function or blood flow, and, when necessary, adequate images can be obtained with the patient supine and the detector viewing the kidneys through the table.

It is now customary to give a small fractional dose of a ^{99m}Tc cortical agent for renal localization and positioning followed by intravenous injection of the major portion of the patient dose of this agent for blood flow studies. The rapid sequence scintiphotographs of blood flow show first the appearance of the agent in the abdominal aorta, followed by the kidneys and the spleen at about the same time, and, much later, the liver. Renal blood flow is sufficient that the kidneys are seen as well-defined images with much less tracer in surrounding structures. Normal renal blood flow distribution will cause the kidney image to appear about as bright as the aorta at the level of the kidney. This type of study can be used to determine vascularity in any renal mass lesion. A corresponding cold area on the ^{99m}Tc blood flow study suggests a lack of vascularity, and, if spherical, a cyst. A mass lesion that is well labeled by ^{99m}Tc in the blood flow study would suggest a vascular tumor, usually a renal cell carcinoma. Vascular tumors often fill at a time differing from the time of renal cortical filling. A renal cell carcinoma is often better visualized during the blood flow study than is the remainder of the renal cortex, particularly in the frequent instance where the tumor mass causes relative ischemia surrounding the region of the tumor. This may be due to a direct pressure effect from the neoplasm or to the invasion of vascular structures, particularly the renal vein. On the other hand, simple cysts tend to cause discrete spherical defects without other disturbance of renal cortical blood flow. Therefore, in static studies, the cortex around a cyst is generally better labeled than the cortex around a neoplasm. An apparent cyst with poorly labeled cortex surrounding it suggests necrosis of a renal cell carcinoma and formation of a cyst—a frequent occurrence.

After the blood flow information is obtained, the renal cortical agent may be used immediately to obtain a urogram since some of the tracer will be filtered and not reabsorbed, appearing in the urine. Early scintiphotographs immediately after injection of the technetium-labeled agents also offer an opportunity to define avascular spaces adjacent to or within the kidney versus vascularity in the background and in the kidney before tracer diffuses into extravascular spaces. This may be particularly important in identifying exophytic renal cysts that protrude from the kidney cortex without sufficient disruption of the cortex to cause a defect in the kidney image. After an hour or more, the ^{99m}Tc cortical agents are cleared from the calyces and renal pelvis, leaving only tracer in the cortex. This affords an excellent opportunity to obtain high resolution images of the kidney cortex, showing small details such as scars, masses, or other lesions which displace normal cortical tissue. The amount of the agent in the cortex relative to other areas of the kidney cortex or the other kidney is related to renal blood flow. When there are focal lesions in the kidney, it often becomes important to obtain special views using oblique orientation or even a different collimator such as a single pinhole collimator which increases spatial resolution of the scintillation camera and may be used to enlarge somewhat the renal size in the field of view.

Iodide-131 hippurate imaging studies are extremely useful even though the images contain fewer data points than is the case with the newer renal cortical labeling agents. With the patient remaining in exactly the same position as that used for the static scintiphotographs, a series of photographs is obtained using a constant exposure time, beginning immediately after peripheral intravenous injection of the hippurate dose. By keeping photographic parameters—including exposure time—constant throughout the series of hippurate scintiphotographs, all the photographs will be comparable. A simultaneous recording of count rate over each kidney provides radioisotope renograms. If renal function is normal, serial hippurate scintiphotographs are usually obtained with a 2- to 4-minute exposure time, but with decreased function it may be best to obtain exposures of as long as 10 minutes each to record significant numbers of counts in each photograph. After extreme reduction of renal function, there is usually insufficient uptake of renal cortical agents to allow renal visualization, whereas slow accumulation of hippurate often does progress without loss of counts from the kidney. In hippurate studies of uremic patients, renal cortical labeling eventually becomes sufficient so that considerable information can be obtained about kidney structure and function from these images alone. Delayed views may even show enough detail of the renal pelvis and ureters to rule out obstructive problems in the severely uremic patient.

Hippurate appearance in the kidneys is dependent initially upon renal blood flow. When blood levels fall as a result of renal accumulation and other extravascular loss, renal accumulation of hippurate slows. As the rate of accumulation is exceeded by hippurate loss through urine drainage from the kidney, the radioactivity count rate over the kidney peaks and then falls. Hippurate scintiphotographs show the location of radioactivity in the kidney during these phases of hippurate excretion. The simultaneously recorded renogram tracing is somewhat different from the conventional renogram obtained with a probe detector. The gamma camera counts are usually obtained from a proportionately greater area surrounding each kidney (each half of the 10 inch diameter field of view) than is detected by a conventional probe counter. Consequently, the content of radioisotope detected from vascular spaces is somewhat greater in the scintillation camera renogram than in a probe-counted renogram. Interpretation of hippurate scintiphotographs is performed both by observing whether the rate of hippurate accumulation and excretion is within normal limits and by comparing the function of the 2 kidneys or part of one kidney with other tissue in the same kidney. Generally speaking, if there is no dilatation of intrarenal drainage structures nor obstruction of urine drainage, the most frequent cause of regional or unilateral decrease of renal function is renal ischemia. Most other causes of decreased renal function will result in generalized changes affecting both kidneys equally—as is usually seen in glomerular nephritis, pyelonephritis, acute tubular necrosis, vasculitis, and other causes of generalized reduction of renal function. When ischemia is present, not only is the accumulation of hippurate in the kidneys slowed but there is increased reabsorption of water by the ischemic tubules, causing decreased urine volume from the area of ischemic renal cortex and a prolongation of the transit time of hippurate through the cortex. The result is that the scintiphotographs will show late labeling of the ischemic kidney when normal renal cortex in the same patient has completely cleared the hippurate it accumulated. During the drainage phase of a hippurate study, various obstructive problems are easily demonstrated. Even with abdominal compression in the prone position, the normal kidney is rapidly emptied of labeled urine by ureteral peristalsis. Fifteen minutes after injection, the kidney usually contains less than the number of counts detected at the maximum count rate. Postvoiding residual urine volume in the bladder can be readily estimated by scintiphotographs, and cine studies can be used to detect and evaluate vesicoureteral reflux. Urine reflux from the bladder can be easily differentiated from the trace amounts of radiopharmaceutical remaining in the ureter.

This extensive renal evaluation can be performed in about 40 minutes if there are no significant abnormalities but may take an hour or more if there are major abnormalities. Depending upon patient tolerance for a complicated procedure, this evaluation can be considerably shortened and tailored to the clinical situation.

EXAMPLES OF CLINICAL UTILIZATION OF RADIONUCLIDE IMAGING STUDIES

The value of nuclear medicine methods in the investigation of renal structure and function can be best appreciated by a review of common clinical findings. Examples both of older studies dating back to as early as 1964 and of more recent studies using newer radiopharmaceuticals and the latest equipment have been selected to demonstrate the wide variety of clinical problems that may be efficiently detected and diagnosed by radionuclide-imaging methods.

Fig 8–3 illustrates 2 uses of mercurial diuretic labeling of the kidney to demonstrate a gross abnormality of kidney structure or position. Fig 8–3A

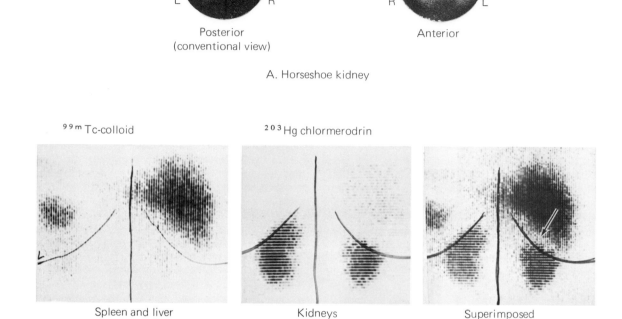

²⁰³Hg chlormerodrin

L   R   R   L

Posterior   Anterior
(conventional view)

A. Horseshoe kidney

⁹⁹ᵐTc-colloid   ²⁰³Hg chlormerodrin

Spleen and liver   Kidneys   Superimposed

B. Suprarenal mass (adrenal carcinoma)

Figure 8–3. Technics of kidney structure imaging. Until approximately 1972, mercurial diuretic agents were most commonly used for renal structure imaging by the scintillation camera *(A)* or by rectilinear scanning *(B).* These images illustrate several principles of radionuclide imaging. In the horseshoe kidney study, the band connecting the lower poles of the kidneys is better seen in the anterior view since there is no interposition of the vertebral masses which would absorb gamma rays and prevent detection of the band of tissue connecting the 2 kidneys when viewed from the posterior view. The rectilinear scans demonstrate that one organ can be imaged using one agent and another organ can be studied at the same time using a second radiopharmaceutical which has a different gamma radiation energy from the first.

shows that a horseshoe kidney is more easily identified in an anterior view because the isthmus is better visualized when the gamma radiation passes through the low-density tissues anteriorly rather than the spinal column posteriorly. The spine absorbs sufficient gamma radiation so that the narrow band of renal cortex connecting the kidneys is difficult to appreciate on the posterior view, although the condition may be suggested by the external contours of the images which appear separate in the posterior view and by the renal axes which lack the normal inclination.

Generally speaking, most renal imaging studies with radionuclides are obtained with the patient prone and the kidneys viewed posteriorly. In this position, with the application of mid and lower abdominal compression, the kidneys assume a somewhat different position than that seen on the accustomed supine intravenous urograms. In the prone position, the liver shape changes, with formation of a space above the right kidney, permitting this kidney to move cephalad.

Fig 8–3B demonstrates kidney position evaluation with a rectilinear scan for demonstration of a suprarenal tumor in the space between the upper pole of the right kidney and the liver. In such combination scans, one radiopharmaceutical is used to label one organ and another to label the second organ, so that a space between the 2 organs is outlined by the labeled organs.

Figs 8–4 and 8–5 demonstrate scintiphoto studies in which vascular tumors are differentiated from nonvascular tumors involving the kidney. When the renal cortex is the site of a tumor, there are 2 ways in which a defect in a static renal cortical image may be produced. Normal cortex may be displaced from a tumor site, or there may be interference with the mechanism of tissue labeling, or both (Fig 8–4). For normal tissue labeling to occur after intravenous introduction of a radiopharmaceutical, blood flow to the area must be normal and the tissue that accumulates the label must have the appropriate metabolic activity. Renal masses will then appear in a scan or scintiphoto

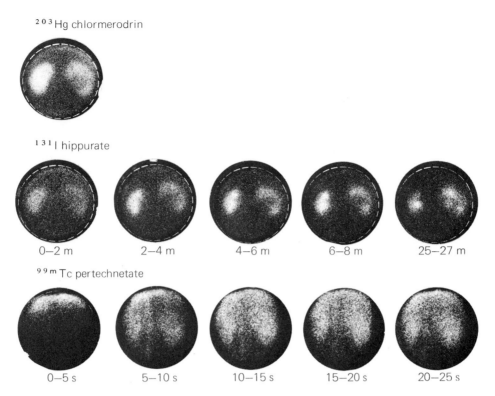

Figure 8—4. Renal cell carcinoma. A typical triple renal examination shows alterations in kidney structure, function, and blood flow typical of renal cell carcinoma. This tumor has invaded the renal vein, causing abnormal renal hemodynamics. The tumor has caused a distinct defect in the cortex of the right kidney (chlormerodrin photograph) that is subsequently shown to be the site of normal or increased blood flow (pertechnetate photograph). There is decrease of chlormerodrin localization in the kidney cortex affected by the tumor, reduction in the rate of hippurate accumulation and prolongation of hippurate transit time due to increased free water reabsorption. s = seconds; m = minutes.

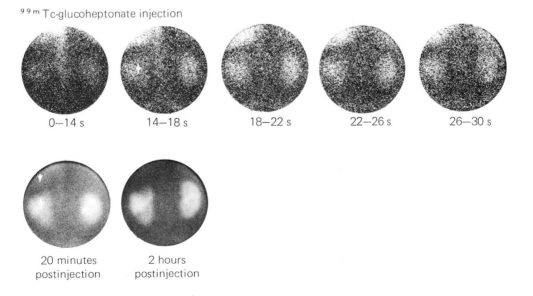

Figure 8—5. Renal cyst. Evaluation of this renal cyst was performed using a single radiopharmaceutical to obtain both blood flow and structure studies. The area above the left kidney and below the spleen image is seen to remain relatively free of blood content of radioactivity during a blood flow study, and a defect of the upper pole of the kidney is clearly defined after localization of the gluconate in the cortex of the kidney. Typically, a renal cyst does not interfere with blood flow to the remainder of the cortex of the affected kidney. s = seconds.

as "cold areas," with absent or reduced labeling surrounded by labeled cortex. Typically, a cyst (Fig 8–5) will be seen as a discrete spherical defect which is not associated with decreased localization of tracer in the cortex adjacent to the cyst. Carcinomas tend to cause much more extensive changes in the kidney, with large, irregular areas of decreased perfusion in the region of the neoplasm. An irregularly shaped renal cortex due to fetal lobulations would be labeled in its entirety since it is composed of normal parenchyma.

To evaluate vascularity of a focal defect, the patient is given a rapid peripheral intravenous injection of a ^{99m}Tc-labeled radiopharmaceutical and a series of 4-second scintiphotographs is obtained. If the lesion is seen to be vascularized, it is presumed to be a neoplasm. After the rapid sequence of blood flow pictures is obtained, an immediate 1-minute exposure using greatly diminished dot intensity on the scintillation camera oscilloscope will produce an image of high quality (high data density) showing the renal vascular pool prior to localization of the label in extravascular spaces. This method can be particularly valuable in differentiating those renal neoplasms that are less well vascularized, particularly the transitional cell carcinomas.

It is essential that the relative positions of the patient and the camera detector be kept constant for each radiopharmaceutical used, so that regional findings with one radiopharmaceutical can be precisely compared with findings by others. For this reason, it is best to avoid changing collimators by using a medium energy collimator for the entire study when ^{131}I hippurate is used.

The camera study is limited by the spatial resolution of the instrument for the number of counts detected. This is a function of of the density radioactivity in the area studied, intrinsic resolution of the detector system, and lack of renal motion during the study. In practice, it may not be possible to visualize renal lesions much less than 1 inch in diameter, although much smaller lesions can theoretically be identified. Comparable spatial resolution can be achieved if a scanning instrument is used rather than a camera, but the study is limited to static imaging. Hippurate excretion evaluation and blood flow imaging require a stationary detector to record dynamic events, ie, a scintillation camera.

The scintiphoto renogram provides an opportunity to determine the presence of regional renal ischemia causing renal vascular hypertension. Fig 8–6 shows the sequential use of 3 radiopharmaceuticals for

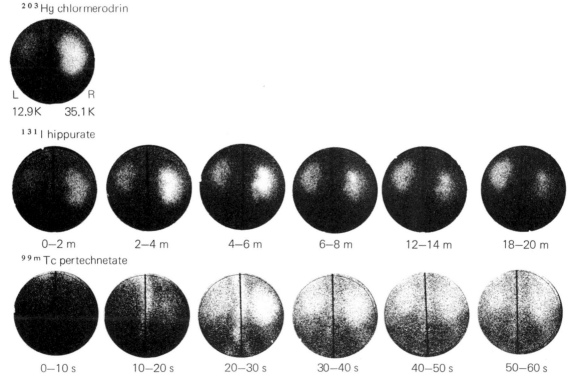

Figure 8–6. Renovascular hypertension secondary to arteriosclerotic disease. Typical of renovascular hypertension, the left kidney has diminished uptake of chlormerodrin as a result of reduced renal blood flow which is confirmed in the blood flow study. There is slowed rate of accumulation of hippurate in this small kidney and a prolongation of transit time of hippurate through the cortex secondary to increased water reabsorption, so that the latter part of the hippurate study shows cortical retention of hippurate at a time when the normal kidney shows only a slight degree of retention in a superior calyceal system and normal clearance of hippurate from other areas. s = seconds; m = minutes.

this purpose. Precise patient positioning was accomplished using chlormerodrin labeling of the renal cortex. Any areas of decreased perfusion tend to have diminished chlormerodrin labeling. Next, the patient is studied with iodide-131 hippurate and a series of scintiphotos with identical photographic exposures is obtained to show accumulation and then drainage of labeled urine from the kidneys. Hippurate is seen to accumulate less rapidly in an ischemic kidney or in an area of regional renal ischemia. The hallmark of renal vascular ischemia is not the slow accumulation of radioactivity, since that occurs also in other disorders that affect renal function adversely; it is the presence of a prolonged hippurate transit time through the ischemic cortical area when other parts of the same kidney—or the other kidney—show normal transit times. The prolonged transit time results from increased water reabsorption by the ischemic area and consequent delayed washout of label from the kidney. When this occurs in the presence of normal function in other areas, it strongly suggests renovascular ischemia. Such late labeling must be differentiated from obstruction. Direct definition of ischemia may be obtained from a blood flow study performed with any of the ^{99m}Tc-labeled agents. A triple renal evaluation can therefore confirm ischemia by 3 different types of radionuclide localization, but the etiologic significance of ischemia in causing hypertension is confirmed only by the hippurate study. The hippurate study therefore defines a characteristic physiologic abnormality similar to findings of the Howard, Stamey, or Rappaport tests. These other tests all require ureteral catheterization and detection of changes in solute concentration or urine volume after admixture of urine from the whole kidney, and this method of collection may mask changes present in regional renal ischemia that can be defined by scintiphotography.

The transplanted kidney study illustrated in Fig 8–7 is an example of several uses of hippurate renography by the scintillation camera. First, this study evaluates the success of the vascular and ureteral anastomoses in the period immediately following transplantation. Good early labeling of the entire renal cortex attests to normal perfusion. If urine is seen to drain normally, patency of the ureteral anastomosis is confirmed. Second, the transplant renogram often demonstrates reduction of function which may be generalized in a rejection reaction, acute tubular necrosis, or other similar processes. Focal decrease of hippurate labeling may be observed if there is regional ischemia, partial infarction, or other local change. The rate at which hippurate is accumulated and subsequently drained characterizes progressive changes in renal function with change in rejection activity or other processes. Last, the hippurate scintiphoto study of a transplanted kidney may show slow hippurate transit through a kidney, allowing high data density scintiphotos or even scans of the renal cortex. In uremia this often allows better renal visualization than the static images obtained with other agents.

In evaluation of renal trauma, radioisotopic studies are useful in the diagnosis of extrarenal hematoma, renal lacerations, reduction of renal function secondary to contusion, or urine extravasation. Fig 8–8 demonstrates the abnormalities seen in a case of simple renal contusion and the clearing of this abnormality 2 weeks later. The hippurate study is particularly useful in demonstrating extravasation of urine either due to trauma or after surgery, as illustrated in Fig 8–7. Small concentrations of extravasated dye which are completely inapparent on simultaneous intravenous urograms are readily visualized using the tracer technics.

The hippurate gamma-imaged urogram is also useful in studying the renal pelvis, ureters, and bladder. In renal obstructive disease, the renogram often defines structures well enough to provide a general idea of the severity of the obstruction without having to perform retrograde urography or other involved procedures. Gamma-imaged urograms may obviate the need for retrograde studies in patients hypersensitive to contrast media since the iodide content of radioiodinated hippurate is insufficient to cause iodide sensitivity. Other uses would include screening uremic patients for obstructive uropathy, evaluation of male infants, follow-up of surgically corrected obstruction for patency and functional status, and evaluations for ureteral

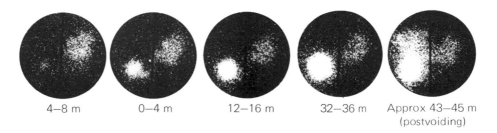

4–8 m   0–4 m   12–16 m   32–36 m   Approx 43–45 m
(postvoiding)

Figure 8–7. Cadaver transplant urine extravasation with voiding. After intravenous administration of I-131-hippurate, accumulation occurs in a transplanted kidney with generalized and localized reductions of accumulation related to rejection reaction or acute tubular necrosis. In this example the kidney is functioning, with considerable excretion of urine into the bladder, but obvious extravasation of urine occurs when the patient attempts to void. The hippurate study is particularly sensitive in detection of minor amounts of urine extravasation that would ordinarily require retrograde studies for detection and even then would be quite difficult to detect. m = minutes.

¹³¹I hippurate

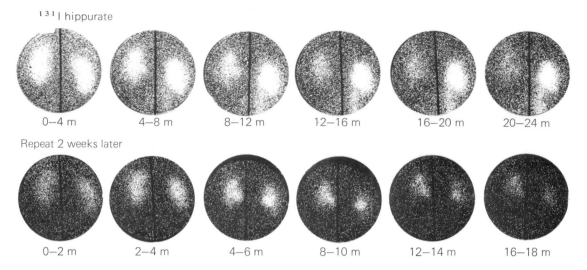

0–4 m   4–8 m   8–12 m   1·2–16 m   16–20 m   20–24 m

Repeat 2 weeks later

0–2 m   2–4 m   4–6 m   8–10 m   12–14 m   16–18 m

Figure 8–8. Renal trauma. This patient was evaluated with serial I-131-hippurate studies since the patient was allergic to contrast media. Actually, the hippurate study is a most sensitive way to serially evaluate kidney function and can be used efficiently for this purpose after trauma. Here the right kidney and ureter show delay of hippurate drainage and retention within the ureter immediately after flank injury but complete clearing of abnormality 2 weeks after the initial study. There was never any evidence of extravasation of urine. m = minutes.

reflux. Fig 8–9 demonstrates a study for ureteral reflux where the reflux occurred only during micturition. This study was done without catheterization of the patient since the tracer utilized was that excreted after peripheral intravenous injection. The study was performed approximately one-half hour after injection of ^{131}I-hippurate, when most of the hippurate had been excreted and the ureters were relatively free of radioactivity.

While definition of individual calyceal structure and other fine detail is not even within an order of magnitude of the resolution available on a conventional radiographic study, a gamma photo study is sufficient for many clinical purposes. It presents enough detail so that more complicated studies may not be required. An important advantage of these radiopharmaceuticals is the generally low radiation absorbed doses to which the patient may be exposed by serial studies. In particular, the ^{131}I-hippurate

studies cause exceedingly low renal and whole body radiation exposure after use of the conventional dose of this agent in the presence of normal renal function.

OTHER RADIONUCLIDE IMAGING PROCEDURES USEFUL IN UROLOGY

Bone scanning and tumor scanning are 2 other radionuclide imaging procedures which have relatively frequent applications in urology. Both tests are best performed by a combination of whole body imaging technics and spot views of suspicious areas. These procedures are performed after intravenous administration of the tracer and then a delay to allow for tracer localization. In bone scanning with the technetium-labeled agents described in Table 8–1, the interval

Left Ureteral Reflux with Voiding
(Anterior View of Bladder after ^{99m}Tc-DTPA Excretion)

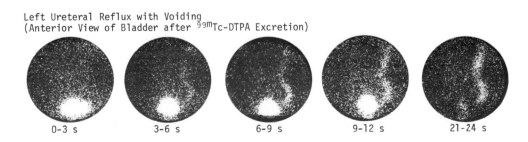

0-3 s   3-6 s   6-9 s   9-12 s   21-24 s

Figure 8–9. Left ureteral reflux with voiding. After the bladder is filled from renal excretion of an intravenously administered radionuclide, ureteral reflux studies may be obtained without catheterization. The patient was simply asked to void with the camera viewing the anterior aspect of the bladder and ureteral area in a sitting position. Ureteral reflux can be seen to occur beginning at 3–6 seconds as the bladder contracts and becomes maximum after voiding is completed. s = seconds.

postinjection before scanning is performed is generally 2 hours. The patient is asked to empty his bladder prior to scanning since a significant portion of the tracer is excreted in the urine. The bone-seeking tracer localizes in areas of bone mineral turnover in normal bone, but in particular will localize in areas of reactive bone formation stimulated by the presence of neoplasm, inflammation, or bone repair. The bone scan is typically much more efficient in detecting early metastatic neoplastic involvement of bone than are conventional x-ray studies. Since both prostatic and renal cell carcinoma have a marked tendency toward early bone metastasis, bone scans are frequently advis-

able in the work-up of these patients prior to planning definitive treatment. Fig 8–10 illustrates an evaluation for metastatic renal cell carcinoma using a conventional dual probe whole body scanner and, for comparison, the same illustration shows metastatic prostatic carcinoma imaged with a newer radiopharmaceutical, ^{99m}Tc-pyrophosphate, and a new whole body imaging modification of the scintillation camera. There is obvious improvement of the spatial resolution of small lesions in the ^{99m}Tc-pyrophosphate study with the scanning adaptation of the scintillation camera. These bone scans can be used both for detection of lesions prior to their appearance in x-ray

Metastatic renal cell carcinoma

Metastatic prostatic carcinoma

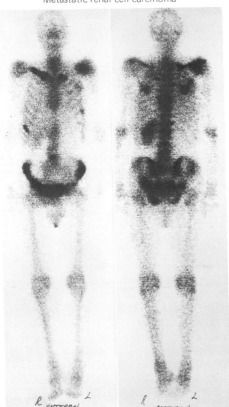

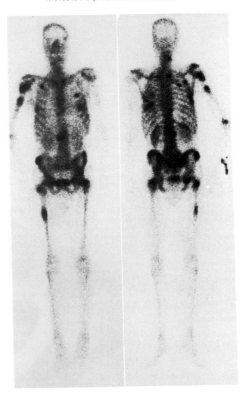

(Obtained with dual-probe rectilinear scanner)

(Obtained with whole body imaging modification of scintillation camera)

Figure 8–10. Whole body bone scanning. Whole body bone scanning can be accomplished using either conventional rectilinear scanners, usually with dual probes and image minification to fit the entire body on a single x-ray film, or with a whole body imaging adaptation of the scintillation camera, which also employs image minification. Illustrated here are bone scans using both methods and technetium-99m-pyrophosphate bone scanning agent. The metastatic renal cell carcinoma scan shows extensive pelvic metastases as well as right clavicular, left shoulder, and several rib metastases. It should be noted that the scans obtained with a dual probe whole body scanner are usually shown with the right side to the viewer's left in both the anterior and posterior view. This is done so that they can be readily superimposed. With whole body imaging adaptations of the scintillation camera, it is conventional to show a "fluoroscopic view" placing the patient's left on the viewer's left in a posterior view. In the illustration of metastatic prostatic carcinoma, there are numerous pelvic, spine, rib, and long bone metastases. It should be noted that the kidneys and bladder show in bone scans, except for the surgical absence of the left kidney in the renal cell carcinoma patient, and that urologic diagnoses are frequently obtained from bone scans.

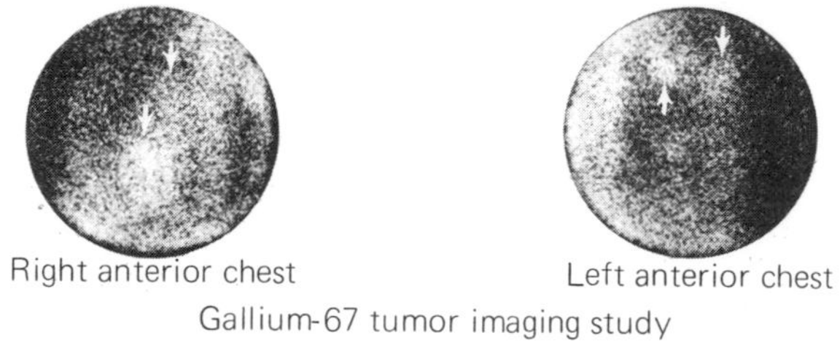

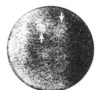

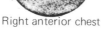

Right anterior chest   Left anterior chest
Gallium-67 tumor imaging study

Figure 8—11. Testicular carcinoma metastatic to the lungs, evaluated with gallium-67 tumor imaging. Several agents have a propensity to accumulate in tumors and abscesses. After intravenous administration, whole body scans at 48—72 hours postinjection will show gallium-67 localization in the liver, to a lesser extent in bone, and to a slight extent in soft tissues, as well as in any site of neoplasm or abscess that has the characteristic of accumulating this tracer. The method is useful for detection of metastases of testicular and other urologic neoplasms for preoperative staging. Illustrated here are several areas of gallium uptake in the lungs and mediastinum consistent with metastasis.

surveys and for evaluation of response of lesions to therapy. If therapy succeeds in causing a bony lesion to heal, there will be lessened accumulation of tracer in a scan compared to control scans.

Fig 8—11 demonstrates tumor scanning with ^{67}Ga-citrate. This is administered intravenously and the scan is done 48—72 hours later when blood levels have decreased to very low concentrations of tracer. A bowel preparation is required prior to scanning because some bowel secretion of the tracer will interfere with evaluation of the abdominal and pelvic areas. Radiogallium localizes in a wide variety of neoplastic lesions and also in abscesses, and even in kidneys involved with active pyelonephritis. The technic may therefore be used to detect both occult neoplasms and occult abscesses or infection. Concentrations of the tracer tend to be greater in abscesses than in neoplastic lesions, and with abscesses there is less opportunity for interference with detection of the lesions by normal uptake of gallium in structures such as the liver, spleen, bones, and gut which always show some gallium localization. Tumor localization may be somewhat more difficult to identify in the abdomen, but the procedure has been considered useful in staging testicular tumors, where it has been reported to be more efficient than lymphography. Because of the greater uptake in abscesses, these scans can be performed only 4 hours after intravenous administration of the radiogallium, compared to the 48—72 hours required for differentiation of neoplastic lesions.

THE RADIOISOTOPE RENOGRAM

The radioisotope renogram is an older method for radioisotopic evaluation of the kidney. It is still useful as a screening test or for serial function evaluations. The renogram consists of recording radioactive count rate over each kidney as a function of time to produce tracings representing function in each kidney. The familiar renogram should be more readily understood after the foregoing discussion of renal scintiphotography.

In essence, the renogram consists of 3 parts which may be described as the vascular phase, the function phase, and the drainage phase. The vascular phase is simply the period during which the count rate rapidly rises in each kidney with the initial appearance of the radioiodinated hippurate in the intravascular spaces of the kidney and prior to similar labeling of other surrounding organs. The vascular phase is best understood by referring to scintiphotos of pertechnetate appearance in the kidneys. During the function phase of the renogram, the increase of count rate over the kidneys is nearly linear. The hippurate blood level is almost constant for the first few minutes after postinjection mixing, and the cortex extracts hippurate from the blood at a constant rate for 3—8 minutes after injection of the hippurate until drainage of urine from the kidney begins to occur. As this drainage continues, it exceeds the rate of accumulation of hippurate, and the count rate tracing begins to decrease. A normally hydrated prone patient with normal urine drainage will show peaking of count rate at 3—8 minutes and then a fall of count rate to less than half of the maximum within 15 minutes. In the sitting position, the peak occurs somewhat earlier and the fall is more rapid. Because a conventional renogram detector has a limited field of view, extrarenal blood levels make a smaller contribution to the renogram count rate tracing than is the case when the scintillation camera is used to produce a renogram in conjunction with scintiphotography. Fig 8—12 summarizes the several abnormalities which may be detected by conventional radioisotope renography using iodide-131 hippurate. The renogram is a valuable study in laboratories where it is used frequently and norms are well established. An entirely normal renogram is an excellent assurance that no major problem exists in the kidney.

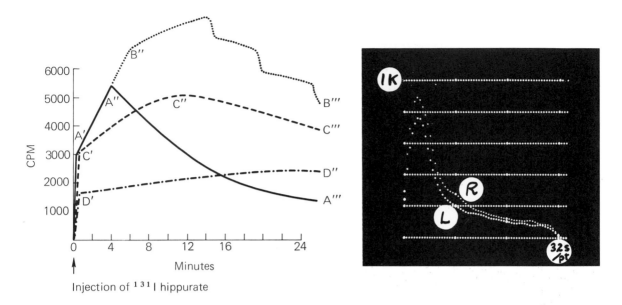

Figure 8—12. Summary of several abnormalities detected by radioisotope renography using iodide-131 hippurate. CPM = counts per minute. ***Solid line:*** Normal renogram idealized as O—A′—A″—A‴. O—A′ = vascular phase. Initial vascular labeling detected. A′—A″ = function phase. Hippurate accumulation by renal cortical cells recorded. A″—A‴ = drainage phase. Drainage exceeds accumulation; count rate decreases. ***Dotted line:*** Renogram of mild obstruction. O—A′ = no change from normal. A′—B″ = accumulation of counts prolonged in function phase. B″—B‴ = poorly defined broad peak and slowed drainage phase. Steps down in count rate suggest intermittent flow. ***Dashed line:*** Renogram of renovascular ischemia, normal renovascular volume. O—C′ = vascular labeling delayed but similar in amount to normal. C′—C″ = decreased function; decreased rate of accumulation. C″—C‴ = increased water reabsorption; decreased urine volume; slowing of hippurate drainage. ***Dash-dotted line:*** Renogram typical of severe ischemia or nephritis and reduced function. O—D′ = delayed and reduced vascular labeling. D′—D″ = extreme slowing of hippurate accumulation; little drainage. The finding of normal function in one kidney and of abnormal function in the other kidney would indicate that renograms O—C‴ or O—D″ are related to unilateral disease typical of renovascular ischemia which may be functionally significant in causing hypertension. Finding of bilateral and symmetric renogram abnormality would indicate a generalized renal disease which, in terms of the renogram, could be glomerulonephritis, pyelonephritis, acute tubular necrosis, or the result of renal vascular disease. A normal renogram has been illustrated for comparison with the diagram of possible abnormalities.

CLEARANCE METHODS

Although radiopharmaceuticals and gamma detection procedures are currently used more as a research tool than as a general diagnostic procedure in the study of renal clearance, these methods offer considerable promise in clinical practice. In particular, the radioiodinated iothalamate test of glomerular filtration is reproducible and easy to perform, requiring only a single blood sample and a determination of count rate decrease in an intravascular space defined by a probe collimator. Hippurate clearance determinations provide information about renal blood flow, but they are less reproducible except in the presence of reduced renal function. Radioisotopic determinations are much simpler than the chemical determinations of the standard clearance evaluation materials, inulin and para-aminohippurate. Evaluation of renal hemodynamics by these methods will no doubt become a much more frequently used clinical tool.

•   •   •

General References

Hine GJ (editor): *Instrumentation in Nuclear Medicine.* Academic Press, 1967.

Maxwell MH & others: Radioisotope renogram in renal arterial hypertension. J Urol 100:376, 1968.

Morris JG & others: The diagnosis of renal tumors by radioisotope scanning. J Urol 97:40, 1967.

Pistema DD, McDougall R, Kriss JP: Screening for bone metastases. JAMA 231:46, 1975.

Powell MR: Evaluation of kidney structure and function by radioisotope imaging. Page 447 in: *Clinical Uses of Radionuclides: Critical Comparison with Other Techniques.* AEC Symposium Series No. 27. US Atomic Energy Commission, 1972.

Rosenthal J: Ortho-iodohippurate-I-131 kidney scanning in renal failure. Radiology 78:298, 1966.

Seminars in Nuclear Medicine. Vol 4, Nos. 1 and 2, Jan and April, 1974.

Shuler SE: The scintillation camera in pediatric renal disease. Am J Dis Child 120:115, 1970.

9...
Instrumental Examination of the Urinary Tract

PRELIMINARY PROCEDURES

Aseptic Technic

Instruments must be prepared and used in an aseptic manner. Metal sounds and rubber or plastic catheters can be autoclaved. Optical instruments are gas sterilized. Soaking instruments in antiseptic solutions is inadequate.

The glans penis should be washed thoroughly with soap and water or an antiseptic solution. The vulva must be cleansed and the labia held apart as the instrument is introduced.

It should be pointed out that because of the presence of bacteria in the distal urethra it is impossible to pass an instrument in a completely sterile manner. Secondary cystitis rarely occurs, however, unless there is residual urine in the bladder.

Lubrication of Urethra

Catheters and other instruments must not be passed into the urinary tract without proper lubrication. In women, it is sufficient to dip the instrument in the lubricant. In men, however, such a procedure is inadequate because the meatus removes the lubricant and the instrument then passes over a relatively dry mucous membrane. The male urethra can be lubricated only by instilling at least 15 ml of a sterile water-soluble lubricant. This is best accomplished with a syringe which has a rubber bulb on one end. It should have a blunt tip so that it does not have to be passed down the urethra. Oils (eg, mineral oil or olive oil) must not be used, since fatal oil emboli have resulted from their use (Fig 16–12). The syringe serves not only to introduce the column of lubricant into the canal but also, by virtue of the constant, steady pressure required, to overcome the normal tone of the external sphincter muscle. This resistance may be increased if the patient is apprehensive. Inexperienced instrumentalists frequently have difficulty introducing catheters against the force of this spasm, and this has resulted in many false diagnoses of "urethral stricture."

Anesthesia

A barbiturate administered 30–45 minutes before instrumentation allays apprehension. As an alternative

measure, morphine, 8 mg, or a similar narcotic can be given intravenously 5–10 minutes before the instrument is inserted. Titration of the patient by intravenous injection of a tranquilizing drug such as diazepam (Valium Injectable) is also effective. Inject it slowly, and stop when the patient exhibits drowsiness.

Local anesthesia is indicated before instrumentation, although this is less effective in men than in women. The female urethra is best anesthetized by introducing a solution of 10% cocaine on a cotton applicator and leaving it in the canal for 5 minutes. With this technic, instrumentation is almost without discomfort. In men, really effective anesthetic agents (ie, cocaine) cannot be instilled for they are easily absorbed through the posterior urethra and prostate into the circulatory system and may cause sudden collapse and even death. Less toxic drugs must therefore be used, and these are usually less efficient. They may be incorporated into the lubricating jelly. These solutions or jellies are retained in the urethra by placing a clamp on the glans for 5 minutes. Useful anesthetic agents include 2% lidocaine (Xylocaine) and 0.5% dyclonine (Dyclone).

General anesthesia should be used if the patient is apprehensive or if biopsy or other painful manipulations are necessary. Thiopental is ideal for short cystoscopic procedures, but spinal anesthesia may prove more useful if x-rays are to be taken, since the patient can be asked to cooperate by holding his breath at the proper time. Explosive agents (eg, ether) are contraindicated if electrocoagulation is to be employed.

Warning to Patient

Instrumentation is always uncomfortable and may be painful. It is essential to warn all patients that this discomfort will occur and to warn men that the discomfort will be greater as the instrument passes through the prostatic urethra. No movement should be rough or abrupt; pick up the instrument slowly, introduce it gently, and advance it gradually. Failure to do these things will cause distrust and apprehension on the part of the patient. Spasm of the external sphincter may develop, in which case instrumentation is made more difficult or even impossible.

Calibration & Size of Instruments

Instruments are most commonly calibrated in the USA according to the French (F) scale. Each number

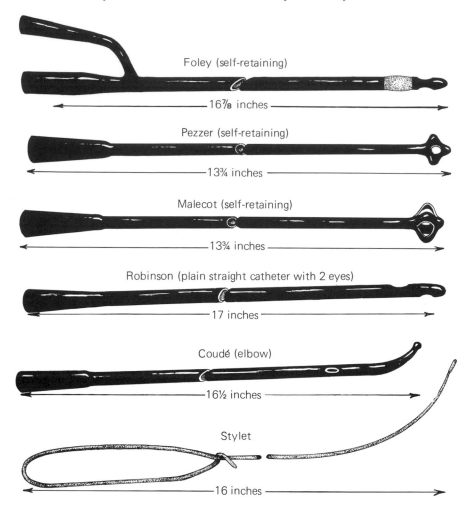

Figure 9—1. Types of catheters; catheter stylet.

on the scale equals 0.33 mm. Therefore, a 30F sound has a diameter of 10 mm.

Each number on the American (A) and English (E) scales equals 0.5 mm; the English scale is 2 numbers less than the American. Hence, 10 mm = 30F = 20A = 18E; and 6 mm = 18F = 12A = 10E.

THE CATHETER

Catheters are used for diagnostic purposes to explore the urethra for stenoses or injury, to discover residual urine in the bladder after voiding, and to introduce contrast medium into the bladder. They are used therapeutically to relieve urinary retention.

Types & Sizes of Catheters (Fig 9—1)

Soft rubber catheters should be used in most instances since they cause less trauma and are easier to manipulate past enlarged prostatic lobes than less flexible instruments. If for any reason a soft rubber catheter fails to pass (eg, it may impinge on the base of a lobe which occupies most of the posterior part of the bladder neck), a stiffer silk-woven coudé (elbow) catheter (which has a bent tip) should be tried. If the catheter is to be left in place (indwelling), a self-retaining (balloon) catheter should be utilized. It may be necessary or advantageous to leave a plain catheter (Robinson) in the bladder; it must then be taped in place (Fig 9—3).

In general, it is a mistake to try to pass small catheters in men (12—14F); they lack body and are apt to coil up at the external sphincter. Catheterization is really less traumatic and more successful if instruments of adequate size (20—22F) are used. The larger catheters are also better suited for exploring the urethra for stricture. The urethra of a girl age 6 will easily accept a 14F catheter. The urethra of a boy of the same age will take a 12F catheter.

Technic of Catheterization

A. In Men: After proper cleansing and anesthesia,

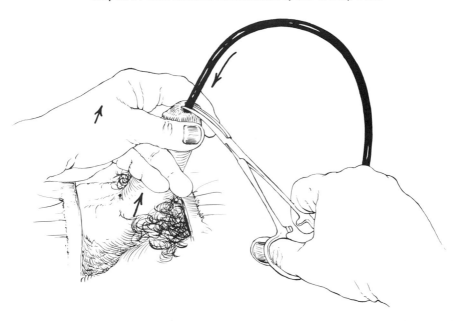

Figure 9–2. Technic of catheterization. A sterile water-soluble lubricant is first instilled into the urethra by means of a bulb syringe. The penis is drawn taut with one hand. The catheter, held near its tip with a sterile clamp, is introduced into the urethra; the other end of the catheter is held between the fourth and fifth fingers of the hand holding the clamp. The clamp is then moved up on the catheter and the catheter introduced farther into the urethra.

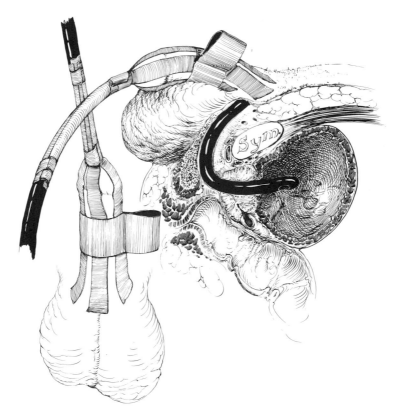

Figure 9–3. Taping the plain catheter in place in the male. Four strips of half-inch adhesive tape are placed on the penis and catheter. They are bound to the catheter by 2 pieces of half-inch tape just distal to the glans and at the point where they terminate on the catheter. A piece of 1-inch tape is placed about the midpenis in such a manner that a loop is formed which will separate if erection occurs.

the catheter can be manipulated with a sterile-gloved hand. It is simpler, however, to grasp the catheter near its tip with a sterile clamp and to hold the other end of the catheter between the fourth and fifth fingers of the same hand. The catheter can then be advanced with the clamp without being touched by the unsterile hand (Fig 9–2). The penis must be stretched taut with the other hand to eliminate urethral redundancy.

If an impassable stricture is encountered, it will be necessary to dilate the urethra with sounds (Fig 9–4) or with filiforms and followers (Figs 9–5 and 9–6).

If a stylet is used (Fig 9–1), the lumen of the catheter should be lubricated before the stylet is inserted; otherwise the stylet will be difficult to remove after passage of the instrument. The technic of passing a catheter with a stylet is similar to that for passing sounds. The catheter should be drawn taut over the stylet so that its tip cannot become dislodged, pass out through the "eye" of the catheter, and traumatize the urethra.

Do not partially withdraw the styleted catheter and then readvance it. The resulting drag on the catheter may allow the tip of the stylet to protrude through the distal opening of the catheter and cause urethral injury. At times it is helpful to guide stiff instruments with a finger in the rectum. When the catheter has been successfully passed, the stylet is removed.

B. In Women: A short metal catheter is more satisfactory than other types since it can be manipulated with one hand while the other holds the labia apart. Rubber catheters can also be used. Those made of glass are contraindicated; small cracks or chips may abrade the mucosa. A self-retaining (Foley) catheter can be used if constant drainage is indicated. A Pezzer or Malecot catheter introduced on a catheter stylet is also satisfactory. A plain catheter can be used for this purpose by taping it to the labial area (after shaving).

METAL SOUNDS

Metal (stainless steel or nickel-plated steel) sounds may be used instead of catheters to explore the urethra for stenoses. Their major use, however, is in the treatment of stricture.

Technic of Passing a Sound
A. In Men: With the penis stretched taut and the instrument held almost horizontally (over the groin), the tip of the sound is introduced into the urethra. When the tip reaches the bulb (at the external sphincter), the handle is brought to the vertical position, which usually enables the tip to pass through the sphincter. Moving the handle to the horizontal position (parallel to the thighs) causes the sound to advance into the bladder (Fig 9–4).

The first sound passed should be a 24F, even though the patient says he has a narrow stricture. This size has a broad tip which will not perforate a friable urethral wall and is therefore ideal for urethral exploration. If a 24F sound cannot be passed, smaller sounds can be tried. If a 20F will not pass, do not use the smaller sizes, for their tips are relatively sharp and may pierce the urethral wall. In this instance, use filiforms and followers, which are much safer (Figs 9–5 and 9–6).

B. In Women: Because of the short and relatively straight canal of the female urethra, the passage of sounds is quite simple in women. Significant stricture is rare, although moderate stenoses are commonly found and are often the cause of chronic or recurrent cystitis, particularly in little girls.

FILIFORMS & FOLLOWERS

Filiforms and followers are the instruments of choice for dilating narrow strictures. Catheterizing followers may be used to catheterize men with narrow strictures.

Types & Sizes
Filiforms are made of woven silk or plastic material and must be quite pliable. Useful sizes are 3–6F. Numerous filiform tips are available, but the coudé and corkscrew types are most useful. The free end of the filiform is equipped with a female thread.

The follower may be made of metal or of woven pliable silk. Useful sizes are 8–30F. It may be solid or it may be hollow to allow simultaneous catheterization. Its end has a male thread which may be easily screwed into the filiform.

Technic of Passing Filiforms
After lubricant jelly has been instilled into the urethra, the filiform is introduced. If it is arrested, it must be partially withdrawn, rotated, and readvanced. If this fails, one or more filiforms should be added and all manipulated in turn. When one finally passes down to its hilt without resistance, its tip has entered the bladder. The appropriate follower is then screwed into the filiform in a clockwise direction and advanced down the urethra (Figs 9–5 and 9–6).

BOUGIES À BOULE

These olive-tipped bougies (Fig 9–7) are useful in calibrating the urethra, particularly in little girls (see Chapter 28). Bougies of increasing size should be used until one passes with some resistance. On withdrawal, there will be a snap as the bougie's broad shoulders pass through the stenotic area.

Example of a sound

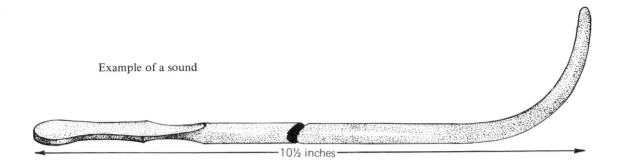

10½ inches

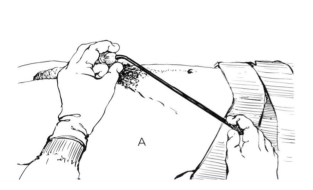

A

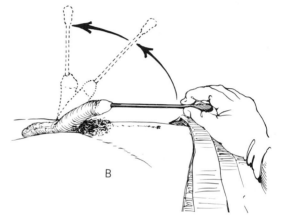

B

After proper urethral lubrication, the tip of the sound enters the urethra. The sound is in the horizontal position over the groin.

The penis is pulled taut on the sound, which is advanced down the urethra and moved simultaneously to the midline; its handle is gradually moved to the vertical position.

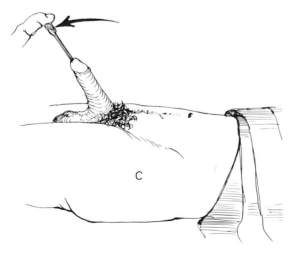

C

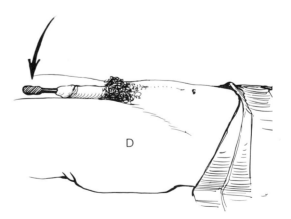

D

The sound will usually pass through the external urinary sphincter if pressure is exerted on the handle at right angles to its shaft with one finger.

When the sound has passed all the way into the bladder it should be possible to rotate it freely. (The curved part of the sound is lying free in the vesical cavity.)

Figure 9–4. Passing a sound through the male urethra.

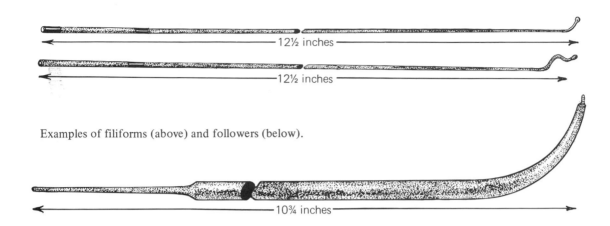

Examples of filiforms (above) and followers (below).

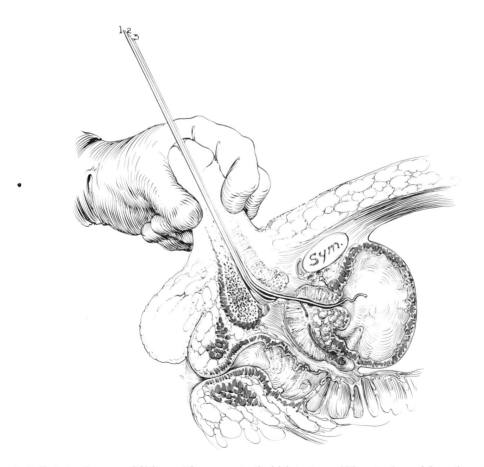

Figure 9—5. Technic of passage of filiforms. After proper urethral lubrication, a filiform is advanced down the urethra; the penis is held taut. If the filiform is arrested at any point, it is partially withdrawn, rotated, and advanced again. If it still fails to pass, 2 or more filiforms are inserted into the urethra. Each filiform in turn is advanced, withdrawn, rotated, and readvanced. One of them will usually pass to the bladder. (Passing of follower is shown in Fig 9—6.)

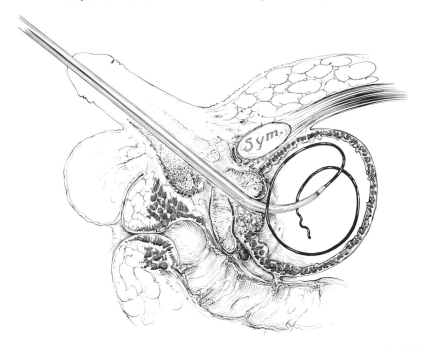

Figure 9–6. Passing the follower. When a filiform passes into the bladder, a small follower is screwed into the filiform and advanced to the bladder, using the same technic as for passage of a sound (Fig 9–5).

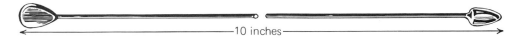

Figure 9–7. Bougie à boule.

CYSTOMETER

The cystometer is a diagnostic instrument which measures the tone of the detrusor in relation to the volume of fluid in the bladder. It evaluates both normal and pathologic physiology of bladder function and contributes much to the management of the patient suffering from vesical dysfunction secondary to disease or trauma of the nervous system. A simple cystometer is illustrated in Fig 9–8.

Technic

The apparatus is so arranged that the zero mark on the manometer is level with the symphysis pubis. Care should be taken that all air is removed from the tubing. As sterile water or normal saline solution is slowly introduced (60–120 drops/minute) into the indwelling catheter, the intravesical pressure is measured on the manometer. As each 50 ml are added, the pressure on the manometer is recorded in relation to the total volume of fluid introduced. The patient is asked to describe all sensations experienced, including the desire to void. These remarks are recorded at the appropriate points on the cystometrogram. When a strong involuntary urge to void occurs, this pressure should be noted.

CYSTOSCOPY & PANENDOSCOPY

Useful Instruments

Many instruments have been devised for the visual inspection of the bladder and urethra, but the 2 most useful are the cystoscope and the panendoscope. They come in sizes varying between 12–26F; therefore, even very young patients may be examined.

A. Cystoscope: The cystoscopic view is largely at right angles to the shaft of the instrument. It has a wide-angle lens and is therefore best for inspection of the bladder. It visualizes the prostatic urethra only fairly well and the distal (and female) urethra not at all.

B. Panendoscope: The panendoscope has a smaller field of vision; its view is almost in line with the shaft of the instrument. Therefore, the portion of the bladder near the bladder neck cannot be seen unless a "retrograde" lens is used with it. This instrument, however, is excellent for visualization of the urethra distal to the neck of the bladder. These instruments, then, complement each other.

Uses

A. Diagnostic Uses: Complete endoscopic studies are among the most precise diagnostic tests in all medicine.

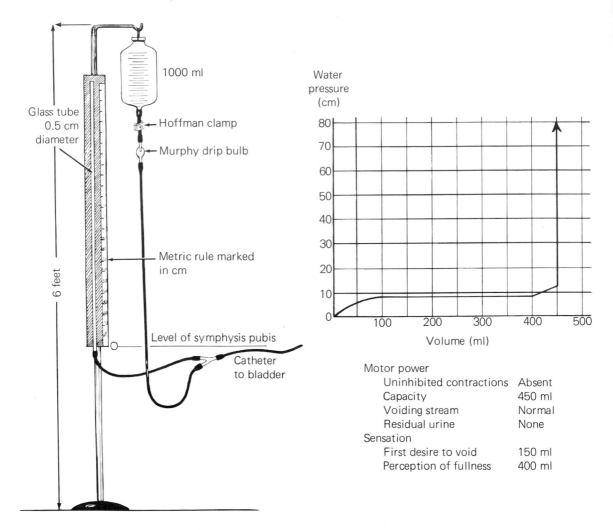

Figure 9—8. Cystometer and normal cystogram. The pressure in the normal bladder remains at about 8—15 cm of water until capacity (350—500 ml) is reached, at which time the intravesical pressure rises sharply to or above 100 cm of water. Involuntary voiding then occurs around the catheter. No uninhibited contractions occur, and there is no residual urine. A spastic neurogenic bladder (Fig 19—6) exhibits uninhibited contractions as demonstrated by transient increases in intravesical pressure as fluid is introduced into the bladder. In either case, involuntary voiding around the catheter occurs at relatively low volumes (50—300 ml). The tone of the flaccid neurogenic bladder (Fig 19—8) is impaired. Thus, intravesical pressure remains low (6—10 ml), there are no uninhibited contractions, and no final involuntary voiding pressure develops even when the bladder is filled with 500 or even 1000 ml of water; vesical capacity is increased.

1. Direct inspection—The cystoscope and pandendoscope make possible visualization of the bladder wall for such diseases as tumor, stone, and ulcer. The configuration and position of the ureteral orifices are of paramount importance when vesicoureteral reflux is suspected. The degree of obstruction from an enlarged prostate and urethral stricture, polyp, or tumor may be seen. Biopsy of neoplasms can be made.

2. "Sterile" urine specimen, relative renal function—Through these instruments clean specimens of urine can be taken from the bladder for bacteriologic study. Catheters can be passed to the renal pelves for the collection of urine specimens and the separate measurement of renal function (ie, PSP test).

3. Radiography—Through these ureteral catheters, radiopaque material can be introduced so that perfect "casts" of the calyces, pelves, and ureters can be observed on x-ray films.

4. Reflux—The presence of vesicoureteral reflux can be ascertained by filling the bladder with sterile water to which indigo carmine or methylene blue dye has been added. After the patient voids, cystoscopy is performed. If blue fluid is seen emanating from a ureteral orifice, reflux has been demonstrated.

B. Therapeutic Uses: Many diseases of the bladder and urethra lend themselves to transurethral treatment. Tumors can be biopsied and resected. Ureteral stones can be manipulated.

Major Indications for Cystoscopy or Panendoscopy & Ureteral Catheterization

These technics are indicated for the evaluation of hematuria, chronic or recurrent urinary infection, unexplained urologic symptoms (eg, enuresis, frequency), and evaluation of congenital anomalies, which are very commonly found in the genitourinary tract. They are useful also in any clinical situation in which excretory urograms have suggested pathologic change but have not furnished all the information necessary for definitive diagnosis and treatment.

Contraindications to Cystoscopy or Panendoscopy

Cystoscopy and panendoscopy are contraindicated in acute urinary tract infection (trauma may exacerbate the infection) and in the presence of severe symptoms of prostatic obstruction, since trauma may produce just enough edema of the bladder neck to cause complete urinary retention. Of course, if cystoscopy must be done, this risk must be taken.

RESECTOSCOPE & LITHOTRITE

Resectoscope

The resectoscope is a commonly used visual instrument with which transurethral resection of the prostate or of vesical carcinoma is performed.

Lithotrite

The lithotrite allows the urologist to crush smaller vesical calculi transurethrally.

REACTIONS TO INSTRUMENTATION

Urethra & Bladder
(Sounds, Cystoscopy)

Some bleeding is to be expected in men. Burning on urination and frequency may be noted because of trauma to the mucous membrane. Acute urinary retention may develop in men suffering from moderate prostatism. This may be due to edema from the instrumentation. Exacerbation of lower tract infection may occur. Epididymitis may develop if prostatocystitis is present. "Urethral chill" (which is really due to bacteremia from an infected prostate traumatized by instrumentation or vesicoureteral reflux) may occur.

Ureters & Kidney
(Ureteral Catheterization, Urography)

Nausea, vomiting, and abdominal cramps are often experienced from overdistention of the renal pelves with radiopaque material. Renal and ureteral pain and colic (from overdistention) or ureteral edema (from trauma) may ensue. Bleeding may occur if the tip of a catheter pierces the renal parenchyma. Exacerbation of kidney infection may develop, or new infection may be introduced. Temporary anuria is rare; it may be caused by excessive ureteral edema from instrumentation or sensitivity to the urographic medium.

●　　●　　●

References

Preliminary Procedures

Bodner H & others: Sodium methohexol amnesia for urethral instrumentation. J Urol 110:208, 1973.

Getzoff PL: A safe and effective topical anesthetic for office cystoscopy. J Urol 99:118, 1968.

Ulm AH, Wagshul EC: Pulmonary embolization with an oily medium. New England J Med 263:137, 1960.

The Catheter

Desautels RE: The causes of catheter-induced urinary infections and their prevention. J Urol 101:757, 1969.

Desautels RE: Managing the urinary catheter. Geriatrics 29:67, 1974.

Cystometer

Marshall S: A disposable cystometer. J Urol 91:458, 1964.

Cystoscopy & Panendoscopy

Amar AD, Chabra K: Reduction of radiation exposure of children during urologic diagnosis including a nonradiographic method of demonstrating vesicoureteral reflux. Pediatrics 35:960, 1965.

10 . . .
Urinary Obstruction & Stasis

Because of their damaging effect on renal function, obstruction and stasis of urinary flow are among the most important of urologic disorders. Either leads eventually to hydronephrosis, a peculiar type of atrophy of the kidney which may terminate in renal insufficiency or, if unilateral, complete destruction of the organ. Furthermore, obstruction leads to infection, which causes additional damage to the organs involved.

Etiology

Congenital anomalies, more common in the urinary tract than in any other organ system, are most commonly obstructive. In adult life, many types of acquired obstruction can occur.

A. Congenital: The common sites of congenital narrowing are just inside the external urinary meatus in little girls, posterior urethral valves, and the ureterovesical and ureteropelvic junctions. Another congenital cause of urinary stasis is damage to sacral roots 2–4 as seen in spina bifida and myelomeningocele. Vesicoureteral reflux causes both vesical and renal stasis (see Chapter 11).

B. Acquired: Acquired obstructions are numerous and may be primary in the urinary tract or secondary to extraurologic lesions which invade or compress the urinary passages. Among the common causes are (1) urethral stricture secondary to infection or injury; (2) benign prostatic hyperplasia or cancer of the prostate; (3) vesical tumor involving the bladder neck or one or both ureterovesical orifices; (4) local extension of cancer of the prostate or cervix into the base of the bladder, occluding the ureters; (5) compression of the ureters at the pelvic brim by metastatic nodes from malignancy of the prostate or cervix; (6) ureteral stone; and (7) pregnancy.

Neurogenic dysfunction affects principally the bladder. The upper tracts are damaged secondarily by ureterovesical obstruction or reflux and, often, complicating infection. Severe constipation in women and children can cause bilateral hydroureteronephrosis from compression of the lower ureters.

Elongation and kinking of the ureter secondary to vesicoureteral reflux commonly leads to ureteropelvic obstruction and hydronephrosis. Unless a voiding cystourethrogram is obtained in all children having this lesion, the primary cause may be missed and improper treatment applied.

Pathogenesis & Pathology

Obstruction and neurovesical dysfunction have the same effects upon the urinary tract. These changes can best be understood by considering (1) the effects upon the lower tract (distal to the bladder neck) of severe external urinary meatal stricture and (2) the effects upon the mid tract (bladder) and upper tract (ureter and kidney) of benign prostatic hyperplasia.

A. Lower Tract: Hydrostatic pressure proximal to the obstruction causes dilatation of the urethra. The wall of the urethra may become thin, and a diverticulum may form. If the urine becomes infected, spontaneous urethral rupture with urinary extravasation may occur. The prostatic ducts may become widely dilated (Fig 24–4).

B. Mid Tract: In the earlier stages (compensatory phase), the muscle wall of the bladder becomes thickened. With decompensation, it may be thinned and, therefore, weakened.

1. Stage of compensation—In order to balance the increasing urethral resistance, the bladder musculature hypertrophies. Its thickness may double. Complete emptying of the bladder is thus made possible.

Little more than hypertrophied muscle may be seen microscopically, although the effects of infection are often superimposed. In case of secondary infection, there may be edema of the submucosa, which may be infiltrated with plasma cells, lymphocytes, and polymorphonuclear cells.

At cystoscopy, surgery, or autopsy, visual evidence of this compensation is demonstrated in the following ways (Fig 10–1):

a. Trabeculation of the bladder wall—The wall of the distended bladder is normally quite smooth. With hypertrophy, individual muscle bundles stand out taut and give a coarsely interwoven appearance to the mucosal surface. The trigonal muscle and the interureteric ridge, which normally are only slightly raised above the surrounding tissues, respond to obstruction by hypertrophy of their smooth musculature. The ridge then becomes a prominent structure. This trigonal hypertrophy causes increased resistance in the intravesical ureteral segments due to accentuated downward pull upon them. It is this mechanism that causes relative stenosis of the ureterovesical junctions leading to hydroureteronephrosis. In the presence of significant residual urine, which further stretches the ureterotri-

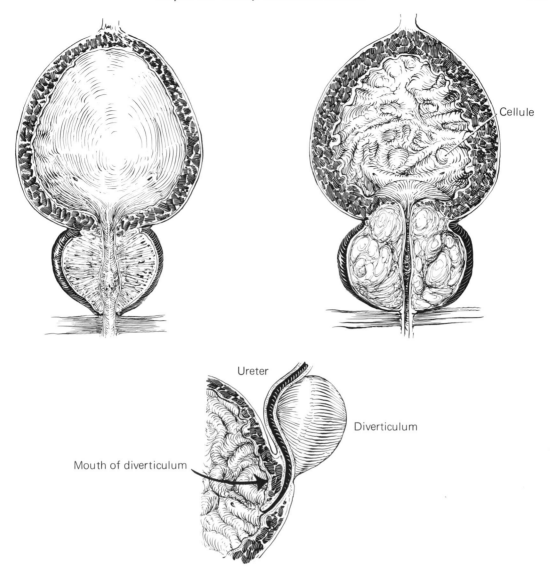

Figure 10–1. Changes in the bladder developing from obstruction. *Above left:* Normal bladder and prostate. *Above right:* Obstructing prostate causing trabeculation, cellule formation, and hypertrophy of the interureteric ridge. *Below:* Marked trabeculation (hypertrophy) of the vesical musculature; diverticulum displacing left ureter.

gonal complex, obstruction increases. (A urethral catheter will relieve this somewhat; definitive prostatectomy leads to reduction of trigonal hypertrophy with relief of the ureterovesical obstruction.)

b. Cellules–Normal intravesical pressure is about 30 cm of water at the beginning of micturition. Pressures 2–4 times as great may be reached by the trabeculated (hypertrophied) bladder in its attempt to force urine past the obstruction. This pressure tends to push mucosa between the superficial muscle bundles, causing the formation of small pockets, or cellules (Fig 10–1).

c. Diverticula–If cellules force their way entirely through the musculature of the bladder wall, they be-

come diverticula, which may be embedded in perivesical fat or covered by peritoneum, depending upon their location. They have no muscle wall and are therefore unable to expel their contents into the bladder efficiently even after the primary obstruction has been removed. When this occurs, secondary infection is difficult to eradicate, and surgical removal of the diverticula may be required. If a diverticulum pushes through the bladder wall on the anterior surface of the ureter, the ureterovesical junction will become incompetent. (See Chapter 11.)

d. Mucosa–In the presence of acute infection, the mucosa may be reddened and edematous. This may lead to temporary vesicoureteral reflux in the presence

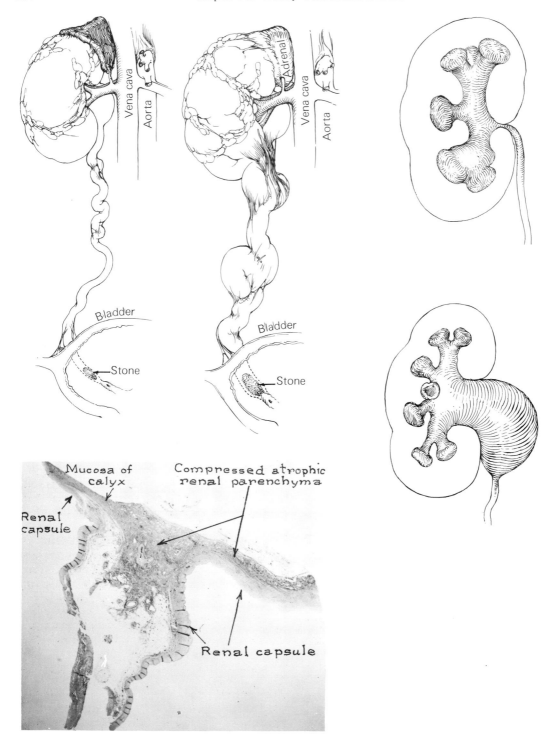

Figure 10–2. Mechanisms and results of obstruction. *Above left:* Early stage. Elongation and dilatation of ureter due to mild obstruction. *Above center:* Later stage. Further dilatation and elongation with kinking of the ureter; fibrous bands cause further kinking. *Below left:* Photomicrograph of advanced hydronephrosis. Thin layer of renal parenchyma covered by fibrous capsule. *Above right:* Intrarenal pelvis. Obstruction transmits all back pressure to parenchyma. *Below right:* Extrarenal pelvis, when obstructed, allows some of the increased pressure to be dissipated by the pelvis.

of a "borderline" junction. The chronically inflamed membrane may be thinned and pale.

2. Stage of decompensation—The compensatory power of the bladder musculature varies greatly. One patient with prostatic enlargement may have only mild symptoms of prostatism but a large obstructing gland that can be palpated rectally and observed cystoscopically; another may suffer acute retention and yet have a gland of normal size on rectal palpation and what appears to be only a mild obstruction cystoscopically.

In the face of progressive urethral obstruction, possibly aggravated by prostatic infection with edema or by congestion from lack of intercourse, decompensation of the detrusor may occur, resulting in the presence of residual urine after voiding. The amount may range up to 500 ml or more.

C. Upper Tract:

1. Ureter—In the early phases of obstruction, intravesical pressure, even when it is increased, is not transmitted to the ureters and renal pelves because of the competence of the ureterovesical "valves." (A true valve is not present; the ureterotrigonal unit, by virtue of its intrinsic structure, resists the retrograde flow of urine.) Eventually, with decompensation of the ureterotrigonal complex, the valvelike action may be lost, vesicoureteral reflux occurs, and the increased intravesical pressure is then transmitted to the renal pelves.

Secondary to the back pressure from reflux or obstruction from the hypertrophied and stretched trigone or a ureteral stone, the ureteral musculature thickens in its attempt to push the urine downward by increased peristaltic activity (stage of compensation). This causes elongation and some tortuosity of the ureter (Fig 10–2). At times this change becomes marked; bands of fibrous tissue develop which on contraction further angulate the ureter so that secondary ureteral stenosis develops. Under these circumstances, removal of the obstruction below may not prevent the kidney from undergoing complete destruction from the acquired ureteral obstruction.

Finally, because of increasing pressure, the ureteral wall becomes attenuated and therefore loses all of its contractile power (stage of decompensation). Dilatation may be so extreme that the ureter resembles a loop of bowel (Figs 10–3 and 11–7, top right).

2. Kidney—The pressure within the renal pelvis is normally close to zero. When this pressure increases because of obstruction or reflux, the pelvis and calyces dilate. The degree of hydronephrosis which develops depends upon the duration, degree, and site of the obstruction. The higher the obstruction, the greater the effect upon the kidney. If the renal pelvis is entirely intrarenal and the obstruction is at the ureteropelvic junction, all the pressure will be exerted upon the parenchyma. If the renal pelvis is extrarenal, a ureteropelvic stenosis will exert only part of the resulting pressure on the parenchyma. The pelvis, being embedded in fat, dilates more readily, thus "decompressing" the calyces (Fig 10–2).

In the earlier stages, the pelvic musculature undergoes compensatory hypertrophy in its effort to force

urine past the obstruction. Later, however, the muscle becomes attenuated (and decompensated).

The progression of hydronephrotic atrophy is as follows:

(1) The earliest changes in the development of hydronephrosis are seen in the calyces. The end of a normal calyx (as seen on a urogram, Fig 6–6) is concave because of the papilla which projects into it; with a chronic increase in intrapelvic pressure, it becomes flattened and then convex (clubbed) as a result of ischemia, necrosis, and absorption of the papilla. The parenchyma between the calyces is affected to a lesser extent.

This spotty atrophy is caused by the nature of the blood supply of the kidney. The arterioles are "end arteries"; therefore, ischemia is most marked in the areas farthest from the interlobular arteries. As the back pressure increases, hydronephrosis progresses, with the cells nearest the main arteries exhibiting the greatest resistance.

This increased pressure is transmitted up the tubules. The tubules become dilated, and their cells atrophy from ischemia.

(2) Only in unilateral hydronephrosis are the advanced stages of hydronephrotic atrophy seen. Eventually the kidney is completely destroyed and appears as a thin-walled sac filled with clear fluid (water and electrolytes) or pus (Fig 10–4).

If obstruction is unilateral, the increased intrarenal pressure will cause some suppression of renal function on that side. The closer the intrapelvic pressure approaches the glomerular filtration pressure (30–40 mm Hg), the less urine can be secreted. Glomerular filtration rate and renal plasma flow are reduced. Concentrating power is gradually lost. The urine urea:creatinine concentration ratio is low when compared to that of the normal kidney.

Hydronephrotic atrophy is an unusual type of pathologic change. Other secretory organs (eg, the submaxillary gland) cease secreting when their ducts are obstructed. This causes primary (disuse) atrophy. The completely obstructed kidney, however, continues to secrete urine. (If this were not so, hydronephrosis could not occur, since it depends upon increased intrarenal pressure.) As urine is excreted into the renal pelvis, fluid and, particularly, soluble substances are reabsorbed, either through the tubules or the lymphatics. This has been demonstrated by injecting PSP into the obstructed renal pelvis. It disappears (is reabsorbed) in a few hours and is excreted by the other kidney. Other evidence is the fact that the markedly hydronephrotic kidney does not contain urine in the true sense; only water and a few salts are present.

Functional impairment in unilateral hydronephrosis, as measured by PSP or excretory urograms, will be greater and will increase faster than that seen in bilateral hydronephrotic kidneys showing comparable damage on urography. As unilateral hydronephrosis progresses, the normal kidney undergoes compensatory hypertrophy of its nephrons (renal counterbalance), thereby assuming the function of the diseased kidney

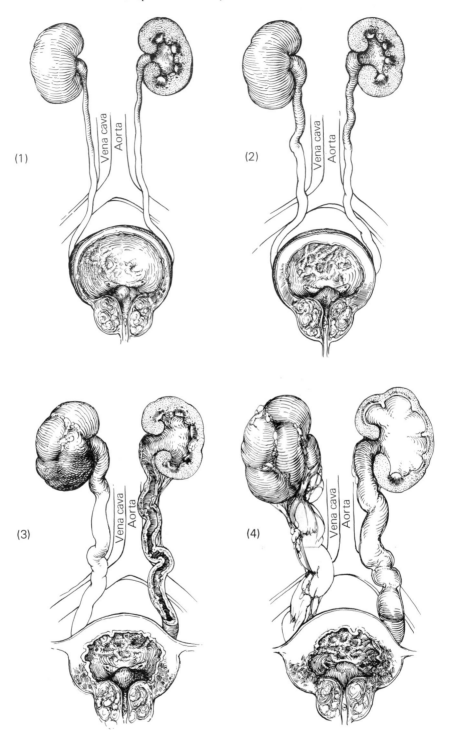

Figure 10–3. Pathogenesis of bilateral hydronephrosis. Progressive changes in bladder, ureters, and kidneys from obstruction of an enlarged prostate: thickening of bladder wall, dilatation and elongation of ureters, and hydronephrosis.

in order to maintain normal total renal function. For this reason, successful anatomic repair of the ureteral obstruction of such a kidney may not only fail to improve its powers of waste elimination but the kidney may even continue to lose function.

If both kidneys are equally hydronephrotic, a strong stimulus is continually being exerted on both to maintain maximum function. This is also true of a solitary hydronephrotic kidney. Consequently, the return of function in these kidneys after repair of their obstructions is at times remarkable.

Physiologic Explanation of Symptoms of Bladder Neck Obstruction

The following hypothesis has been brought forward to explain the syndrome known as "prostatism" which occurs with progressive vesical obstruction:

The bladder, like the heart, is a hollow muscular organ which receives fluid and forcefully expels it. And, like the heart, it reacts to an increasing work load by going through the successive phases of compensation and finally decompensation.

Normally, contracture of the detrusor muscle and the trigone pulls the bladder neck open and forms a funnel through which the urine is expelled. The intravesical pressure generated in this instance varies between 20–40 cm of water; this force further widens the bladder neck.

With bladder neck obstruction, hypertrophy of the vesical musculature develops, allowing intravesical pressure to rise to 50–100 cm or more of water in order to overcome the increased urethral resistance. Despite this, the encroaching prostate appears to interfere with the mechanisms which ordinarily open the internal orifice. In addition, the contraction phase may not last long enough for all of the urine to be expelled; "exhaustion" of the muscle occurs prematurely. The refractory phase then sets in, and the detrusor is temporarily unable to respond to further stimuli. A few minutes later, voiding may again be initiated and completed.

A. Compensation Phase:

1. Stage of irritability—In the earliest stages of obstruction of the bladder neck, the vesical musculature begins to hypertrophy. The force and size of the urinary stream remain normal because the balance is maintained between the expelling power of the bladder and urethral resistance. During this phase, however, the bladder appears to be hypersensitive. As the bladder is distended, the need to void is felt. In the individual with a normal bladder these early urges can be inhibited, and the bladder relaxes and distends to receive more urine. However, in the patient with hypertrophied detrusor, the contraction of the detrusor is so strong that it virtually goes into spasm, producing the symptoms of an irritable bladder. The earliest symptoms of bladder neck obstruction, therefore, are urgency (even to the point of incontinence) and frequency, both day and night.

2. Stage of compensation—As the obstruction increases, further hypertrophy of the muscle fibers of

the bladder occurs and the power to empty the bladder completely is thereby maintained. During this period, in addition to urgency and frequency, the patient notices hesitancy in initiating urination while the bladder develops contractions strong enough to overcome resistance at the bladder neck. The obstruction causes some loss in the force and size of the urinary stream, and the stream becomes slower as vesical emptying nears completion (exhaustion of the detrusor as it nears the end of the contraction phase).

B. Decompensation Phase: If vesical tone becomes impaired or if urethral resistance exceeds detrusor power, some degree of decompensation (imbalance) occurs. The contraction phase of the vesical muscle becomes too short to completely expel the contents of the bladder, and residual urine is the result.

1. Acute decompensation—The tone of the compensated vesical muscle can be temporarily embarrassed by rapid filling of the bladder (high fluid intake) or by overstretching of the detrusor (postponement of urination though the urge is felt). This may cause increased difficulty of urination, with marked hesitancy and the need for straining to initiate urination; a very weak and small stream; and termination of the stream before the bladder completely empties (residual urine). Acute and sudden complete urinary retention may also occur.

2. Chronic decompensation—As the degree of obstruction increases, a progressive imbalance between the power of the bladder musculature and urethral resistance develops. Therefore, it becomes increasingly more difficult to expel all the urine during the contraction phase of the detrusor. The symptoms of obstruction become more marked. This residuum gradually increases, thus diminishing the functional capacity of the bladder. Progressive frequency of urination is noted. On occasion, as the bladder decompensates, it becomes overstretched and attenuated. It may contain 1000–3000 ml of urine. It loses its power of contraction, and overflow (paradoxical) incontinence results.

Clinical Findings

A. Symptoms:

1. Lower and mid tract (urethra and bladder)—Symptoms of obstruction of the lower and mid tract are typified by the symptoms of urethral stricture, benign prostatic hyperplasia, neurogenic bladder, and tumor of the bladder involving the vesical neck. The principal symptoms are hesitancy in starting urination, lessened force and size of the stream, terminal dribbling; hematuria, which may be initial with stricture, total with prostatic obstruction or vesical tumor; burning on urination, cloudy urine (complicating infection), and acute urinary retention.

2. Upper tract (ureter and kidney)—Symptoms of obstruction of the upper tract are typified by the symptoms of congenital ureteral stenosis or ureteral or renal stone. The principal complaints are pain in the flank radiating along the course of the ureter, gross total hematuria (from stone), gastrointestinal symptoms, chills, fever, burning on urination, and cloudy

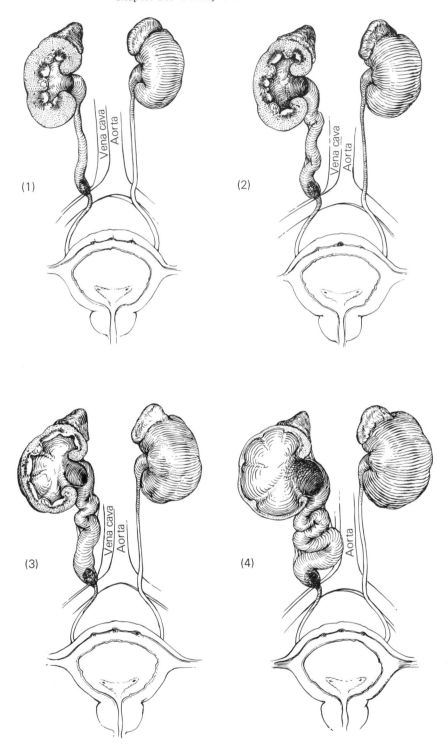

Figure 10—4. Pathogenesis of unilateral hydronephrosis. Progressive changes in ureter and kidney secondary to obstructing calculus. As the right kidney undergoes gradual destruction, the left kidney gradually enlarges (compensatory hypertrophy).

urine with onset of infection, which is the common sequel to obstruction or vesicoureteral reflux. Nausea, vomiting, loss of weight and strength, and pallor are due to uremia secondary to bilateral hydronephrosis.

Obstruction of the upper tract may be silent even when uremia supervenes.

B. Signs:

1. Lower and mid tract—Palpation of the urethra may reveal induration about a stricture. Rectal examination may show atony of the anal sphincter (damage to the sacral nerve roots) or benign or malignant enlargement of the prostate. Vesical distention may be found.

Although observation of the force and caliber of the urinary stream affords a rough estimate of maximum flow rate, the rate can be measured accurately with a urine flowmeter or, even more simply, by the following technic: Have the patient begin to void. When observed maximum flow has been reached, interpose a container to collect the urine, and simultaneously start a stopwatch. When urine flow begins to fade, remove the container and stop the watch. The flow in milliliters per second can then be calculated. The normal maximum urine flow rate is 15 ml or more per second. Flow rates associated with an atonic neurogenic bladder (diminished detrusor power), urethral stricture, or prostatic obstruction (increased urethral resistance) may be as low as 3–5 ml/second. A cystometrogram will differentiate between these 2 causes of impaired flow rate. After definitive treatment of the cause, flow rate should return to normal.

In the presence of a vesical diverticulum or vesicoureteral reflux, although detrusor power is normal, the urinary stream may be impaired because of the diffusion of intravesical pressure into the diverticulum and vesicoureteral junctions as well as the urethra. Excision of the diverticulum or repair of the vesicoureteral junctions leads to efficient expulsion of urine via the urethra.

2. Upper tract—An enlarged kidney may be discovered by palpation or percussion. Renal tenderness may be elicited if infection has supervened. Cancer of the cervix may be noted; it may invade the base of the bladder and occlude one or both ureteral orifices, or its metastases to the iliac lymph nodes may compress the ureters. A large pelvic mass (tumor, pregnancy) can displace and compress the ureters. Children with advanced urinary tract obstruction (usually due to posterior urethral valves) may develop ascites. Rupture of the renal fornices allows leakage of urine which passes into the peritoneal cavity through a tear in the peritoneum.

C. Laboratory Findings: Anemia may be found secondary to chronic infection or in advanced bilateral hydronephrosis (stage of uremia). Leukocytosis is to be expected in the acute stage of infection. Little if any elevation of the white blood count accompanies the chronic stage.

Large amounts of protein are usually not found in the obstructive uropathies. Casts are not common from hydronephrotic kidneys. Microscopic hematuria may indicate renal or vesical infection, tumor, or stone. Pus cells and bacteria may or may not be present.

In the presence of unilateral hydronephrosis, the PSP test will be normal because of the contralateral renal hypertrophy. Suppression of the PSP indicates bilateral renal damage, residual urine (vesical or bilateral ureterorenal), or vesicoureteral reflux.

In the presence of significant bilateral hydronephrosis, urine flow through the renal tubules is slowed. Thus, urea is significantly reabsorbed but creatinine is not. Blood chemistry therefore reveals a urea:creatinine ratio well above the normal 10:1 relationship.

D. X-Ray Findings: (Fig 10–5.) A plain film of the abdomen may show enlargement of renal shadows, calcific bodies suggesting ureteral or renal stone, or metastases to the bones of the spine or pelvis. If metastases are present in the spine, they may be the cause of spinal cord damage (neurogenic bladder). If osteoblastic, cancer of the prostate is almost certainly the cause.

Excretory urograms will reveal almost the entire story unless renal function is severely impaired. They are more informative when obstruction is present because the opaque material is retained. These urograms will demonstrate the degree of dilatation of the pelves, calyces, and ureters. The point of ureteral stenosis will be revealed. Segmental dilatation of the lower end of a ureter implies the possibility of vesicoureteral reflux (Fig 11–6), which can be revealed by cystography. The accompanying cystogram may show trabeculation as an irregularity of the vesical outline and may show diverticula. Vesical tumors, nonopaque stones, and large intravesical prostatic lobes may cause radiolucent shadows. A film taken immediately after voiding will show residual urine. Few tests that are as simple and inexpensive give the physician so much information.

Retrograde cystography shows changes of the bladder wall caused by distal obstruction (trabeculation, diverticula) or demonstrates the obstructive lesion itself (enlarged prostate, posterior urethral valves, vesical neoplasm). If the ureterovesical valves are incompetent, ureteropyelograms will be obtained by reflux (Fig 6–8).

Retrograde urograms may show better detail than the excretory type, but care must be taken not to overdistend the passages with too much opaque fluid; small hydronephroses can be made to look quite large. The degree of ureteral or ureterovesical obstruction can be judged by the degree of delay of drainage of the radiopaque fluid instilled.

E. Isotope Scanning: In the presence of obstruction, the radioisotope renogram may show depression of both the vascular and secretory phases and a rising rather than a falling excretory phase due to retention of the radiopaque urine in the renal pelvis.

The ^{131}I activity recorded on the gamma camera will reveal poor uptake of the isotope, slow transport of the isotope through the parenchyma, and accumulation of scintillations in the renal pelvis. (See Chapter 8.)

F. Instrumental Examination: Exploration of the urethra with a catheter or other instrument is a valu-

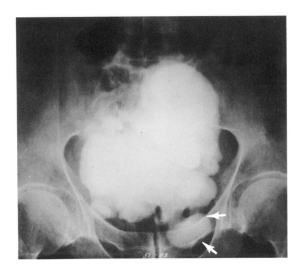

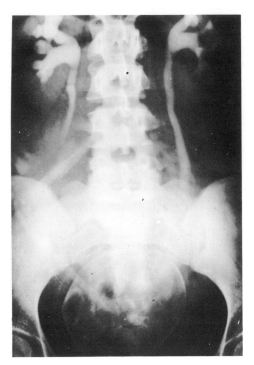

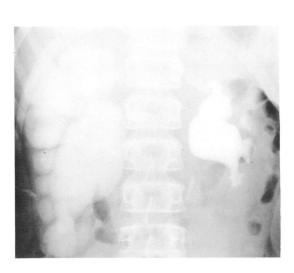

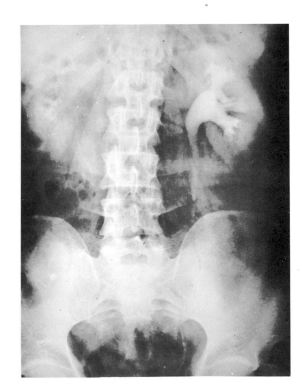

Figure 10–5. Changes in bladder, ureters, and kidneys caused by obstruction. ***Above left:*** Cystogram showing benign prostatic enlargement and multiple diverticula. Arrows point to femoral hernia which probably developed as a result of straining to urinate. ***Above right:*** Pregnancy. Significant dilatation and elongation of upper right ureter due to compression at the pelvic line. Left side normal. ***Below left:*** Excretory urogram, 70 minutes after injection. Advanced right hydronephrosis secondary to ureteropelvic obstruction. Mild ureteropelvic obstruction on left. ***Below right:*** Stone in right ureter (see arrow) with mild hydronephrosis.

able diagnostic measure. Passage may be blocked by a stricture or tumor. External sphincter spasm may make passage difficult. Passage of the catheter immediately after voiding allows estimation of the amount of residual urine in the bladder. Residual urine is common in bladder neck obstruction (enlarged prostate), cystocele, and neurogenic bladder. Even though the urinary stream may be markedly impaired with urethral stricture, residual urine is usually absent.

Measurement of vesical tone by means of cystometry is helpful in diagnosing the neurogenic bladder and in differentiating between bladder neck obstruction and vesical atony.

Inspection of the urethra and bladder by means of cystoscopy and panendoscopy may reveal the primary obstructive agent. Catheters may be passed to the renal pelves and urine specimens obtained. Measurement of the function of each kidney may be done (PSP test), and retrograde ureteropyelograms can be made.

Differential Diagnosis

A thorough examination usually leaves no doubt about the diagnosis. The differential diagnosis under these circumstances is rarely difficult. If seemingly simple infection does not respond to medical therapy, or if infection recurs, obstruction or vesicoureteral reflux is the probable cause and complete study of the urinary tract is indicated.

Complications

Stagnation of urine leads to infection, which then may spread throughout the entire urinary system. Once established, infection is difficult and at times impossible to eradicate even after the obstruction has been relieved.

Often the invading organisms are urea-splitting (proteus, staphylococci). This causes the urine to become alkaline, in which case calcium salts precipitate and form bladder or kidney stones more easily.

If both kidneys are affected, the result may be renal insufficiency. Secondary infection increases renal damage.

Pyonephrosis is the end stage of a severely infected and obstructed kidney. The kidney is functionless and is filled with thick pus. At times, a plain film of the abdomen may show an air urogram caused by gas liberated by infecting organisms.

Treatment

A. Relief of Obstruction: Treatment of the main causes of obstruction and stasis is described in detail elsewhere: benign prostatic hyperplasia, cancer of the prostate, neurogenic bladder, ureteral stone, posterior urethral valves, and ureteral stenosis.

1. Lower tract obstruction (distal to the bladder)—With patients in whom secondary renal or ureterovesical damage (reflux in the latter) is minimal or nonexistent, correction of the obstruction is sufficient. If significant reflux is demonstrated, "triple voiding" should be instituted once a day. This consists of voiding with strain; walking around, voiding with strain; walking around and then voiding again. This technic will usually empty the entire urinary tract completely, thus increasing the chances of sterilizing the urine and keeping it sterile. However, if there is considerable hydronephrosis in addition to reflux, drainage of the bladder by indwelling catheter or other means of diversion (eg, loop ureterostomy) is indicated in order to preserve or improve renal function. If, after many months of drainage, reflux persists, surgical repair of the incompetent intravesical portion of the ureter should be done.

2. Upper tract obstruction (above the bladder)—If tortuous, kinked, dilated, or atonic ureters have developed secondary to lower tract obstruction (so that they are themselves obstructive), vesical drainage will not protect the kidneys from further damage; the urine proximal to the obstruction must be diverted by nephrostomy or ureterostomy. The kidneys then may regain some function. Over a period of many months, the ureter may become less tortuous and less dilated; its obstructive areas may open up. If radiopaque material instilled into the nephrostomy tube passes readily to the bladder, it may be possible to remove the nephrostomy tube. If obstruction or reflux persists, surgical repair is indicated. Permanent urinary diversion (eg, ureteroileal conduit) may be necessary.

If one kidney has been badly damaged, as measured by tests of function and urography, nephrectomy may be necessary.

B. Eradication of Infection: Once the obstruction is removed, every effort should be made to eradicate infection. If it has been severe and prolonged, antibiotics may fail to sterilize the urinary tract.

Prognosis

No simple statement can be made about the prognosis in this group of patients. The outcome depends upon the cause, site, degree, and duration of the obstruction. The prognosis is also definitely influenced by complicating infection, particularly if it has been present for a long time.

If renal function is fair to good, if the obstruction or other causes for stasis can be corrected, and if complicating infection can then be eradicated, the prognosis is generally excellent.

•   •   •

References

Almgård LE, Fernström I: Percutaneous nephropyelostomy. Acta radiol (diag) 15:288, 1974.

Aron B, Tessler A, Morales P: Angiography in hydronephrosis. Urology 2:231, 1973.

Belman AB, King LR: Vesicostomy: Useful means of reversible urinary diversion in selected infants. Urology 1:208, 1973.

Berdon WE & others: Hydronephrosis in infants and children: Value of high dosage excretory urography in predicting renal salvageability. Am J Roentgenol 109:380, 1970.

Better OS & others: Studies on renal function after relief of complete unilateral ureteral obstruction of three months' duration in man. Am J Med 54:234, 1973.

Blackard CE, Nicolaidis AN, Johnston JD: Modified loop cutaneous ureterostomy. J Urol 110:291, 1973.

Bourne RB: Intermittent hydronephrosis as a cause of abdominal pain. JAMA 198:1218, 1966.

Bredin HC & others: The surgical correction of congenital ureteropelvic junction obstructions in normally rotated kidneys. J Urol 111:460, 1974.

Bryan PJ, Azimi F: Ultrasound in diagnosis of congenital hydronephrosis due to obstruction of pelviureteric junction. Urology 5:17, 1975.

Chovnick SD: Anterior sacral meningocele as a cause of urinary retention. J Urol 106:371, 1971.

Cook GT: Appendiceal abscess causing urinary obstruction. J Urol 101:212, 1969.

Culp DA: Acute urinary retention. Postgrad Med 31:252, 1962.

Edelmann CM Jr, Spitzer A: The maturing kidney: A modern view of well-balanced infants with imbalanced nephrons. J Pediat 75:509, 1969.

Engel RME: Permanent urinary diversion in childhood: Indications and types. Urology 3:178, 1974.

Fayad MM & others: The ureterocalyceal system in normal pregnancy: A study using isotope renography and intravenous pyelography. Acta obst gynec scandinav 52:69, 1973.

Ghoneim MA, Ashamallah A: Further experiences with the rectosigmoid bladder. Brit J Urol 46:511, 1974.

Glen ES: Spontaneous intraperitoneal rupture of hydronephrosis. Brit J Urol 41:414, 1969.

Green N, Fingerhut AG, French S: Mechanism of renovascular backflow: A pathophysiologic study. Radiology 92:531, 1969.

Guyer PB, Delany D: Urinary tract dilatation and oral contraceptives. Brit MJ 4:588, 1970.

Halpern GN, King LR, Belman AB: Transureteroureterostomy in children. J Urol 109:504, 1973.

Hawtrey CE & others: Clinical experience with loop nephrostomy for urinary diversion. J Urol 112:36, 1974.

Herwig KR: Pyohydronephrosis: Diagnosis with selective renal angiography. J Urol 109:964, 1973.

Hutch JA, Tanagho EA: Etiology of non-occlusive ureteral dilatation. J Urol 93:177, 1965.

Johnston JH: The presentation of management of neonatal obstructive uropathies. Postgrad MJ 48:486, 1972.

Kelalis PP: Urinary diversion in children by the sigmoid conduit: Its advantages and limitations. J Urol 112:666, 1974.

Kelalis PP & others: Ureteropelvic obstruction in children: Experiences with 109 cases. J Urol 106:418, 1971.

Kelalis PP, McLean P: The treatment of diverticulum of the bladder. J Urol 98:349, 1967.

Kendall AR, Karafin L: Intermittent hydronephrosis: Hydration pyelography. J Urol 98:653, 1967.

Kornitzer AD, Olsson CM: Methods of urinary diversion. Geriatrics 29:85, Sept 1974.

Krohn AG & others: Compensatory renal hypertrophy: The role of immediate vascular change in its production. J Urol 103:564, 19740.

Leary DJ Jr & others: Preoperative aortography in hydronephrosis. J Urol 107:542, 1972.

Leff LO, Smith JP: Achalasia in children and adults. Urology 2:139, 1973.

Marshall S: Urea-creatinine ratio in obstructive uropathy and renal hypertension. JAMA 190:719, 1964.

Michaelson G: Percutaneous puncture of the renal pelvis, intrapelvic pressure and the concentrating capacity of the kidney in hydronephrosis. Acta med scandinav, Suppl 559, 1974.

Morillo MM: Intravesical pressure before and after surgery for bladder neck obstruction. J Urol 91:361, 1964.

Newling DWW, Heslop RW, Kille JN: Pelviureteral obstruction: Results of the Anderson-Hynes pyeloplasty procedure. J Urol 111:12, 1974.

Olsson CA, Moyer JD, Chute R: Oral diuretics and renal pain: A provocative test. J Urol 108:25, 1972.

Perlmutter AD, Patil J: Loop cutaneous ureterostomy in infants and young children: Late results in 32 cases. J Urol 107:655, 1972.

Preissig RS, Barry WF Jr, Lester RG: The increased incidence of carcinoma of the colon following ureterosigmoidostomy. Am J Roentgenol 121:806, 1974.

Rose JS & others: B-mode sonographic evaluation of abdominal masses in the pediatric patient. Am J Roentgenol 120:691, 1974.

Saxton CS, Ogg CS, Cameron JS: Needle nephrostomy. Brit M Bull 28:210, 1972.

Schmidt JD & others: Complications, results and problems of ileal conduit diversions. J Urol 109:210, 1973.

Sholem SL, Lattimer JK, Uson AC: Further experience with loop cutaneous ureterostomy to save badly damaged kidneys. J Urol 111:827, 1974.

Shopfner CE: Urinary tract pathology associated with constipation. Radiology 90:865, 1968.

Smart WR: Chapter 55 in: *Urology,* 3rd ed. Campbell MF, Harrison JH (editors). Saunders, 1970.

Stephens FD: Idiopathic dilatations of the urinary tract. J Urol 112: 819, 1974.

Stephens FD: Treatment of megaloureters by multiple micturition. Australian New Zealand J Surg 27:130, 1957.

Tanagho EA, Meyers FH: Trigonal hypertrophy: A cause of ureteral obstruction. J Urol 93:678, 1965.

Tanagho EA, Smith DR, Guthrie TH: Pathophysiology of functional ureteral obstruction. J Urol 104:73, 1970.

Thompson IA, Bruns TNC: Neonatal ascites: A reflection of obstructive disease. J Urol 107:509, 1972.

Tsingoglou S, Dickson JAS: Lower urinary obstruction in infancy: A review of lesions in 165 cases. Arch Dis Childhood 47:215, 1972.

Walsh PC & others: Percutaneous antegrade pyelography in hydronephrosis: Preoperative assessment. Urology 1:537, 1973.

Wedge JJ, Grosfeld JL, Smith JP: Abdominal masses in the newborn: 63 cases. J Urol 106:770, 1971.

Zincke H, Malek RS: Experience with cutaneous and transureterouretostomy. J Urol 111:760, 1974.

11...
Vesicoureteral Reflux

Under normal circumstances, the ureterovesical junction allows urine to enter the bladder but prevents urine from regurgitating into the ureter, particularly at the time of voiding. In this way, the kidney is protected from high pressure in the bladder and from contamination by infected vesical urine. When this valve is incompetent, although some degree of hydroureteronephrosis may ensue, the chance for the development of urinary infection is significantly enhanced and pyelonephritis is then inevitable. With few exceptions, pyelonephritis—acute, chronic, or healed—is secondary to vesicoureteral reflux.

ANATOMY OF THE
URETEROVESICAL JUNCTION

An understanding of the causes of vesicoureteral reflux requires a knowledge of the anatomy of the ureterovesical valve. Anatomic studies performed by Hutch (1972) and by Tanagho and Pugh (1963) are incorporated into the following discussion (Fig 11–1).

Mesodermal Component

This structure, which arises from the Wolffian duct, is made of 2 parts which are innervated by the sympathetic nervous system:

A. The Ureter and the Superficial Trigone: The smooth musculature of the renal calyces, pelvis, and extravesical ureter is composed of helically oriented fibers. So constituted, they can undergo peristaltic activity. As these fibers approach the vesical wall, they are reoriented into the longitudinal plane. The ureter passes obliquely through the vesical wall; the intravesical ureteral segment is thus composed of longitudinal muscle fibers only and therefore cannot undergo peristalsis. As these smooth muscle fibers approach the ureteral orifice, those that form the roof swing dorsally and join the fibers that form the floor of the ureter. They then spread out and join those muscle bundles from the other ureter and also continue caudally, thus forming the superficial trigone, which then passes over the neck of the bladder, ending at the verumontanum in the male and just inside the external urethral orifice in the female. Thus, the ureterotrigonal complex is one

structure. Above the ureteral orifice, it is tubular; below that point, it is flat.

B. Waldeyer's Sheath and the Deep Trigone: Beginning at a point about 2–3 cm above the bladder, an external layer of longitudinal smooth muscle surrounds the ureter. These fibers pass through the vesical wall, to which they are connected by a few detrusor fibers. As this muscular sheath enters the vesical lumen, its roof fibers also diverge to join their floor fibers, which then spread out, joining muscle bundles from the contralateral ureter and forming the deep trigone which ends at the bladder neck.

Endodermal Component

The vesical detrusor muscle bundles are intertwined and run in various directions. However, as they converge upon the internal orifice of the bladder, they tend to become oriented into 3 layers:

A. Internal Longitudinal Layer: This layer continues into the urethra submucosally and ends just inside the external meatus in the female and at the caudal end of the prostate in the male.

B. Middle Circular Layer: This layer is thickest anteriorly and stops at the vesical neck.

C. Outer Longitudinal Layer: These muscle bundles take a circular and spiral course about the external surface of the female urethra and are incorporated within the peripheral prostatic tissue in the male. They constitute the true vesicourethral sphincter.

The vesical detrusor muscle is innervated by the parasympathetic nerves (S2–4).

PHYSIOLOGY OF THE
URETEROVESICAL JUNCTION

While many investigators had suspected that normal trigonal tone tended to occlude the intravesical ureter, it remained for Tanagho & others (1965) to prove it. Using nonrefluxing dogs, they demonstrated the following:

(1) Interruption of the continuity of the trigone resulted in reflux. An incision was made in the trigone 3 mm below the ureteral orifice, resulting in an upward and lateral migration of the ureteral orifice with short-

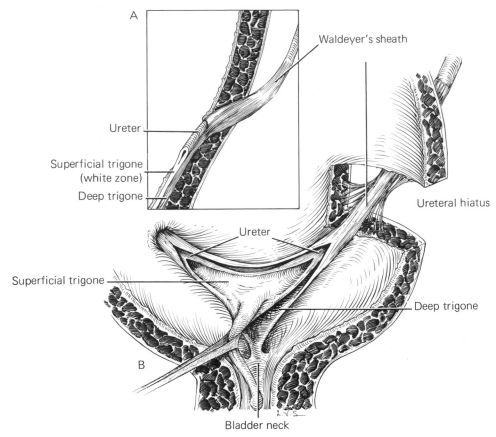

The ureteral muscle extends downward and becomes the superficial trigone.

Waldeyer's sheath extends downward and becomes the deep trigone.

Figure 11–1. Normal ureterotrigonal complex. *A:* Side view of ureterovesical junction. Waldeyer's muscular sheath invests the juxtavesical ureter and continues downward as the deep trigone, which extends to the bladder neck. The ureteral musculature becomes the superficial trigone, which extends to the verumontanum in the male and stops just short of the external meatus in the female. *B:* Waldeyer's sheath is connected by a few fibers to the detrusor muscle in the ureteral hiatus. This muscular sheath, inferior to the ureteral orifices, becomes the deep trigone. The musculature of the ureters continues downward as the superficial trigone. (Redrawn and modified, with permission, from Tanagho & Pugh: The anatomy and function of the ureterovesical junction. Brit J Urol 35:151, 1963.)

ening of the intravesical ureter. Reflux was demonstrable. After the incision healed, reflux ceased.

(2) Unilateral lumbar sympathectomy resulted in paralysis of the ipsilateral trigone. This led to lateral and superior migration of the ureteral orifice and reflux.

(3) Electrical stimulation of the trigone caused the ureteral orifice to move caudally, thus lengthening the intravesical ureter. This maneuver caused a marked rise in resistance to flow through the ureterovesical junction. Ureteral efflux of urine ceased. The intravenous injection of epinephrine caused the same reaction. On the other hand, isoproterenol caused the degree of occlusion to drop below normal. If, however, the trigone was incised, electrical stimulation of the trigone or the administration of epinephrine failed to increase ureteral occlusive pressure.

(4) During gradual filling of the bladder, intra-

vesical pressure increased but little, whereas the pressure within the intravesical ureter rose progressively—due, apparently, to increasing trigonal stretch. A few seconds before the expected sharp rise in intravesical pressure generated for voiding, the closure pressure in the intravesical ureter rose sharply and was maintained for 20 seconds after detrusor contracture had ceased. This experiment demonstrated that ureterovesical competence is independent of detrusor action and is governed by the tone of the trigone, which, just before voiding, contracts vigorously and thus helps to open and funnel the vesical neck. At the same time, significant pull is placed upon the intravesical ureter, thus occluding it during the period when intravesical pressure is high. During the voiding phase, there is naturally no efflux of ureteral urine.

One may liken this function to the phenomenon of the Chinese thimble: the harder the finger (trigone) pulls, the tighter the thimble (intravesical ureter). Contrariwise, a deficient pull may lead to incomplete closure of the ureterovesical junction.

It was concluded from these experiments that normal ureterotrigonal tone prevents vesicoureteral reflux. Electrical or pharmacologic stimulation of voiding caused increased occlusive pressure in the intravesical ureter and increased resistance to flow down the ureter. Contrariwise, incision or paralysis of the trigone led to reflux. The theory that ureterovesical competence was maintained by intravesical pressure crushing the intravesical ureter against its backing of detrusor muscle was thereby disproved.

Biopsy of the trigone (and the intravesical ureter) in patients with primary reflux revealed marked deficiency in the development of its smooth muscle (Fig 11–2). Electrical stimulation of such a trigone caused only a minor contraction of the ureterotrigonal complex. This work led to the conclusion that the common cause of reflux, particularly in children, is congenital attenuation of the ureterotrigonal musculature.

THE ETIOLOGY OF REFLUX

The major cause of vesicoureteral reflux is attenuation of the trigone and its contiguous intravesical ureteral musculature. Any condition that shortens the intravesical ureter may also lead to reflux, but this is less common. Familial vesicoureteral reflux has been observed by a number of authors. It appears to be a genetic trait.

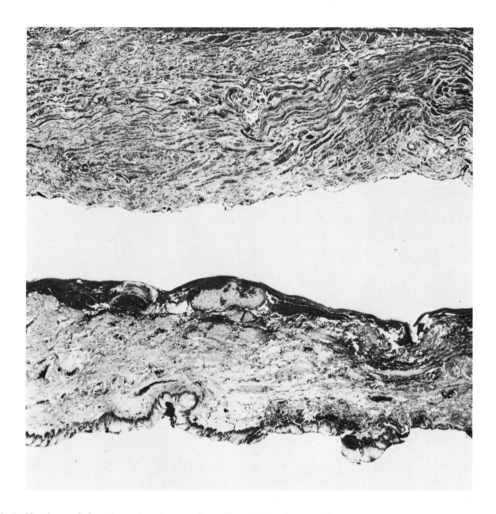

Figure 11–2. Histology of the trigone in primary reflux. ***Above:*** Normal trigone demonstrating wealth of closely packed smooth muscle fibers. ***Below:*** The congenitally attenuated trigonal muscle that accompanies vesicoureteral reflux. Note absence of inflammatory cells. (Reproduced, with permission, from Tanagho & others: Primary vesicoureteral reflux: Experimental studies of its etiology. J Urol 93:165, 1965.)

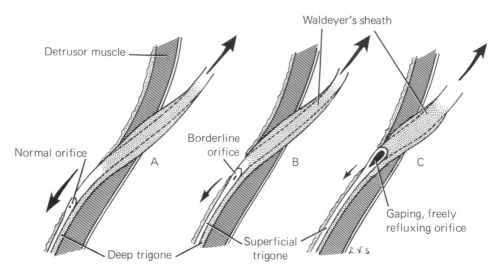

Figure 11—3. The effect of trigonal tone on the competency of the ureterovesical junction. *A:* Normal ureterotrigonal complex. Normal upper ureteral and ureterotrigonal muscles exert equal pull as shown by arrows. Trigonal tone occludes ureteral orifice and protects length of intravesical ureteral segment. *B:* Trigonal musculature moderately attenuated. The occlusive force on the orifice is subnormal and the tone and peristaltic action of the normal upper ureter may cause some cephalad migration of the ureter, thus decreasing the length of the intravesical ureter. This is a "borderline" valve that may reflux if the bladder becomes infected. *C:* Severe attenuation of intravesical-trigonal musculature. Little occlusive force exerted on ureteral orifice. Lumbar ureteral muscle has pulled the ureteral orifice up to the ureteral hiatus. Valve action is destroyed, and low-pressure reflux occurs.

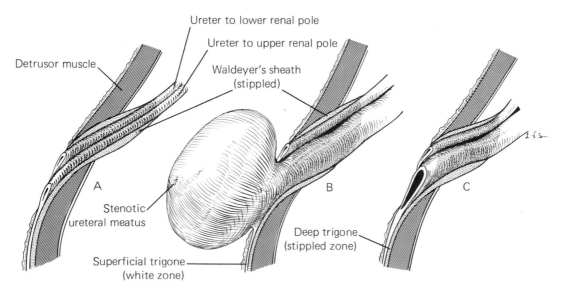

Ureteral and superficial trigonal
muscles are one and the same.

Waldeyer's and deep trigone are stippled
because they are one and the same.

Figure 11—4. Ureteral duplication and ureterocele as causes of vesicoureteral reflux. *A:* Ureteral duplication showing juxtavesical and intravesical ureters encased in common sheath (Waldeyer's). The superior ureter, which always drains the lower renal pole, has a shorter intravesical segment; in addition, it is somewhat devoid of muscle. It therefore tends to allow reflux. *B:* Duplication with ureterocele that always involves caudal ureter which drains upper renal pole. Pinpoint orifice is obstructive, causing hydroureteronephrosis. Resulting wide dilatation of ureter and ureteral hiatus shortens the intravesical segment of the other ureter, often causing it to reflux. *C:* Resection of ureterocele allows reflux into that ureter.

Congenital Causes

A. Trigonal Weakness ("Primary Reflux"): This is by far the most common cause of ureteral regurgitation. It is most often seen in little girls, though it is observed occasionally in boys. Reflux in adults—usually women—probably represents the same congenital defect. Weakness of one side of the trigone leads to decrease in the occlusive pressure in the ipsilateral intravesical ureter. Diffuse ureterotrigonal weakness causes bilateral reflux.

In the normal state, the intravesical ureterotrigonal muscle tone exerts a downward pull whereas the extravesical ureter tends to pull cephalad (Fig 11–3). If trigonal development is deficient, not only is its occlusive power diminished but the ureteral orifice tends to gravitate upward toward the ureteral hiatus. The degree of this retraction relates to the degree of incompetence of the junction. If the ureteral orifice lies over the ureteral hiatus in the bladder wall (so-called golf-hole orifice), it is completely incompetent. The degree of incompetency is judged by the findings on excretory urography and on cystography and the cystoscopic appearance of the ureteral orifices.

B. Ureteral Abnormalities:

1. Complete ureteral duplication—(Fig 11–4.) The intravesical portion of the ureter to the upper renal segment is usually of normal length, whereas that of the ureter to the lower pole is abnormally short; this orifice is commonly incompetent. However, Stephens (1964) has demonstrated that the musculature of the superiorly placed orifice is attenuated, and this further contributes to its weakness.

2. Ectopic ureteral orifice—A single ureter or one of a pair may open well down on the trigone, at the vesical neck, or in the urethra. In this instance, vesicoureteral reflux is the rule. This observation makes it clear that the length of the intravesical ureter is not the sole factor in reflux. Stephens (1964) has observed that such intravesical ureteral segments are usually devoid of smooth muscle. Thus, it has no occlusive force.

3. Ureterocele—A ureterocele involving a single ureter rarely allows reflux, but this lesion usually involves the ureter that drains the upper pole of a duplicated kidney. Since the ureteral orifice is obstructed, the intramural ureter becomes dilated. This increases the diameter of the ureteral hiatus, thus further shortening the intravesical segment of the other ureter, which therefore may become incompetent. Resection of the ureterocele usually causes its ureter to reflux freely as well.

Vesical Trabeculation

Occasionally, a heavily trabeculated bladder may be associated with reflux. The causes include the spastic neurogenic bladder and severe obstruction distal to the bladder. These lesions, however, are associated with trigonal hypertrophy as well; the resultant extra pull on the ureterotrigonal muscle tends to protect the junction from incompetency. In a few such cases, however, the vesical mucosa may protrude through the ureteral hiatus just above the ureter, thus forming a diverticulum or saccule (Fig 11–5). The resulting dilatation of the hiatus shortens the intravesical segment; reflux may then occur.

Edema of the Vesical Wall Secondary to Cystitis

As noted above, valves vary in their degrees of incompetency. A "borderline" junction may not allow reflux when the urine is sterile, but the edema involving the trigone and intravesical ureter associated with cystitis may impair valvular function, in which case

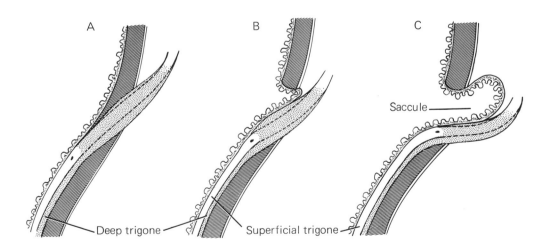

Figure 11–5. The effect of trabeculation of the bladder on the ureterovesical junction. *A:* Trabeculated bladder caused by upper motor neuron lesion or vesical neck obstruction. Normal and competent ureterovesical junction protected from reflux by hypertrophied trigonal muscle. *B:* High intravesical voiding pressure forces a nipple of vesical mucosa into the ureteral hiatus. This has the effect of shortening the intravesical ureter; reflux may occur. *C:* A large saccule or diverticulum may form with complete destruction of valvular action. (Modified from Hutch & Amar: *Vesicoureteral Reflux.* Volume 7, *Encyclopedia of Urology.* Springer, 1968.)

secondary pyelonephritis may ensue. After cure of the infection, cystography again reveals no reflux. It is believed that a completely normal junction will not decompensate even under these circumstances.

It has been shown that pyelonephritis of pregnancy is associated with vesicoureteral reflux. Many of these women give a history of urinary tract infections during childhood. The implication is that they "outgrew" their reflux at puberty but that if bacteriuria becomes established during pregnancy their "borderline" valves may become incompetent. This may be enhanced by the hormones of pregnancy that may contribute to a further loss of tone of the ureterotrigonal complex. After delivery, the reflux is usually no longer demonstrable (Hutch & Amar, 1972).

Eagle-Barrett (Prune Belly) Syndrome

This is a relatively rare condition in which there is failure of normal development of the abdominal muscles and the smooth muscle of the ureters and bladder. Bilateral cryptorchism is the rule. At times, talipes equinovarus and hip dislocation are also noted. Because of deficiency of the smooth muscle of the ureterotrigonal complex, reflux is to be expected; advanced hydroureteronephrosis is therefore found.

Iatrogenic Causes

Certain operative procedures may lead to either temporary or permanent ureteral regurgitation.

A. Prostatectomy: With any type of prostatectomy, the continuity of the superficial trigone is interrupted at the vesical neck. If the proximal trigone moves upward, temporary reflux may occur. This mechanism may account for the high fever (even bacteremia) that is sometimes observed when the catheter is finally removed. Fortunately, in 2–3 weeks the trigone again becomes anchored and reflux ceases.

B. Wedge Resection of the Posterior Vesical Neck: This procedure, often performed in conjunction with plastic revision of the vesical neck for supposed vesical neck stenosis or dysfunction, may also upset trigonal continuity and allow reflux.

C. Ureteral Meatotomy: Ureteral meatotomy occasionally is followed by reflux if it is extensive. Fortunately, however, limited incision of the roof of the intravesical ureter divides few muscle fibers since they have left the roof to join those fibers on the floor. Wide resection in the treatment of vesical neoplasm is often followed by ureteral regurgitation.

D. Resection of Ureterocele: If the ureteral hiatus is widely dilated, this procedure is often followed by reflux.

Contracted Bladder

A bladder that is contracted secondary to interstitial cystitis, tuberculosis, radiotherapy, carcinoma, or schistosomiasis may be associated with ureteral reflux.

COMPLICATIONS OF VESICOURETERAL REFLUX

Vesicoureteral reflux damages the kidney through one or both of 2 mechanisms: (1) pyelonephritis and (2) hydroureteronephrosis.

Pyelonephritis

Vesicoureteral reflux is one of the common contributing factors leading to the development of cystitis, particularly in females. In the presence of vesicoureteral reflux, the bacteria reach the kidney. In the face of reflux, the urinary tract cannot empty itself completely and the infection is perpetuated. (See Pathogenesis, p 141, for a discussion of this phenomenon.)

Hydroureteronephrosis

Some degree of dilatation of the ureter, renal pelvis, and calyces is usually observed in association with reflux. Its degree may be extreme (Fig 11–7). Such changes are often seen in the absence of infection in the male because of the relatively long segment of sterile urethra in that sex. Sterile reflux is less damaging than infected reflux.

Intravesical pressure is transmitted through the incompetent ureteral orifice. This back pressure is quite high at the time of voiding. Furthermore, the ureteropelvic and ureterovesical junctions are less distensible than the rest of the ureter. Either junction may have trouble passing the volume of normal urinary secretion plus the refluxed urine; functional obstruction may result. The common cause of ureteropelvic and ureterovesical "obstruction" is vesicoureteral reflux. Such changes indicate the need for cystography.

THE INCIDENCE OF REFLUX

Incompetency of the ureterovesical junction is an abnormal condition. Peters and others found no reflux in 66 premature infants; Lich and co-workers found none in 26 infants studied during the first 2 days of life. Leadbetter and others noted normal cystograms in 50 adult males. (See Smith, 1970, reference.)

The incidence of vesicoureteral reflux is 50% in children with urinary tract infection but only 8% in adults with bacteriuria. This discrepancy is explained by the fact that the female child usually has pyelonephritis whereas the adult female usually has cystitis only. The concept that bacteriuria implies the presence of pyelonephritis must be condemned.

The fairly competent ("borderline") valve only refluxes during an acute attack of cystitis. Since cystography is only performed in this group after the infection has been eradicated, the incidence of reflux is abnormally low. On the other hand, in patients whose excretory urograms reveal significant changes typical of healed pyelonephritis, reflux is demonstrable in 85%.

When infection associated with reflux occurs during the first few weeks of life, many are septic and uremic. Most are boys who have posterior urethral valves. After the age of 6 months, the female:male ratio of infection with reflux is 10:1.

CLINICAL FINDINGS

A story compatible with acute pyelonephritis implies the presence of vesicoureteral reflux. This is most commonly seen in females, particularly little girls. Persistence of recurrent "cystitis" should suggest the possibility of reflux. Often, in these instances, the patient has an asymptomatic low-grade pyelonephritis.

Symptoms Related to Reflux

A. Symptomatic Pyelonephritis: The usual symptoms in the adult are chills and high fever, renal pain, nausea and vomiting, and symptoms of cystitis. In children, only fever and vague abdominal pains and sometimes diarrhea are apt to be experienced.

B. Asymptomatic Pyelonephritis: The patient may have no symptoms whatsoever. The incidental finding of pyuria and bacteriuria may be the only clue. This merely points up the need for a proper urinalysis in all children.

C. Symptoms of Cystitis Only: In these patients, the bacteriuria is resistant to antimicrobials, or, if bacteriuria clears, relapse quickly occurs. These patients may have reflux with asymptomatic chronic pyelonephritis.

D. Renal Pain on Voiding: Surprisingly, this is a rare complaint in the refluxing patient.

E. Uremia: The last stage of bilateral reflux is uremia due to destruction of the renal parenchyma by hydronephrosis or pyelonephritis (or both). The patient may often adjust to renal insufficiency and may appear quite healthy. Many renal transplants are performed in patients whose kidneys have deteriorated secondarily to reflux and accompanying infection. Early diagnosis, based upon careful urinalysis, would lead to the proper diagnosis in childhood. Progressive pyelonephritis is, with few exceptions, a preventable disease.

F. Hypertension: In the later stages of atrophic pyelonephritis, a significant incidence of hypertension is observed.

Symptoms Related to the Underlying Disease

The clinical picture is often dominated by the signs and symptoms of the primary disease.

A. Urinary Tract Obstruction: The little girl may be noted to have hesitancy in initiating the urinary stream and an impaired or intermittent stream secondary to spasm of the periurethral striated muscle (see Distal Urethral Stenosis, Chapter 28). In males, the

urinary stream may be slow as a result of posterior urethral valves (infants) or prostatic enlargement (men over 50).

B. Spinal Cord Disease: The patient may have a serious neurogenic disease such as paraplegia, quadriplegia, multiple sclerosis, or meningomyelocele. Symptoms may be limited to those of neurogenic bladder: incontinence of urine, urinary retention, and vesical urgency.

Physical Findings

During an attack of acute pyelonephritis, renal tenderness may be elicited. Absence of such a finding does not rule out chronic renal infection.

Palpation and percussion of the suprapubic area may reveal a distended bladder secondary to obstruction or neurogenic disease.

The finding of a hard midline mass deep in the pelvis in a male infant is apt to represent a markedly thickened bladder caused by posterior urethral valves.

Examination may reveal a neurologic deficit compatible with a paretic bladder.

Laboratory Findings

The most common complication, particularly in the female, is infection. Bacteriuria without pyuria is not uncommon. In the male, because of his long, sterile urethra, the urine may be normal.

PSP excretion will be diminished in the face of uremia. The curve, even when renal function is normal, may be "flat" because some of the first half-hour excretion may be refluxed back up to the kidneys; with gross bilateral reflux, the total PSP may be alarmingly low. The serum creatinine may be elevated in the advanced stage of renal damage, but it may be normal even when the degree of reflux and hydronephrosis is marked (Fig 11–7, above right). The PSP test is the superior screening test in this instance.

X-Ray Findings

The plain film may reveal evidence of spina bifida, meningomyelocele, or absence of the sacrum, thus pointing to a neurologic deficit. Even in the face of vesicoureteral reflux, excretory urograms may be normal, but usually one or more of the following clues to the presence of reflux may be noted (Fig 11–6): (1) A persistently dilated lower ureter. (2) Areas of dilatation in the ureter. (3) Ureter visualized throughout its entire length. (4) Presence of hydroureteronephrosis with a narrow juxtavesical ureteral segment. (5) Changes of healed pyelonephritis: calyceal clubbing with narrowed infundibula or cortical thinning.

The presence of ureteral duplication suggests the possibility of reflux into the lower pole of the kidney. In this instance, hydronephrosis or changes compatible with pyelonephritic scarring may be noted. Abnormality of the upper segment of a duplicated system can be caused by the presence of an ectopic ureteral orifice with reflux or by obstruction secondary to a ureterocele.

Reflux is diagnosed by demonstrating its exist-

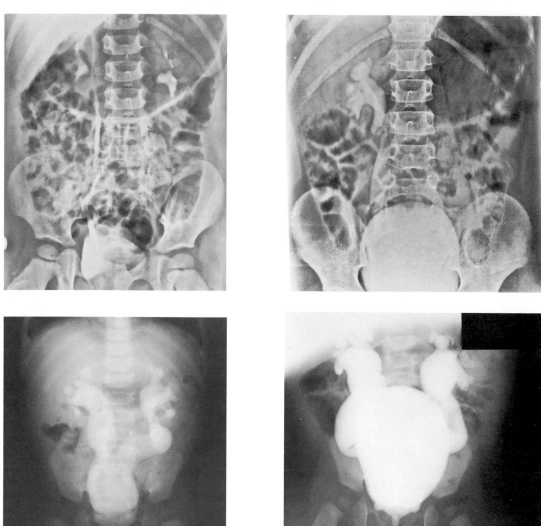

Figure 11–6. Excretory urogram with changes that imply right vesicoureteral reflux. *Top left:* Excretory urogram showing normal right urogram and a ureter which is mildly dilated and remains full through its entire length. The ureteral change implies reflux. *Top right:* Cystogram demonstrates the reflux. Note, now, the degree of dilatation of the ureter, pelvis, and calyces. *Bottom left:* Excretory urogram shows bilateral ureterohydronephrosis with pyelonephritic scarring. These findings imply the presence of reflux. *Bottom right:* Voiding cystourethrogram. Free reflux bilaterally.

ence with one of the following technics: simple or delayed cystography, voiding cystourethrography, or voiding cinefluoroscopy. A radionuclide technic can be used. One mCi of ^{99m}Tc is instilled into the bladder along with sterile solution. The gamma camera will reveal ureteral reflux.

Amar (1966) has shown that reflux can be demonstrated by filling the bladder with sterile water containing 5 ml of indigo carmine per 100 ml. The patient then voids. The bladder is thoroughly flushed out with sterile water. The ureteral orifices are viewed cystoscopically for blue-tinged efflux. This technic protects the patient from radiation exposure, and its efficiency is equal to that of voiding cystourethrography. In general, reflux that is demonstrated only with voiding implies a more competent valve than that which allows low-pressure regurgitation. As has been pointed out, failure to demonstrate reflux on one study does not rule out intermittent reflux.

The voiding phase of the cystogram may reveal changes compatible with distal urethral stenosis with secondary spasm of the voluntary periurethral muscles in the female child (Fig 28–1) or changes in the small boy that are diagnostic of posterior urethral valves.

Instrumental Examination

A. Urethral Calibration: In females, urethral calibration, using bougies à boule, should be done. Distal urethral stenosis is almost routinely found in little girls suffering from urinary infection. Destruction of the

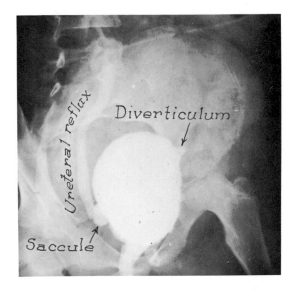

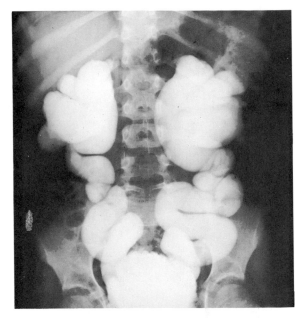

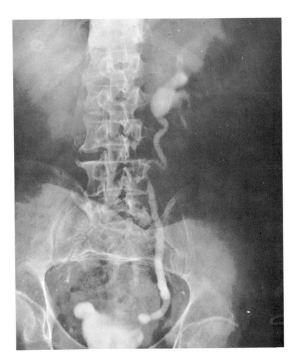

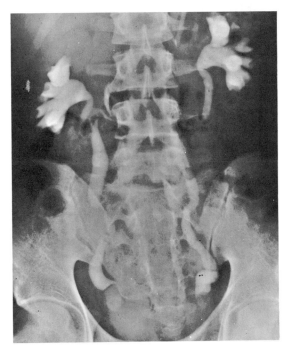

Figure 11–7. Cystograms revealing vesicoureteral reflux. *Above left:* Saccule at right ureterovesical junction. *Above right:* Meningomyelocele. Reflux with severe bilateral ureterohydronephrosis; serum creatinine, 0.6 mg/100 ml; PSP excretion, 5% in 1 hour. *Below left:* Postprostatectomy patient with reflux on left and bilateral saccules. *Below right:* Ten-year-old boy with meningomyelocele. Bladder has been emptied. Impairment of drainage at ureterovesical junctions is demonstrated. (Courtesy of JA Hutch.)

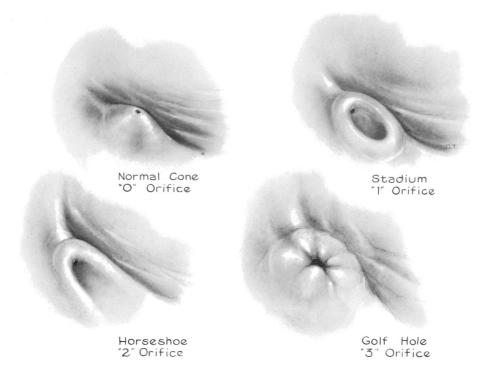

Normal Cone
"O" Orifice

Stadium
"I" Orifice

Horseshoe
"2" Orifice

Golf Hole
"3" Orifice

Figure 11—8. Cystoscopic appearance of the normal ureteral orifice and three degrees of incompetency of the ureterovesical junction. (Reproduced, with permission, from Lyon, Marshall, & Tanagho: The ureteral orifice: Its configuration and competency. J Urol 102:504, 1969.)

ring is an important step in improving the hydrodynamics of voiding: lowered intravesical voiding pressure and the abolition of vesical residual urine (see Chapter 28). Less commonly, urethral stenosis is discovered in the adult female. It, too, should be treated.

B. Cystoscopy: Most little girls with reflux have smooth-walled or only slightly trabeculated bladders. Evidence of chronic cystitis may be noted. Ureteral duplication may be seen. A ureterocele may be evident. An orifice may be found to be ectopic at the bladder neck or even in the urethra. As the bladder is filled, a small diverticulum may form on the roof of the ureteral orifice (Fig 11—5). These findings imply the possibility of reflux. The major contribution of cystoscopy is to allow study of the morphology of the ureteral orifice and its position in relation to the vesical neck (Fig 11—8).

1. Morphology—The normal ureter has the appearance of a volcanic cone. The orifice of a slightly weaker valve looks like a football stadium; an even weaker one has the appearance of a horseshoe with its open end pointing toward the vesical neck. The completely incompetent junction has a "golf-hole" orifice which lies over the ureteral hiatus.

2. Position—By and large, the more defective the appearance of the ureteral orifice, the farther from the vesical neck it lies. The degree of retraction of the orifice reflects the degree of ureterotrigonal deficiency.

DIFFERENTIAL DIAGNOSIS

Functional (nonocclusive) vesicoureteral obstruction may cause changes similar to those suggesting the presence of reflux on excretory urography. Multiple cystograms fail to show reflux. Tanagho and others (1970) have shown that this congenital obstruction is due to a heavy layer of circularly oriented smooth muscle fibers surrounding the ureter at this point. Its action is sphincteric.

Significant obstruction distal to the vesical neck leads to hypertrophy of both the detrusor and trigonal muscles. The latter exert an exaggerated pull upon the intravesical ureter, thus causing functional obstruction (see Tanagho & Meyers, 1965). Ureterohydronephrosis is therefore to be expected; vesicoureteral reflux is uncommon.

Other lesions that may cause ureterohydronephrosis without reflux include low ureteral stone, ureteral occlusion by cervical or prostatic cancer, urinary tract tuberculosis, and schistosomiasis.

TREATMENT

It is impossible to give a concise and definitive discourse on the treatment of vesicoureteral reflux because of the many factors involved and because there is no unanimity of opinion among urologists on this subject. In general, probably more than half of children with primary reflux can be controlled by nonsurgical means and the rest will require some form of operative procedure. Adults exhibiting reflux will usually require vesicoureteroplasty.

Medical Treatment

A. Indications: The child with primary reflux (attenuated trigone) who has fairly normal upper tracts on urographic study and whose ureterovesical valves on cystoscopy appear fair to good has an excellent chance of "outgrowing" the defect, particularly if cystograms show only transient or "high-pressure" reflux.

The male child with posterior urethral valves may cease to reflux once these valves are destroyed.

The adult female who occasionally develops acute pyelonephritis following intercourse but whose urine quickly clears on antimicrobial therapy will probably be controlled if she takes steps to prevent vesical infections (see Treatment, p 163). This is particularly true if, when her urine is sterile, reflux cannot be demonstrated on cystography. The maintenance of sterile urine will allow her "borderline" valve to remain competent.

B. Methods of Treatment: Destruction of the ring of distal urethral stenosis in little girls, or posterior urethral valves in boys, has an excellent chance of reducing voiding intravesical pressure, abolishing vesical residual urine and reflux.

Definitive treatment of the urinary infection with bactericidal drugs should be given, followed by chronic suppressive therapy for 6 months or more.

Triple voiding. Since vesicoureteral reflux prevents the urinary tract from emptying itself completely, thus destroying the vesical defense mechanism, triple voiding once a day is helpful if the child is old enough to be trained. When reflux is present, the bladder empties itself on voiding, but some urine ascends to the kidneys and then returns to the bladder. Voiding again a few minutes later will push less urine into the ureters. A third voiding will usually completely empty the urinary tract. Thus, the patient's own natural resistance can operate to a maximum degree.

Children with reflux often have thin-walled bladders and do not perceive the normal urge to void when the bladder is full. Further detrusor tone is lost with overfilling, thus contributing to residual urine. Such children should "void by the clock" every 3–4 hours whether they have the urge or not. Vesical residual urine may then be minimized.

The infant female with markedly dilated upper urinary tracts may be tided over by means of an indwelling urethral catheter. Over a period of months, the ureteral dilatation and elongation may regress; renal function is protected. At a convenient and strategic time, more definitive therapy can then be accomplished.

C. Evaluation of Success of Medical Treatment:

Urinalysis should be done at least once a month for a year or more. Maintenance of sterile urine is an encouraging sign.

Cystograms should be repeated every 4–6 months, hoping for disappearance of the reflux. Excretory urography should be ordered at 6 and 12 months to be sure that renal deterioration does not occur.

About half of children with reflux will be successfully cured by medical means.

Surgical Treatment

A. Indications: Reflux caused by the following abnormalities will not disappear spontaneously: (1) ectopic ureteral orifice, (2) ureteral duplication, (3) ureterocele associated with ureteral duplication and reflux into the uninvolved ureter, (4) "golf-hole" ureteral orifice, and (5) low-pressure reflux with significant hydroureteronephrosis.

Surgery is indicated (1) if it is not possible to keep the urine sterile and reflux persists; (2) if acute pyelonephritis recurs despite a strict medical regimen and chronic suppressive antimicrobial therapy; (3) if there is increased renal damage as portrayed by serial excretory urograms; or (4) if reflux persists for 1 year after institution of therapy.

B. Types of Surgical Therapy: Surgical treatment may require preliminary urinary diversion to improve renal function and to allow dilated ureters to regain tone. Later, definitive relief of obstruction (eg, posterior urethral valves) and ureterovesicoplasty can be performed at the optimum time. Some patients with irreversible lesions causing reflux (eg, meningomyelocele) or badly damaged and atonic ureters may require permanent diversion of the urine (ie, ureteroileocutaneous anastomosis).

1. Temporary urinary diversion—If drainage of refluxed urine into the bladder is free, cystostomy (or an indwelling urethral catheter in girls) may prove helpful. If the ureters are dilated and kinked, a redundant loop can be brought to the skin. The ureter is opened at this point and urine collected into an ileostomy bag. Later, the loop can be resected and its ends anastomosed. Ureteral reimplantation can then be done. Nephrostomy may be necessary if ureteral redundancy is absent.

2. Permanent urinary diversion—If it is felt that successful ureterovesicoplasty cannot be accomplished, a Bricker type of diversion is indicated. If renal function is poor and the ureters are widely dilated and atonic, uretero-cutaneous diversion may be the procedure of choice.

3. Other surgical procedures—

a. If reflux is unilateral and the kidney badly damaged and the other kidney is normal, nephrectomy is indicated.

b. If one renal pole of a duplicated system is essentially functionless, heminephrectomy with removal of its entire ureter should be done. If there is moderate hydronephrosis of one renal pole with duplication, an alternative is anastomosis of the dilated ureter or pelvis to the normal ureter or pelvis. The remainder of the dilated refluxing ureter should be removed.

c. In the face of unilateral reflux, anastomosis of the lower end of the refluxing ureter into the side of its normal mate (transuretero-ureterostomy) has a few proponents.

4. Definitive repair.

Definitive Repair of Ureterovesical Junction (Ureterovesicoplasty)

A. **Principles of Repair**: (Tanagho, 1970.)

1. Resect the lower 2—3 cm of the ureter whose muscle is underdeveloped.

2. Free up enough extravesical ureter so that an intravesical segment 2.5 cm long can be formed.

3. Place the intravesical ureter in a submucosal position.

4. Suture the wall of the new ureteral orifice to the cut edge of the trigonal muscle.

B. **Types of Operation**: The following procedures satisfy the above principles and have afforded success in a high percentage of cases: The advancement operation (Hutch, 1963; Glenn and Anderson, 1967), and the Politano-Leadbetter (1958) and the Paquin (1959) operations.

If the ureters are unduly tortuous, the redundant portions must be resected. If widely dilated, their lower ends must be tailored to a more normal size.

C. **Results of Ureterovesicoplasty**: About 93% of patients no longer show reflux after uretero-vesicoplasty. About 3% develop ureterovesical stenosis which requires reoperation. At least 75% will have and maintain sterile urine without antimicrobials 3—6 months after surgery. Many patients in whom bacteriuria persists have cystitis only. Febrile attacks cease. This has been demonstrated by finding that the renal urines collected by ureteral catheters are sterile. These are impressive results considering that only the most severe and advanced cases are submitted to surgical repair, and they exceed by far the cure rates reported when only antimicrobials are used (10—15%). This operation is rightly considered one of the most significant accomplishments of modern urology.

PROGNOSIS

In patients with reflux who are judged to have fairly competent valves, conservative therapy as outlined above is highly successful in the cure of the reflux and therefore infection.

Patients with very incompetent ureterovesical valves subjected to surgical repair also have an excellent prognosis. A few children, however, have such badly damaged urinary tracts when finally submitted to diagnostic procedures that little help other than permanent urinary diversion can be offered.

•   •   •

References

Amar AD: Cystoscopic demonstration of vesicoureteral reflux: Evaluation in 250 patients. J Urol 95:776, 1966.

Amar AD: Reimplantation of completely duplicated ureters. J Urol 107:230, 1972.

Amar AD: Vesicoureteral reflux associated with congenital bladder diverticulum in boys and young men. J Urol 107:966, 1972.

Amar AD: Vesicoureteral reflux in adults: A 12-year study of 122 patients. Urology 3:184, 1974.

Amar AD, Singer B: Vesicoureteral reflux: A 10-year study of 280 patients. J Urol 109:999, 1973.

Arap S & others: The extra-vesical antireflux plasty. Urol Internat 26:241, 1971.

Bischoff PF: Problems in treatment of vesicoureteral reflux. J Urol 107:133, 1972.

Burkholder GV, Harper RC, Beach PD: Congenital absence of the abdominal muscles. Am J Clin Path 53:602, 1970.

Burko H, Rhamy RK: Lower urinary tract problems related to infection: Diagnosis and treatment. P Clin North America 17:233, 1970.

Carter TC, Tomskey GC, Ozog LS: Prune-belly syndrome: Review of 10 cases. Urology 3:279, 1974.

Cattolica EV: Renal scarring and primary reflux in adults. Urology 4:397, 1974.

Conway JJ & others: Detection of vesicoureteral reflux with radionuclide cystography: A comparison study with roentgenographic cystography. Am J Roentgenol 115:720, 1972.

Cremin BJ: The urinary tract anomalies associated with agenesis of the abdominal walls. Brit J Radiol 44:767, 1971.

Devine PC & others: Vesicoureteral reflux in children: Indications for surgical and nonsurgical treatment. Urology 3:315, 1974.

Fair WR & others: Urinary tract infections in children. 1. Young girls with non-refluxing ureters. Western J Med 121:366, 1974.

Fehrenbaker LG, Kelalis PP, Stickler GB: Vesicoureteral reflux and ureteral duplication in children. J Urol 107:862, 1972.

Filly RA & others: Urinary tract infections in children. 2. Roentgenologic aspects. Western J Med 121:374, 1974.

Garrett RA, Schlueter DP: Complications of antireflux operations: Causes and management. J Urol 109:1002, 1973.

Geist RW, Antolak SJ Jr: The clinical problems of children with sterile ureteral reflux. J Urol 108:343, 1972.

Glenn JF, Anderson EE: Distal tunnel ureteral reimplantation. J Urol 97:623, 1967.

Gonzales ET, Leitner WA, Glenn JF: An analysis of various modes of therapy for vesicoureteral reflux. Internat Urol Nephrol 4:235, 1972.

Govan DE & others: Urinary tract infections in children: 3. Treatment of ureterovesical reflux. Western J Med 121:382, 1974.

Haran PJ, Darling DB, Fisher JH: The excretory urogram in

children with ureterorenal reflux. Am J Roentgenol 99:585, 1967.

Harley LM, Chen Y, Rattner WH: Prune belly syndrome. J Urol 108:174, 1972.

Hendren WH: Complications of megaureter repair in children. J Urol 113:228, 1975.

Hendren WH: Reoperation for the failed ureteral reimplantation. J Urol 111:403, 1974.

Hodson CJ: The radiological contribution toward the diagnosis of chronic pyelonephritis. Radiology 88:857, 1967.

Hutch JA: The mesodermal component: Its embryology, anatomy, physiology and role in prevention of vesicoureteral reflux. J Urol 108:406, 1972.

Hutch JA: Ureteric advancement operation: Anatomy, technique, and early results. J Urol 89:180, 1963.

Hutch JA, Amar AD: *Vesicoureteral Reflux and Pyelonephritis*. Appleton-Century-Crofts, 1972.

Hutch JA, Smith DR, Osborne R: Review of a series of ureterovesicoplasties. J Urol 100:285, 1968.

Kogan SJ, Freed SZ: Postoperative course of vesicoureteral reflux associated with benign obstructive prostatic disease. J Urol 112:322, 1974.

Leadbetter GW Jr: Skin ureterostomy with subsequent ureteral reconstruction. J Urol 107:462, 1972.

Lome LG, Williams DI: Urinary reconstruction following temporary cutaneous ureterostomy diversion in children. J Urol 108:162, 1972.

Lyon RP, Marshall S, Tanagho EA: The ureteral orifice: Its configuration and competency. J Urol 102:504, 1969.

Lyon RP: Renal arrest. J Urol 109:707, 1973.

Lytton B, Weiss RM, Berneike RR: Ipsilateral ureteroureterostomy in the management of vesicoureteral reflux in duplication of the upper urinary tract. J Urol 105:507, 1971.

MacGregor M: Pyelonephritis lenta: Consideration of childhood urinary infection as the forerunner of renal insufficiency in later life. Arch Dis Childhood 45:159, 1970.

Miller HC, Caspari EW: Ureteral reflux as genetic trait. JAMA 220:842, 1972.

Moore CCM: Vesicoureteral reflux in childhood. MJ Australia, 1: 569, 1974.

Mounger EJ, Scott EVZ: Surgical correction of vesicoureteral reflux. J Urol 108:347, 1972.

Paquin AJ Jr: Ureterovesical anastomosis: The description and evaluation of a technique. J Urol 82:573, 1959.

Politano VA, Leadbetter WF: An operative technique for correction of vesicoureteral reflux. J Urol 79:932, 1958.

Rees RWM: The effect of transurethral resection of the intravesical ureter during the removal of bladder tumours. Brit J Urol 41:2, 1969.

Rolleston GL, Maling TMJ, Hodson CJ: Intrarenal reflux and the scarred kidney. Arch Dis Childhood 49:531, 1974.

Rose JS, Glassberg KI, Waterhouse K: Intrarenal reflux and its relationship to renal scarring. J Urol 113:400, 1975.

Sala NL, Rubi RA: Ureteral function in pregnant women. 5. Incidence of vesicoureteral reflux and its effect upon ureteral contractility. Am J Obst Gynec 112:871, 1972.

Salvatierra O Jr, Kountz SL, Belzer FO: Primary vesicoureteral reflux and end-stage renal disease. JAMA 226:1454, 1973.

Savage DCL & others: Covert bacteriuria of childhood: A clinical and epidemiological study. Arch Dis Childhood 43:8, 1973.

Schmidt JD & others: Vesicoureteral reflux: An inherited lesion. JAMA 220:821, 1972.

Servadio C, Nissenkorn I, Baron J: Radioisotope cystography using ^{99m}Tc sulfur colloid for the detection and study of vesicoureteral reflux. J Urol 111:750, 1974.

Siegel SR, Sokoloff B, Siegel B: Asymptomatic and symptomatic urinary tract infection in infancy. Am J Dis Child 125:45, 1973.

Smith DR: Vesicoureteral reflux and other abnormalities of the ureterovesical junction. Chapter 10 in: *Urology*, 3rd ed. Campbell MF, Harrison JH (editors). Saunders, 1970.

Stephens FD: Intramural ureter and ureterocele. Postgrad MJ 40:179, 1964.

Stephens FD: Treatment of megaloureters by multiple micturition. Australian New Zealand J Surg 27:130, 1957.

Stickler GB & others: Primary interstitial nephritis with reflux: A cause of hypertension. Am J Dis Child 122:144, 1971.

Tanagho EA: Surgical revision of the incompetent ureterovesical junction: A critical analysis of techniques and requirements. Brit J Urol 42:410, 1970.

Tanagho EA: Ureteral tailoring. J Urol 106:194, 1971.

Tanagho EA, Guthrie TH, Lyon RP: The intravesical ureter in primary reflux. J Urol 101:824, 1969.

Tanagho EA, Hutch JA, Miller ER: Diagnostic procedures and cinefluoroscopy in vesicoureteral reflux. Brit J Urol 38:435, 1966.

Tanagho EA, Meyers FH: Trigonal hypertrophy: A cause of ureteral obstruction. J Urol 93:678, 1965.

Tanagho EA, Pugh RCB: The anatomy and function of the ureterovesical junction. Brit J Urol 35:151, 1963.

Tanagho EA, Smith DR, Guthrie TH: Pathophysiology of functional ureteral obstruction. J Urol 104:73, 1970.

Tanagho EA & others: Primary vesicoureteral reflux: Experimental studies of its etiology. J Urol 93:165, 1965.

Timothy RP, Decter A, Perlmutter AD: Ureteral duplication: Clinical findings and therapy in 46 children. J Urol 105:445, 1971.

Udall DA & others: Transureteroureterostomy. Urology 2:401, 1973.

Urinary tract infection in newborn. Brit MJ 3:542, 1972.

Waldbaum RS, Marshall VF: The prune belly syndrome: A diagnostic therapeutic plan. J Urol 103: 668, 1970.

Warren MM, Kelalis PP, Stickler GB: Unilateral ureteroneocystostomy: The fate of the contralateral ureter. J Urol 107:466, 1972.

Weber AL, Weylman WT: Evaluation of vesicoureteral reflux by intravenous pyelography and cinecystography. Radiology 87:489, 1966.

Welch KJ, Kearney GP: Abdominal muscular deficiency syndrome: Prune belly. J Urol 111:693, 1974.

Williams DI: The natural history of reflux. Urol Internat 26:350, 1971.

Williams GL & others: Vesicoureteric reflux in patients with bacteriuria in pregnancy. Lancet 2:1202, 1968.

Zel G, Retik AB: Familial vesicoureteral reflux. Urology 2:249, 1973.

12...
Nonspecific Infections of the Urinary Tract

The "nonspecific" infections of the genitourinary tract are a group of diseases having similar manifestations and caused by the gram-negative rods (eg, *Escherichia coli, Proteus vulgaris*) and gram-positive cocci (staphylococci and streptococci). They are to be distinguished from infections caused by "specific" organisms, each of which causes a clinically unique disease (eg, tuberculosis, gonorrhea, actinomycosis). In acute infections, a single organism is usually found; mixed infections are often seen in chronic stages.

By far the most common invaders are the gram-negative bacteria, particularly *E coli*. Others in this group are *Enterobacter aerogenes, Proteus vulgaris* and *P mirabilis,* and *Pseudomonas aeruginosa. Streptococcus faecalis* and *Staphylococcus aureus* are found on occasion. A pure coccal infection may suggest renal stone.

These infections can involve any of the urinary organs (or genital organs in the male) and can spread from a given locus to any or all of the others. Renal infections are of the greatest importance because of the parenchymal destruction caused by them.

Identification of the type of bacteria (ie, rods or cocci) may be important in the empirical selection of medication.

PATHOGENESIS

Four Main Pathways of Entry Into the Urinary Tract

It is not always possible to trace the mode of entry of bacteria into the genitourinary tract. There are 4 major possibilities.

A. Ascending Infection: There is increasing evidence that ascending infection is the most common cause of urinary tract infection. The incidence of urinary infection—judged by age group and sex—permits certain inferences. Urosepsis is common from birth to age 10. At least 80% of these affect the female, and the incidence of pyelonephritis is relatively high. New infections are seldom seen from this age until age 20, at which time urinary infection again becomes common. Again, the great majority affect women, and the incidence parallels the years of sexual activity. This high incidence appears to be related to the short urethra of the female, which often harbors urinary pathogens which migrate from the perineum to the vaginal vestibule. Most of these infections involve the bladder only. At age 60 and beyond, the incidence of infection again increases; and because bladder neck obstruction and the inevitable vesical residual urine commonly affect males of this age, most of these patients are men. Secondary pyelonephritis in this latter group is uncommon.

These data strongly support the inference that the most common route of infection is up the urethra, particularly in the female. Pyelonephritis is quite common in very young people and is usually associated with demonstrable vesicoureteral reflux. Infection in older men is usually secondary to prostatitis or obstruction with or without reflux.

B. Hematogenous Spread: This is an uncommon pathway of bacterial invasion of the kidneys, prostate, and testes. During the course of many infections elsewhere in the body, bacteria are apt to enter the bloodstream; in fact, this may occur in a healthy person. These invaders are usually destroyed by normal body processes; however, if the number of bacteria is great, if they are virulent, and particularly if the field is receptive (eg, renal stone), infection of the genitourinary tract may occur. In experimental animals, intravenous injection of urinary pathogens only leads to pyelonephritis if the ureter is temporarily obstructed or the kidney traumatized. It seems conceivable that ureteral or ureteropelvic obstruction or vesicoureteral reflux could prepare the ground for hematogenous pyelonephritis by this mechanism.

The most obvious examples of renal infection via hematogenous invasion are tuberculosis (metastatic from the lungs) and renal carbuncle (metastatic from skin infection). Conversely, in the course of acute infections of the kidney or prostate, bacteria often enter the bloodstream.

C. Lymphogenous Spread: There is firm evidence that infection can spread to the urinary tract through the lymphatic channels, but this probably occurs rarely. A few investigators believe that infections spread from the large bowel to the urinary tract through the lymphatics. Others think that cervicitis may cause vesical or renal infection by the spread of bacteria via the periureteral lymph vessels. Bloodstream infections of lymphatic origin are also a theoretical possibility.

D. Direct Extension From Another Organ: Intraperitoneal abscesses (appendiceal abscess, diverticulitis of the sigmoid) may involve and infect the urinary organs (bladder).

Factors Contributing to Infection

Other factors which contribute to the establishment of bacteria in the genitourinary organs include the following:

A. Stasis and Obstruction: Bacteria are better able to gain a foothold if there is stasis or obstruction as seen with distal urethral stenosis in little girls, enlarged prostate, and vesicoureteral reflux. Under these circumstances, pathogenic urethral bacteria ascending to the bladder become established in the bladder because the vesical defense mechanism is made inoperative by the presence of vesical residual urine.

Constipation in children has been related to urinary tract infection of both sexes (Neumann & others). Many have great difficulty voiding. When the constipation is relieved, most of the children cease having infections.

B. Presence of a Foreign Body: A kidney containing a stone is apt to become infected even in the absence of obstruction. A foreign body introduced into the bladder (eg, indwelling catheter) will lead to infection. Such objects seem to lower the normal resistance to successful invasion by bacteria.

C. General Body Resistance: Resistance may be lowered in the course of debilitating illnesses and during periods of chronic or excessive fatigue, in which case infection gains a foothold more easily. Diabetes predisposes to urinary infection.

Organs & Pathways of Infection Within the Urinary Tract (Fig 12–1)

A. Kidney: It is becoming increasingly clear that the most common cause of renal infection is vesicoureteral reflux. Reflux is found in association with most instances of atrophic pyelonephritis. Hematogenous invasion is a rare route of infection.

B. Bladder: The bladder may become involved by bacteria descending from the kidney or, more commonly, ascending from the urethra or prostate. Direct bloodstream invasion of the bladder is undoubtedly rare. Lymphogenous spread from cervical or uterine infection seems possible. Infections of the bowel may spread to the bladder by contiguity (diverticulitis of the sigmoid colon).

C. Prostate: The prostate is most commonly infected by ascent of the urethral flora, whose numbers are increased in urethritis. Hematogenous invasion is a possibility.

D. Urethra: The urethra in both sexes usually becomes infected by ascending bacteria. These infections are usually nonvenereal. Deep ascent of these bacteria may cause cystitis and, if there is ureteral reflux, pyelonephritis. Infection may also descend to the urethra from prostate or bladder.

E. Epididymis: Infection usually reaches the epididymis by descent (reflux of urine) along the vas or the perivasal lymphatics from an infected prostate.

F. Testis: The testis is commonly invaded hematogenously by bacteria (pneumococci, brucellae, etc) or viruses (mumps, etc). Occasionally it becomes infected by direct extension from epididymal inflammation (both tuberculous and nonspecific).

Relation of Symptoms to Onset of Infection

If lower tract symptoms precede the onset of chills, fever, and renal pain, a primary (ascending) urologic infection is probably present. In this instance, vesicoureteral reflux should be suspected. If, however, the systemic symptoms precede the complaints referable to the lower urinary tract, metastatic infection or spread from some other area of infection may have occurred. In the latter instance, the extraurologic focus must be identified if possible.

Correlation of Factors that Cause & Perpetuate Urinary Tract Infections

The cause of urinary tract infections and their perpetuation can now be explained on a scientific basis. With few exceptions, the offending organism ascends the urethra and gains a foothold in the presence of vesical residual urine. The complication of pyelonephritis implies incompetency of the ureterovesical junction.

A. Source of Bacteria: Years ago, Helmholz showed that, with few exceptions, bacteria are found in significant numbers only in the distal 3–4 cm of the male urethra. Furthermore, it is unusual to find urinary pathogens in the male urethra. It is for these reasons that bladder or kidney infection develops late or not at all in males even in the presence of significant vesical residual urine (posterior urethral valves, enlarged prostate). It may be that anything that slows the voiding flow rate might allow further ascent of bacteria in males so that the organisms finally reach the bladder.

In the female, however, the short urethra presents an entirely different problem. Cox and co-workers studied the urethral flora in women. In those without a history of urinary tract infections, 50% had bacteria in the proximal one-fourth of the urethra; of these bacteria, 27% were urinary pathogens. These organisms have their source in the perineum. In a group of women suffering from recurrent infections, 77% had bacteria in the proximal 1 cm of the urethra and 55% of the organisms were pathogenic to the urinary tract. Unfortunately, successful eradication of the urinary infection is not accompanied by sterilization of the urethra. The same organism may remain, in which case the next infection is caused by that bacterium; or a new pathogen may become established and cause a new infection.

These findings readily explain the common but mistaken observation that urinary infections are "difficult to cure." Infection usually is eradicated, but new infections develop in a high percentage of cases (Turck & others). Certainly, a new organism represents a new

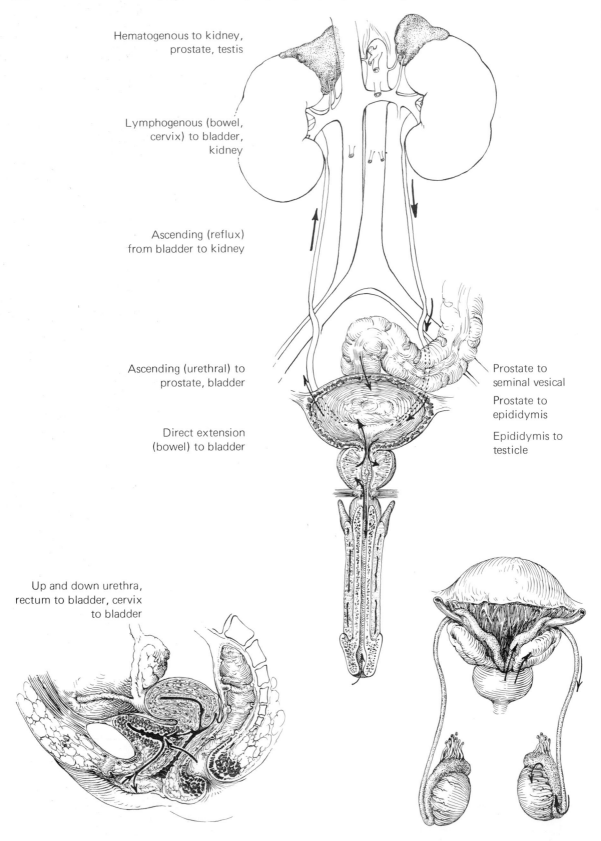

Hematogenous to kidney, prostate, testis

Lymphogenous (bowel, cervix) to bladder, kidney

Ascending (reflux) from bladder to kidney

Ascending (urethral) to prostate, bladder

Direct extension (bowel) to bladder

Prostate to seminal vesical

Prostate to epididymis

Epididymis to testicle

Up and down urethra, rectum to bladder, cervix to bladder

Figure 12—1. Routes of infection in the genitourinary tract.

infection, but the reappearance of the same bacterium does not necessarily imply relapse. The nature of the urethral flora governs the bacteriologic findings in the urine. Measures to correct vesical outlet obstruction (posterior urethral valves, distal urethral stenosis in little girls) usually stop recurrent urinary infection, but the pathogenic urethral bacteria are still present.

We may say, then, that with few exceptions the bacteria infecting the bladder ascend from the urethra.

B. The Vesical Defense Mechanism: Clinical experience demonstrates that the bladder has an intrinsic defense against bacteria. It is impossible to pass a catheter to the bladder without carrying bacteria into the bladder, but cystitis secondary to this procedure is rare unless there is vesical residual urine. Cox and Hinman (Hinman, 1968) showed that, though significant numbers of bacteria were introduced into the bladders of normal young men by catheter, all had sterile urine within 72 hours without the use of antimicrobials. A similar observation was made in a group of women who required indwelling catheters for some days following certain gynecologic operations. Without the use of antimicrobials, their urine became sterile spontaneously. They were able to show experimentally that a bladder that completely empties itself seldom becomes infected. Complete voiding washes out most of the bacteria. Those few left in a film of urine on the vesical mucosa are killed. The implication is that the mucosa represents the intrinsic vesical defense mechanism against bacteria.

C. Factors Causing Perpetuation of Urinary Infection: The urinary tract that completely empties itself at the time of voiding tends to remain sterile even though bacteria ascend to the bladder. If, however, there is some urologic abnormality which defeats this normal mechanism, the bacteria not only gain a foothold but the infection is perpetuated.

1. Vesical residual urine—Any defect that causes residual urine contributes to persistence of infection. Such diseases include neurogenic bladder, urethral obstruction, enlarged prostate, and cystocele. Although drugs may fail to keep the urine sterile, correcting the urologic disease will often cause the urine to clear spontaneously. If it does not, antimicrobials will then usually bring about cure.

2. Foreign bodies in the bladder—Even though meticulous hygiene and antibiotic coverage are practiced when an indwelling catheter is in place, after 10–21 days bacteriuria is almost always found. It cannot be eradicated until the catheter is removed. Following certain gynecologic operations, it has been customary to leave a urethral catheter in place for 3–10 days, and infection in such cases was almost inevitable. Recently, enthusiasm has developed for draining the bladder suprapubically with a small (8–10F) plastic catheter. The majority do not become infected, and spontaneous sterilization of the urine occurs on removal of the catheter. The remaining 10% respond promptly to antimicrobials. The presence of a stone in the bladder will cause infection to persist.

3. Vesicoureteral reflux—At the time of voiding,

in the presence of vesicoureteral reflux, the bladder usually empties itself completely but some urine is forced into the ureter and kidney. Within a few minutes after voiding, this urine drains back to the bladder; in essence, the patient has not emptied the bladder. This defeats the vesical defense mechanism.

4. Urethrovesical reflux—In a child who suffers from spasm of the external periurethral sphincter caused by distal urethral stenosis (Tanagho & Miller), the proximal urethra becomes distended with voiding. The turbulent flow of urine in this segment washes urinary pathogens back into the bladder, which never quite empties itself (Hinman, 1966). Cystitis supervenes. In some adult women, periodic spasm of the external sphincter occurs as a result of anxiety or tension. This, too, may cause urethral bacteria to ascend to the bladder.

5. Residual urine in the upper urinary tract—Any disease causing retention of urine in the renal pelvis (ureteral stone, ureteropelvic junction obstruction) will perpetuate infection once it gains a foothold.

6. Foreign bodies in the kidney—Once renal infection ensues, the presence of a stone will tend to defeat efforts to sterilize the urine.

NONSPECIFIC INFECTIONS OF THE KIDNEYS

ACUTE PYELONEPHRITIS

The term "pyelonephritis" is used because infections of the renal pelvis alone ("pyelitis") do not occur; however, it is the "nephritis" that is important.

Bacteria can reach the kidney through the bloodstream, or they may travel up a ureter which has an incompetent ureterovesical valve. The latter mechanism is by far the most common. It has been shown that vesicoureteral reflux may occur during acute cystitis but ceases when the infection has been cured. This explains the onset of secondary pyelonephritis. If obstruction, reflux, or stasis is present, the chances for the bacteria to gain a foothold are increased. These factors also tend to perpetuate the infection.

One-third of pregnant women with pyelonephritis will exhibit reflux. After termination of the pregnancy, reflux disappears. It is for this reason that the not uncommon bacteriuria seen in pregnancy (6% incidence) is potentially dangerous.

Pathology

A. Gross: The kidney may be greatly enlarged as a result of edema. The surface may be dull. On cut section, the sharp demarcation between cortex and medulla is lost; multiple small abscesses may be visible. The pelvic mucosa is often injected and roughened.

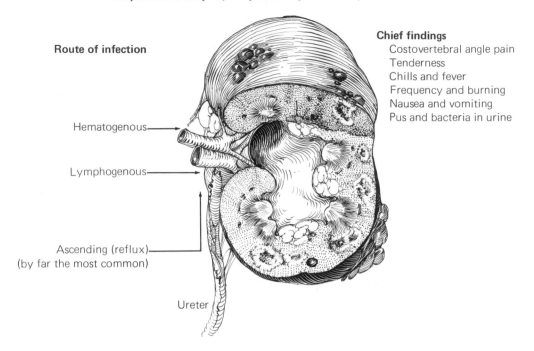

Route of infection

Hematogenous——

Lymphogenous——

Ascending (reflux)——
(by far the most common)

Ureter

Chief findings
Costovertebral angle pain
Tenderness
Chills and fever
Frequency and burning
Nausea and vomiting
Pus and bacteria in urine

Figure 12—2. Pathogenesis of acute pyelonephritis.

B. Microscopic: There is diffuse or spotty inflammation characterized by leukocytic infiltration, edema, and small hemorrhagic areas. The tubular epithelium may desquamate if the infection is severe. The glomeruli are much less involved; in fact, they are peculiarly immune to inflammatory change except in the most severe cases.

Pathogenesis (Fig 12—2)

With few exceptions, acute pyelonephritis develops from infection in the bladder through the mechanism of vesicoureteral reflux. If the ureterovesical junction, anatomically and physiologically, is of "borderline" quality, cure of the infection will cause the "valve" to revert to competency; a cystogram taken at this time will fail to reveal reflux. When the junction is grossly abnormal, response to antimicrobial therapy may be slow; sterilization of the urine may not be possible. Even in the presence of sterile urine, reflux persists. This inability to completely empty the urinary tract makes the vesical defense mechanism inoperative; recurring infections are, therefore, to be expected.

If the urine becomes sterile, the renal lesion has been healed, although new infections may occur. Some of these patients may become afebrile, although bacteriuria persists. This represents the asymptomatic stage of chronic pyelonephritis.

Each acute infection leads to healing by scar. The kidney becomes smaller and its edge irregular. In the past, these radiographic findings have been called "chronic pyelonephritis." This is not correct since these scars represent evidence of previous infections and such a patient may have had sterile urine for many

years. The x-ray, then, is of no help in judging whether active infection exists, although the findings of bacteriuria and reflux imply the presence of chronic pyelonephritis.

Clinical Findings

A. Symptoms: At the onset, there is a severe constant ache over one or both kidneys (flank and back) due to the distention of the renal capsule caused by edema. The pain may radiate to the lower abdominal quadrant. Young children seldom complain of localized renal pain, which is apt to be reflected as ill-localized abdominal discomfort. Symptoms of cystitis develop: frequency, nocturia, urgency, and burning on urination. The patient is quite prostrated and usually suffers from nausea and vomiting.

B. Signs: The patient appears to be quite sick. Intermittent high fever with chills is to be expected. The pulse rate is, however, the best index of the severity of the infection. If the infection is due to *E coli*, the pulse rate may be only 90/minute; with staphylococci, it may reach 140. Tenderness is present over the affected kidney, which is usually not palpable because of muscle spasm. Fist percussion over the costovertebral angle will be quite painful. Abdominal distention may be marked and rebound tenderness may be present, suggesting an intraperitoneal lesion. Auscultation usually reveals a quiet intestine.

C. Laboratory Findings: The white blood count may reach 40,000/μl, and the neutrophil count is elevated. The sedimentation rate is increased. The urine is usually cloudy, shows a little protein, and contains large amounts of pus and bacteria. A few red cells may also be noted. Quantitative cultures will be positive and may be helpful in treatment of refractory infections, in which case sensitivity studies should be done. Renal function as measured by specific gravity of urine or PSP will be only slightly affected unless there is overwhelming sepsis with bilateral multiple cortical abscesses or necrotizing papillitis. Serial blood cultures should be done on any patient with urinary tract infection who has chills and fever since bacteremia is not uncommon in such cases.

D. X-Ray Findings: A plain film of the abdomen may show some obliteration of the renal shadow due to edema of the kidney and perinephric fat. Suspicious calcifications (stones) should be sought. Excretory urograms during the acute stage usually show little diminution in function, although the pelvis and calyces on the affected side may be small because of secretion of a small volume of urine as compared to the uninvolved kidney. These films are most valuable in surveying the tract for the presence of obstruction or possible vesicoureteral reflux. When the infection is severe, the involved kidney may be enlarged, show a decreased nephrogram effect on the immediate film, and reveal little or no calyceal radiopaque material. After appropriate therapy, the urograms return to normal (Davidson & Talner, 1973).

While cystography might reveal vesicoureteral reflux during the acute stage of infection, such an examination is contraindicated at this time. Excretory urography and cystography should be done later after the infection is controlled.

Differential Diagnosis

Pancreatitis causes pain, which may be posterior, and its position and degree may be confused with that of pyelonephritis. Serum amylase, however, will be elevated and pyuria will not be found.

Basal pneumonia may cause pain in the subcostal area, but it is usually pleuritic in type. Examination of the chest should make that diagnosis.

Acute appendicitis or acute disease of the gallbladder may be suspected if the patient's pain is largely anterior and if there is muscle spasm and rebound tenderness in the right upper or lower quadrants. Careful palpation over the kidney should reveal some tenderness, and proper urinalysis should be definitive.

Acute diverticulitis of the descending colon may cause pain in the left flank. Usually, however, a history of change in bowel habits may be elicited. The urine is normal. A barium enema will reveal evidence of changes in the bowel.

Herpes zoster affecting the somatic segments of the renal area (T12, L1) can simulate pain arising from the kidney. However, the pain is superficial, and skin hypersensitivity can be demonstrated. The onset of the typical skin changes of shingles will settle the problem.

Complications

If diagnosis is delayed and treatment inadequate, the infection may become chronic. This is particularly true if vesicoureteral reflux is present. The chronic form is seldom recognized because it is usually silent and because few or no pus cells are found in the urine. The bacteria can be found, however, if they are diligently sought for. The chronic infection may lead to (1) renal insufficiency; (2) secondary arteriolar sclerosis, which may cause renal ischemia and, in turn, hypertension; or (3) stone formation and further renal damage.

Bacteremia or septicemia of renal origin may develop in the acute stage of fulminating pyelonephritis and may cause infection or even multiple cortical abscesses of the other kidney. Metastatic abscesses may develop in other organs. Bacteremic shock is occasionally seen, especially when gram-negative rods invade the bloodstream.

In the late stage of infected hydronephrosis or pyonephrosis, particularly in diabetic patients, gas may be liberated in the kidney, leading to an air urogram on the plain film. The mortality rate from this type of sepsis is significant.

Prevention

Pyelonephritis in the male infant implies the presence of significant urinary obstruction (eg, posterior urethral valves). Excretory urography and, when indicated, retrograde cystography—or even endoscopy—should be done once the first infection is controlled.

Renal infection in a little girl suggests the presence of vesicoureteral reflux. Intravenous urograms and a voiding cystourethrogram are therefore essential. Treatment of the accompanying distal urethral stenosis will improve vesical hydrodynamics and lessen the chance for the development of cystitis. If there is no cystitis, there can be no pyelonephritis.

Pyelonephritis in an adult female suggests incompetency of the ureterovesical segment. Radiologic study is indicated. Steps should be taken to prevent the onset of cystitis (see section on prevention of acute cystitis).

Infection of the kidney in the male is usually secondary to obstruction, eg, by ureteral stone or an enlarged prostate. Such lesions should be sought and treated.

Treatment

A. Specific Measures: Urine should first be obtained for microscopy, cultures, and sensitivity tests. Based upon the findings gained from the stained smear of the sediment, a relatively nontoxic drug, chosen empirically, should be started. Preferably it should afford both a high urine and tissue concentration (eg, one of the tetracyclines, ampicillin). Ureteral obstruction may have to be relieved by cystoscopic means. This may mean extraction of a ureteral stone or temporary drainage with an indwelling ureteral catheter, as in acute ureteral obstruction due to pregnancy or to extrinsic pressure on the ureter from cancer.

If other methods fail, surgical treatment of obstruction may be necessary (eg, removal of a ureteral stone).

B. General Measures: Pain must be relieved by

appropriate drugs. Vesical irritability can be minimized by alkalinizing the urine (which may require 12–20 g/day of sodium bicarbonate) or by giving an antispasmodic such as belladonna or atropine with phenobarbital. Bed rest is definitely indicated during the acute phase of the infection. Adequate urinary output (1000 ml/day) should be maintained, but indiscriminate forcing of fluids only leads to urinary dilution of the antimicrobial drug being administered. Nausea and vomiting may necessitate the administration of parenteral fluids.

C. Failure of Response: If no clinical improvement occurs in 48–72 hours, either the wrong drug is being used or obstruction or stasis is present. Obtain excretory urograms, and look for changes suggesting vesicoureteral reflux or obstruction. Obtain a report on the culture and sensitivity tests and switch to an appropriate bactericidal drug, observing the usual precautions against toxicity.

D. Follow-Up Care: Even after clinical response, the urinary sediment must be examined for pathogens periodically for 2 months. Absence of symptoms is not proof of cure, nor is lack of pus cells in the urine.

Prognosis

The prognosis is good if the response to antibiotics is complete, ie, if all infecting organisms are eliminated. If obstruction or reflux is present but is not discovered, recurrences are to be expected. Persistence of bacteriuria requires explanation. Estimation of vesical residual urine, excretory urograms, and cystograms must then be done.

CHRONIC PYELONEPHRITIS

Etiology & Pathogenesis

The term "chronic pyelonephritis" implies the persistent presence of bacteria in the kidney. An outdated medical tenet states that once a kidney becomes infected it is difficult to cure by medical means. The implication is that renal infection is not often curable by the administration of appropriate drugs as are infections of the lungs, meninges, and other organs and structures. It has become increasingly clear that if the urine of such a patient can be rendered sterile, another attack represents a new infection. The failure of medical treatment is readily explained by the omission of a proper urologic work-up seeking evidence of stasis of urine and, particularly, vesicoureteral reflux. The cure rate of recurrent or chronic pyelonephritis is at least 80% if refluxing ureterovesical valves are corrected by medical means or by surgery, whereas medical treatment alone permanently cures only 40–50% of a similar group of patients. The cure of a disease requires understanding of its cause.

The source of the bacteria is, with few exceptions, the urethra; they ascend to the bladder with ease, particularly in females following sexual inter-

course. If the ureterovesical valves are entirely normal, the infection is confined to the bladder. In the presence of a "borderline" valve, acute cystitis may cause such a valve to become temporarily incompetent, thus causing pyelonephritis. Cure by antibiotics again leads to competency of the ureterovesical junction. If the vesical urine can be kept sterile, pyelonephritis is prevented. If, however, the ureterovesical junction is grossly abnormal, bacteria in the bladder reach the kidney and, since the infection is then perpetuated, true chronic pyelonephritis persists. Recent observations have made it clear that healed or atrophic pyelonephritis, portrayed on x-rays, is usually associated with vesicoureteral reflux.

In the absence of reflux, hematogenous pyelonephritis may occur secondary to ureteral obstruction or the presence of a renal stone. Again, treatment of the cause must be considered if infection is to be permanently relieved.

It should be pointed out that "chronic pyelonephritis" cannot be diagnosed on urograms. Evidence of scarring may be noted, but this represents healing from previous infections and tells us nothing about the presence or absence of renal bacteriuria. These changes should be read as "healed pyelonephritis."

Pathology

Grossly, the kidney is of normal size or small, depending upon the stage and duration of the disease. The capsule is pale and strips poorly. The surface of the kidney is often pitted and depressed; scarred areas are usual. The cut surface may show fairly well defined cortical and medullary zones, but in a more advanced stage the tissues may be pale and scarred. The pelvic mucosa is pale and fibrotic (Fig 12–3).

Microscopically, the parenchyma is diffusely infiltrated with plasma cells and lymphocytes. The tubules show varying stages of degeneration; some may show considerable dilatation and may contain proteinaceous casts. The glomeruli may be fibrosed, even hyalinized. Considerable thickening of arteries and arterioles is obvious. Not infrequently, the kidney will show areas of acute as well as varying degrees of healed disease.

It is often stated that evidence of pyelonephritis is found in 10–15% of autopsies. As diagnostic criteria for this entity are tightened, the incidence is now considered to be in the range of 1–2% (Freedman).

Many instances of xanthogranulomatous pyelonephritis have been reported. The kidney is usually functionless. It is enlarged, often nodular, and may suggest carcinoma. Sheets of lipid-filled histiocytes, plasma cells, and lymphocytes in a fibrous stroma are microscopically visible; these signs may be confused with those of renal cancer even after radiographic study.

Clinical Findings

A. Symptoms: Except during acute exacerbations, there are apt to be few symptoms. There may be mild discomfort over the kidney and some degree of vesical irritability. These, however, may be entirely absent. Vague gastrointestinal complaints may be noted, particularly in children. Unexplained low-grade fever or anemia may be the only clue to the presence of disease. Hypertension is common, particularly in children (Still & Cotton, 1967).

When acute exacerbations occur, localized renal pain may be present and the patient may complain of vesical symptoms. This clinical picture may be misinterpreted as a recurrent acute infection rather than an acute stage of chronic infection.

If the disease is advanced and bilateral (atrophic pyelonephritis), the presenting symptoms may be those of uremia.

B. Signs: There are usually no physical findings unless exacerbation is present, in which case some degree of localized renal tenderness may be elicited. Hypertension may be discovered.

C. Laboratory Findings: Anemia may be found, especially if the patient is uremic. The white blood count may be elevated during an acute stage but otherwise is usually normal.

The urinary sediment may or may not contain white cells, but some bacteria can almost always be demonstrated in the stained smear or culture. The degree of seriousness of an infection cannot be gauged by numbers of pus cells or organisms.

Quantitative cultures should be obtained and sensitivity tests performed.

Some type of renal function test should be done. If the PSP is low, bilateral renal damage, residual urine, or reflux should be suspected.

D. X-Ray Findings: A plain film of the abdomen may show that one or both kidneys are small (atrophic). Evidence of stone may be noted. Excretory urograms may be normal, but changes are usually seen that suggest scarring from repeated attacks of renal infection (small kidney; indentations of the lateral borders, representing scars; narrowing of the infundibula where they join the pelvis; dilatation and roughening of the calyces; and delayed excretion and poor concentration of the medium; see Figs 12–3 and 12–4). Dilatation or fullness of the ureter may imply the presence of vesicoureteral reflux (Fig 11–6).

Retrograde urograms will show similar changes. Voiding cystourethrography demonstrates vesicoureteral reflux in at least half of patients with scarred kidneys.

E. Instrumental Examination: On cystoscopy the bladder wall may show evidence of chronic infection. Abnormal configuration and position of a ureteral orifice may be compatible with a refluxing ureterovesical junction. Stained smears and cultures of vesical and renal urine specimens will place the site of infection accurately. Only in this way can the presence of active renal infection be established. Renal function tests (PSP) will measure function of each kidney separately. Diminution may be noted in advanced disease.

Differential Diagnosis

Recurrent acute cystitis may cause symptoms identical to those of a mild attack of pyelonephritis. A history of recurrent attacks of vesical irritability associated with bacteriuria indicates the need for excretory urograms and possibly cystograms. These should allow differentiation.

Chronic cystitis can only be differentiated from chronic pyelonephritis by the absence of renal infection as demonstrated by ureteral catheterization. Urograms are normal in cystitis but show evidence of scarring in pyelonephritis.

Tuberculosis may mimic chronic pyelonephritis perfectly. The absence of bacteria on the methylene blue stain or culture of sediment containing pus cells should suggest tuberculosis. Further bacteriologic studies will confirm this. Urography may reveal parenchymal calcifications and motheaten (ulcerated) calyceal changes which are typical of tuberculosis.

Xanthogranulomatous pyelonephritis and cancer of the kidney may be confused on urography. The former is usually functionless, whereas the latter can almost always be visualized by means of excretory urography. Angiography or an isotope scan (see Chapter 8) should differentiate the two.

Complications

A. Unilateral Infection: In the atrophic stage, hypertension may develop due to renal ischemia from severe arteriolar sclerosis. During the stage of exacerbation, bacteremia may occur with involvement of the other kidney.

B. Bilateral Infection: In the late stage of bilateral renal infection, the incidence of hypertension is high. The end stage is often uremia.

C. General: Stone formation is enhanced in the presence of urea-splitting organisms, which produce an alkaline urine, since calcium salts are less soluble in an alkaline medium.

Prevention

Recurrent or chronic renal infection is usually secondary to vesicoureteral reflux or obstruction. (See section on prevention of acute pyelonephritis.)

Treatment

The finding of pus and bacteria in the urine does not establish the diagnosis of pyelonephritis. The most common cause of these abnormal elements is acute or chronic cystitis, particularly in adults.

A. Specific Measures:

1. Medical—Intensive chemotherapeutic and antibiotic therapy is needed. The choice of drug depends upon antimicrobial sensitivity tests prepared from cultures of the urine. The drug should be given for 2–3 weeks. This should be followed by suppressive therapy for months or years. Suitable drugs include the sulfonamides, methenamine plus a urinary acidifier, or nitrofurantoin. Palmer has shown that the severely involved kidney fails to concentrate many drugs because of tubular damage, thus lessening their effectiveness.

2. Local—The eradication of chronic prostatic infection or the treatment of a urethral stricture may contribute to the ultimate control of the renal infection.

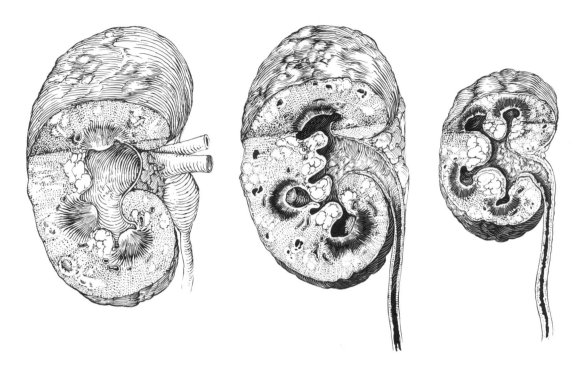

Figure 12–3. Progressive pathologic changes in kidney resulting from repeated attacks of acute pyelonephritis with progressive scarring. *Left:* Early stage of focal parenchymal scarring. *Center:* Progressive scarring with narrowing of the necks of the calyces, which therefore become dilated (Fig 12 4). *Right:* End stage of recurrent pyelonephritis (stage of atrophy).

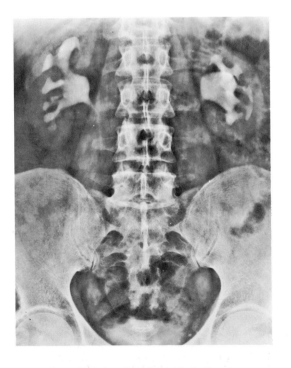

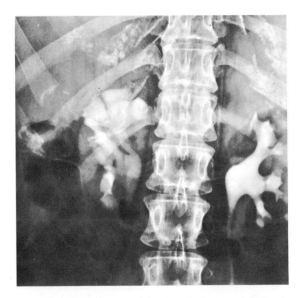

Figure 12–4. Healed pyelonephritis. *Left:* Excretory urogram showing flattening and clubbing of the calyces; edge of renal shadow close to ends of the calyces. These changes reflect numerous past episodes of acute pyelonephritis. *Right:* Excretory urogram showing marked atrophy of parenchyma of right kidney with calyces of upper pole extending to renal capsule. Left kidney normal.

3. Surgical—Correction of obstructive lesions may be indicated. If vesicoureteral reflux has been demonstrated and sterilization of the urine cannot be gained or maintained, repair of the ureterovesical junction must be considered. If one kidney is badly damaged, nephrectomy may be the procedure of choice.

B. Treatment of Complications: If the disease is bilateral and function is impaired (loss of concentrating power), a urine output of 1000–1500 ml is necessary to facilitate the removal of metabolic waste products. If hypertension is present in association with a unilateral atrophic kidney (and provided the other kidney functions perfectly), nephrectomy should be considered.

Prognosis

If the diagnosis is delayed until both kidneys are badly scarred, only medical therapy is indicated in the hope of conserving what functioning tissue is left. Dialysis or even renal transplantation may become necessary (see Chapter 24). Fortunately, repair of the incompetent ureterovesical junction leads to permanent sterilization of the urine in a high percentage of patients with chronic pyelonephritis.

BACTEREMIC SHOCK

Etiology

The genitourinary tract is one of the common sources of bacteremia. Bacteremia may develop spontaneously following obstruction (eg, an infected kidney suddenly occluded by a calculus) or instrumentation of an infected prostatic urethra, or vesical bacteria may be forced up through incompetent ureterovesical valves under the hydrostatic pressure of an irrigating solution.

There is an increased incidence of bacteremia wherever antibiotics are used indiscriminately. Patients receiving immunosuppressive drugs (eg, renal transplantation) and those with diabetes, cirrhosis, cancer, burns, peritonitis, and septic abortion are at greater risk. An increased incidence of serratia and candida sepsis has have been noted in septic shock.

Shock is caused by cardiac decompensation or inadequate circulating blood volume. It reflects a failure of blood flow to the cells; the hypotension is secondary. Perhaps 30% of patients with gram-negative bacteriuria will go into shock. The immediate cause is liberation of endotoxin from the walls of dead bacteria. Septic shock is relatively rare in gram-positive infections since these organisms liberate an exotoxin.

Pathogenesis & Pathology

Shock due to trauma or heart failure causes constriction of the precapillary sphincters (increased peripheral resistance) and is associated with decreased cardiac output. Shock caused by gram-negative bacteremia initially reflects increased peripheral resistance, but in most cases this rapidly progresses to decreased peripheral resistance and increased cardiac output. It seems that—though capillary resistance persists—it is overcome by the opening of arteriovenous shunts which deprive cells of both oxygen and nutrition. The postcapillary sphincters remain closed. Plasma and, to a lesser extent, red cells leak into the interstitial tissues because of increased hydrostatic pressure, leading to diminished circulating blood volume. Patients with bacteremic shock who have a low cardiac output probably have suffered prior myocardial damage; this group, therefore, has a poorer prognosis.

The heart and brain suffer relatively less anoxia than other tissues and organs, for vasoconstriction does not occur in these vital organs. Cerebral anoxia is manifested by apathy or even stupor. The anoxic myocardium may fail.

The liver normally converts lactate to pyruvate. In shock, this process is impaired and serum lactic acid rises. This implies diminution of hepatic blood flow. Diminished renal blood flow results in oliguria with retention of water and salt. If treatment is delayed, acute tubular necrosis may supervene.

Disseminated intravascular coagulation is always present in shock. This diffuse coagulation consumes large numbers of platelets, fibrinogen, and other clotting factors, thus depleting the blood of normal coagulating power. Hemorrhages are common, particularly from the gastrointestinal tract. Ischemia of gastric mucosa may also lead to bleeding. Damage to the reticuloendothelial system will lower the host's resistance to bacteria.

The most serious lesions occur in the lungs. There is a decrease in surfactant; edema or even hemorrhage into the intra-alveolar septa occurs, leading to increased pulmonary compliance. Fibrin thrombi and even hyaline membranes may be noted. Loss of plasma from congested capillaries contributes to interstitial edema. Because of sludging, disseminated intravascular coagulation may develop throughout the body, but particularly in the lungs. When peripheral and visceral capillaries open up as a consequence of definitive treatment, this sludged material is filtered by the lungs, which may be overwhelmed.

Perhaps 20–40% of the alveoli become nonfunctioning because of the development of these lesions. Their blood receives no oxygen, and venous admixture occurs. For this reason, Pa_{O_2} is low (50–60 mm Hg) despite the addition of O_2 to the inspired air. Because of shunting across the capillary beds throughout the body, the partial pressure of O_2 in the veins approaches that in the arterial tree, thus reflecting serious tissue anoxia.

Anoxia leads to an increase in respiratory rate. CO_2 is blown off, leading to respiratory alkalosis. As anoxia persists, anaerobic metabolism develops, leading to the accumulation of lactic acid and metabolic acidosis. Cellular damage and even death of cells ensues.

The most common cause of death in septic shock is pulmonary failure (shock lung). The problem, then, is to immediately attack the cause of the shock (ie, bacteremia) and the shock itself.

Clinical Findings

A. Symptoms: The patient develops fever ranging from 38.5–40 °C (101–104 °F) and associated chills. Early, he may be anxious; later, apathy develops. There is evidence of bacterial infection (eg, urinary tract, peritoneum). There is often a history of urethral instrumentation a few hours previously.

B. Signs: Cloudy mentation is usual when hypotension supervenes. Peripheral cyanosis with a moist, pale skin is present. Respirations are shallow and rapid. The pulse is rapid and thready. The blood pressure is in the range of 70/40 mm Hg, or 25 mm Hg below the hypertensive patient's normal systolic pressure. Capillary refill of the nail beds is prolonged. Oliguria is to be expected. Some hours may pass, however, before hypotension develops.

C. Laboratory Findings: The white count is elevated, with a shift to the left. The number of platelets is diminished because of consumption coagulopathy. The PCV is usually increased owing to loss of plasma into the interstitial tissues. Blood volume studies may be misleading. Because of diminished renal blood flow, urine specific gravity is increased, and the ratio of serum BUN to creatinine may exceed the normal 10:1 ratio. In most instances, the ECG will suggest the diagnosis of myocardial infarction, but these changes merely reflect diminished coronary artery blood flow. There is an increase in the blood levels of fatty acids and glucose.

Since the source of the bacteremia is often the urinary tract, pyuria and bacteriuria may be found. Urine cultures and serial blood cultures with sensitivity testing are mandatory. *E coli* is the most common offender.

Since pulmonary insufficiency is the rule, frequent estimates of arterial pH and P_{aO_2} as well as serum electrolytes are necessary. Serum lactate levels (normal, 0.44–1.8 mM/liter) are important in estimating prognosis. Values of 5 mM/liter or more are associated with a high mortality rate and reflect the degree of tissue anoxia. On the other hand, a progressive decrease in the serum lactate level following therapy is a most encouraging sign.

If possible, the cardiac index should be measured. A high output improves prognosis. Estimation of peripheral resistance is helpful. Progressive increase from an initial low level after therapy has been instituted implies increased tissue oxygenation via opening capillaries.

D. X-Ray Findings: A chest film may show diffuse alveolar infiltrates which may progress to complete consolidation as part of "shock lung."

Differential Diagnosis

Simple bacteremia is accompanied by chills and fever, but hypotension and oliguria do not occur. This is particularly true of coccal infections. Secondary heart failure may lead to hypotension, thus obscuring the diagnosis. Estimation of central venous pressure will facilitate differentiation (see below).

Acute cardiac failure, especially when secondary to myocardial infarction, may cause sudden hypotension. Evidence of overwhelming infection is absent.

Hypovolemic shock may be caused by marked dehydration (eg, vomiting, diarrhea) or hemorrhage. Symptoms and signs of infection are absent. Basically, the treatment of this condition is the same as that of bacteremic shock, ie, restoration of circulating blood volume.

Complications

The primary infection may not respond to antibiotic therapy. Prolonged hypoxia and hypotension may lead to acute renal tubular necrosis or myocardial infarction. Heart failure may ensue. Hemorrhages from bowel ulceration or disseminated intravascular coagulation (consumptive coagulopathy) may develop. The most serious complication is, however, acute respiratory failure. Even though infection is conquered and the microcirculatory lesion is improved, irreversible and progressive pulmonary damage may lead to death.

Prevention

If urologic instrumentation is necessary, the urine should first be sterilized. There is no convincing evidence that prophylactic antibiotic therapy reduces the incidence of bacteremia.

If an indwelling catheter is necessary, aseptic technic must be used in its passage. A closed drainage system should be used to decrease the chances of ascent of bacteria to the bladder, but the development of bacteriuria is inevitable. Careful intermittent catheterization markedly decreases the incidence of infection but creates a problem of availability of personnel to perform the procedure.

Treatment

Since early diagnosis and immediate treatment significantly influence prognosis, the clinician must be on the alert for this impending catastrophe. If a patient at risk—eg, one undergoing urethral instrumentation—is observed to develop anxiety or lethargy, fever, rapid and shallow respiration, and an accelerated, thready pulse, the possibility of bacteremia with impending shock should be considered and preventive measures instituted. Begin appropriate antibiotic therapy immediately and give 1 liter of crystalloid or (preferably) colloid solution IV. An intravenous bolus of a corticosteroid should be administered (see below).

If the patient is in shock, the aim of treatment is to combat the infection, restore circulating blood volume, and improve the perfusion of vital organs (heart, brain, and lungs). Abscesses must be drained. With septic abortion, hysterectomy must be considered. An obstructing ureteral stone should be removed or bypassed by catheter.

A. Specific Measures:

1. Initial step—

a. Insert a urethral catheter to monitor urine flow.

b. Introduce a small plastic catheter into the superior vena cava or right atrium so that central venous pressure can be estimated. Its position should be checked by x-ray. Pressures of 0–4 cm of water imply poor filling of the heart due to diminished circulating blood volume; levels of 6–12 cm of water are compatible with adequate filling of the right heart but can occur if both cardiac failure and diminished blood volume are present. A pressure above 15 cm of water is diagnostic of heart failure. The central venous pressure affords a rough estimate of blood volume.

2. **Antibiotics**—If the organism from the primary site has been identified and sensitivity tests have been obtained, the best drug or combination of drugs should be administered. If the offending organism has not yet been identified, gram-negative bacillary infection should be assumed. Empiric therapy should be begun immediately. Gentamicin is the drug of choice. Give 1.5 mg/kg IM every 8 hours. Kanamycin plus cephalothin or chloramphenicol is also efficacious. Subsequent bacteriologic reports may suggest the use of other antimicrobial drugs. If oliguria or renal failure is present, less frequent administration will be necessary. (See Table 12–1.)

3. **Steps to improve circulating blood volume and perfusion of vital organs**—
a. **Parenteral fluids**—If the central venous pressure is low, immediately begin infusion of a crystalloid solution (eg, normal saline or Ringer's injection). The hematocrit will probably be elevated because of selective loss of plasma from the engorged capillaries. Colloid solutions should be administered as soon as possible because more than 75% of crystalloids and water enter the extravascular space. The colloids include low molecular weight dextran, pooled plasma (risk of hepatitis), blood, or albumin (5% solution). Their oncotic pressure tends to draw plasma back into the capillaries, thus lessening tissue and cellular edema and helping to wash sludged red and white cells and platelets into the general circulation. Low molecular weight dextran decreases blood viscosity and combats platelet adhesiveness. These fluids can be pushed until the central venous pressure approaches 12–14 cm of water, care being taken to seek signs of cardiac overload.

Even though the central venous pressure is within the normal range, a test loading dose of 500 ml of a crystalloid or colloid solution should be rapidly infused. An immediate rise in pressure of 5 cm of water suggests that more fluid administration may lead to heart failure. If the patient tolerates this amount, additional fluid should be given. An increase in secretion of urine as determined by hourly measurements of output and clearing mentation are favorable signs even though the peripheral blood pressure rises only moderately or not at all. Evidence of improving tissue perfusion is far more important than an increase in peripheral blood pressure.

In most instances, antibiotic therapy plus correction of the diminished circulating blood volume is all that is needed for complete recovery.

B. **Glucocorticoids**—If the above steps do not result in significant improvement within 3–4 hours, corticosteroids should be administered in pharmacologic doses (20–50 times physiologic doses). These agents appear to protect the cellular mitochondrial membrane from rupturing and releasing lysosomal enzymes that would destroy the cell. They may also preserve the integrity of small vessels and decrease adhesiveness of platelets. In addition, they may have an inotropic effect. Since the antibiotics continually kill the bacteria, there is a constant liberation of endotoxin. Evidence suggests that corticosteroids protect the capillaries from the action of endotoxin. Give one of the following as a bolus IV: dexamethasone (Decadron), 3–6 mg/kg; methylprednisolone succinate (Solu-Medrol), 15–30 mg/kg; or hydrocortisone sodium succinate (Solu-Cortef), 50–150 mg/kg. Repeat this dose every 4–6 hours. These drugs can be given for as long as 3 or even 4 days and then stopped abruptly without apparent harm.

c. **Vasodilators**—If, after restoration of circulating blood volume and the administration of corticosteroids, significant improvement has not occurred, the use of vasodilators should be considered.

(1) **Alpha-adrenergic blocking agent**—Phenoxybenzamine (Dibenzyline) blocks the vasoconstricting action of the catecholamines, which are circulating in large amounts during shock. The usual dose is 1 mg/kg in 100 ml of saline given over a period of 2 hours. Since it is a long-acting drug, titration cannot be done.

(2) **Beta-adrenergic stimulating agent**—Isoproterenol decreases venous pooling and arterial tone and increases venous return. In addition, this drug has both inotropic and chronotropic effects. Overdose may lead to tachycardia and arrhythmias. 2.5–5 mg of the drug are added to 500 ml of 5% dextrose in water, and the infusion is run at a rate of about 1 ml/minute. If there is no change in central venous pressure, pulse pressure, or urine output, the rate of drip should be increased.

Before either adrenergic drug is used, blood volume must first be corrected (central venous pressure at 12–15 cm of water). Even then the central venous pressure may drop, necessitating immediate further infusion of colloids or crystalloid solutions.

d. **Vasopressors**—Vasopressors are rarely indicated except to support coronary artery flow in the late stages of shock. The patient who is already in shock has vasospasm from excessive amounts of circulating catecholamines. Such a drug merely treats the blood pressure cuff but causes further tissue anoxia.

4. **Support of vital organs**—
a. **Lungs**—The pulmonary complications of shock are the most serious since they interfere with normal oxygenation of the blood. Oxygen (5–8 liters/minute) should be administered by mask and a nasal tube, though significant increase in Pa_{O_2} is seldom seen because of blood admixture. Intubation or tracheostomy may be necessary, so that assisted or controlled ventilation can be accomplished if the Pa_{O_2} remains at 60 mm Hg or below. An attempt should be made to raise the Pa_{O_2} to 70–90 mm Hg and hold the Pa_{CO_2} between 32–40 mm Hg. The treatment of heart failure may reduce pulmonary edema, thus improving aeration.

b. Heart—Steps taken to raise the central venous pressure will improve cardiac output. Immediate digitalization is necessary in the face of heart failure. Vasodilators seem to have an inotropic effect, as do the corticosteroids also. Acidosis has a deleterious effect upon the myocardium. Appropriate treatment ($NaHCO_3$ given IV) is indicated.

c. Kidneys—In the early stage of shock, oliguria usually develops. Aggressive infusion of fluids usually corrects this defect. It may be further improved by corticosteroids and vasodilating drugs. If these measures fail, give a diuretic, eg, furosemide (Lasix), 20–40 mg IV. Should this fail to increase urine flow, assume the presence of acute tubular necrosis and limit fluids thereafter.

5. Other measures—

a. Problems in fluid and electrolyte balance are to be expected—particularly hyperkalemia due to leakage of K^+ from the anoxic cell as Na^+ enters it. Cell death further liberates K^+, and lactic acidosis, which develops in shock, causes further loss of potassium from the cell. (Banked whole blood contains 10–30 mEq of K^+ per liter.) Treat the acidosis with intravenous $NaHCO_3$ and give 200 ml of 50% glucose containing 20 units of insulin. Sodium polystyrene sulfonate (Kayexalate) enemas (50 g in 200 ml of glucose) every 4 hours may prove efficacious. Dialysis may be necessary. Constant ECG monitoring is essential.

b. Disseminated intravascular coagulation (DIC) contributes to circulatory and respiratory failure, especially the latter. The infusion of low molecular weight dextran, in addition to expanding circulating blood volume, decreases the viscosity of blood. One to 2 units should be given the first day and 1 unit per day thereafter. If blood studies show evidence of consumption coagulopathy or if hemorrhagic phenomena develop, give heparin, 1000–2000 units IV every 4–6 hours. Periodic measurements of blood clotting are necessary. Improvement in pulmonary function may supervene.

Prognosis

Prompt diagnosis and the immediate institution of treatment afford a fairly good prognosis. Encouraging signs include clearing mentation, establishment of good urine flow, control of fever, and increasing Pa_{O_2}. The most serious sign is progressive pulmonary failure. High levels of serum lactate are also of great concern. If, however, there is underlying lethal disease (eg, leukemia), the mortality rate approaches 85%. In favorable cases, particularly those of urologic origin, the survival rate approaches 85%.

NECROTIZING PAPILLITIS
(Papillary Necrosis)

Etiology

This is an uncommon type of renal inflammation, though Harrow believes that the necrosis is primary and the infection secondary. Formerly, it was usually a complication of pyelonephritis in diabetes or in patients suffering from urinary obstruction. Today, most patients with papillitis give a history of excessive and prolonged ingestion of analgesics containing phenacetin and aspirin for the relief of migraine or arthritic pain. Patients with sickle cell trait may develop papillary necrosis. The combination of infection and vesicoureteral reflux may also cause this lesion. The association of papillary necrosis and cirrhosis has been cited. Papillary necrosis appears to be caused by ischemic necrosis of the papilla or the entire pyramid, leading to the diagnostic urographic changes. A few cases have been reported in infancy, though most are seen in women with migraine.

Pathogenesis & Pathology (Figs 12–5 and 12–6)

The disease is usually bilateral; a few or all of the calyces may become progressively more severely involved. While most patients have pyelonephritis as well, a few are found to have sterile urine. This latter group has associated chronic interstitial nephritis which is seen in association with analgesic abuse.

Some degree of renal atrophy secondary to infection may be noted. In fact, in adults, only 2 renal lesions will cause shrinking of the kidney in a period of a few weeks: an acute vascular lesion and acute papillary necrosis. Simple pyelonephritis in the adult will not cause this phenomenon. One or more papillae are absent. The line of demarcation is shaggy. Retained or calcified papillae may be found free in the pelvis. Infiltration of neutrophils, small round cells, and plasma cells is microscopically visible at the site of papillary slough. Changes typical of chronic pyelonephritis are usually evident. In the case of analgesic abuse, the interstitial tissues are infiltrated by fibrous tissue and round cells (chronic interstitial nephritis). Severe ischemia of the pyramids may be noted.

Clinical Findings

A. Symptoms: In the rare fulminating type of papillitis, severe sepsis may come on abruptly. Renal pain may be noted. Oliguria with uremic coma may develop rapidly, culminating in death. More commonly, the patient complains of symptoms of chronic cystitis, often with exacerbations of pyelonephritis. Attempts at sterilization of the urine usually fail. Recurrent renal colic may be experienced as sloughed papillae are passed. Known sickle cell trait, vesicoureteral reflux, diabetes, cirrhosis, or a history of prolonged use of analgesics (6–60 pills a day for years) may be significant.

B. Signs: In acute papillitis, fever is high and prostration marked. Renal tenderness may be noted. In the

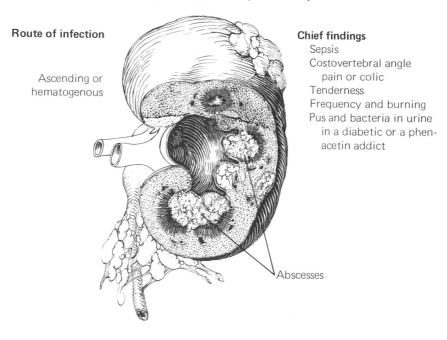

Route of infection

Ascending or
hematogenous

Chief findings
Sepsis
Costovertebral angle
   pain or colic
Tenderness
Frequency and burning
Pus and bacteria in urine
   in a diabetic or a phen-
   acetin addict

Abscesses

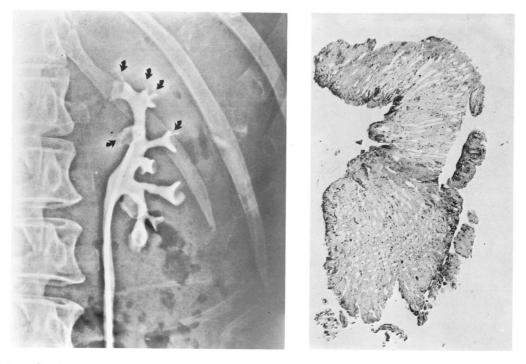

Figure 12–5. Papillary necrosis. *Above:* Pathogenesis. *Left:* Arrows point to "cracks" into parenchyma in a patient in the earliest stage of papillitis (medullary type). *Right:* Papilla passed spontaneously in urine, recovered by patient. (Reduced 30% from × 10.)

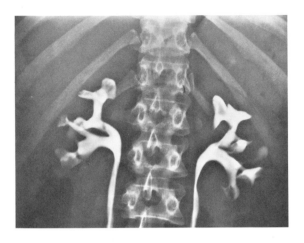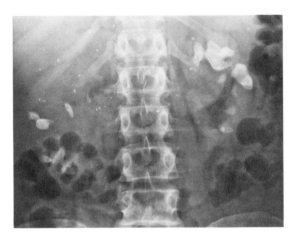

Figure 12—6. Papillary necrosis. *Left:* Retrograde urogram showing papillary necrosis. Calyces seem enlarged because of sloughed papillae. "Negative" shadows in upper medial calyces and in lowest calyces on left represent sloughed papillae. *Right:* (Same patient 5 years later.) Multiple renal stones caused by calcification of retained sloughed papillae. The papillae are represented by the relatively translucent centers in peculiarly shaped stones.

chronic form, no abnormal signs are usually elicited. At the time of febrile flare-up, renal tenderness may be found.

C. Laboratory Findings: In the fulminating form, the white blood count is significantly elevated. Urinalysis reveals pyuria and bacteriuria. Blood cultures may be positive. Shock may ensue. Glycosuria and acidosis will be noted in the uncontrolled diabetic. Progressive azotemia is to be expected.

Most of the patients in the chronic phase have infected urine. Anemia may be found in association with renal insufficiency. PSP excretion is usually depressed, often below 30% in one-half hour. At this level, tests of nitrogen retention will be elevated.

D. X-Ray Findings: Satisfactory excretory urograms in the uremic patient may only be obtained by infusing increased amounts of radiopaque material. In the earliest stages, before papillary slough, the urograms may show no anatomic abnormality. Later, ulceration of the central portion of a papilla (medullary necrosis; Fig 12—5) or delineation of cavities, caused by sloughed papillae, may be seen (Fig 12—6). "Negative" shadows representing retained papillae may be noted. During the later phase, irregular calcified bodies containing radiolucent centers (the papillae) are diagnostic.

If uremia is of such severity as to preclude excretory urography, retrograde urography must be performed. Retrograde urography will either establish the diagnosis or will reveal a urologic lesion that may be amenable to therapy.

Differential Diagnosis

Uncomplicated diabetic coma can be diagnosed on the basis of blood glucose and serum electrolytes. Treatment of the coma should cause prompt response. If bilateral necrotizing papillitis is present as a complication, the diabetic patient will not improve under

insulin therapy; progressive renal impairment will be observed, and death from renal failure and sepsis may ensue. Patients with acute pyelonephritis are not so prostrated, nor does acute renal failure develop.

Bilateral renal cortical abscesses secondary to bacteremia may simulate acute papillitis clinically. Both may show progressive loss of renal function. Urograms made early in the course of either disease may be normal or may show evidence of chronic infection. After 2 or 3 weeks, when the necrotic papillae have sloughed, the urographic demonstration of necrotizing papillitis is diagnostic.

Complications

If the patient with bilateral papillary necrosis recovers, persistent chronic pyelonephritis is usually seen; bacteriuria resists antimicrobial therapy.

If the sloughed papillae are not passed down the ureter, they may undergo peripheral calcification. The clinical picture is then compatible with nephrolithiasis or ureterolithiasis.

Prevention

Because of the relatively high incidence of papillitis in diabetics and cirrhotics, careful urinalyses and periodic urine cultures should be obtained whether symptoms of urologic infection are present or not. Infection, once discovered, should be treated vigorously. Pharmaceutical compounds containing aspirin and particularly phenacetin should be considered nephrotoxic; their long-term and persistent use must be condemned. If the patient stops taking these drugs, renal function may improve to some extent.

Treatment

A. Specific Therapy: Intensive treatment with an appropriate antibiotic is indicated, although the results have been disappointing insofar as sterilization of the urine is concerned. The choice of drug depends upon the type of bacteria found in the urine and the results of antibiotic sensitivity studies.

B. General Measures: Diabetes must be carefully controlled. The aspirin or phenacetin addict must stop taking the drug.

C. Surgical Therapy: If the disease is unilateral and fulminating (as demonstrated by physical examination, urography, and renal function tests) and if drug therapy does not result in prompt improvement, nephrectomy must be considered. This procedure must be undertaken with caution, however, since the other kidney may later become involved. If a sloughed papilla should obstruct a ureter, it can usually be removed by cystoscopic manipulation (Jameson & Heal, 1973).

Prognosis

The rare fulminating form is rapidly fatal. Patients with the chronic type usually do fairly well. Although renal function may be depressed, progressive uremia is unusual if chronic suppression with antimicrobial drugs is instituted.

RENAL CARBUNCLE

Etiology

Renal carbuncle is due to a unilateral hematogenous infection complicating a pyogenic skin lesion.

The infecting organism is usually hemolytic *Staphylococcus aureus.*

Pathogenesis & Pathology (Fig 12–7)

Although a diffuse acute pyelonephritis may be simultaneously present, the infection is usually localized in a single zone of the parenchyma. Development of a multilocular abscess takes place as necrosis advances. The abscess may rupture, giving rise to a perinephric abscess.

Clinical Findings

A. Symptoms: Renal carbuncle may have an abrupt onset with well-localized symptoms associated with marked sepsis, or its course may be mild with no symptoms other than low-grade fever.

B. Signs: In the acute case, the localized signs are flank tenderness and possibly a palpable mass, as well as, at times, edema of the skin of the costovertebral area. In mild cases, few signs may be discovered over the affected kidney.

C. Laboratory Findings: If staphylococci are the cause, the urine is free of formed sediment (cells, bacteria, etc) and cultures are negative until the abscess breaks into the pelvis. The white count is high, with an absolute increase in polymorphonuclear neutrophils. If there are chills and fever, blood cultures should be obtained.

D. X-Ray Findings: The plain film may show an enlarged kidney or absence of renal shadow. The psoas shadow may be obliterated. The abscess may be seen as

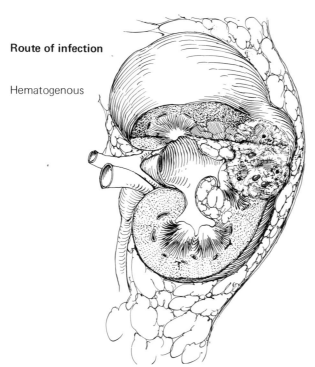

Route of infection

Hematogenous

Chief findings
Fever (high or low grade)
Costovertebral angle pain
Tenderness or no localizing
    signs or bladder symptoms
Normal urine

Figure 12–7. Pathogenesis of renal carbuncle.

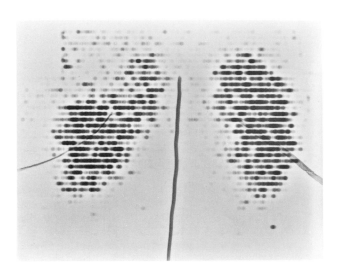

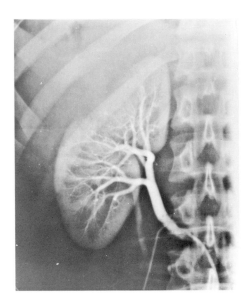

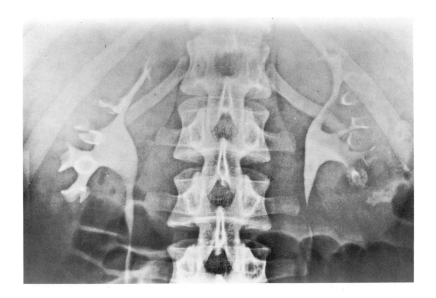

Figure 12–8. Renal carbuncle. *Above left:* Renal scan revealing absence of functional renal tissue in superolateral portion, right kidney. *Above right:* Selective renal angiogram, same patient, showing avascular mass in superolateral portion, right kidney. Surgical diagnosis: renal carbuncle. *Below:* Excretory urogram. Elongation of upper calyx, right kidney. Carbuncle was a complication of measles.

a bulge of the external contour of the kidney. Excretory or retrograde urograms often demonstrate a space-occupying lesion. Angiography will reveal an avascular mass (Fig 12–8).

E. Isotope Scanning: The rectilinear scan will depict a space-occupying lesion (Fig 12–8). The Anger camera scan will show an avascular space-occupying lesion with technetium compounds. These findings are also compatible with simple cyst. (See Chapter 8.)

Differential Diagnosis

In acute pyelonephritis, the urinary sediment shows pus and bacteria (usually rods). No space-occupying lesion is seen on urography.

Acute cholecystitis may resemble renal carbuncle. The presence of a tender and palpable gallbladder may make the diagnosis. Radiographic visualization of the gallbladder and kidneys should be definitive.

Acute appendicitis may be confused with renal carbuncle since renal pain often radiates to the lower abdominal quadrant. However, signs and symptoms in the flank should suggest renal disease. Excretory urograms make the diagnosis.

Since x-ray findings of a space-occupying lesion of the kidney can be due to one of 3 diseases (tumor, cyst, or carbuncle), the differentiation may be impossible until the kidney is explored surgically.

Complications

Bacteremia with general sepsis; rupture of carbuncle leading to perinephric abscess.

Treatment

A. Specific Measures: If the clinical diagnosis of renal carbuncle is made, the patient should be intensively treated with a drug—or combination of drugs—most likely to kill *S aureus*. (Choose a penicillin that is resistant to β-lactamase.) If cocci are present in the urine, sensitivity tests will prove invaluable. If the abscess does not respond, surgical drainage of the carbuncle is the treatment of choice; but if it is small and limited to one renal pole, heminephrectomy may be feasible. Nephrectomy may at times be necessary.

B. General Measures: Pain should be relieved by appropriate drugs and heat to the flank. An adequate urinary output must be maintained.

C. Treatment of Complications: Perinephric abscess requires surgical drainage.

Prognosis

Administration of the appropriate drug early in the course of the disease usually aborts the infection. If diagnosis is late or treatment inadequate, surgical intervention may be necessary.

PERINEPHRIC ABSCESS

Etiology

Perinephric abscess can be secondary to a staphylococcal infection of the kidney but is usually a complication of an advanced chronic nonspecific renal infection.

Pathogenesis & Pathology (Fig 12–9)

Perinephric abscess lies between the renal capsule and the perirenal (Gerota's) fascia. The staphylococcal type probably originates from rupture of a small renal cortical abscess or, less commonly, from a renal carbuncle. The primary renal lesion may heal although the perinephric abscess progresses.

Perinephric cellulitis and abscess, however, usually complicate severe chronic renal infection such as calculous pyonephrosis or infected hydronephrosis. The presumption is that spontaneous extravasation of infected material occurs. In this instance, pus and bacteria (usually gram-negative rods) are found in the urine.

Perirenal abscesses may become quite large. When advanced, they tend to point over the iliac crest (Petit's triangle) posterolaterally.

Clinical Findings

A. Symptoms: In the more common type (secondary to advanced chronic renal infection), a history of prolonged or recurrent urinary infection may be elicited. In the staphylococcal type, there is often a history of a skin infection a few weeks before the onset of symptoms. Malaise may be mild or severe, depending upon the virulence of the invading organism. Pain in the flank varies in degree. The patient may discover a tender mass in the renal area.

B. Signs: Fever may be low-grade or septic. Marked tenderness over the kidney and in the costovertebral angle is usually found. A large mass may be felt or percussed in the flank. Some rebound tenderness may be elicited. The diaphragm on the affected side may be high and fixed. Ipsilateral pleural effusion is common. Scoliosis of the spine, with its concavity to the affected side, is usually seen. This is due to spasm of the psoas muscle, which also causes the patient to lie with the ipsilateral leg flexed on the abdomen. Edema of the skin over the abscess may be evident. Minimal edema is best demonstrated by having the patient lie on a rough towel for a few minutes.

C. Laboratory Findings: Anemia may be found. The white count may be markedly or only slightly elevated. The sedimentation rate is usually accelerated. The urine may be free of pus and bacteria if the renal organism is a staphylococcus. If the abscess is secondary to other chronic renal disease, pus and bacteria (usually rods) are found. Renal function tests are usually normal except in the face of chronic bilateral renal disease.

D. X-Ray Findings: A plain film of the abdomen typically shows evidence of a mass in the flank. The

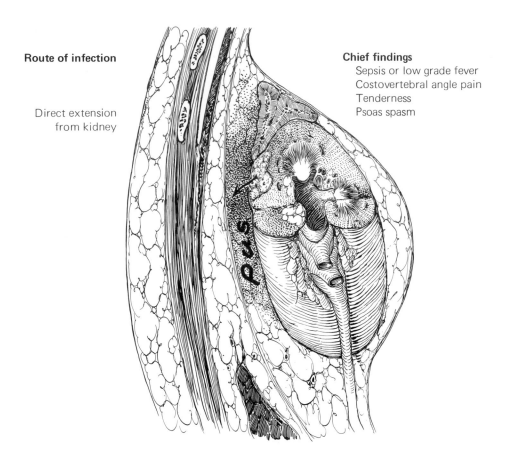

Route of infection

Direct extension
from kidney

Chief findings
Sepsis or low grade fever
Costovertebral angle pain
Tenderness
Psoas spasm

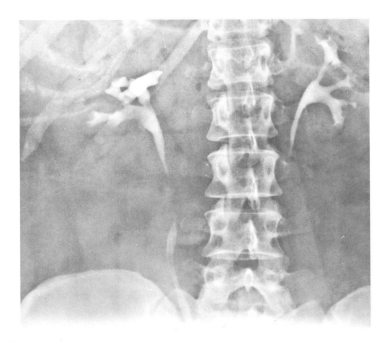

Figure 12–9. Perinephric abscess. ***Above:*** Pathogenesis. ***Below:*** Excretory urogram showing lateral displacement of lower pole of right kidney, scoliosis of spine, and absence of right psoas shadow. Note compression of upper right ureter by abscess.

renal and psoas shadows are obliterated because of neighboring edema. Scoliosis of the spine with its concavity to the affected side is usually seen. The presence of a calcific body in this area should suggest an abscess secondary to calculous pyonephrosis.

Excretory urograms may show delayed visualization due to parenchymal disease. Changes suggesting a space-occupying lesion (eg, carbuncle) may be noted, but evidence of advanced hydronephrosis or calculous pyonephrosis is most commonly seen. Lack of mobility of the kidney with change in position of the patient or with respiration strongly suggests a diagnosis of acute or chronic perinephritis. The entire kidney or only one pole may be displaced laterally by the abscess (Fig 12–9).

A barium enema may show displacement of the bowel anteriorly, laterally, or medially.

A chest film may demonstrate an elevated diaphragm on the ipsilateral side, and fluoroscopy often shows fixation on respiration. Some free pleural fluid and disk atelectasis may be seen.

Retrograde urograms may be necessary if the excretory films are equivocal.

Differential Diagnosis

Chronic renal infection may cause many of the symptoms which accompany perinephric abscess: fever, localized pain, and tenderness. The urine shows evidence of infection. The plain abdominal x-ray and excretory urograms should reveal a clearly defined renal shadow; the psoas shadow should be present and the spine straight. Urographic evidence of chronic pyelonephritis may be seen.

Infected hydronephrosis may cause fever and localized pain and tenderness and may account for the presence of a mass in the flank. The urine is infected. Excretory urograms should make the differentiation.

Paranephric abscess is a collection of pus external to the perirenal fascia and is often secondary to inflammatory disease of the spine (eg, tuberculosis). Many of the signs of perinephric abscess may be seen on a plain x-ray film, but the finding of a bone lesion in the low thoracic area should suggest the proper diagnosis. Urograms are normal.

Complications

Rarely, the perinephric abscess may point just above the iliac crest posterolaterally or extend downward into the iliac fossa and inguinal region. It can cross the spine within the perirenal fascia and involve the other side, but this, too, is rare.

Considerable ureteral compression from the abscess may develop, giving rise to hydronephrosis. Even after drainage of the abscess, ureteral stenosis may develop during the healing process.

Prevention

Since most instances of perinephric abscess complicate a pyelonephritic kidney, its removal should be considered.

Treatment

A. Specific Measures: In the stage of perinephritis, resolution of the infection, when due to staphylococci, may be expected when proper antibiotics are used. When a frank abscess is present, surgical drainage through the flank is indicated. If the cause is primary renal disease (eg, calculous pyonephrosis, infected hydronephrosis), nephrectomy may be indicated. Whether this should be done at the time of drainage of the abscess or later depends upon the judgment of the surgeon.

B. General Measures: In the early stages, local heat may be helpful in relieving pain and muscle spasm.

C. Follow-Up Care: Even though the kidney itself is normal, excretory urograms must be obtained 2 or 3 months after drainage of the abscess to be sure ureteral stenosis has not developed.

Prognosis

If the abscess is uncomplicated by primary renal disease and if proper treatment is used, the prognosis is good. Removal of the kidney may be necessary if the organ is badly damaged.

NONSPECIFIC INFECTIONS OF THE URETER

Isolated infection of the ureter does not occur. Although ureteritis accompanies pyelonephritis, the former contributes few symptoms and is clinically of little importance. In the presence of chronic renal and ureteral infection, the ureteral wall may become fibrotic. This may lead to stricture formation or interfere with normal peristalsis. Except in these unusual circumstances, cure of the renal infection leads to resolution of ureteral inflammation.

NONSPECIFIC INFECTIONS OF THE BLADDER

ACUTE CYSTITIS

Etiology

Cystitis is far more common in the female than in the male. In the female, cystitis is caused by ascent of bacteria from the urethra. The symptoms of cystitis usually develop 36–48 hours after sexual intercourse. It is for this reason that the patient seldom recognizes this association. Many women state that they have difficulty in urinating (eg, hesitancy and slow stream), but careful questioning will usually reveal that voiding is free most of the time. The obstructive symptoms are therefore not suggestive of urethral stenosis; they must arise from periodic spasm of the striated periurethral sphincter, ordinarily caused by anxiety and tension. Under these circumstances, there is wide dilatation of the proximal urethra, leading to turbulent urinary flow that washes the flora of the deep urethra into the bladder. Cystitis, of course, also accompanies the rare hematogenous renal infection. Lymphogenous spread from an infected cervix seems possible but must be rare.

In man, cystitis is always secondary to some other factor: infection in the prostate or kidney or residual urine associated with the enlarged prostate. The presence of a vesical calculus or an ulcerated vesical neoplasm is often complicated by cystitis.

Infections of the bowel (eg, diverticulitis, appendiceal abscess) may involve the bladder by contiguity.

Pathogenesis & Pathology

The infected bladder, unless it is constantly insulted by an infected prostate or kidney or contains residual urine, tends to heal spontaneously. Particularly with the use of modern antibiotic therapy, acute infection usually resolves without residual structural or functional injury.

In acute cystitis, the bladder either is diffusely reddened or contains multiple foci of submucosal hemorrhage. The mucosa is edematous; its surface may be covered by a purulent membrane. Superficial ulcers are occasionally seen. The muscularis is usually not involved. Microscopically, in addition to the edema, some desquamation of the mucosa occurs. Dilatation of capillaries is striking. Leukocytic infiltration is present and may extend into the muscle. Temporary ureteral reflux through a "borderline" ureterovesical junction may occur, thus leading to secondary acute pyelonephritis.

Clinical Findings

A. Symptoms: Symptoms include burning on urination, urgency to the point of incontinence, frequency and nocturia, and often hematuria, which is usually terminal (on the toilet tissue). Fever is low-grade or absent unless prostatic or renal infection is present. Urinary complaints predominate; little malaise occurs. There may be mild low backache or suprapubic discomfort.

In women, the attack usually follows intercourse ("honeymoon cystitis"). In men, a quiescent prostatitis may be activated by considerable sexual excitement and alcoholic indulgence and thus cause secondary cystitis. A preceding urethral discharge (either nonspecific or gonorrheal) may imply the presence of prostatitis. With nonspecific urethritis in men, it seems possible that these microorganisms might ascend to the prostate or bladder.

In children, most instances of cystitis really represent chronic pyelonephritis because of the high incidence of reflux at this age. There is a group of children who develop symptoms of acute hemorrhagic cystitis which has been shown to be caused by adenovirus type 11 or 21. It is a self-limiting disease.

A history of recurrent attacks of cystitis suggests the presence of unrecognized prostatitis or residual urine, exacerbations of chronic cystitis or pyelonephritis, or, most commonly in women, ascent of bacteria in association with sexual intercourse.

Cyclophosphamide (Cytoxan) not infrequently causes acute cystitis with hemorrhage. Although stopping the drug may be followed by resolution, in a few instances cystectomy has been necessary as a lifesaving procedure. In association with this vesical inflammation, vesicoureteral reflux may develop.

B. Signs: Examination of the abdomen is usually normal. Tenderness is occasionally found over the bladder. The presence of a tender epididymis points to prostatitis as an obvious cause for the cystitis. Rectal examination may reveal a relaxed anal sphincter, suggesting neurogenic dysfunction and the presence of residual urine. In men, the prostate may be enlarged, firm, and tender—even hot. (These findings are compatible with acute prostatitis.) Not until the acute phase of the infection has abated should the gland be massaged to prove the presence of infection, since the following complications can occur: bacteremia with pyelonephritis, acute epididymitis, and prostatic abscess.

Pelvic examination may reveal acute urethritis (nonspecific or gonorrheal), urethral diverticulum, vaginitis (including trichomonal vaginitis), or cystocele (with residual urine) as causes of cystitis. The urethra may be markedly tender. Infection in Skene's glands should be sought. Vaginal discharge should be examined bacteriologically. A partially imperforate hymen or urethrohymenal fusion should be sought.

C. Laboratory Findings: The white blood count is usually elevated. Urinalysis shows pus cells and bacteria; red blood cells may be present. In acute infection, great amounts of pus are common. (In chronic disease, little or no pus is found.) Renal function is not affected.

D. X-Ray Findings: X-rays are not indicated unless stasis or renal infection is suspected. They may be needed, however, if the patient fails to respond to adequate therapy for the cystitis or if infection is recurrent; obstruction, vesicoureteral reflux, tuberculosis, or calculus may be the cause.

E. Instrumental Examination: Cystoscopy is contraindicated during the acute phase. It should be done 7–10 days later, however, if hematuria has been noticed; an ulcerating vesical neoplasm, stone, or foreign body may be found.

Differential Diagnosis

Chronic prostatitis may cause similar symptoms, yet the urine may be normal. Prostatic massage will reveal pus in the secretion.

Allergic cystitis may have an abrupt onset. A few pus cells and monocytes are found. No bacteria are seen on the stained smear. A history of ingestion of food which has caused a similar reaction in the past may be elicited. Allergy to certain spermatocidal jellies may cause vesical irritability. A history of other allergies may be helpful.

Acute exacerbation of a chronic bladder infection may simulate a new infection, for chronic cystitis often causes no symptoms. Such exacerbation usually resists routine treatment, thereby suggesting the presence of chronic disease. Cystoscopy will be of help in differentiation.

The psychosomatic cystitis syndrome may cause symptoms similar to those of acute cystitis. However, urinalysis shows no evidence of infection. A history of recurrent attacks precipitated by anxiety or emotional upset can usually be obtained (see Chapter 34).

Tuberculous cystitis may be differentiated by the finding of "sterile" pyuria on the stained smear or on culture. Tubercle bacilli usually are demonstrable on an acid-fast stain or on culture. There is no response to adequate therapy for a nonspecific infection. This should cause the physician to be suspicious.

Neoplasm involving the bladder may be primary or due to direct extension from the colon or cervix. With invasion and ulceration, infection is inevitable and will not respond to antibiotics. Since this is an indication for cystoscopy, the diagnosis will become obvious.

Many children, reacting to the detergents in bubble bath, may complain of symptoms suggesting cystitis. Urinalysis shows no infection.

Complications

Acute pyelonephritis is a common complication of ascending acute cystitis in little girls because of the relatively high incidence of vesicoureteral reflux in this age group. It is relatively rare in the adult.

Prevention

In women who are suspected of suffering recurrent attacks of cystitis following intercourse, postcoital voiding with vigor followed by a similar effort the next morning will abolish infections in 80% of cases. If this is ineffective, give 1 g of a sulfonamide or 100 mg of nitrofurantoin orally at the time of vigorous voiding. Landes & others (1970) have observed a marked decrease in incidence of recurrent cystitis in women following application of povidone-iodine (Betadine) ointment to the periurethral area following the last voiding in the evening and the first voiding in the morning.

Treatment

A. Specific Measures: Nitrofurantoin, ampicillin, penicillin G, nalidixic acid, and the tetracyclines are the most useful drugs for the treatment of acute cystitis. The sulfonamides are also efficacious and the least expensive. If they fail to sterilize the urine within 2 weeks, a thorough urologic investigation is indicated. In women who suffer from recurrent attacks of cystitis following intercourse, postcoital voiding and the administration of 1 g of a sulfonamide, 100 mg of nitro-

furantoin, or 400,000 units of penicillin G by mouth immediately after coitus and a similar dose the next morning will usually prevent further trouble. Application of povidone-iodine (Betadine) ointment to the periurethral area following the last voiding in the evening and the first voiding in the morning has been reported to cause a marked decrease in the incidence of recurrent cystitis in women (see Landes reference, p 176).

B. General Measures: The irritable bladder may be sedated by one of the following measures:

1. Alkalinization of the urine—It may be necessary to give 16–20 g of sodium bicarbonate. Fruit juices are also helpful.

2. Antispasmodics—Many of the antispasmodics used in the treatment of gastrointestinal disorders are useful. Tincture of belladonna or atropine combined with phenobarbital may afford relief.

3. Local heat—Hot sitz baths may ease severe pain and spasm. An adequate fluid intake is desirable, but forcing of fluids is not necessary and only increases the patient's urinary frequency. Further, it decreases the concentration of the antimicrobial drug in the urine.

4. Hymenotomy—Urethrohymenal fusion or incomplete hymenal perforation should be treated appropriately.

Prognosis

In the absence of stasis, acute cystitis resolves promptly with proper medical therapy. No vesical injury should result. If the infection recurs, the underlying cause must be determined.

CHRONIC CYSTITIS

Etiology & Pathogenesis

Chronic infection of the bladder is often secondary to chronic infection of the upper tract. It may also be due to residual urine, ureteral reflux, or urethral stenosis. Too frequently it is the result of incomplete treatment of simple acute cystitis. The most common cause of pyuria and bacteriuria is cystitis. The presence of these abnormal urinary constituents is not pathognomonic of pyelonephritis, which must be proved by thorough urologic examination.

Pathology

In the chronic stage, the mucosa is often pale and appears thinned. Ulceration is rare. The surface may be studded with cysts (cystitis cystica). Capacity is diminished if fibrosis of the detrusor is extensive. Pericystic fibrosis is a rare complication. Microscopic section usually shows thinning of the epithelium. The submucosa and muscle layers are infiltrated with fibroblasts, small round cells, and plasma cells.

Clinical Findings

A. Symptoms: Complaints may be those of constant or recurrent mild vesical irritability, or there may be none at all. In men, chronic cystitis may be secondary to chronic prostatitis but is more often due to obstruction distal to the bladder with residual urine. In women, it may persist because of chronic urethritis or residual urine (eg, cystocele, urethral stenosis). In both males and females, chronic kidney infection is often the cause. Symptoms suggesting such disease should be sought.

B. Signs: Renal tenderness (infection) or enlargement (hydronephrosis) may be noted. A distended bladder may be found. Examination of the external genitalia in the male is usually noncontributory. Rectal examination may demonstrate impaired tone of the anal sphincter, which suggests detrusor weakness related to neurogenic bladder. Prostatic enlargement, cancer, or infection may be discovered. Pelvic examination may show cervicitis, vaginitis, or inflammation of Skene's or Bartholin's glands. Palpation of the urethra may reveal a mass which, when pressure is applied to it, causes pus to exude from the meatus. This finding is typical of urethral diverticulum

C. Laboratory Findings: The blood count is usually not remarkable. If anemia is present, something other than bladder infection is the cause. In many instances few or no pus cells are found; nevertheless, the stained smear or culture reveals bacteria.

Renal function tests in simple chronic cystitis are normal. If the excretion of PSP is depressed, it means either bilateral renal damage (obstruction or infection), reflux, or vesical residual urine. In either case, such a finding is an important clue suggesting further search for the cause of chronicity.

D. X-Ray Findings: A plain film of the abdomen may reveal a large kidney (hydronephrosis) or a small one (atrophic pyelonephritis). An excretory urogram shows no abnormality in uncomplicated cystitis. However, since a significant number of cases of chronic cystitis are secondary to upper urinary tract infection or vesical residual urine, this examination should always be performed. Renal calcification suggesting stone or tuberculosis may be seen.

This examination may reveal hydronephrosis due to ureteral obstruction or changes compatible with healed pyelonephritis. The cystogram may demonstrate trabeculation of the bladder wall, suggesting obstruction distal to the bladder. Ureteral reflux may be observed. The film taken after voiding may reveal residual urine. Retrograde urograms may be required.

E. Instrumental Examination: The passage of a large catheter (22F) may reveal a urethral stricture or residual urine. Either can perpetuate chronic infection.

Cystoscopy will demonstrate the degree of a cystocele or prostatic obstruction. Ulceration of the vesical wall may be seen (tuberculosis); foreign bodies may be found. Panendoscopy may reveal the orifice of a urethral diverticulum.

Ureteral catheterization for relative renal function studies and separate urine specimens for bacteriologic survey may be needed to determine the source of the infection and the presence of ureteral obstruction.

Differential Diagnosis

Chronic prostatitis may cause symptoms of cystitis, but the finding of pus in the prostatic secretion makes the diagnosis.

Since chronic pyelonephritis is often without symptoms referable to the kidneys, thorough urologic investigation (including a voiding cystourethrogram) is needed to establish the cause of the infection in all cases of chronic cystitis.

Tuberculosis of the kidney and bladder is a chronic disease which may mimic chronic cystitis in every way. Certain findings should suggest the presence of tuberculosis: (1) "sterile" pyuria on a stained smear or culture of urinary sediment, (2) lack of response to the usual antibiotics, (3) evidence of a renal lesion by urography, (4) the finding of acid-fast organisms by smear or culture, and (5) ulceration of the bladder wall, with biopsy positive for tuberculosis.

Emotional tension as a cause of chronic bladder symptoms should be suspected if urinalysis is normal and emotional instability is noted. (See Chapter 34.)

Senile urethritis in women past the menopause commonly causes symptoms suggesting chronic cystitis. Urinalysis is normal, and the appearance of the vaginal mucosa is typical of senile change.

Interstitial cystitis causes frequency, nocturia, and suprapubic pain when the contracted bladder becomes full. The urine is free of pus cells and bacteria. Cystoscopy reveals the typical vesical contracture, and when the bladder is overdistended the mucosa on the dome may split and bleed.

Irradiation cystitis may occur following radiotherapy of tumors in the region of the bladder (eg, cancer of the cervix). The urine may become infected if vesical ulceration develops. The history of previous x-ray or radium therapy as well as the cystoscopic finding of a pale, edematous, or telangiectatic vesical mucosa and, at times, ulceration make the differentiation. Biopsy may be indicated to rule out neoplasm.

Chronic urethritis in women may also cause longstanding symptoms suggestive of chronic cystitis. The urine, however, is negative. Panendoscopy will reveal inflammation of the urethral mucosa. Some urethral stenosis is usually found as well.

Complications

Renal infection may occur either because of an incompetent ureterovesical valve or, rarely, by the hematogenous route. Occasionally, fibrosis of the bladder wall may cause contracture with loss of capacity. Stenosis of the intramural portion of the ureters or vesicoureteral reflux may develop, whereupon hydronephrosis follows.

Prevention

Most cases are secondary to vesical residual urine (eg, cystocele, enlarged prostate). Treatment designed to improve vesical emptying is indicated.

Treatment

A. Specific Measures: One of the less expensive,

less toxic drugs should be tried first (eg, a sulfonamide or nitrofurantoin); if it fails to cure the infection, further drug therapy should be based on the results of sensitivity tests. Antibiotic treatment must be intensive and prolonged (3–4 weeks). Even under these conditions, therapy is often unsuccessful. Chronic antimicrobial suppression treatment (eg, sulfonamides, methenamine with an acidifier) should then be instituted.

Thorough studies are essential in order to identify the underlying cause of the infection (eg, urethral stenosis, prostatitis). Unless these conditions are corrected, treatment will be unsatisfactory.

B. General Measures: Since symptoms of vesical irritability are usually not as severe as those which accompany acute infection, they can usually be relieved by the measures listed on p 157.

Prognosis

Simple drug therapy often fails to eradicate the infection unless steps are taken to treat the cause (eg, enlarged prostate, chronic prostatitis, chronic urethritis in the female).

NONSPECIFIC INFECTIONS OF THE PROSTATE GLAND

ACUTE PROSTATITIS & PROSTATIC ABSCESS

Etiology

Acute prostatic infection may be hematogenous or may occur as a result of ascent of bacteria up the urethra. It is seen occasionally in childhood and has been observed in the neonatal period. A chronic quiescent prostatic infection can become acute following too vigorous prostatic massage or urethral instrumentation.

Pathogenesis & Pathology

Acute bacterial prostatic infection is usually complicated by acute cystitis and even by acute urinary retention. It may resolve (especially with proper medication), or, rarely, it may progress to abscess formation. Microscopic examination of the acutely infected gland reveals diffuse leukocytic infiltration; abscesses may be noted. Edema is marked. Similar changes are found also in the seminal vesicles, for these are usually involved when the prostate is infected.

Granulomatous prostatitis is a second form of acute prostatitis. It, too, is usually a febrile disease at onset and is usually associated with pyuria. Resolution is slow, and the gland becomes hard. It can, therefore, suggest carcinoma. Microscopically, a granulomatous reaction is noted. The stroma is infiltrated with polymorphonuclear leukocytes, lymphocytes, plasma cells, and multinucleated giant cells. The stroma shows in-

creased fibrosis. Many of the acini have ruptured, releasing prostatic secretion into the connective tissue. It is thought that this is the cause of the severe inflammatory reaction.

Towfighi & others (1972) find many eosinophils in the tissues as well as a frequent history of allergic phenomena.

Clinical Findings

A. Symptoms: Vesical irritability (burning, frequency, urgency, nocturia) may be extreme. Hematuria may be present; it is usually initial or terminal but may be total. Purulent urethral discharge may be noted. There may be perineal aching or low back pain. Moderate to high fever is usual. Cloudy urine is to be expected. Symptoms may have developed during an acute upper respiratory infection, following the extraction of infected teeth, or after urethral instrumentation. Swelling of the gland may cause urinary retention.

B. Signs: The patient ordinarily is not prostrated, but fever may be high. Urethral discharge may be present. Rectal examination reveals an exquisitely tender, enlarged, "hot" prostate. It may be quite firm. Fluctuation means abscess formation. The prostate should not be massaged while acutely inflamed. After the acute phase is over, however, massage is indicated both for diagnosis and treatment.

In the granulomatous form, the prostate may persist in its enlargement and become quite indurated, thus simulating carcinoma. Three to 6 months may be required for resolution.

C. Laboratory Findings: The white blood count is usually elevated in the range of $20,000/\mu l$. Urinalysis shows pus and bacteria on stain and culture. Sensitivity tests should be done. Prostatic secretion should be subjected to culture and sensitivity tests, though the cultures are usually negative.

D. Instrumental Examination: Instrumentation is contraindicated during the acute stage. The only exception to this rule is to relieve acute urinary retention due to prostatic edema or abscess. If an abscess is suspected, the diagnosis may be established by perineal needle puncture.

Differential Diagnosis

Acute pyelonephritis may also be marked by severe vesical irritability. The backache with prostatitis is usually sacral, whereas in pyelonephritis it is in the lumbar area. Rectal examination should establish the diagnosis of acute prostatitis.

Amicrobic pyuria may cause exactly the same symptoms as acute prostatitis. Urinalysis or culture, however, reveals no demonstrable organisms in amicrobic pyuria. Rectal findings also help in differentiation.

Acute congestive prostatitis (prostatosis), often due to lack of sexual activity, may cause perineal, back, and testicular pain as well as urethral discharge. The prostate may be swollen and moderately tender. There are, however, no symptoms of vesical irritability and no fever. Massage of the prostate will produce copious secretion, often containing pus cells, with prompt cessation of symptoms.

Carcinoma of the prostate may be confused with subsiding granulomatous prostatitis. Perineal or transrectal needle biopsy may be indicated.

Complications

Acute urinary retention may occur from swelling of the gland. If an abscess forms, it may rupture spontaneously into the urethra, rectum, or perineum. Acute pyelonephritis may occur by the hematogenous route. This is particularly apt to happen if the prostate is massaged or if instrumentation is done during the acute stage. Acute epididymitis is not uncommon. It too is apt to occur from prostatic manipulation or instrumentation during the acute stage.

Prevention

Prostatic massage should be part of the physical examination of all men. The discovery and treatment of asymptomatic prostatitis may prevent the later development of an acute process. Too vigorous prostatic massage may lead to exacerbation of a chronic infection.

In the presence of bacteriuria, the urine should be sterilized before catheterization or endoscopy is done.

Treatment

A. Specific Measures: Only 3 antimicrobials are active in prostatic tissue: erythromycin, oleandomycin, and trimethoprim. Since the bacteria are usually gram-negative rods, a combination of a sulfonamide (sulfamethoxazole) and trimethoprim (co-trimoxazole) should be administered. The dose is 1 g orally twice a day for 10–14 days. The urine (and the acute symptoms) should respond in a few days. After subsidence of the acute symptoms and the development of sterile urine, the prostate should be massaged to note the pus content and to obtain material for culture.

Instrumentation is contraindicated at first unless urinary retention occurs. If a frank abscess develops, drainage by perineal needle in addition to antimicrobial medication may lead to resolution. Surgical perineal drainage or transurethral unroofing of the abscess may be necessary.

Granulomatous prostatitis may respond to corticosteroids.

B. General Measures: Perineal pain may require analgesics; sitz baths may afford some relief and may hasten resolution of the inflammation. Vesical irritability can be relieved by antispasmodics. Bed rest is essential. An adequate fluid intake is needed.

Prognosis

The prognosis is good if antibiotic therapy is instituted. If treatment is inadequate, the infection may become chronic and more difficult to eradicate.

CHRONIC PROSTATITIS

Etiology

Chronic prostatitis usually develops as a result of invasion of bacteria from the urethra. It may also have a hematogenous source. Inadequate treatment of acute prostatitis may lead to the chronic form. It may develop secondary to cystitis or pyelonephritis. A few cases of coccidioidal granuloma of the prostate have been reported.

Pathogenesis & Pathology

An acute or subacute prostatic infection may become chronic. Chronic infection may rarely lead to contracture of the bladder neck. Function (eg, potency, fertility) is not impaired.

Chronic prostatic infection usually causes the gland to be firmer than normal as a result of fibrosis. The ducts may contain pus; their lining cells may degenerate. Similar changes are found in the seminal vesicles, for these are usually involved when the prostate is infected.

Clinical Findings

A. Symptoms: There are usually no symptoms. Most men with chronic prostatitis have no reason to suspect it. A few men may note an aching or "fullness" in the perineum, low back pain, or an unexpected low-grade fever. Urethral discomfort with ejaculation may be felt.

Symptoms accompanying a mild exacerbation may include urethral discharge (which may be the only symptom) and symptoms of cystitis. If the patient has symptoms of prostatic obstruction, these may suddenly increase as a result of swelling of the gland. Acute epididymitis may occur; this usually signifies that prostatitis exists.

Other symptoms which are often incorrectly attributed to prostatitis include infertility (uncomplicated chronic prostatitis rarely causes sterility), impotence (exceedingly rare if it occurs at all), and such psychosomatic complaints—usually associated with sexual difficulties—as nervousness, insomnia, and emotional tension.

B. Signs: Epididymitis is usually caused by prostatitis, though reflux of sterile urine down the vas may cause a type of chemical epididymitis. Rectal examination may reveal a normal, boggy, or indurated prostate. There may be areas of fibrosis. Crepitation may sometimes be felt if stones are present. Massage of the prostate will produce secretion which contains pus. A few pathogens may be found on culture, but sensitivity tests have not proved helpful (Mears & Stamey, 1968). The degree of tenderness is of little help in diagnosis, since tenderness is generally determined by the pain threshold of the patient and the degree of apprehension from which he suffers.

C. Laboratory Findings: Urethral discharge should be examined both unstained (trichomonads, lecithin bodies from the prostate) and stained. The white blood count is generally normal unless an exacerbation or complication (epididymitis) is present. The urine may contain pus and bacteria. The PSP test is normal unless there is a silent bilateral renal disease (infection) or residual urine (bladder neck obstruction).

D. X-Ray Findings: Plain films or excretory urograms will be normal unless there are complications (eg, prostatic enlargement, urethral stricture, chronic pyelonephritis).

E. Instrumental Examination: Instrumentation is not indicated unless there is evidence of complications (eg, prostatic enlargement, urethral stricture, upper tract infection).

Differential Diagnosis

Symptoms of acute or chronic urethritis may suggest prostatitis, but the prostatic secretions in those instances will be clear.

Cystitis may be confused with prostatitis, but one must remember that cystitis in men is always secondary to renal or prostatic infection or residual urine. Again, examination of the prostatic secretion will make the differentiation.

Diseases of the anus (eg, fissure, thrombosed hemorrhoid) may cause perineal pain and, at times, urinary urgency, but proper examination of this area should make the correct diagnosis.

Complications

Acute or chronic cystitis may occur secondary to prostatic infection. Pyelonephritis by the hematogenous route may develop from exacerbation of the prostatic infection. Acute epididymitis may follow physical strain, prostatic massage, or urethral instrumentation. An exacerbation of the infection may occur spontaneously or after prostatic massage or urethral instrumentation. Contracture of the bladder neck caused by fibrosis of the prostatic parenchyma is occasionally seen. If so, there are symptoms of prostatism and, at times, residual urine.

Prevention

Vigorous treatment of acute prostatitis may prevent the development of chronic disease. Since prostatitis is often secondary to urethral infection, appropriate treatment of both nonspecific and gonorrheal urethritis is indicated.

Treatment

A. Specific Measures: Bacterial prostatitis is resistant to medical treatment. A complicating cystitis will often respond rapidly to the commonly used antimicrobials (eg, sulfonamides, nitrofurantoin), but Mears & Stamey (1968), Stamey & others (1970), and Madsen & others (1968) find that the usual chemotherapeutic drugs do not reach the prostate even when adequate serum and urine levels are achieved. Since trimethoprim is the only drug that does enter the prostate in significant concentration and is effective against coliform bacilli, trimethoprim-sulfamethoxazole (Bactrim, Septra; co-trimoxazole), 1 g twice a day, should be administered for 10–14 days. Drach (1974) suggests a course of 28 days, but even then some relapses occur and it may be necessary to keep the patient on chronic suppressive antimicrobial drugs to prevent recurrent cystitis. A prostatic massage every 2 weeks may promote drainage. Intercourse should therefore be encouraged. Mears & Stamey (1972) have suggested that transurethral prostatic resection may be indicated in recalcitrant cases to remove the infected tissue.

B. General Measures: Daily sitz baths may hasten resolution of the infection.

Prognosis

Although chronic prostatic infection causes little harm in itself, the complications arising from it are important. This points up the need for routine prostatic massage with microscopic examination of the secretion in all men so that silent chronic prostatitis may be discovered and treated.

NONSPECIFIC INFECTIONS OF THE SEMINAL VESICLES

Almost all infections of the prostate involve the seminal vesicles as well, but it is doubtful if seminal vesiculitis contributes any specific symptoms. Infection of the seminal vesicles without prostatitis probably does not occur. For these reasons, seminal vesiculitis is covered in the discussion of prostatic infections.

NONSPECIFIC INFECTIONS OF THE MALE URETHRA*

ACUTE URETHRITIS

Etiology

Acute urethritis is usually an ascending infection, but it can be caused by an infection descending from an infected prostate. Both gram-negative rods and gram-positive cocci are occasionally found. In most cases, however, stained smears or cultures of the secretion are usually negative for bacteria. No particular microorganism has yet been incriminated. In normal controls, 27% of young men harbor T-mycoplasmas. In those with urethral discharge, 76% have this organism. After treatment of the nonspecific urethritis, only 28%

---

*See Chapter 14 for nonspecific infection of the female urethra and for gonorrheal urethritis.

have positive cultures for this organism (McChesney & others, 1973). *Mycoplasma hominis* is also often found. It should be pointed out that the mycoplasmas are normal inhabitants of both the vagina and urethra in both sexes. Whether they are truly the etiologic agents is moot. Chlamydia is also suspect. Trichomonads occasionally cause urethritis.

Pathogenesis & Pathology

Urethritis may ascend to the prostate and bladder. If urethritis is severe enough, a periurethral abscess may form and urethral stricture may then develop, but this is rare. In the acute stage of infection, the mucosa is red, edematous, and covered with a purulent exudate. It may be ulcerated. Microscopic examination shows marked edema and infiltration by leukocytes, plasma cells, and lymphocytes. Capillaries are markedly dilated. The glands of Littré may be engorged or plugged by masses of pus cells.

Acute urethritis in the female is seldom seen except in association with gonorrhea.

Clinical Findings

A. Symptoms: Urethral discharge is the leading symptom; it may be quite as profuse as that seen with gonorrhea. There may be a constant itching or burning sensation in the urethra. Burning on urination may be noted.

The onset of symptoms often seems to be related to intercourse. Symptoms may develop a few days thereafter, or the interval may be longer. A history of intercourse during menstruation, when the vaginal bacterial flora is increased, may be obtained. Usually, however, no obvious cause can be discovered.

B. Signs: The discharge may be profuse or scanty, thick and purulent, thin or mucoid. The lips of the meatus are often red, edematous, and everted.

C. Laboratory Findings: The discharge must be examined unstained and stained. Wet preparations may show trichomonads or may reveal lecithin bodies (typical of prostatic secretion). Rods and cocci may be found on the stained slide, but in most instances no bacteria are seen; this raises the question of possible infection with T-strain mycoplasmas or chlamydiae. This step is the important one in differentiating nonspecific urethritis from gonorrheal urethritis. Cultures may be necessary in doubtful cases. Sensitivity tests are of little help in treatment.

If no discharge is available at the time of examination, the first portion of the voided urine will contain "subclinical" discharge. This should be centrifuged and the sediment examined as discharge.

The midstream specimen of urine will be free of pus and bacteria unless complications (prostatitis, cystitis) are present.

D. Instrumental Examination: Instrumentation is contraindicated during the acute stage. Later, however, the passage of a sound will rule out urethral stricture as a cause of the urethritis.

Differential Diagnosis

Gonorrheal urethritis often causes the same symptoms. The stained smear makes the differentiation.

Amicrobic pyuria may start with acute urethritis but is also associated with severe symptoms of acute cystitis. Sterile pyuria and discharge are the rule.

Trichomonal urethritis is differentiated by microscopic identification of the motile organisms, though cultures of prostatic secretion or the ejaculate are much more rewarding.

Nonspecific prostatitis is often accompanied by urethral discharge. The absence of pus in the prostatic secretion differentiates the 2 conditions.

Complications

Prostatitis or cystitis may occur by direct extension. These complications are usually caused, however, by the passage of instruments or the use of forceful urethral irrigations.

Periurethral abscess may develop, but this also is usually a complication of injudicious urologic treatment. The abscess may rupture into the urethra or may drain through the skin. The complications of periurethral abscess are urinary fistula and urethral stricture caused by the fibrosis in the healing process.

Prevention

Acute urethritis may develop from an indwelling urethral catheter made of latex. Use the smallest catheter that is practical, preferably coated with (or made of) silicon. Since nonspecific urethritis due to chlamydiae is usually transmitted by intercourse, empirical treatment of the partner should be considered if that group of organisms is the suspected offender.

Treatment

A. Specific Measures: Although antimicrobial therapy is not often spectacular, the combination of a sulfonamide and either tetracycline or erythromycin seems to afford the best result. They are efficacious for both chlamydial and T-strain mycoplasmal infections.

Prostatitis is often the cause of urethral discharge. Prostatic massage is contraindicated in the early stages of acute urethritis; if prostatitis is present, massage may exacerbate its symptoms. However, massage is indicated after a few days for differential diagnostic purposes (silent chronic prostatitis). A course of massage is indicated if prostatitis is found.

B. General Measures: Experience has shown that intercourse should be temporarily discontinued since it prolongs the acute phase of the disease.

Prognosis

Acute nonspecific urethritis is at times difficult to eradicate (see Chronic Urethritis, below). Underlying causes (eg, prostatitis, urethral stricture) must be sought. Fortunately, little harm is done organically by this disease although it does cause the patient considerable anxiety.

CHRONIC URETHRITIS

Etiology

Chronic urethral infection may represent the end stage of an incompletely healed acute urethritis or may be an infection which has spread from a chronic prostatitis or has developed at the point of urethral stricture. One or more types of pyogenic organisms are usually found.

The urethral discharge may develop in men who have had no intercourse for months. Others, after a period of abstinence followed by sexual activity (frequently accompanied by moderate alcoholic intake), may develop discharge even though a condom has been used. Recurrent discharge is often a symptom of psychosexual trouble and is probably caused by psychic overstimulation of the glands of Littré. In this instance, pus cells are absent from the secretion.

Pathogenesis & Pathology

In chronic urethritis, the mucosa is usually granular and often appears dull but may be reddened. Microscopically, one sees lymphocytes, plasma cells, and a few leukocytes; fibroblasts are increased.

Clinical Findings

A. Symptoms: Urethral discharge is the primary symptom. It varies in amount and consistency and may appear and disappear spontaneously. The discharge may only be noticed before the first urination after waking. Some urethral irritation may be noted which is not usually related to urination. If there are symptoms of vesical irritability, prostatitis or cystitis is probably present. Psychosexual problems may be uncovered.

B. Signs: The discharge may or may not be present at the time of examination. Prostatic examination may reveal a gland which is boggy and congested or, conversely, firm, even containing fibrotic nodules. It may be normal on palpation. Many cases of chronic urethritis are secondary to chronic prostatitis.

C. Laboratoray Findings: The unstained discharge should be examined for lecithin bodies and in saline for trichomonads. Culture (if available) should be done if trichomoniasis is suspected. The former suggests a prostatic source for the urethral secretions. The discharge should be stained with methylene blue and with Gram's stain. Nonspecific organisms (rods and cocci) and gonococci should be sought. Quite often, no bacteria are seen at all; this suggests infection with mycoplasma or chlamydia or a psychosomatic reaction. Cultures may be needed in equivocal cases.

If no discharge is present at the time of examination, the first part of the voided urine can be centrifuged since it contains the pus cells, microorganisms, and mucus that make up the discharge. It is then examined in the same manner as the discharge itself. A less satisfactory technic that is sometimes used is to give the patient slides on which he can place any discharge for later examination.

The midstream specimen of urine should be free of pus and bacteria unless complications are present (eg, cystitis).

D. Instrumental Examination: The passage of a sound may be arrested by a urethral stricture, which may prove to be an important factor in producing the discharge. Panendoscopy will visualize the inflamed urethral wall. It may demonstrate a urethral tumor or a diverticulum containing pus.

Differential Diagnosis

Gonorrheal urethritis develops 2–5 days following exposure. The discharge is usually profuse and purulent. The stained smear tells the story. If any doubt exists, cultures can be made.

Reiter's symdrome is characterized by iritis and arthritis as well as urethritis. The discharge is usually free of bacteria. The infective agent is not established but is thought to be one of the chlamydiae.

Trichomonal urethritis is difficult to diagnose because the organism is often hard to demonstrate in a wet preparation. Culture of prostatic secretion or the ejaculate is necessary.

Complications

The urethral infection can ascend to the prostate or bladder, but this is not usual unless instrumentation is done injudiciously.

Prevention

See under Acute Urethritis.

Treatment

The usual chemotherapeutic and antibiotic drugs do not usually cure the disease, but they should be tried. A combination of a sulfonamide and an antibiotic such as one of the tetracyclines or erythromycin may prove helpful.

A congested or infected prostate requires periodic massage. A urethral stricture must be dilated. Sexual problems should be resolved if possible. This may require psychiatric referral.

Prognosis

The disease itself is not harmful, although urinary tract complications occasionally develop from it. The psychologic effect is usually the most serious result of the infection.

NONSPECIFIC INFECTIONS OF THE EPIDIDYMIS

ACUTE EPIDIDYMITIS

Etiology

There are 3 common causes of epididymitis: (1) Preexisting prostatitis, or prostatic infection introduced by an interval or indwelling urethral catheter. (2) Prostatectomy, particularly the transurethral type, where the ejaculatory ducts are laid open in the prostatic fossa. The hydrostatic pressure with voiding or with physical strain may force urine (which may contain bacteria for 8–12 weeks after the operation) down the vas. The infection may also reach the epididymis through the perivasal lymphatics. (3) Reflux of sterile urine down the vas deferens will lead to a chemical epididymitis. Recurrent epididymitis in a young boy suggests the possibility of ureteral drainage into a seminal vesicle. Recurrent epididymitis has been described in a few patients with sarcoidosis.

Pathogenesis & Pathology

In its early stages, epididymitis is a cellular inflammation (cellulitis). It starts in the vas deferens and descends to the lower pole of the epididymis. The initial symptoms may be pain in the groin and even in the flank secondary to the vasitis.

In the acute stage, the epididymis is swollen and indurated. The infection spreads from the lower to the upper pole. On section, small abscesses may be seen. The tunica vaginalis often secretes serous fluid (inflammatory hydrocele), and this fluid may contain pus. The spermatic cord becomes thickened. The testis becomes swollen secondarily from passive congestion but rarely becomes involved in the inflammation.

Microscopically, changes grade from edema and infiltration with leukocytes, plasma cells, and lymphocytes to actual abscess formation. The tubular epithelium may show necrosis. Resolution may be complete without residual injury, but peritubular fibrosis often develops, occluding the ducts. If bilateral, it may result in sterility.

Clinical Findings

A. Symptoms: Epididymitis often follows severe physical strain such as lifting a heavy object. It may develop after considerable sexual excitement. The trauma of urethral instrumentation may initiate the complication. It is not uncommon after prostatectomy. Prostatitis is usually the underlying cause.

Pain develops rather suddenly in the scrotum. It may radiate along the spermatic cord and even reach the flank. The pain is generally quite severe and the epididymis exquisitely sensitive. Swelling is rapid and may cause the organ to become twice the size of normal in the course of 3 or 4 hours. The temperature may reach 40 °C (104 °F). Urethral discharge may be noted. Symptoms of cystitis with cloudy urine may accompany the painful swelling.

B. Signs: There may be tenderness over the groin (spermatic cord) or in the lower abdominal quadrant on the affected side. The scrotum is enlarged. The overlying skin may be reddened. If abscess is present, the skin may appear dry, flaky, and thinned; it may rupture spontaneously. If seen early, the enlarged, indurated, tender epididymis may be distinguished from the testis. After a few hours, however, the testis and epididymis become one mass.

The spermatic cord is thickened by edema. Hydrocele secondary to the inflammation may develop within a few days. Urethral discharge may be seen.

Palpation of the prostate may reveal changes suggesting acute or chronic prostatitis. The gland should not be massaged during the acute phase, since the epididymitis may be made worse.

C. Laboratory Findings: The white blood count often reaches 20,000–30,000/μl. Urethral discharge, if present, should be examined both unstained and stained. Urinalysis may or may not reveal evidence of infection.

Differential Diagnosis

Tuberculous epididymitis is usually not painful. The epididymitis is usually distinguishable from the testis on palpation. "Beading" of the vas may be noted. Induration of the prostate and a thickened ipsilateral seminal vesicle are compatible with tuberculosis. The finding of a "sterile" pyuria by smear and of tubercle bacilli on culture will establish the diagnosis.

Testicular tumor is almost always painless; on occasion, however, because of internal hemorrhage, there may be sudden distention of the tunica albuginea which will cause pain. The mass may be found to be separate from a normal epididymis. Prostatic examination and urinalysis will be normal. If doubt exists, urinary chorionic gonadotropins should be measured, although only 15% of testicular tumors elaborate this substance. If testicular tumor cannot be ruled out, orchiectomy should be done.

Torsion of the spermatic cord is usually an affliction of children just before puberty, although it is occasionally seen in men. Epididymitis occurs in an older age group. In the early phase of torsion, the examiner may palpate the epididymis anterior to the testis. The testis is apt to be retracted. Later, however, the testis and epididymis become one enlarged, tender mass. Prehn's sign may be helpful in differentiation: if pain is relieved when the scrotum is gently lifted onto the symphysis, the pain is due to epididymitis; if pain is increased, torsion is the more probable diagnosis. If torsion cannot be ruled out, the testis should be explored.

Torsion of the appendages of the testis or epididymis is a rare disease of prepuberal boys. These pedunculated bodies may twist, causing localized pain and swelling. If seen early, a tender nodule is felt at the upper pole of the testicle; the epididymis is normal. Later, the entire testis becomes swollen, making the differential diagnosis between epididymitis and torsion of the cord or rudimentary appendages difficult. Early surgery is necessary in this instance, for torsion of the cord must receive prompt treatment.

Testicular trauma may simulate acute epididymitis in every way, but the history of the injury and the absence of pyuria will help in differentiation.

Mumps orchitis is usually accompanied by parotitis. There are no urinary symptoms, and the urinary sediment is free of pus cells and bacteria.

Complications

Abscess formation may occur but is rare unless urethral instrumentation or prostatic massage has been done. The abscess may drain spontaneously through the scrotum or may require surgical drainage.

Epididymal abscess may extend into and destroy the testis (epididymo-orchitis), but this is rare.

Prevention

Once the process has subsided, the presence of prostatitis should be sought and, if present, treated. Recurrent acute attacks may indicate the need for ipsilateral vasoligation.

Treatment

A. Specific Measures: If the patient is seen within 24 hours after onset, the disease may be almost completely aborted by infiltrating the spermatic cord just above the testicle with 20 ml of 1% procaine hydrochloride or other local anesthetic agent, thereby obtaining complete anesthesia. Fever usually falls abruptly. Pain may disappear almost completely. The inflammatory mass may resolve in a few days rather than the usual 2 or 3 weeks. If one injection does not afford relief, it should be repeated the next day.

Antibiotics are helpful but not curative. Secondary cystitis will usually clear quickly.

After the epididymitis has subsided (usually 2 or 3 weeks), treatment of the prostatitis is indicated.

B. General Measures: Bed rest is necessary during the acute phase (3–4 days). Support for the enlarged heavy testicle partially relieves the discomfort. Scrotal supporters are too small; the more roomy athletic supporter, lined with cotton, is best.

Analgesics should be used as necessary to combat pain. Local heat usually affords comfort and probably hastens resolution of the inflammatory process. The sitz bath is a useful means of applying heat to the infected prostate and epididymis. If, as sometimes happens, heat increases the pain, an ice bag should be used instead.

Sexual excitement or physical strain (eg, with defecation) may exacerbate the infection and must therefore be controlled.

Prognosis

Almost all acutely inflamed epididymides resolve spontaneously, although it may take 1 or 2 weeks before all pain is gone and 4 weeks or longer for the epididymis to approach normal size and consistency. Complications are not common, although sterility is always a threat if the disease is bilateral.

CHRONIC EPIDIDYMITIS

Chronic epididymitis is the irreversible end stage of a severe acute epididymitis which has been followed by frequent mild attacks.

In chronic epididymitis, fibroplasia has caused induration of the organ. Microscopically, the scarring is so marked that tubular occlusion is usually seen. The tissues are infiltrated with lymphocytes and plasma cells.

There are usually no symptoms except during a mild exacerbation, at which time there may be some degree of local discomfort. The patient may notice a lump in the scrotum.

The epididymis is thickened and somewhat enlarged. It may or may not be tender. It is easily distinguished from the testis on palpation. Often the spermatic cord is thickened and at times the diameter of the vas is increased. The prostate may be firm or contain areas of fibrosis. Its secretion will usually contain pus.

Urinalysis may show infection secondary to prostatitis.

Tuberculous epididymitis mimics nonspecific chronic epididymitis in every way. Beading of the vas, thickening of the ipsilateral seminal vesicle, and the finding of "sterile" pyuria and tubercle bacilli in the urine will make the diagnosis of tuberculous epididymitis. Cystoscopy may reveal vesical ulcers; urograms are of further help.

Testicular tumor may present with a "lump in the testicle." Palpation will show either a thickened epididymis or a hard, insensitive testis (tumor).

Tumors of the epididymis are very rare. Differentiation from chronic epididymitis may ultimately be made only by the pathologist.

If chronic epididymitis is bilateral, sterility is to be expected.

Little benefit can be derived from the administration of antibiotics alone. The prostatitis which is often present must be treated. If prostatic massages cause exacerbation of the epididymal infection, vasoligation should be done during a quiescent interval. The prostatitis can then be treated. Epididymectomy may at times be necessary.

Except for recurring pain and the threat of infertility in bilateral involvement, chronic epididymitis is of little consequence. Once the stage of fibrosis is reached, nothing can be done to resolve it.

NONSPECIFIC INFECTIONS OF THE TESTIS

ACUTE ORCHITIS

Etiology

The testis may become inflamed from a hematogenous source. Orchitis may occur with any infectious disease (eg, coxsackievirus infection, dengue). Patients with mumps parotitis excrete the virus in the urine.

Therefore, it would appear that a complicating mumps epididymo-orchitis may also be a descending infection. The edema which develops probably leads to death of the spermatogenic cells from ischemia. Primary infection of an epididymis may involve its testis by direct extension.

Pathogenesis & Pathology

Grossly, in nonspecific orchitis, the testis is much enlarged, congested, and tense. On section, small abscesses may be noted. Microscopically, there is edema of the connective tissue with diffuse neutrophilic infiltration. The seminiferous tubules also show involvement; necrosis is present. In the healed stage, the seminiferous tubules are embedded in fibrous tissue. On histologic study they may show considerable atrophy. The interstitial cells are usually preserved.

Mumps is the most common cause of inflammation of the testis, which occurs only after puberty. It is usually unilateral but may be bilateral. Grossly, the testis is much enlarged and bluish in color. On section, because of the interstitial reaction and edema, the tubules do not extrude. Microscopically, edema and dilatation of blood vessels are noted. Neutrophils, lymphocytes, and macrophages are abundant. Tubular cells show varying degrees of degeneration. In the healed stage, the testis is small and flabby. Microscopic study in this instance shows marked tubular atrophy, although the Leydig cells are usually normal in appearance. The epididymis usually shows similar changes.

Clinical Findings

A. Symptoms: Onset is sudden, with pain and swelling of the testicle. The scrotum becomes reddened and edematous. There are no urinary symptoms, as are often seen with epididymitis. Fever may reach 40 °C (104 °F), and prostration may be marked.

B. Signs: The parotitis of mumps may be present, or evidence of other infectious disease may be found. One or both testes may be enlarged and very tender. The epididymis cannot be distinguished from the testis on palpation. The scrotal skin may be reddened. An acute transilluminating hydrocele may develop.

C. Laboratory Findings: The white blood count is usually elevated. Urinalysis is usually normal, although some protein may be found. Abnormal renal function is found in all patients with mumps. Microhematuria and proteinuria are common. The specific virus can be found in the urine. Later, renal function and urine return to normal.

Differential Diagnosis

Acute epididymitis, when seen early, will be obvious because the involvement is solely epididymal. Later, this sign will become obscure. Urethral discharge, pyuria, and absence of a generalized infectious disease should point to epididymitis.

Torsion of the spermatic cord may present difficulties in differentiation. In torsion, the epididymis may be felt anterior to the testis during the early stages. Absence of infection tends to rule out orchitis.

Complications

In one-third to one-fourth of patients, the involved testis becomes infertile due to irreversible damage to spermatogenic cells. Androgenic function, however, is usually maintained.

Prevention

The incidence of mumps orchitis may possibly be lessened by administering mumps convalescent serum, 20 ml, during the incubation period or very early in the disease. Mumps-attenuated virus vaccine is highly effective and safe and is recommended for all susceptible persons over age 1. Routine administration of estrogens or corticosteroids to all postpuberal males who develop mumps has been suggested as a prophylactic against orchitis. However, there seems to be little evidence that this practice is effective.

Treatment

A. Specific Measures: Appropriate antibiotics are helpful in controlling some infections but are of no value in the treatment of mumps orchitis. Infiltration of the spermatic cord just above the involved testis with 20 ml of 1% procaine sometimes causes rapid resolution of the swelling and thereby relieves pain. There is evidence that this may protect spermatogenic activity as well by improving blood supply.

B. General Measures: Bed rest is necessary. Local heat is helpful and may relieve the pain. Support to the organ affords some comfort. An athletic supporter containing cotton padding is useful even when the patient is in bed.

Prognosis

Destruction of spermatogenic cells is to be feared, particularly if the disease is bilateral. This is one of the causes of infertility. The acute phase lasts about 1 week. Noticeable atrophy may be observed in 1 or 2 months

CHEMOTHERAPEUTIC & ANTIBIOTIC TREATMENT OF NONSPECIFIC INFECTIONS

Factors Which Influence the Choice of Drug

A. Type of Organism: To avoid relapses and chronicity, drugs or drug combinations should be employed which are capable of rapidly killing the infecting organisms. Selection of the proper drug for treating urinary tract infections depends upon (1) stained smear of sediment or discharge, (2) quantitative culture, and (3) antibiotic sensitivity tests. The stained smear differentiates cocci from bacilli and so is of value as a nonspecific guide in the immediate empirical selection of a drug. Quantitative urine culture should be used as a basis for drug therapy only if a significant

Table 12–1. Antibiotic dosage in renal failure.*

	Principal Mode of Excretion or Detoxification	Approximate Half-Life in Serum		Proposed Dosage Regimen in Renal Failure		Significant Removal of Drug by Dialysis (H = Hemodialysis; P = Peritoneal Dialysis)
		Normal	Renal Failure*	Initial Dose†	Give Half of Initial Dose at Interval Of	
Penicillin G	Tubular secretion	0.5 hour	6 hours	6 gm IV	8–12 hours	P yes, H no
Ampicillin	Tubular secretion	1 hour	8 hours	6 gm IV	8–12 hours	H yes, P no
Carbenicillin	Tubular secretion	1.5 hours	16 hours	4 gm IV	12–18 hours	H, P yes
Methicillin	Tubular secretion	0.5 hour	6 hours	6 gm IV	8–12 hours	H, P no
Cephalothin	Tubular secretion	0.8 hour	8 hours	4 gm IV	18 hours	H, P yes
Cephalexin	Tubular secretion and glomerular	1 hour	15 hours	2 gm orally	8–12 hours	H, P yes
Cefazolin	filtration	2 hours	30 hours	2 gm IM	24 hours	H, P yes
Streptomycin	Glomerular filtration	2.5 hours	3–4 days	1 gm IM	3–4 days	H, P yes‡
Kanamycin	Glomerular filtration	3 hours	3–4 days	1 gm IM	3–4 days	H, P yes‡
Gentamicin	Glomerular filtration	2.5 hours	2–4 days	3 mg/kg IM	2–3 days	H, P yes‡
Vancomycin	Glomerular filtration	6 hours	6–9 days	1 gm IV	5–8 days	H, P yes
Polymyxin B	Glomerular filtration	5 hours	2–3 days	2.5 mg/kg IV	3–4 days	P yes, H no
Colistimethate	Glomerular filtration	3 hours	2–3 days	5 mg/kg IM	3–4 days	P yes, H no
Tetracycline	Glomerular filtration	8 hours	3 days	1 gm orally or 0.5 gm IV	3 days	H, P no
Chloramphenicol	Mainly liver	3 hours	4 hours	1 gm orally or IV	8 hours	H, P poorly
Erythromycin	Mainly liver	1.5 hours	5 hours	1 gm orally or IV	8 hours	H, P poorly
Clindamycin	Glomerular filtration and liver	2.5 hours	4 hours	600 mg IV or IM	8 hours	H, P no

*Modified and reproduced, with permission, from Krupp & Chatton (editors): *Current Medical Diagnosis & Treatment 1975.* Lange, 1975.

†Considered here to be marked by creatinine clearance of 10 ml/minute or less.

‡For a 60-kg adult with a serious systemic infection. The "initial dose" listed is administered as an intravenous infusion over a period of 1–8 hours, or as 2 intramuscular injections during an 8-hour period, or as 2–3 oral doses during the same period.

number of organisms are identified. Culture identification is a more accurate guide to antimicrobial therapy than a stained smear and is therefore indicated for acutely ill patients or those with symptoms of chronic infection.

B. Organ Infected: The usual acute vesical infection might be treated with a sulfonamide or nitrofurantoin, whereas a patient with acute renal infection might do better with ampicillin or a cephalosporin.

C. Severity of Infection: The patient suffering from an overwhelming infection (eg, bacteremia) should be given the most effective antibiotic or combination of antibiotics to which the bacteria are sensitive. It is essential that the drug afford high serum and tissue levels as well (eg, gentamicin).

D. Stage of Infection: Acute infections tend to be self-limiting; therefore, the less toxic drugs may suffice (eg, tetracyclines, nitrofurantoin). Chronic infections may require treatment with the most effective drug as

shown by sensitivity testing (eg, kanamycin, colistimethate).

E. Side Reactions: The soluble sulfonamides are the least toxic of the antimicrobial agents. If circumstances warrant, side reactions must be risked (skin reaction from penicillin, bowel upset, proctitis, or vulvitis from the tetracyclines). A history of drug sensitivity should be taken into consideration in evaluating the drug to be used.

Antibiotic Sensitivity Tests

In general urologic office practice, sensitivity tests (and, therefore, cultures) are not indicated in the majority of cases. The stained smear of the urinary sediment affords some knowledge about the infecting organism. In most cases, empirical selection of drugs is effective. Exceptions include patients with chills and fever (with possible bacteremia) and those suspected of having chronic pyelonephritis.

Sensitivity tests are indicated in the care of those patients who are septic. Though it is now clear that the urinary concentration of the drug is of prime importance, the usual disks used in testing indicate which drug or drugs will have a bacteriostatic or bactericidal effect in the urine. (The only exception to this rule is the disk measuring sensitivity to penicillin G.) There is a reasonably good correlation between disk and tube dilution tests.

Heretofore, most authorities agreed that the efficacy of a drug was measured by its concentration in blood and tissues and the specific sensitivity of the bacteria to the drug. On this basis, the "urinary antiseptics" (nitrofurantoin, nalidixic acid, and methenamine mandelate) would have no place in the treatment of parenchymal (renal) infections. Stamey, Govan, & Palmer (1965), however, believe that renal infections involve the renal medulla rather than the cortex. Therefore, the concentration of the drug in the urine is the important factor. This would account for the fact that the "urinary antiseptics" and penicillin G are efficacious in the treatment of pyelonephritis. These studies further show that the administration of penicillin G by mouth affords a very high concentration in the urine and that many gram-negative rod infections respond best to this drug or to nitrofurantoin.

Dosage of Drugs

Most antimicrobial drugs are excreted by the kidneys and appear in the urine in much higher concentration than in the tissues. Although small doses give sufficient concentration in the urine to suppress bacteria, such "urinary doses" are undesirable in the treatment of acute urinary infection. Antimicrobials should be given in standard therapeutic dosage or in dosage which ensures bacteriostatic or bactericidal action as determined by sensitivity tests. Since much of the effect of drugs depends upon their concentration in the urine, fluids should not be forced beyond 2000 ml/day.

In the presence of renal insufficiency, care must be taken in the dosage of the drug prescribed (Table 12–1). The following drugs should not be used: (1) nitrofurantoin (peripheral neuropathy), (2) nalidixic acid (liver and CNS toxicity), (3) methenamine (acidosis), cephaloridine (renal toxicity), and the tetracyclines (liver damage).

Duration of Treatment & Follow-Up

Drugs should be administered for at least 14 days (often for much longer) to give the greatest chance for permanent cure of acute or chronic infections. Bacteriologic urine cultures and stained smears should be obtained at 1, 4, and 8 weeks after completion of treatment.

If bacteriuria persists and thorough examination fails to reveal an organic cause, chronic suppressive therapy should be instituted. One might give a sulfonamide, 0.5 g twice a day, or nitrofurantoin, 50 mg twice a day. It may be necessary to continue this regimen for months or years.

The Use of Antimicrobials During Pregnancy

Among the drugs ordinarily used to combat urinary tract infections, the following may have a deleterious effect upon the newborn child: streptomycin (eighth nerve deafness), chloramphenicol (the "gray syndrome," which may be lethal), sulfonamides (kernicterus), and tetracyclines (inhibition of bone growth, discoloration of teeth, and hypoplastic enamel which may lead to caries). Tetracycline is most dangerous after the fourth month of pregnancy. The others cause damage during the first trimester.

ANTIMICROBIAL DRUGS

Sulfonamides

The soluble sulfonamides are bacteriostatic, have a wide antibacterial spectrum, are inexpensive, and cause few significant side reactions other than skin rash and fever. They are quite useful in acute infections where toxicity is not marked. The sulfonamides which are most soluble in urine are sulfisoxazole (Gantrisin), sulfamethizole (Thiosulfil), and trisulfapyrimidines, a combination of 3 different sulfonamides. At least 4 g/day should be given, and treatment should be continued for 14 days or more. The long-acting sulfonamides, if used in therapeutic dosage, cause a significant incidence of skin reactions; sulfonamide crystalluria may develop. No instances of crystalluria have been reported following use of the soluble sulfonamides. They offer no advantage over the more soluble preparations and are contraindicated in children, in whom a number of instances of Stevens-Johnson syndrome have been reported following their use.

The sulfonamides are useful for additional therapy after an adequate course of one of the antibiotics has been given. In chronic pyelonephritis which has proved resistant to antibiotic treatment, small doses of sulfonamides (0.5 g 2 or 3 times a day) can be given for months or years to suppress infecting bacteria.

Kass has shown that prophylactic administration of a sulfonamide (0.5 g 2 or 3 times a day) sharply reduces the incidence of pyelonephritis in pregnancy in women who are found to have bacteriuria.

Sulfonamide-Trimethoprim (Co-trimoxazole)

This combination acts synergistically since each drug affects bacteria in a different manner. Each tablet (Bactrim, Septra) contains 400 mg of sulfamethoxazole and 80 mg of trimethoprim. The dose is 2 tablets twice daily. In the United States, the FDA has limited the use of this drug combination to the treatment of chronic infections. It should not be used in children under 2 years of age and is contraindicated during pregnancy. It is quite ineffective against pseudomonas but other gram-negative organisms seem to be quite sensitive to the drug. It appears to be at least as effective as ampicillin and superior to the sulfonamides used alone. In a patient with impaired renal function, the dose must be modified. If the creatinine clearance is 15–30 ml/minute, give 1 tablet twice daily. The drug is not recommended if renal function is below that level. Trimethoprim is the only drug effective against gram-negative rods that develops high concentrations in the prostate.

Penicillins

Penicillin G is a bactericidal drug which has been used chiefly in coccal infections. At least 2 million units per day should be given intramuscularly. For overwhelming infections, millions of units should be administered intravenously.

Oral penicillin G is quite efficacious in the treatment of cystitis in the female since it affords a very high urine concentration. *Escherichia coli* and *Proteus mirabilis* are particularly sensitive. The dose is 800,000 units 4 times a day on an empty stomach.

Ampicillin is a broad-spectrum penicillin which is exceedingly active against *E coli* and *P mirabilis* and, to a lesser extent, against enterococci. The average dose is 500 mg every 6 hours. It can also be given intravenously or intramuscularly. Hetacillin is converted to ampicillin in vivo; there is no clear-cut indication for its use.

Carbenicillin is active against proteus (particularly *P mirabilis*), *E coli*, and *Pseudomonas aeruginosa.* The dose is 12–30 g/day IV. Carbenicillin indanyl sodium is administered by mouth. The dose is 0.5–1 g (1–2 tablets) every 6 hours.

β-Lactamase (penicillinase)-producing staphylococci are resistant to penicillin G but usually respond to a group of penicillins that are unaffected by β-lactamase. In severe infections, give methicillin, nafcillin, or cloxacillin, 8–16 g/day IV. For milder infections, dicloxacillin, nafcillin, or cloxacillin can be given orally. The dose is 1–3 g/day.

Cephalosporins

These semisynthetic drugs, while most effective in the treatment of infections caused by β-lactamase-resistant staphylococci, are bactericidal against *E coli,* some of the klebsiella-enterobacter group, and *P mirabilis.* They are usually ineffective against *Ps aeruginosa, Proteus vulgaris,* and enterococci.

The cephalosporins can cause bone marrow depression and thrombocytopenia. Skin rash is not uncommon. Cephalothin and 2 new cephalosporins, cephapirin and cefazolin, exhibit little or no renal toxicity, but cephaloridine does, particularly in the presence of impaired renal function (Fair, 1972). These drugs must be used parenterally. The dose is 2–4 g IV every 6 hours. Cephaloridine can also be given IM; the dose is 0.5–1 g every 6 hours.

Cephalexin is an effective oral cephalosporin. The dose is 1–2 g/day in divided doses. It should be taken on an empty stomach. Cephaloglycin, another oral preparation, has little to recommend it.

Tetracyclines

A number of tetracyclines are available, but the ones that are most useful in the treatment of urinary tract infections are those that afford a high concentration in the urine. Chlortetracycline, oxytetracycline, and tetracycline are bacteriostatic agents. All 3 may be useful in both bacillary (gram-negative) and coccal (gram-positive) infections. The dosage is 1–4 g/day divided into 4 doses. The tetracyclines are inactivated if taken with milk or iron medication. In acute infections, treatment should be continued for 10–14 days. These drugs can be given parenterally if the patient is severely ill. For chronic pyelonephritis, it may be necessary to give these drugs for 1 month. Even then, only suppression of the infection may be obtained. "Outdated" tetracycline may cause a syndrome typified by potassium depletion.

With renal impairment, the usual dose of the tetracyclines is apt to cause a further degree of azotemia. In such instances, the dose should be decreased. Administration of these drugs later than the fourth month of gestation may lead to dental caries in the infant. Prolonged administration to children causes discoloration of the teeth.

Chloramphenicol

Chloramphenicol is a potent bacteriostatic drug, but it should be reserved for those patients suffering from serious disease due to an organism that is more likely to respond to chloramphenicol than to other drugs, as shown by sensitivity tests. It has hematopoietic toxicity which may not reveal itself until 2 months after its use. This is most apt to occur in patients with hepatic or renal insufficiency. Serial reticulocyte counts should be done. Optic neuritis has been reported as a complication in a few children. Two to 4 g/day are given in divided doses. Chloramphenicol should not be used during the first 2 months of life.

Aminoglycosides

A. Neomycin and Kanamycin: These bactericidal drugs are similar in action and toxicity, although kanamycin is less toxic than neomycin. They are effective in the treatment of infections caused by gram-negative rods (but not *Ps aeruginosa*). Because these drugs are nephrotoxic and may affect the eighth nerve (deafness) as well as cause skin rashes, they should be employed only to combat the most serious infections. This risk is increased if renal function is impaired.

Neomycin and kanamycin are poorly absorbed from the intestinal tract, and parenteral administration is necessary. The dose is 1–2 g/day IM in divided doses, though kanamycin can be given intravenously.

B. Gentamicin: This drug is similar to kanamycin but shows some differences in antibacterial activity. It is particularly useful in severe infections caused by *E coli,* pseudomonas, proteus, serratia, and klebsiella-enterobacter. Enterococci are resistant. The dose is 1–3 mg/kg/day IM in 3 equal doses for 7–10 days. Evidence of toxicity involving the kidneys and the eighth nerve must be sought, especially when renal insufficiency is present. If nephrotoxicity occurs, renal function usually returns to pretreatment levels on cessation of the drug.

Table 12—2. Antibiotic and chemotherapeutic agents.

	Route	Adult Dose*	Pediatric Dose*	Minimum ℞ (days)	Toxic Side-Effects (See manufacturer's brochure.)
Sulfonamides	Oral	2 g stat, then 4 g/day	120–150 mg/kg/day	10–14	Skin rash, fever, nausea and vomiting. Rarely, hematopoietic effects and nephrotoxicity. Crystalluria not a problem with water-soluble sulfonamides.
Trimethoprim-sulfamethoxazole	Oral	1g (2 tablets) twice daily	Trimethoprim, 10 mg/kg/day, and sulfamethoxazole, 50 mg/kg/day	10–14	Nausea and vomiting, bone marrow depression, allergic reactions. Crystalluria (sulfamethoxazole) very rare.
Penicillins Penicillin G	IV	Several million units daily	20–500 thousand units/kg/day. Newborn: 50,000 units/kg every 8–12 hours. Adolescents: 5–60 million units	7–14	Skin rashes, fever, anaphylaxis, superinfection, nausea and vomiting, diarrhea. Neurotoxicity with very high doses.
	IM	0.6–5 million units every 4–6 hours	20–50 thousand units/kg/day		
	Oral	3.2 million units	100–400 thousand units per dose in 5 doses before meals		
Amoxicillin	Oral	0.75–1 g/day	20–40 mg/kg/day		
Ampicillin	Oral	2–6 g/day	50–150 mg/kg/day		
Carbenicillin Disodium	IV	250–500 mg/kg/day	500–600 mg/kg/day		
Indanyl sodium	Oral	4–8 tablets/day	500–1000 mg/kg/day		
Methicillin	IV or IM	8–16 g/day	200–300 mg/kg/day		
Nafcillin	IV or IM	6–12 g/day	50–250 mg/kg/day		
	Oral	1–3 g/day			
Cloxacillin	Oral	1–3 g/day	50–100 mg/kg/day		
Dicloxacillin	Oral	1–3 g/day	25–50 mg/kg/day		
Cephalosporins Cephaloridine	IV or IM	4 g/day	30–50 mg/kg/day	7–10	Anaphylaxis, fever, skin rashes, hemolytic anemia, granulocytopenia. Renal toxicity (cephaloridine).
Cephalothin	IV	8–16 g/day	60–150 mg/kg/day		
Cephapirin	IV or IM	2–6 g/day	40–80 mg/kg/day		
Cefazolin	IV or IM	0.75–1.5 g/day	25–50 mg/kg/day		
Cephalexin	Oral	2 g/day	50–100 mg/kg/day		
Tetracycline group Tetracycline, chlortetracycline, oxytetracycline	Oral IV	1–4 g/day 0.5–2 g/day	20–40 mg/kg/day 12 mg/kg/day	10–14	Fever, skin rash, nausea and vomiting, diarrhea. Adverse effect upon teeth of fetus and child.
Chloramphenicol	Oral	1–4 g/day	50–100 mg/kg/day	10–14	Nausea, vomiting, diarrhea, anemia. Aplastic anemia (rare).
	IV	1–4 g/day	100–150 mg/kg/day		
Kanamycin	IV	1–2 g/day	15 mg/kg/day	10	Nephrotoxicity, ototoxicity (auditory).
	IM	1–2 g/day	15–20 mg/kg/day		

Table 12—2 (cont'd). Antibiotic and chemotherapeutic agents.

	Route	Adult Dose*	Pediatric Dose*	Minimum ℞ (days)	Toxic Side-Effects (See manufacturer's brochure.)
Gentamicin	IM	1–3 mg/kg/day	5–7 mg/kg/day	7–10	Nephrotoxicity, ototoxicity.
Polymyxin	IV or IM	2.5 mg/kg/day	3.5–5 mg/kg/day	7–10	Paresthesias, dizziness, nephrotoxicity.
Colistimethate	IM	5 mg/kg/day	5–10 mg/kg/day		
Nitrofurantoin tabs	Oral	0.4 g/day	5–7 mg/kg/day	7–14	Nausea and vomiting, skin rash, pulmonary infiltration, neurotoxicity (rare).
Crystals	Oral	0.4 g/day	5–7 mg/kg/day		
Sodium	IV	180–360 mg/day			
Methenamine with acidifier					
Methenamine hippurate	Oral	2 g/day	20 mg/kg/day	7–14	Vesical irritation.
Methenamine mandelate	Oral	4 g/day	50 mg/kg/day		
Methanamine sulfosalicylate	Oral	4 g/day	50 mg/kg/day		
Nalidixic acid	Oral	4 g/day	50 mg/kg/day	7	Nausea and vomiting, skin rashes.

*In divided doses unless otherwise noted.

Trade Names and Available Preparations of Drugs Listed in the Table

Sulfonamides (various mfrs)
Tablets, 0.5 g
Oral suspension, 0.5 g/5 ml
Soluble preparations include sulfisoxazole, sulfamethazole, and trisulfapyrimidines.

Trimethoprim-sulfamethoxazole (Bactrim, Septra)
Tablets containing trimethoprim, 80 mg, and sulfamethoxazole, 400 mg.

Penicillins
Amoxicillin (Larocin, Amoxil)
Capsules, 250 and 500 mg
Oral suspension, 250 mg/5 ml
Pediatric drops, 50 mg/ml
Ampicillin (Omnipen, Penbritin, Polycillin)
Capsules, 250 and 500 mg
Oral suspension, 125 mg/5 ml and 250 mg/5 ml
Injectable solutions, 125, 250, 500, and 1000 mg
Carbenicillin disodium (Geopen, Pyopen)
Injectable solutions, 1, 2, and 5 g
Carbenicillin indanyl sodium (Geocillin)
Tablets, 382 mg
Cloxacillin sodium (Orbenin, Tegopen)
Capsules, 125 and 250 mg
Granules (suspension), 125 mg/5 ml
Dicloxacillin monohydrate (Dynapen, Veracillin)
Capsules, 125 and 250 mg
Methicillin (Dimocillin, Staphcillin)
Injectable solution, 1, 4, and 6 g
Nafcillin (Unipen)
Capsules, 250 mg
Oral solution, 125 and 250 mg/5 ml
Injectable solution, 0.5, 1, and 2 g

Penicillin G potassium (various mfrs)
Tablets, 50, 100, 200, 250, 400, 500, and 800 thousand units and 1 million units
Soluble tablets, 50, 100, 200, 250, and 400 thousand units
Oral solution, 100, 125, 200, 250, 400, and 500 thousand units per 5 ml
Injectable solutions, 0.2–20 million units

Cephalosporins
Cephalexin (Keflex)
Capsules, 250 and 500 mg
Oral suspension, 125 and 250 ml/5 ml
Cephaloridine (Loridine)
Injectable solution, 0.5 and 1 g
Cephalothin sodium (Keflin)
Injectable solution, 1, 2, and 4 g
Cephapirin (Cefadyl)
Injectable solution, 1, 2, and 4 g
Cefazolin sodium (Ancef, Kefzol)
Injectable solution, 0.25, 0.5, and 1 g

Tetracyclines
Chlortetracycline (Aureomycin)
Capsules, 250 mg
Oxytetracycline (Terramycin)
Capsules, 125 and 250 mg
Pediatric drops, 100 mg/ml
Syrup, 125 mg/5 ml
Tetracycline (various mfrs)
Capsules, 250 and 500 mg
Syrup, 125 mg/5 ml

Trade Names and Available Preparations of Drugs Listed in the Table (cont'd)

Chloramphenicol (Chloromycetin)
    Capsules, 50, 100, and 250 mg
    Oral suspension, 150 mg/5 ml

Kanamycin-neomycin group
    Kanamycin sulfate (Kantrex)
      Injectable solution, 0.75 (pediatric), 0.5, and 1 g
    Neomycin (various mfrs)
      Injectable solution, 0.5 and 5 g

Gentamicin (Garamycin)
    Injectable solution, 10 and 40 mg/ml

Polymyxin group
    Colistimethate (Coly-Mycin)
      Injectable solution, 20 and 150 mg
    Polymyxin B sulfate (Aerosporin)
      Injectable solutions, 500,000 units

Nitrofurantoins
    Nitrofurantoin (various mfrs)
      Tablets, 50 and 100 mg
      Oral suspension, 25 mg/5 ml
    Nitrofurantoin crystals (Macrodantin)
      Capsules, 25, 50, and 100 mg
    Nitrofurantoin sodium (Furadantin)
      Solution, 180 mg

Methenamine with acidifier
    Methenamine hippurate (Hiprex, Urex)
      Tablets, 1 g
    Methenamine mandelate (Mandelamine)
      Tablets, 0.25, 0.5, and 1 g
    Methenamine sulfosalicylate (Hexalet)
      Tablets, 0.5 and 1 g

Nalidixic acid (NegGram)
    Capsules, 250 and 500 mg
    Oral suspension, 250 mg/5 ml

Table 12–3. Antimicrobial spectra of chemotherapeutic and antibiotic agents in urinary tract infections.

	Sulfonamides	Trimethoprim-Sulfamethoxazole	Penicillins — Penicillin G	Penicillins — Methicillin, Cloxacillin, Etc	Penicillins — Amoxicillin, Ampicillin	Penicillins — Carbenicillin	Cephalosporins	Tetracyclines	Chloramphenicol	Amino-glycosides — Neomycin, Kanamycin	Amino-glycosides — Gentamicin	Polymyxin, Colistimethate	Urinary Antiseptics — Nitrofurantoin	Urinary Antiseptics — Methenamine With Acidifier	Nalidixic Acid
Bacilli															
E coli	+	++	++		++	+	++	+	+	++	++	+	+	±	+
Klebsiella		+			+		+	±		++	++	+	+		+
Enterobacter	±	+					+	±	+	++	++	+	+	±	+
Serratia						±				++	++			±	
P mirabilis	±	+	++		++	+	+	±	+	+	+		±	±	±
P vulgaris and others		±				++	±	±	+	++	+			±	±
Ps aeruginosa						++	±	+	+	+	++	++			
Cocci															
Str haemolyticus	±		++	±	+		+	+	+					±	
Str faecalis (enterococcus)	±		±		++ C		+	±		++ C			+		
S aureus	±		++	±	+		++	±	±	+					
β-Lactamase-producing				++			+		±						

    ++ = Drugs of choice   ± = Moderate effect
    + = Alternate drugs   C = Drugs used in combinations

Polymyxin B & Colistimethate (Polymyxin E)

These closely related bactericidal drugs have some nephrotoxic effect, but nephrotoxicity does not commonly occur when renal function is normal (though a few instances of acute tubular necrosis due to a hypersensitivity reaction have been reported). Few other drugs are more effective against *Ps aeruginosa*. They are useful for coliform organisms but are not effective in the treatment of *P vulgaris* infections. If renal function is impaired, the usual dose should be reduced by half. If urinalysis reveals hematuria, casts, or protein, these signs will disappear when the drug is withdrawn. Both drugs are administered intramuscularly. The average dose for both is 2.5–5 mg/kg/day in divided doses. The injection of polymyxin is painful. Colistimethate, which contains a local anesthetic, is the drug of choice. For intravenous therapy, polymyxin B sulfate, 3.5 mg/kg/day, is preferable. Toxic effects include renal impairment, paresthesias, and dizziness. These disappear on cessation of the drug.

URINARY ANTISEPTICS

Nitrofurantoin

The usual disk sensitivity test is useful even though this drug causes no measurable serum or tissue level for it does reflect sensitivity to its concentration in the urine, which is of paramount importance in the cure of most infections of the urinary tract. Since blood and tissue levels of the drug are insignificant, it should not be used for serious infections. The dose is 100 mg 4 times a day. The effects are enhanced if the pH of the urine is below 5.5. To suppress chronic infection, 50 mg can be given 2 or 3 times a day. Nitrofurantoin is not effective against indole-producing proteus or *Ps aeruginosa* infections. Sodium nitrofurantoin can be injected intravenously if the patient is unable to take it by mouth. This produces adequate levels in the urine. The intravenous dose is 180–360 mg/day in divided doses. The drug is not recommended for chil-

dren. The chronic use of this drug in the uremic patient is contraindicated; it may cause a severe and progressive polyneuritis. Instances of allergic pneumonitis associated with fever and cough have been reported. Resolution occurs when the drug is stopped.

Methenamine With Organic Acid

Methenamine is one of the oldest drugs used in the treatment of urinary tract infections. The addition of mandelic, sulfosalicylic, or hippuric acid affords an acid urine which in itself is bacteriostatic. In order to be efficacious, methenamine mandelate or sulfosalicylate must be given in a dose of 3–6 g/day in divided doses. The recommended dose of methenamine hippurate is 1 g twice a day. The pH of the urine should be 5.5 or lower, and the urinary output should be limited to 1000 ml/day in order to afford an adequate concentration of formaldehyde. The pH can be checked by the patient with nitrazine paper; additional acidification may be necessary. Ascorbic acid, 1 g 4 times a day, is an efficient acidifier. Formaldehyde, the active bacteriostatic agent liberated in the urine, may cause vesical irritability or even hematuria. Use of the acidified methenamines is contraindicated in the face of renal insufficiency; acidosis may occur.

Methenamine is a useful drug for prolonged suppressive therapy, but the full dosage should be prescribed. Should the dose be cut in half, not only is there less methenamine available but less urinary acidification as well, thus negating its effect.

Nalidixic Acid

Nalidixic acid is a naphthyridine derivative which is effective against gram-negative rods with the exception of *Ps aeruginosa*. It is ineffective against enterococci. It has been shown that bacteria develop resistance to nalidixic acid rather rapidly, so it does not lend itself to chronic suppressive therapy. The recommended dose is 4 g/day in divided doses. Toxic symptoms include skin rash, nausea, drowsiness, and, rarely, convulsions. False-positive tests for urinary 17-ketosteroids and glucose occur when this drug is present in the urine.

●   ●   ●

References

Pathogenesis

Bergström T: Sex differences in childhood urinary tract infection. Arch Dis Childhood 47:227, 1972.

Cattell WR & others: Periurethral enterobacterial carriage in pathogenesis of recurrent urinary infection. Brit MJ 4:136, 1974.

Corriere JN Jr, McClure JM III, Lipschultz LI: Contamination of bladder urine by urethral particles during voiding: Urethrovesical reflux. J Urol 107:399, 1972.

Cox CE: The urethra and its relationship to urinary tract infection: The flora of the normal female urethra.

South MJ 59:621, 1966.

Cox CE, Lacy SS, Hinman F Jr: The urethra and its relationship to urinary tract infection. 2. The urethral flora of the female with recurrent urinary infection. J Urol 99:632, 1968.

Elkins IB, Cox CE: Perineal, vaginal and urethral bacteriology of young women. 1. Incidence of gram-negative colonization. J Urol 111:88, 1974.

Fass RJ, Klainer AS, Perkins RL: Urinary tract infection: Practical aspects of diagnosis and treatment. JAMA 225:1509, 1973.

Glynn AA, Brumfitt W, Howard CJ: K antigens of *Esche-*

richia coli and renal involvement in urinary tract infections. Lancet 2:514, 1971.

Heidrick WP, Mattingly RF, Amberg JR: Vesicoureteral reflux in pregnancy. Obst Gynec 29:571, 1967.

Hinman F Jr: Bacterial elimination. J Urol 99:811, 1968.

Hinman F Jr: Mechanism for the entry of bacteria and the establishment of urinary tract infection in female children. J Urol 96:546, 1966.

Hodson CJ, Wilson S: Natural history of chronic pyelonephritic scarring. Brit JM 2:191, 1965.

Hutch JA, Ayers RD, Noll LE: Vesicoureteral reflux as cause of pyelonephritis of pregnancy. Am J Obst Gynec 87:478, 1963.

Hutch JA, Miller ER, Hinman F Jr: Perpetuation of infection in unobstructed urinary tracts. J Urol 90:88, 1963.

Leadbetter G Jr, Slavin S: Pediatric urinary tract infections: Significance of vaginal bacteria. Urology 3:581, 1974.

Mattingly RF, Moore DE, Clark DO: Bacteriologic study of suprapubic bladder drainage. Am J Obst Gynec 114:732, 1972.

Neumann PZ, de Domenico IJ, Nogrady MB: Constipation and urinary tract infection. Pediatrics 52:241, 1973.

Simon RD: Pinworm infestation and urinary tract infection in young girls. Am J Dis Child 128:21, 1974.

Stamey TA: The role of introital enterobacteria in recurrent urinary infections. J Urol 109:467, 1973.

Stamey TA, Pfau A: Urinary infections: A selective review and some observations. California Med 113:16, Dec 1970.

Stamey TA, Sexton CC: The role of vaginal colonization with enterobacteriaceal in recurrent urinary infections. J Urol 113:214, 1975.

Stephens SD: Urologic aspects of recurrent urinary tract infection in children. J Pediat 80:725, 1972.

Tanagho EA, Miller ER: Abnormal voiding and urinary tract infection. Internat Urol Nephrol 4:165, 1972.

Turck, M, Ronald AR, Petersdorf RF: Relapse and reinfection in chronic bacteriuria. The correlation between site of infection and pattern of recurrence in chronic bacteriuria. New England J Med 278:422, 1968.

Nonspecific Infections of the Kidneys

Beachley MC, Ranninger K, Roth F-J: Xanthogranulomatous pyelonephritis. Am J Roentgenol 121:500, 1974.

Bontemps S, Bryk D: Pyonephrosis with pneumoureteropyelogram. J Urol 109:160, 1973.

Cha EM & others: Xanthogranulomatous pyelonephritis. Urology 3:159, 1974.

Costas S: Renal and perirenal emphysema. Brit J Urol 44:311, 1972.

Davidson AJ, Talner LB: Urographic and angiographic abnormalities in adult-onset acute bacterial nephritis. Radiology 106:249, 1973.

Freedman LR: Chronic pyelonephritis at autopsy. Ann Int Med 66:697, 1967.

Harris RE, Gilstrap LC III: Prevention of recurrent pyelonephritis during pregnancy. Obst Gynec 44:637, 1974.

Heptinstall RH: Pathology of end-stage kidney disease. Am J Med 44:656, 1968.

Hinman F Jr, Hutch JA: Atrophic pyelonephritis from

utereal reflux without obstructive signs. J Urol 87:230, 1962.

Hodson CJ: The radiological contribution toward the diagnosis of chronic pyelonephritis. Radiology 88:857, 1967.

Jensen MM: Viruses and kidney disease. Am J Med 43:897, 1967.

Kessler WO & others: Gallium-67 scans in the diagnosis of pyelonephritis. Western J Med 121:91, 1974.

Kimmelstiel P: The nature of chronic pyelonephritis. Geriatrics 19:145, 1964.

Little PJ: The incidence of urinary infection in 5000 pregnant women. Lancet 2:925, 1966.

Mosley JG: A case of emphysematous pyelonephritis. Brit J Surg 60:495, 1973.

Palmer JM: Differential antibiotic excretion in unilateral structural pyelonephritis. Western J Med 120:363, 1974.

Saunders CD, Corriere JN Jr: The inability to diagnose chronic pyelonephritis on the excretory urogram in adults. J Urol 111:560, 1974.

Smith JF: The diagnosis of the scars of chronic pyelonephritis. J Clin Path 15:522, 1962.

Stephens SD: Urologic aspects of recurrent urinary tract infection in children. J Pediat 80:725, 1972.

Still Jl, Cotton D: Severe hypertension in childhood. Arch Dis Childhood 42:34, 1967.

Symposium on pyelonephritis. J Infect Dis 120:1, 1969.

Thomas V, Shelokov A, Forland M: Antibody-coated bacteria in the urine and the site of urinary-tract infection. New England J Med 290:588, 1974.

Zinner SH, Kass EH: Long-term (10 to 14 years) follow-up of bacteriuria of pregnancy. New England J Med 285:820, 1971.

Bacteremic Shock

Baue AE: The treatment of septic shock: A problem intensified by advancing science. Surgery 65:850, 1969.

Beller FK, Douglas GW: Thrombocytopenia indicating gram-negative infection and endotoxemia. Obst Gynec 41:521, 1973.

Blaisdell FW: Pathophysiology of the respiratory distress syndrome. Arch Surg 108:44, 1974.

Blaisdell FW, Schlobohm RM: The respiratory distress syndrome: A review. Surgery 74:251, 1973.

Bredenberg CE & others: Respiratory failure in shock. Ann Surg 169:392, 1973.

Cristy JH: Treatment of gram-negative shock. Am J Med 50:77, 1971.

Crowder JG, Gilkey GH, White AC: *Serratia marcescens* bacteremia: Clinical observations and studies of precipitin reactions. Arch Int Med 128:247, 1971.

Feller I & others: Diagnosis and treatment of postoperative bacterial sepsis. S Clin North America 52:1391, 1972.

Fossard DP, Kakkar VV: The limulus test in experimental and clinical endotoxaemia. Brit J Surg 61:798, 1974.

Gowen GF: Interpretation of central venous pressure. S Clin North America 53:649, 1973.

Hanson GC: Septicaemic shock: Report of three cases: A review of diagnosis and management. Postgrad MJ 50:288, 1974.

James PM Jr, Meyers RT: Central venous pressure monitoring: Misinterpretation, abuses, indications and a new technic. Ann Surg 175:693, 1973.

Johnson AOB, Clark RG: Malpositioning of central venous catheters. Lancet 2:1395, 1972.

Lillehei RC & others: The pharmacologic approach to the treatment of shock: 1. Defining traumatic, septic, and cardiogenic shock. Genetics 27:73, July 1972. 2. Diagnosis of shock and plan of treatment. Genetics 27:81, Aug 1972.

Marcus AJ: Heparin therapy for disseminated intravascular coagulation. Am J Med Sc 264:365, 1972.

McGovern VJ: The pathophysiology of gram-negative septicaemia. Pathology 4:265, 1972.

McHenry MC, Hawk WA: Bacteremia caused by gram-negative bacilli. M Clin North America 58:623, 1974.

Milligan GF & others: Pulmonary and hematologic disturbances during septic shock. Surg Gynec Obst 138:43, 1974.

Myerowitz RL, Medeiros AA, O'Brien TF: Bacterial infection in renal homotransplant recipients. Am J Med 53:308, 1972.

Nishijima H & others: Hemodynamic and metabolic studies on shock associated with gram-negative bacteremia. Medicine 52:287, 1972.

Preston FE & others: Intravascular coagulation and *E coli* septicaemia. J Clin Path 26:120, 1973.

Putman CE, Minagi H, Blaisdell FW: The roentgen appearance of disseminated intravascular coagulation (DIC). Radiology 109:13, 1973.

Roberts JM, Laros RK Jr: Hemorrhagic and endotoxic shock: A pathophysiologic approach to diagnosis and management. Am J Obst Gynec 110:1041, 1971.

Rodrigues RJ, Wolff WI: Fungal septicemia in surgical patients. Ann Surg 180:741, 1974.

Rosenbaum RW, Hayes MF Jr, Matsumoto T: Efficacy of steroids in the treatment of septic and cardiogenic shock. Surg Gynec Obst 136:914, 1973.

Schumer W, Sperling R: Shock and its effect on the cell. JAMA 205:215, 1968.

Weil MH, Shubin H: The "VIP" approach to the bedside management of shock. JAMA 207:337, 1969.

Weil MH, Shubin H: Treatment of shock caused by bacterial infections. California Med 119:7, Nov 1973.

Welch TR, Nogrady MB, Outerbridge EW: Roentgenologic sequelae of neonatal septicemia and urinary tract infection. Am J Roentgenol 18:28, 1973.

Winslow EJ & others: Hemodynamic studies and results of therapy in 50 patients with bacteremic shock. Am J Med 54:421, 1973.

Necrotizing Papillitis

Aspirin and the kidneys. Editorial. Canad MAJ 111:629, 1974.

Bailey RR, Neale TJ, Little PJ: Analgesic nephropathy. New Zealand MJ 79:1053, 1974.

Chrispin AR: Medullary necrosis in infancy. Brit M Bull 28:233, 1973.

Cove-Smith JR, Knapp MS: Sodium handling in analgesic nephropathy. Lancet 2:70, 1973.

Desai S, Libertino JA, Dowd JB: Unilateral acute, fulminating renal papillary necrosis with *Escherichia* septicemia. Urology 2:184, 1973.

Eckert DE, Jonutis AJ, Davidson AJ: The incidence and manifestations of urographic papillary abnormalities in patients with S hemoglobinopathies. Radiol 113:59, 1974.

Edmondson HA, Reynolds TB, Jacobson HG: Renal papillary necrosis with special reference to chronic alcoholism. Arch Int Med 118:255, 1966.

Flaster S, Lome LG, Presman D: Urologic complications of renal papillary necrosis. Urology 5:331, 1975.

Flint LD, Libertino JA, Desai SG: Renal papillary necrosis: Unusual patterns and treatment. J Urol 111:321, 1974.

Gault MH, Blennerhassett J, Muehrcke RC: Analgesic nephropathy: A clinicopathologic study using electron microscopy. Am J Med 51:740, 1971.

Harrow BR: Renal papillary necrosis: A critique of pathogenesis. J Urol 97:203, 1967.

Husband P, Howlett KA: Renal papillary necrosis in infancy. Arch Dis Childhood 48:116, 1973.

Jameson RM, Heal MR: The surgical management of acute renal papillary necrosis. Brit J Surg 60:428, 1973.

Lalli AF: Renal papillary necrosis. Am J Roentgenol 114:741, 1972.

Longacre AM, Popky GL: Papillary necrosis in patients with cirrhosis: A study of 102 patients. J Urol 99:391, 1968.

Macklon AF & others: Aspirin and analgesic nephropathy. Brit MJ 1:597, 1974.

Murray RM: Analgesic nephropathy: Removal of phenacetin from proprietary analgesics. Brit MJ 4:131, 1972.

Nanra RS, Kincaid-Smith P: Papillary necrosis in rats caused by aspirin and aspirin-containing mixtures. Brit MJ 3:559, 1970.

Nogrady MB, Lesk DM: Renal papillary necrosis in the newborn: A case report with roentgenologic documentation of late sequelae. Am J Roentgenol 116:661, 1972.

Poynter JD, Hare WSC: Necrosis in situ: A form of renal papillary necrosis seen in analgesic nephropathy. Radiology 111:69, 1974.

Renal Carbuncle

Craven JD & others: Acute renal carbuncle: The importance of preoperative angiography. J Urol 111: 727, 1974.

Fair WR, Higgins MH: Renal abscess. J Urol 104:179, 1970.

Gadrinab NM, Lome LG, Presman D: Renal abscess: Role of renal arteriography. Urology 2:39, 1973.

Koehler PR: The roentgen diagnosis of renal inflammatory masses—special emphasis on angiographic changes. Radiology 112:257, 1974.

Lyons RW & others: Arteriographic and antibiotic therapy of a renal carbuncle. J Urol 107:524, 1972.

Pederson JF, Hancke S, Kristensen JK: Renal carbuncle: Antibiotic therapy governed by ultrasonically guided aspiration. J Urol 109:777, 1973.

Rabinowitz JG & others: Acute renal carbuncle: The roentgenographic clarification of a medical enigma. Am J Roentgenol 116:740, 1972.

Renal carbuncle. Editorial. Brit MJ 3:63, 1973.

Perinephric Abscess

Love L, Baker D, Ramsey R: Gas producing perinephric abscess. Am J Roentgenol 119:783, 1973.

Meyers MA & others: Radiologic features of extraperitoneal effusions. Radiology 104:249, 1972.

Plevin SN, Balodimos MC, Bradley RF: Perinephric abscess in diabetic patients. J Urol 103:539, 1970.

Simpkins KC, Barraclough NC: Renal cortical abscess, perinephritis and perinephric abscess in diabetes. Brit J Radiol 46:433, 1973.

Nonspecific Infections of the Bladder

Alexander AR, Morrisseau PM, Leadbetter GW Jr: Urethral-hymenal adhesions and recurrent post-coital cystitis: Treatment by hymenoplasty. J Urol 107:597, 1972.

Bailey RR & others: Urinary-tract infection in non-pregnant women. Lancet 2:275, 1973.

Bass HN: "Bubble bath" as an irritant to the urinary tract of children. Clin Pediat 7:174, 1968.

Berkson BM, Lome LG, Shapiro I: Severe cystitis induced by cyclophosphamide: Role of surgical management. JAMA 225:605, 1973.

Corriere JN Jr, Wise MF: Acute cystitis in young women: Diagnosis and treatment. Urology 1:453, 1973.

Fair WR & others: Urinary tract infections in children. 1. Young girls with non-refluxing ureters. Western J Med 121:366, 1974.

Hawtry CE, Williams JJ, Schmidt JD: Cystitis emphysematosis. Urology 3:612, 1974.

Helin I, Okmian L: Haemorrhagic cystitis complicating cyclophosphamide treatment in children. Acta paediat scandinav 62:497, 1973.

Landes RR, Melnick I, Hoffman AA: Recurrent urinary tract infections in women: Prevention by topical application of anatimicrobial ointment to urethral meatus. J Urol 104:749, 1970.

Lapides J & others: Followup on unsterile, intermittent self-catheterization. J Urol 111:184, 1974.

Lewis EL, Griffith TH: Recurring cystourethritis in women: Is an effective therapy available? J Urol 110:544, 1973.

Mufson MA & others: Cause of acute hemorrhagic cystitis in children. Am J Dis Child 126:605, 1973.

Person DA & others: Herpesvirus type 2 in genitourinary tract infections. Am J Obst Gynec 116:993, 1973.

Powell NB & others: Allergy of the lower urinary tract. J Urol 107:631, 1972.

Vosti KL: Recurrent urinary tract infections: Prevention by prophylactic antibiotics after sexual intercourse. JAMA 231:934, 1975.

Chronic Cystitis

See references listed under Nonspecific Infections of the Kidneys.

Nonspecific Infections of the Prostate Gland

Blacklock NJ: Anatomical factors in prostatitis. Brit J Urol 46:47, 1974.

Bourne CW, Frishetti WA: Prostatic fluid analysis and prostatitis. J Urol 97:140, 1967.

Bush I, Orkin LA, Baker S: Steroid therapy in non-specific granulomatous prostatitis. J Urol 92:303, 1964.

Chesley AE, Dow D: Use of trimethoprim-sulfamethoxazole in chronic prostatitis. Urology 2:280, 1973.

Drach GW: Problems in diagnosis of bacterial prostatitis: Gram-negative, gram-positive and mixed infections. J Urol 111:630, 1974.

Drach GW: Trimethoprim/sulfamethoxazole therapy of chronic bacterial prostatitis. J Urol 111:637, 1974.

Chronic prostatitis. Editorial. Brit MJ 3:1, 1972.

Fair WR: Diffusion of menocycline into prostatic secretion in dogs. Urology 3:339, 1974.

Garnes HA: Doxycycline levels in serum and prostatic tissue in man. Urology 1:205, 1973.

Gritti EJ, Cook FE Jr, Spencer HB: Coccidioidomycosis granuloma of the prostate: A rare manifestation of the disseminated disease. J Urol 89:249, 1963.

Madsen PO & others: The nitrofurantoin concentration in prostatic fluid of humans and dogs. J Urol 100:54, 1968.

Mann S: Prostatic abscess in the newborn. Arch Dis Childhood 35:396, 1960.

Mears EM Jr, Stamey TA: Bacteriologic localization patterns in bacterial prostatitis and urethritis. Invest Urol 5:492, 1968.

Mears EM Jr, Stamey TA: The diagnosis and management of bacterial prostatitis. Brit J Urol 44:175, 1972.

Mitchell RJ, Blake JRS: Spontaneous perforation of prostatic abscess with peritonitis. J Urol 107:622, 1972.

Mobley DF: Chronic prostatitis. South MJ 67:219, 1974.

Mobley DF: Erythromycin plus sodium bicarbonate in chronic bacterial prostatitis. Urology 3:60, 1974.

Morrisseau PM, Phillips CA, Leadbetter GW Jr: Viral prostatitis. J Urol 103:767, 1970.

Murnahan GF & others: Chronic prostatitis: An Australian view. Brit J Urol 46:55, 1974.

Nielsen ML, Hansen I: Trimethoprim in human prostatic tissue and prostatic fluid. Scandinav J Urol Nephrol 6:244, 1972.

Nielsen ML, Vestergaard BF: Virological investigations in chronic prostatitis. J Urol 109:1023, 1973.

Pai MG, Bhat HS: Prostatic abscess. J Urol 108:599, 1972.

Smart CJ, Jenkins JD: The role of transurethral prostatectomy in chronic prostatitis. Brit J Urol 45:654, 1973.

Stamey TA, Mears EM Jr, Winningham DG: Chronic bacterial prostatitis and the diffusion of drugs into prostatic fluid. J Urol 103:187, 1970.

Thybo E, Zdravkovic D, Zdravkovic M: Granulomatous prostatitis. Scandinav J Urol Nephrol 7:111, 1973.

Towfighi J & others: Granulomatous prostatitis with emphasis on the eosinophilic variety. Am J Clin Path 58:630, 1972.

Nonspecific Infections of the Male Urethra

Bennett AH, Kundsin RB, Shapiro SR: T-strain mycoplasmas, the etiologic agent of non-specific urethritis: A venereal disease. J Urol 109:427, 1973.

Conger KB: Gonorrhea and nonspecific urethritis. M Clin North America 48:767, 1964.

Dunlop EMC & others: Relation of TRIC agent to "nonspecific" genital infection. Brit J Ven Dis 42:77, 1966.

Hobson D & others: Simplified method for diagnosis of genital and ocular infections with chlamydia. Lancet 2:555, 1974.

Marshall S: The effect of bubble bath on the urinary tract. J Urol 93:112, 1965.

McChesney JA & others: Acute urethritis in male college students. JAMA 226:37, 1973.

McCormack WM & others: The genital mycoplasmas. New England J Med 288:78, 1973.

McCormack WM & others: Sexual activity and vaginal colonization with genital mycoplasmas. JAMA 221:1375, 1972.

Nonspecific Infections of the Epididymis

Carlton CE Jr, Leader AJ: The cystourethrographic demonstration of retrograde urinary flow in the vas deferens as a cause of epididymitis. J Urol 84:123, 1960.

Kiviat MD, Shurtleff D, Ansell JS: Urinary reflux via the vas deferens: Unusual cause of epididymitis in infancy. J Pediat 80:476, 1972.

Lawrence D, Mishkin F: Radionuclide imaging in epididymo-orchitis. J Urol 112:387, 1974.

Megalli M, Gursel E, Lattimer JK: Reflux of urine into ejaculatory ducts as a cause of recurring epididymitis in children. J Urol 108:978, 1972.

Miller HC: Local anesthesia for acute epididymitis. J Urol 104:735, 1970.

Smith DR: Treatment of epididymitis by infiltration of the spermatic cord with procaine hydrochloride. J Urol 46:74, 1941.

Wilson SK, Hagan KW, Rhamy RK: Epididymectomy for acute and chronic disease. J Urol 112:357, 1974.

Winnacker JL & others: Recurrent epididymitis in sarcoidosis. Ann Int Med 66:743, 1967.

Nonspecific Infections of the Testis

Lyon RP, Bruyn HB: Treatment of mumps epididymo-orchitis. JAMA 196:736, 1966.

Riggs S, Sanford JP: Viral orchitis. New England J Med 266:990, 1962.

Utz JP, Houk VN, Alling DW: Clinical and laboratory studies of mumps. 4. Viruria and abnormal renal function. New England J Med 270:1283, 1964.

Chemotherapeutic & Antibiotic Treatment of Nonspecific Infections

Apgar V: Drugs in pregnancy. JAMA 190:840, 1964.

Bennett WM, Singer I, Coggins CJ: A guide to drug therapy in renal failure. JAMA 230:1544, 1974.

Kline AH, Blattner RJ, Lunin M: Transplacental effect of tetracyclines on teeth. JAMA 188:178, 1964.

Lorian V: The mode of action of antibiotics on gram-negative bacilli. Arch Int Med 128:623, 1971.

McCracken GH Jr: Pharmacological basis for antimicrobial therapy in newborn infants. Am J Dis Child 128:407, 1974.

McCracken GH Jr, Eichenwald HF: Anti-microbial therapy: Therapeutic recommendations and a review of the newer drugs. 2. The clinical pharmacology of the newer antimicrobial agents. J Pediat 85:451, 1974.

McCracken GH Jr, Eichenwald HF, Nelson JD: Antimicrobial therapy in theory and practice. 1. Clinical pharmacology. J Pediat 75:742, 1969.

O'Grady F, Brumfitt W: Urinary tract infection. Proceedings of the First National Symposium held in London, April 1968. Oxford Univ Press, 1968.

Parker RH, Fossieck BE Jr: A five-step approach to antimicrobial medication. 2. Urinary tract infections. Geriatrics 29:75, 1974.

Robinson GC, Cambon KG: Hearing loss in infants of tuberculous mothers treated with streptomycin during pregnancy. New England J Med 271:949, 1964.

Stamey TA, Govan DE, Palmer JM: The localization and treatment of urinary tract infections: The role of bactericidal urine levels as opposed to serum levels. Medicine 44:1, 1965.

Symposium on efficacy of antimicrobial and antifungal agents. M Clin North America 54:1077, 1970.

Turck M, Lindemeyer RI, Petersdorf RG: Comparison of single-disc and tube-dilution techniques in determining antibiotic sensitivities of gram-negative pathogens. Ann Int Med 58:56, 1963.

VanOmmen RA: Untoward effects of antimicrobial agents on major organ systems. M Clin North America 58:465, 1974.

Antimicrobial Drugs

Bailey A & others: Cephalexin: a new oral antibiotic. Postgrad MJ 46:157, 1970.

Bailey RR, Koutsaimanis KG: Oral administration of a new carbenicillin in the treatment of urinary tract infection. Brit J Urol 44:235, 1972.

Bailey RR & others: Prevention of urinary-tract infection with low-dose nitrofurantoin. Lancet 2:1112, 1971.

Beirne GJ & others: Acute renal failure caused by hypersensitivity to polymyxin B sulfate. JAMA 202:62, 1967.

Bobrow SN Jaffe E, Young RC: Anuria with acute tubular necrosis associated with gentamicin and cephalothin. JAMA 222:1546, 1972.

Bodner SJ, Koenig MG: Clinical and in vitro evaluation of cephapirin: A new parenteral cephalosporin. Am J Med Sci 263:43, 1972.

Böse W & others: Controlled trial of co-trimoxazole in children with urinary tract infection. Lancet 2:614, 1974.

Brumfitt W, Pursell R: Double-blind trial to compare ampicillin, cephalexin, co-trimoxazole, and trimethoprim in treatment of urinary infection. Brit MJ 2:673, 1972.

Brusch JL & others: An in vitro and pharmacological comparison of amoxicillin and amphicillin. Am J Med Sc 267:41, 1974.

Burton JR & others: Acute renal failure during cephalothin therapy. JAMA 229:679, 1974.

Cederberg Ä & others: Nalidixic acid in urinary tract infections with particular reference to the emergence of resistance. Scandinav J Infect Dis 6:259, 1974.

Chan RA, Benner EJ, Hoeprich PD: Gentamicin therapy in renal failure: A nomogram for dosage. Ann Int Med 76:773, 1972.

Chang N, Giles CL, Gregg RH: Optic neuritis and chloramphenicol. Am J Dis Child 112:46, 1966.

Chattopadhyay B: Trimethoprim-sulfamethoxazole in urinary tract infection due to *Streptococcus faecalis*. J Clin Path 25:531, 1972.

Cosgrove MD, Morrow JW: Ampicillin versus trimethoprim/sulfamethoxazole in chronic urinary tract infection. J Urol 111:670, 1974.

Craig WA, Kunin CM: Trimethoprim-sulfamethoxazole: Pharmacodynamic effects of urinary pH and impaired renal function. Ann Int Med 78:491, 1973.

Dillon ML, Postlewait RW: Cephaloridine in patients with impaired renal function. JAMA 218:250, 1971.

Dorfman LE, Smith JP: Sulfonamide crystalluria: A forgotten disease. J Urol 104:482, 1970.

Ellis FG: Acute polyneuritis after nitrofurantoin therapy.

Lancet 2:1136, 1962.

Fillastre JP & others: Acute renal failure associated with combined gentamicin and cephalothin therapy. Brit MJ 2:396, 1973.

Fulop M, Drapkin A: Potassium-depletion syndrome secondary to nephropathy apparently caused by "outdated tetracycline." New England J Med 272:986, 1965.

Harris MJ, Wise G, Beveridge J: The Stevens-Johnson syndrome and long-acting sulfonamides. Australian Paediat J 2:101, 1966.

Harrison LH, Cox CE: Bacteriologic and pharmacodynamic aspects of nalidixic acid. J Urol 104:908, 1970.

Hodges GR, Perkins RL: Carbenicillin indanyl sodium oral therapy of urinary tract infections. Arch Int Med 131:679, 1973.

Hodges GR, Saslaw S: Experiences with cefazolin: a new cephalosporin antibiotic. Am J Med Sc 265:23, 1973.

Hulbert J: Gram-negative urinary infection treated with oral penicillin G. Lancet 2:1216, 1972.

Kabins SA: Interactions among antibiotics and other drugs. JAMA 219:206, 1972.

Katul MJ, Frank IN: Antibacterial activity of methenamine hippurate. J Urol 104:320, 1970.

Klastersky J & others: Bacteriological and clinical activity of the ampicillin/gentamicin and cephalothin/gentamicin combinations. Am J Med Sc 262:283, 1971.

Klastersky J & others: Effectiveness of the carbenicillin/cephalothin combination against gram-negative bacilli. Am J Med Sc 265:45, 1973.

Kluge RM & others: The carbenicillin-gentamicin combination against *Pseudomonas aeruginosa*. Ann Int Med 81:584, 1974.

Koch-Weser J & others: Adverse reactions to sulfisoxazole, sulfamethoxazole, and nitrofurantoin. Arch Int Med 128:399, 1971.

Kursh ED, Mostyn EM, Persky L: Nitrofurantoin pulmonary complications. J Urol 113:392, 1975.

Lacey RW & others: Trimethoprim-resistant coliforms. Lancet 1:409, 1972.

Laxdal T, Hallgrimsson J: The "grey toddler": Choramphenicol toxicity. Arch Dis Childhood 49:235, 1974.

Lerner PI, Smith H, Weinstein L: Penicillin neurotoxicity. Ann New York Acad Sc 145:310, 1967.

Lincoln K, Lidin-Janson G, Winberg J: Faecal and periurethral flora after administration of sulfonamide, nitrofurantoin and nalidixic acid. Acta Paediat Scandinav 61:643, 1972.

Marks MI, Eickhoff TC: Carbenicillin: A clinical and laboratory evaluation. Ann Int Med 73:179, 1970.

Maxwell D & others: Ampicillin nephropathy. JAMA 230:586, 1974.

McCracken GH Jr: Clinical pharmacology of gentamicin in infants 2 to 24 months of age. Am J Dis Child 124:884, 1972.

McHenry MC & others: Gentamicin dosages for renal insufficiency. Ann Int Med 74:192, 1971.

Miller H, Phillips E: Antibacterial correlates of urine drug levels of hexamethylenetetramine and formaldehyde. Invest Urol 8:21, 1970.

Milman N: Renal failure with gentamicin therapy. Acta med scandinav 196:87, 1974.

Milner RDG & others: Clinical pharmacology of gentamicin in the newborn infant. Arch Dis Childhood 47:927, 1972.

Murphy FJ, Zelman S: Ascorbic acid as a urinary acidifying agent: 1. Comparison with the ketogenic effect of fasting. J Urol 94:297, 1965.

Nelson JD, McCracken GH Jr: The current status of gentamicin for the neonate and young infant. Am J Dis Child 124:13, 1972.

Paisley JW, Smith AL, Smith DH: Gentamicin in newborn infants. Am J Dis Child 126:473, 1973.

Pasternak DP, Stephens BG: Reversible nephrotoxicity associated with cephalothin therapy. Arch Int Med 135:599, 1975.

Phillips ME & others: Tetracycline poisoning in renal failure. Brit MJ 2:149, 1974.

Reeves DS: Sulfamethoxazole/trimethoprim: The first two years. J Clin Path 24:430, 1971.

Regamey C, Gordon RC, Kirby WMM: Cefazolin vs cephalothin and cephaloridine. Arch Int Med 133:407, 1974.

Reeves DS: Sulfamethoxazole/trimethoprim: The first two years. J Clin Path 24:430, 1971.

Reyes MP, Palutke M, Lerner AM: Granulocytopenia associated with carbenicillin: Five episodes in two patients. Am J Med 54:413, 1973.

Ross RR Jr, Conway GF: Hemorrhagic cystitis following accidental overdose of methenamine mandelate. Am J Dis Child 119:86, 1970.

Sanders WE Jr, Johnson JE III, Taggart JG: Adverse reactions to cephalothin and cephapirin: Uniform occurrence on prolonged intravenous administration of high doses. New England J Med 290:424, 1974.

Seneca H: Drug susceptibility/resistance pattern of gram-negative pathogens to seven cephalosporins. Am J Med Sc 266:381, 1973.

Seneca H: Indanyl carbenicillin in chronic recurrent urinary tract infections. J Urol 110:249, 1973.

Seneca H, Uson A, Peer P: Cephalexin in urinary tract infections. J Urol 107:832, 1972.

Smith EK, Williams JD: The use of cephalexin monohydrate in chronic bacteriuria and acute urinary tract infection. Brit J Urol 42:522, 1970.

Stamey TA, Govan DE, Palmer JM: The localization and treatment of urinary tract infections: The role of bactericidal urine levels as opposed to serum levels. Medicine 44:1, 1965.

Stewart DJ: Prevalence of tetracyclines in children's teeth. 2. A resurvey after five years. Brit MJ 3:320, 1973.

Toivonen S & others: Comparison of ampicillin and nalidixic acid in the treatment of urinary infections caused by *E. coli*. Acta med scandinav 195:181, 1974.

Wallerstein RO & others: Statewide study of chloramphenicol therapy and fatal aplastic anemia. JAMA 208:2045, 1969.

Weinstein L, Madoff MA, Samet CM: The sulfonamides. (4 parts.) New England J Med 263:793, 842, 900, 952, 1960.

Whelton A & others: Carbenicillin concentrations in normal and diseased kidneys. Ann Int Med 78:659, 1973.

Wilkowske CJ & others: *Serratia marcescens.* JAMA 214:2157, 1970.

13...
Specific Infections of the Urinary Tract

TUBERCULOSIS

Tubercle bacilli may invade one or more (or even all) of the organs of the genitourinary tract and cause a chronic granulomatous infection which shows the same characteristics as tuberculosis in other organs. Urinary tuberculosis is a disease of young adults (60% of patients are between the ages of 20–40) and is a little more common in males than in females.

Etiology

The infecting organism is *Mycobacterium tuberculosis,* which reaches the genitourinary organs by the hematogenous route from the lungs. The primary site is often not symptomatic or apparent.

The kidney and possibly the prostate are the primary sites of tuberculous infection in the genitourinary tract. All other genitourinary organs become involved either by ascent (prostate to bladder) or descent (kidney to bladder; prostate to epididymis). The testis may become involved by direct extension from epididymal infection.

Pathogenesis (Fig 13–1)

A. Kidney and Ureter: When a shower of tubercle bacilli hits the renal cortex, the organisms may be destroyed by normal tissue resistance. Evidence of this is commonly seen in autopsies of persons who have died of tuberculosis; only scars are found in the kidneys. However, if enough bacteria of sufficient virulence become lodged in the kidney and are not overcome, a clinical infection is established.

Tuberculosis of the kidney progresses slowly; it may take 15–20 years to destroy a kidney in a patient having good resistance to the infection. As a rule, therefore, there is no renal pain and little or no clinical disturbance of any type until the lesion has involved the calyces or the pelvis, at which time pus and organisms may be discharged into the urine. It is only at this stage that symptoms (of cystitis) are manifested. The infection then proceeds to the pelvic mucosa and the ureter, particularly its upper and vesical ends. This may lead to stricture and back pressure (hydronephrosis).

As the disease progresses, a caseous breakdown of tissue occurs until the entire kidney is replaced by cheesy material. Calcium may be laid down in the re-

parative process. The ureter undergoes fibrosis and tends to be shortened and therefore straightened. This change leads to a "golf hole" (gaping) ureteral orifice, typical of an incompetent valve.

B. Bladder: Vesical irritability develops as an early clinical manifestation of the disease as the bladder is bathed by infected material. Tubercles form later, usually in the region of the involved ureteral orifice, and finally coalesce and ulcerate. These ulcers may bleed. With severe involvement, the bladder becomes fibrosed and contracted; this leads to marked frequency. Ureteral reflux or stenosis and, therefore, hydronephrosis may develop. If contralateral renal involvement develops later, it is probably a separate hematogenous infection.

C. Prostate and Seminal Vesicles: The passage of infected urine through the prostatic urethra will ultimately lead to invasion of the prostate and one or both seminal vesicles. There is no local pain.

On occasion, the primary hematogenous lesion in the genitourinary tract is in the prostate. Prostatic infection can extend to the bladder and descend to the epididymis.

D. Epididymis and Testis: Tuberculosis of the prostate can extend along the vas or through the perivasal lymphatics and affect the epididymis. Because this is a slow process, there is usually no pain. If the epididymal infection is extensive and an abscess forms, it may rupture through the scrotal skin, thus establishing a permanent sinus, or it may extend into the testicle.

Pathology

A. Kidney and Ureter: The gross appearance of the kidney with moderately advanced tuberculosis is often normal on its outer surface, although it is usually surrounded by marked perinephritis. Usually, however, there is a soft, yellowish localized bulge. On section, the involved area is seen to be filled with cheesy material (caseation). Widespread destruction of parenchyma is evident. In otherwise normal tissue, small abscesses may be seen. The walls of the pelvis, calyces, and ureter may be thickened, and ulceration appears frequently in the region of the calyces at the point at which the abscess drains. Ureteral stenosis may be complete, causing "autonephrectomy." Such a kidney is fibrosed and functionless. Under these circumstances, the blad-

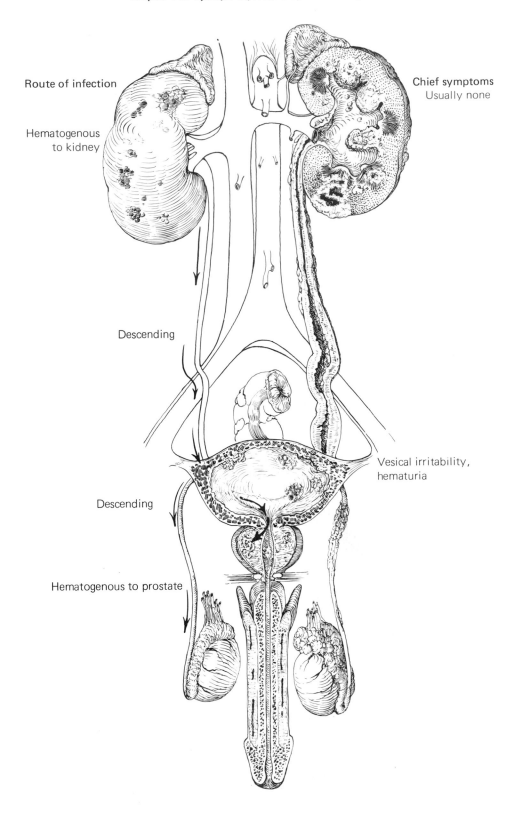

Figure 13—1. Pathogenesis of tuberculosis of the urinary tract.

der urine may be normal and symptoms absent.

Microscopically, the caseous material is seen as an amorphous mass. The surrounding parenchyma shows fibrosis with tissue destruction, small round cell and plasma cell infiltration, and epithelial and giant cells typical of tuberculosis. Acid-fast stains will usually demonstrate the organisms in the tissue. Similar changes can be demonstrated in the wall of the pelvis and ureter.

In both the kidney and ureter, calcification is common. It may be macroscopic or microscopic. Such a finding is strongly suggestive of tuberculosis. Secondary renal stones occur in 10% of patients.

In the most advanced stage of renal tuberculosis, the parenchyma may be completely replaced by caseous substance or fibrous tissue. Perinephric abscess may develop, but this is rare.

B. Bladder: In the early stages, the mucosa may be inflamed, but this is not a specific change. The bladder is quite resistant to actual invasion. Later, tubercles form and can be seen easily, especially through the cystoscope, as white or yellow raised nodules surrounded by a halo of hyperemia. With severe vesical contracture, reflux may occur.

Microscopically, the nodules are typical tubercles. These break down to form deep, ragged ulcers. At this stage the bladder is quite irritable. With healing, fibrosis develops which involves the muscle wall.

C. Prostate and Seminal Vesicles: Grossly, the exterior surface of these organs may show nodules and areas of induration from fibrosis. Areas of necrosis are common. In rare cases, healing may end in calcification. Large calcifications in the prostate should suggest tuberculous involvement.

D. Spermatic Cord, Epididymis, and Testis: The vas deferens is often grossly involved; fusiform swellings represent tubercles. The epididymis is enlarged and quite firm. It is usually separate from the testis, although occasionally it may adhere to it. Microscopically, the changes typical of tuberculosis are seen. Tubular degeneration may be marked.

The testis is usually not involved except by direct extension of an abscess in the epididymis.

Clinical Findings

Tuberculosis of the genitourinary tract should be considered in the presence of any of the following situations: (1) chronic cystitis which refuses to respond to adequate therapy, (2) the finding of pus without bacteria in a methylene blue stain or culture of the urinary sediment, (3) gross or microscopic hematuria, (4) a nontender, enlarged epididymis with a beaded or thickened vas, (5) a chronic draining scrotal sinus, or (6) induration or nodulation of the prostate and thickening of one or both seminal vesicles (especially in a young man). A history of present or past tuberculosis elsewhere in the body should cause the physician to suspect tuberculosis in the genitourinary tract when signs or symptoms are present.

The diagnosis rests upon the demonstration of tubercle bacilli in the urine (acid-fast stain, culture). The extent of the infection is determined by (1) the palpable findings in the epididymides, vasa deferentia, prostate, and seminal vesicles; (2) the renal and ureteral lesions as revealed by excretory urograms; (3) involvement of the bladder as seen through the cystoscope; (4) the degree of renal damage as measured by loss of function; and (5) the presence of tubercle bacilli in one or both kidneys.

A. Symptoms: There is no classic clinical picture of renal tuberculosis. Most symptoms of this disease, even in the most advanced stage, are vesical in origin (cystitis). Vague generalized malaise, fatigability, low-grade but persistent fever, and night sweats are some of the nonspecific complaints. Even vesical irritability may be absent, in which case only proper collection and examination of the urine will afford the clue. Active tuberculosis elsewhere in the body is found in less than half of patients with genitourinary tuberculosis.

1. Kidney and ureter—Because of the slow progression of the disease, the affected kidney is usually completely asymptomatic. On occasion, however, there may be a dull ache in the flank. The passage of a blood clot, secondary calculi, or a mass of debris may cause renal and ureteral colic. Rarely, the presenting symptom may be a painless mass in the abdomen.

2. Bladder—The earliest symptoms of renal tuberculosis may arise from secondary vesical involvement. These include burning, frequency, and nocturia. Hematuria is occasionally found and is of either renal or vesical origin. At times, particularly in a late stage of the disease, the vesical irritability may become extreme. If ulceration occurs, suprapubic pain may be noted when the bladder becomes full.

3. Genital tract—Tuberculosis of the prostate and seminal vesicles usually causes no symptoms. The first clue to the presence of tuberculous infection of these organs is the onset of a tuberculous epididymitis.

Tuberculosis of the epididymis usually presents as a painless or only mildly painful swelling. An abscess may drain spontaneously through the scrotal wall. A chronic draining sinus should be regarded as tuberculous until proved otherwise. In rare cases, the onset is quite acute and may simulate an acute nonspecific epididymitis.

B. Signs: Evidence of extragenital tuberculosis may be found (lungs, bone, lymph nodes, tonsils, intestines).

1. Kidney—There is usually no enlargement or tenderness of the involved kidney.

2. External genitalia—A thickened, nontender, or only slightly tender epididymis may be discovered. The vas deferens often is thickened and beaded. A chronic draining sinus through the scrotal skin is almost pathognomonic of tuberculous epididymitis. In the more advanced stages, the epididymis cannot be differentiated from the testis upon palpation. This may mean that the testis has been directly invaded by the epididymal abscess.

Hydrocele occasionally accompanies tuberculous epididymitis. The "idiopathic" hydrocele should be tapped so that underlying pathologic changes, if pres-

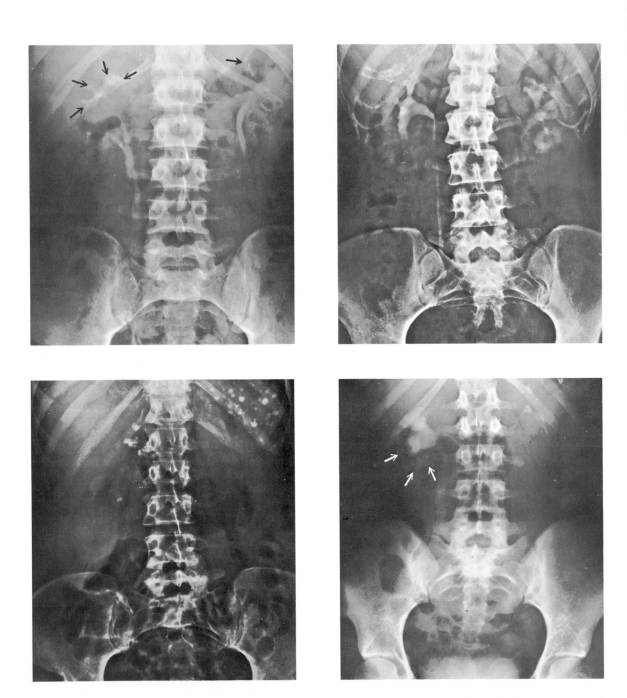

Figure 13–2. Radiologic evidence of tuberculosis. *Above left:* Excretory urogram showing "motheaten" calyces in upper renal poles. Calcifications in upper calyces; right upper ureter is straight and dilated. *Below left:* Plain film showing calcifications in right kidney, adrenals, and spleen (tuberculosis of right kidney and Addison's disease). *Above right:* Excretory urogram showing ulcerated and dilated calyces on the left. *Below right:* Excretory urogram. Dilatation of calyces; upper right ureter dilated and straight. Arrows point to poorly defined parenchymal abscesses.

ent, can be evaluated (epididymitis, testicular tumor).

3. Prostate and seminal vesicles—These organs may be normal to palpation. Ordinarily, however, the tuberculous prostate shows areas of induration, even nodulation. The involved vesicle is usually indurated, enlarged, and fixed. If epididymitis is present, the ipsilateral vesicle usually shows changes as well.

C. Laboratory Findings: Proper urinalysis affords the most important clue to the diagnosis of genitourinary tuberculosis.

1. Persistent pyuria without organisms on culture or on the smear stained with methylene blue means tuberculosis until proved otherwise. Acid-fast stains done on the concentrated sediment from a 24-hour specimen are positive in at least 60% of cases. This must be corroborated by a positive culture.

About 15–20% of patients with tuberculosis have secondary pyogenic infection; the clue ("sterile" pyuria) is thereby obscured. If clinical response to adequate treatment fails and pyuria persists, tuberculosis must be ruled out by bacteriologic and roentgenologic means.

2. Cultures for tubercle bacilli from urine are positive in a high percentage of cases of tuberculous infection. In the face of strong presumptive evidence of tuberculosis, negative cultures should be repeated.

The blood count may be normal or may show anemia in advanced disease. The sedimentation rate is usually accelerated.

Tubercle bacilli may often be demonstrated in the secretions from an infected prostate. Renal function will be normal unless there is bilateral damage: As one kidney is slowly injured, compensatory hypertrophy of the normal kidney develops. It can also be infected with tubercle bacilli, or may become hydronephrotic from fibrosis of the bladder wall (ureterovesical stenosis) or vesicoureteral reflux.

If tuberculosis is suspected, perform the tuberculin test. A positive test, particularly in an adult, is hardly diagnostic; but a negative test in an otherwise healthy patient speaks against a diagnosis of tuberculosis.

D. X-Ray Findings: (Fig 13–2.) A chest film which shows evidence of tuberculosis should cause the physician to suspect tuberculosis of the urogenital tract in the presence of urinary signs and symptoms. A plain film of the abdomen may show enlargement of one kidney or obliteration of the renal and psoas shadows due to perinephric abscess. Punctate calcification in the renal parenchyma may be due to tuberculosis. Renal stones are found in 10% of cases. Calcification of the ureter may be noted, but this is rare (Fig 6–2). Small prostatic stones the size of grape-seeds in the region of the symphysis pubis are ordinarily not due to tuberculosis, but large calcific bodies may be.

Excretory urograms can be diagnostic if the lesion is moderately advanced. The typical changes include (1) a "motheaten" appearance of the involved ulcerated calyces, (2) obliteration of one or more calyces, (3) dilatation of the calyces due to ureteral stenosis from fibrosis, (4) abscess cavities which connect with calyces, (5) single or multiple ureteral strictures, with secondary dilatation, with shortening and therefore straightening of the ureter, and (6) absence of function of the kidney, due to complete ureteral occlusion and renal destruction (autonephrectomy).

If the excretory urograms demonstrate gross tuberculosis in one kidney, there is no need to do a retrograde urogram on that side. In fact, there is at least a theoretical danger of hematogenous or lymphogenous dissemination resulting from the increased intrapelvic pressure. Retrograde urography should, however, be carried out on the unsuspected side as a verification of its normality. This is further substantiated if the urine from that side is free of both pus cells and tubercle bacilli.

E. Instrumental Examination: Thorough cystoscopic study is indicated even when the offending organism has been found in the urine and excretory urograms show the typical renal lesion. This will clearly demonstrate the extent of the disease. Cystoscopy may reveal the typical tubercles or ulcers of tuberculosis. Biopsy can be done if necessary. Severe contracture of the bladder may be noted. A cystogram may reveal ureteral reflux. A clean specimen of urine should also be obtained for further study. Ureteral catheters are then passed to the renal pelves. This will afford urine specimens from each kidney for bacteriologic examination. Relative function of each kidney can be determined with the PSP test. Considerable destruction is necessary, however, before this test shows impairment.

Differential Diagnosis

Chronic nonspecific cystitis or pyelonephritis may mimic tuberculosis perfectly, especially since 15–20% of cases of tuberculosis are secondarily invaded by pyogenic organisms. If nonspecific infections do not respond to adequate therapy, a search for tubercle bacilli should be made. Painless epididymitis points to tuberculosis. Cystoscopic demonstration of tubercles and ulceration of the bladder wall means tuberculosis. Urograms are usually definitive.

Acute or chronic nonspecific epididymitis may be confused with tuberculosis since the onset of tuberculosis is occasionally quite painful. It is rare to have palpatory changes in the seminal vesicles with nonspecific epididymitis, but these are almost routine findings in tuberculosis of the epididymis. The presence of tubercle bacilli in the urine is diagnostic. On occasion, only the pathologist can make the diagnosis by microscopic study of the surgically removed epididymis.

Amicrobic cystitis usually has an acute onset and is often preceded by a urethral discharge. "Sterile" pyuria is found, but tubercle bacilli are absent. Cystoscopy may reveal ulcerations, but these are acute and superficial. Although urograms show mild hydroureter and even hydronephrosis, there is no ulceration of the calyces as seen in renal tuberculosis.

Interstitial cystitis is typically characterized by frequency, nocturia, and suprapubic pain with vesical filling. The urine is usually free of pus. Tubercle bacilli are absent.

Multiple small renal stones or nephrocalcinosis seen by x-ray may suggest the type of calcification seen in the tuberculous kidney. In renal tuberculosis, the calcium is in the parenchyma, although secondary stones are occasionally seen.

Necrotizing papillitis, which may involve all of the calyces of one or both kidneys or, rarely, a solitary calyx, shows calyceal lesions (including calcifications) which simulate those of tuberculosis. Careful bacteriologic studies will fail to demonstrate tubercle bacilli.

Medullary sponge kidneys may show small calcifications just distal to the calyces. The calyces, however, are sharp, and no other stigmas of tuberculosis can be demonstrated.

Complications

A. Renal Tuberculosis: Perinephric abscess may cause an enlarging mass in the flank. A plain film of the abdomen will show obliteration of the renal and psoas shadows. Renal stones may develop if secondary nonspecific infection is present. Uremia is the end stage if both kidneys are involved.

B. Ureteral Tuberculosis: Scarring with stricture formation is one of the typical lesions of tuberculosis and most commonly affects the juxtavesical portion. This may cause progressive hydronephrosis. Complete ureteral obstruction may cause complete nonfunction of the kidney.

C. Vesical Tuberculosis: When severely damaged, the bladder wall becomes fibrosed and contracted. Stenosis of the ureters or reflux occurs, causing hydronephrotic atrophy.

D. Genital Tuberculosis: The ducts of the involved epididymis become occluded. If this is bilateral, sterility results. Abscess of the epididymis may rupture into the testis, through the scrotal wall, or both, in which case the spermatogenic tubules may slough out.

Treatment

Tuberculosis must be treated as a generalized disease. Even when it can be demonstrated only in the urogenital tract, one must assume activity elsewhere. (It is theoretically possible, however, for the primary focus to have healed spontaneously.) This means that basically the treatment is medical. Surgical excision of an infected organ, when indicated, is merely an adjunct to overall therapy.

A. Renal Tuberculosis: A strict medical regimen should be instituted.

The following combination of drugs can be utilized. They should be given for at least 2 years. (1) Cycloserine, sodium aminosalicylic acid (PAS), and isoniazid (INH). (2) Cycloserine, ethambutol, and isoniazid. (3) Rifampin, ethambutol, and isoniazid. The latter is probably the most efficacious. The oral dose of each is as follows: Cycloserine, 250 mg twice daily; PAS, 15 g in divided doses; INH, 300 mg; ethambutol, 1.2 g; rifampin, 600 mg. Sensitivity testing may indicate the use of streptomycin intramuscularly. Administer 1 g/day the first month, 1 g 3 times a week for the next month, and then 1 g twice a week. Since INH may cause peripheral neuropathy, give pyridoxine, 100 mg/day orally.

If, after 3 months, cultures are still positive and gross involvement of the affected kidney is radiologically evident, nephrectomy should be considered. However, this is rarely necessary.

If bacteriologic and radiographic studies demonstrate bilateral disease, only medical treatment can be considered. The only exceptions are (1) severe sepsis, pain, or bleeding from one kidney (may require nephrectomy as a palliative or lifesaving measure); and (2) marked advance of the disease on one side and minimal damage on the other (consider removal of the badly damaged organ).

B. Vesical Tuberculosis: Tuberculosis of the bladder is always secondary to renal or prostatic tuberculosis; it tends to heal promptly when definitive treatment for the "primary" genitourinary infection is given. Vesical ulcers which fail to respond to this regimen may require transurethral electrocoagulation. Vesical instillations of 0.2% monoxychlorosene (Clorpactin) may also stimulate healing.

Should extreme contracture of the bladder develop, it may be necessary to divert the urine from the bladder or perform subtotal cystectomy and anastomose a patch of ileum or sigmoid to the remainder (ileocystoplasty, sigmoidocystoplasty) in order to afford comfort.

C. Tuberculosis of the Epididymis: This is never an isolated lesion; the prostate is always involved and usually the kidney as well. Only rarely does the epididymal infection break through into the testis. Treatment is medical. If after months of treatment an abscess or a draining sinus exists, epididymectomy is indicated.

D. Tuberculosis of the Prostate and Seminal Vesicles: Although a few urologists advocate removal of the entire prostate and the vesicles when they become involved by tuberculosis, the majority opinion is that only medical therapy is indicated. Control can be checked by culture of the semen for tubercle bacilli.

E. General Measures for All Types: Optimum nutrition is no less important in treating tuberculosis of the genitourinary tract than in the treatment of tuberculosis elsewhere. Bladder sedatives may be given for the irritable bladder.

F. Treatment of Complications: Perinephric abscess usually occurs when the kidney is destroyed, but this is rare. The abscess must be drained, and nephrectomy should be done either then or later to prevent development of a chronic draining sinus. Prolonged antimicrobial therapy is indicated. If ureterovesical stricture or reflux develops and causes progressive hydronephrosis of the uninvolved kidney, diversion of the urine by cutaneous ureterostomy, nephrostomy, or replacement of the diseased ureter with a segment of ileum may have to be done to prevent death from uremia. For this reason, serial excretory urograms are necessary even under medical treatment.

Prognosis

The prognosis varies with the extent of the disease and the organs involved, but the overall control rate is 98% at 5 years. The urine must be studied bacteriologically every 6 months for 5 years. Relapse will indicate the need for reinstitution of treatment. Nephrectomy is rarely necessary. In the healing process, ureteral stenosis or vesical contraction may develop. Appropriate surgical intervention may be necessary.

AMICROBIC (ABACTERIAL) CYSTITIS

Amicrobic cystitis is a rare disease of abrupt onset with a marked local vesical reaction. Although it acts like an infectious disease, bacterial search for the usual urinary pathogens is negative. It affects adult men and occasionally children, usually boys.

Etiology

The patient usually gives a history of recent sexual exposure. Mycoplasma and chlamydia organisms have been isolated or suspected as etiologic agents. An adenovirus has been isolated from the urine in children suffering from acute hemorrhagic cystitis.

Pathogenesis & Pathology

Whatever the source and identity of the invader, the disease is primarily manifested as an acute inflammation of the bladder. Vesical irritability is severe and is often associated with terminal hematuria. The mucosa is red and edematous, and superficial ulceration is occasionally seen. A thin membrane of fibrin often lies upon the wall. Similar changes may be noted in the posterior urethra. The renal parenchyma is not involved, although the pelvic and ureteral mucosa may show mild inflammatory changes. Some dilatation of the lower ureters is apt to develop. This may be due to an inflammatory reaction about the ureteral orifices, for these changes regress after successful treatment.

Microscopically, there is nothing specific about the reaction. The mucosa and submucosa are infiltrated with neutrophils, plasma cells, and eosinophils. Submucosal hemorrhages are common; superficial ulceration of the mucosa may be noted.

Clinical Findings

A. Symptoms: All symptoms are local. Urethral discharge, which is usually clear and mucoid but which may be purulent, may be the initial symptom in men. Symptoms of acute cystitis come on abruptly. Urgency, frequency, and burning may be severe. Terminal hematuria is not uncommon. Suprapubic discomfort or even pain may be noted; it is most apt to be present as the bladder fills and is relieved somewhat by voiding. There is no fever or malaise.

B. Signs: Some suprapubic tenderness may be found. Urethral discharge may be profuse or scanty, and purulent or thin and mucoid. The prostate is usu-ally normal to palpation. Massage is contraindicated during the acute stage of urinary tract infection. When done later, infection is usually not present.

C. Laboratory Findings: Some leukocytosis may develop. The urine is grossly purulent and may contain blood as well. Stained smears reveal an absence of bacteria. Routine cultures are uniformly negative. In a few cases, mycoplasma and TRIC agent have been identified, but the significance of this is not yet clear. Search for tubercle bacilli is not successful.

Urethral discharge reveals no bacteria. Renal function is not impaired.

D. X-Ray Findings: Excretory urograms may demonstrate some dilatation of the lower ureters, but these changes regress completely when the disease is cured. The bladder shadow is small because of its markedly diminished capacity. Cystograms may reveal reflux.

E. Instrumental Examination: Cystoscopy is not indicated in the face of acute inflammation of the bladder. It has been done, however, when the diagnosis was obscure and tuberculosis suspected. In such cases it reveals redness and edema of the mucosa. Superficial ulceration may be noted. Bladder capacity is markedly diminished. Biopsy of the wall shows nonspecific changes.

Differential Diagnosis

Tuberculosis causes symptoms of cystitis, which, however, usually come on gradually and become severe only in the stage of ulceration. A painless, nontender enlargement of an epididymis suggests tuberculosis. Although both tuberculosis and amicrobic cystitis produce pus without bacteria, thorough laboratory study will demonstrate tubercle bacilli only in the former. On cystoscopy the tuberculous bladder may be studded with tubercles. The ulcers in this disease are deep and of a chronic type. The changes in amicrobic cystitis are more acute; ulceration, if present, is superficial. Excretory urograms in tuberculosis may show "motheaten" calyces typical of infection with acid-fast organisms.

Nonspecific (pyogenic) cystitis may mimic amicrobic cystitis perfectly, but pathogenic organisms are easily found on a smear stained with methylene blue or on culture.

Cystitis secondary to chronic nonspecific prostatitis occasionally produces pus without bacteria. The findings on rectal examination, the pus in the prostatic secretion, and the response to antibiotics point to the proper diagnosis.

Vesical neoplasm may ulcerate, become infected, and bleed; hence it may mimic amicrobic cystitis. Bacteriuria, however, will be found. In case of doubt, cystoscopy is indicated.

Interstitial cystitis may be accompanied by severe symptoms of vesical irritability. However, it usually affects women past the menopause, and urinalysis is entirely negative except for a few red cells. Cystoscopy should be diagnostic.

Complications

Amicrobic cystitis is usually self-limited. Rarely, secondary contracture of the bladder develops. Under these circumstances, vesicoureteral reflux may be noted.

Treatment

A. Specific Measures: One of the tetracyclines or chloramphenicol, 1 g/day orally in divided doses for 3–4 days, is said to be curative in 75% of cases. Streptomycin, 1–2 g/day IM for 3–4 days, may be tried. Neoarsphenamine is also effective and appears to be the drug of choice. The first dose is 0.3 g IV; subsequent dosage is 0.45 g IV every 3–5 days for a total of 3–4 injections.

Penicillin and the sulfonamides are without effect.

In the cases reported in children, cure occurred spontaneously.

B. General Measures: Bladder sedatives are usually of little help if symptoms are severe. Analgesics or narcotics may prove necessary to combat pain. Hot sitz baths may relieve spasm.

Prognosis

The prognosis is excellent.

CANDIDIASIS

Candida albicans is a yeastlike fungus that is a normal inhabitant of the respiratory and gastrointestinal tracts and the vagina. The intensive use of potent modern antibiotics is apt to disturb the normal balance between normal and abnormal organisms, thus allowing fungi such as candida to overwhelm an otherwise healthy organ. The bladder and, to a lesser extent, the kidneys have proved vulnerable; candidemia has been observed.

The patient may present with vesical irritability or symptoms and signs of pyelonephritis. Fungus balls may be passed spontaneously. The diagnosis is made by observing mycelial or yeast forms of the fungus microscopically in a properly collected urine specimen. The diagnosis may be confirmed by culture. Excretory urograms may show calyceal defects and ureteral obstruction (fungus masses).

Vesical candidiasis usually responds to alkalinization of the urine with sodium bicarbonate. A urinary pH of 7.5 is desired; the dose is regulated by the patient, who checks the urine with indicator paper. Should this fail, amphotericin B should be instilled via catheter 3 times a day. Dissolve 100 mg of the drug in 500 ml of 5% dextrose solution.

If there is renal involvement, irrigations of the renal pelvis with a similar concentration of amphotericin B are efficacious. In the presence of systemic manifestations or candidemia, flucytosine (Ancobon) is the drug of choice. The dose is 100 mg/kg/day orally in divided doses given for 1 week. In the face of serious involvement, give 600 mg IV on the first day and then shift to the oral form of the drug. Amphotericin B (Fungizone) has the disadvantages of requiring parenteral administration and being highly nephrotoxic. It is given intravenously in a dosage of 1–5 mg/day in divided doses dissolved in 5% dextrose. The concentration of the solution should be 0.1 mg/ml.

ACTINOMYCOSIS

Actinomycosis is a chronic granulomatous disease in which fibrosis tends to become marked and spontaneous fistulas are the rule. On rare occasions, the disease involves the kidney, bladder, or testis by hematogenous invasion from a primary site of infection. The skin of the penis or scrotum may become involved through a local abrasion. The bladder may also become diseased by direct extension from the appendix, bowel, or Fallopian tube.

Etiology

Actinomyces israelii (A bovis).

Clinical Findings

There is nothing specifically pathognomonic about the symptoms or signs in actinomycosis. The microscopic demonstration of the organisms, which are visible as yellow bodies called "sulfur granules," makes the diagnosis. If persistently sought for, these may be found in the discharge from sinuses or in the urine. Definitive diagnosis is established by culture.

Urographically, the lesion in the kidney may resemble tuberculosis (eroded calyces) or tumor (space-occupying lesion).

Treatment

Clindamycin is probably the drug of choice. Initially, it should be administered either intramuscularly or intravenously. The daily dose is 1.2–2.7 g in divided doses. Parenteral therapy may be required for 2 or more months, after which 1 g a day may be given by mouth. Penicillin G is also effective. Give 10–20 million units a day for 1 month and then switch to oral penicillin V in similar dosage for 3–6 months or longer. Surgical removal of the infected organ is usually indicated.

Prognosis

Removal of the involved organ (eg, kidney or testis) may be promptly curative. Drainage of a granulomatous abscess may cause the development of a chronic draining sinus. Chemotherapy is helpful.

TRICHOMONIASIS IN THE MALE

Etiology

Trichomonas vaginalis is the most common cause of vaginitis; about 15% of women harbor the organism. It is found not infrequently in the urethra and prostate in men and in the bladder in both sexes. It is transmitted to men by sexual intercourse. The sexual partners of all women with trichomoniasis should be examined for trichomonads.

Clinical Findings

A. Symptoms and Signs: Men harboring the organism may suffer from some degree of urethral itching and discharge which may be thin or purulent, scanty or profuse; at times there is frequency and burning on urination. There are usually, however, no symptoms at all.

B. Laboratory Findings:

1. Urethral discharge, wet preparation—The discharge should be mixed immediately with 1–2 ml of saline or Trichomonas solution and studied microscopically. In about 10% of those whose wives harbor the protozoon, motile trichomonads (about the size of pus cells) are seen. A dried smear should be stained with methylene blue to study the bacterial flora as well, since secondary infection with pyogenic bacteria is common.

2. Urethral scrapings will reveal the organisms microscopically in 75% of cases. Dark-field examination may prove helpful.

3. Urine, wet preparation—The sediment of a centrifuged specimen of urine should be studied for the motile organisms. This is successful in 25% of patients.

4. Prostatic secretion—Motile trichomonads may be discovered in the secretion obtained by prostatic massage.

5. Culture of semen, prostatic secretion, or urethral discharge—If the wet preparations are negative, a suitable culture medium should be inoculated, incubated for 48 hours at 37 °C, and examined microscopically. With this technic, 90% of men whose wives are infected with *Trichomonas vaginalis* will have a positive culture.

6. Urethral discharge stained by the Papanicolaou technic often reveals the organism.

Treatment

Once the diagnosis has been made, a condom should be used during intercourse until treatment has been successful.

Metronidazole (Flagyl), 400 mg orally twice a day, should be administered for 7 days. Davidson finds that giving 1 g for 2 days in divided doses is also efficacious. Nitrimidazine (Naxogin), 250 mg twice a day for 6 days, is equally effective, as is flunidazole, 200 mg 3 times a day for 5 days.

Prognosis

Most trichomonad infections respond promptly to metronidazole or nitrimidazine. Vigorous treatment of the man's sexual partner is imperative.

SCHISTOSOMIASIS
(Bilharziasis)

Schistosoma haematobium, a blood fluke, invades primarily the bladder. Schistosomiasis is endemic and very common in most of Africa and in Madagascar, southern Portugal, Greece, and the Near and Middle East. In some areas, 25–50% of the population are affected. The manifestations of the disease are severe in Egypt but mild in central Africa.

Etiology

The adult female *S haematobium* is a threadlike white worm. The male is about 1 cm and the female 2 cm long. They lodge in the venous plexus of the bladder wall, where the female lays myriads of eggs which occlude the smaller vessels. The eggs are extruded into the bladder and voided with the urine. These eggs are oval and possess a terminal spine. If they are passed into warm fresh water, they hatch and the larvae (miracidia) are freed. If within a few hours they enter a particular freshwater snail, they reach the sporozoite stage, multiplying rapidly and emerging from their host as cercariae (fork-tailed larvae).

If these cercariae find a human host, they penetrate the skin and enter the vascular system. Only those reaching the portal vein survive. In the liver the larvae develop into the adult stage. They then migrate against the bloodstream to the veins of the bladder, and mate. The female lays eggs, and the cycle is repeated. The adult flukes live for many years; untreated, the disease is progressive.

Pathogenesis & Pathology

The eggs with their terminal spines penetrate the wall of the vein with the assistance of muscular contraction. This allows the eggs to be extruded into the vesical cavity. Healing is by scar formation, and the bladder gradually becomes thickened and contracted. The appearance of calcification of the bladder wall is caused by calcium deposition in the shells of the ova. The intramural portions of the ureters may become stenotic, with consequent hydronephrosis. Ureteral reflux is common. With the advent of secondary infection, pericystitis may occur. Ulcerations and papillomatous lesions develop on the vesical mucosa. The incidence of bulky squamous cell carcinomas in patients suffering from schistosomiasis is very high.

The major lesion is in the trigonal area. Mucosal congestion and edema are at first the only findings, but, as the eggs approach the mucosa, "tubercles" are noted which are quite similar to the lesion of tuberculosis. The small yellow nodule represents the egg and

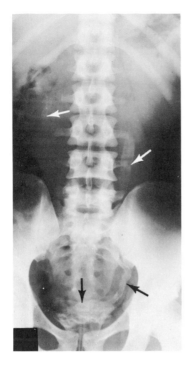 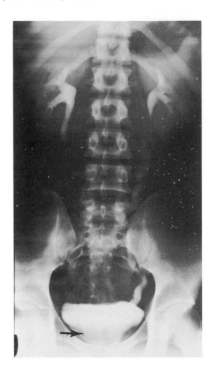

Figure 13–3. Bilharzia. *Left:* Plain abdominal film showing calcification in the ureteral and vesical walls. *Right:* Excretory urogram of the same patient, revealing normal upper tracts. Note calcification in right side of bladder wall.

the specific cellular reaction around it. The egg is surrounded by a zone of hyperemia. Larger nodular and polypoid masses develop later and then break down and ulcerate. At this stage, the eggs are easily found in the urine. In the later stages, fibrosis may be extreme.

Microscopic examination of the bladder wall reveals many eggs surrounded by neutrophils, eosinophils, and foreign body giant cells. Calcified eggs are seen in the submucosa and muscle layer. Later, fibroplastic proliferation dominates the picture.

Clinical Findings

A. Symptoms: Intense itching may be present when the parasites are invading the skin. Generalized symptoms develop in about 1–3 months, when the adult flukes begin to lay eggs. The patient may develop headache, backache, chills, fever, and profuse sweats.

Symptoms of cystitis appear when the bladder wall has become involved. Terminal hematuria is common. If untreated, the bladder symptoms gradually increase in severity. As ulcerations develop, these symptoms may be extreme. Secondary infection exacerbates the symptoms. Calcific incrustation and even stones may form. Markedly contracted bladders are sometimes seen. Renal pain may be experienced as ureteral stenosis or reflux leads to hydronephrosis. Death may occur as a result of uremia or general sepsis.

B. Signs: In the early stages the physical examination is noncontributory. Later, urethral stricture and perineal fistulas may be found. A mass in the flank may be discovered if hydronephrosis is present. Rectal examination may reveal fibrosis of the prostate and base of the bladder. Elephantiasis of the external genitalia may occur as a result of lymphatic obstruction, but this is rare.

C. Laboratory Findings: During the egg-laying stage, leukocytosis is present; eosinophils often outnumber neutrophils. Anemia may be due to blood destruction by the flukes or may be secondary to nonspecific infection or uremia. The urine contains pus, red blood cells, and the eggs of *S haematobium.* These findings establish the diagnosis. Nonspecific pyogenic organisms may also be found. Renal function may be impaired in the presence of ureteral stenosis or vesicoureteral reflux.

D. X-Ray Findings: (Fig 13–3.) Calcifications in the bladder wall or lower ureters may be demonstrated on a plain film of the abdomen. Excretory urograms may show hydroureters and hydronephroses due to vesicoureteral reflux or stenosis. Cystograms may demonstrate a contracted bladder, vesical tumor, or reflux.

E. Instrumental Examination: Urethral strictures may be discovered on attempting the passage of a catheter or other instrument. Cystoscopy may show varying stages of the disease: tubercle formation, nodulation with tubercle formation, widespread ulceration, papillomatous reaction, carcinoma, vesical stones or calcium deposits, and evidence of severe fibrosis and contracture of the bladder wall. Biopsy of the lesions will show the eggs.

Differential Diagnosis

Nonspecific cystitis may be differentiated from schistosomiasis in the early stages since, although no bacteria will be found on a stained smear, eggs will probably be discovered. Nonspecific cystitis will ordinarily respond to antibiotics; schistosomiasis will not. Tuberculous cystitis may be confused with schistosomiasis since the history in both may be the same, neither responds to the usual antibiotics, and, superficially at least, the cystoscopic appearance may be similar (tubercles). Careful urinalysis should demonstrate the eggs in one and tubercle bacilli in the other. Excretory urograms may show the typical renal lesion of tuberculosis. Cystoscopic biopsy gives a positive differentiation.

Amicrobic cystitis has a more abrupt onset than schistosomiasis. In neither disease are bacteria found on stained smear unless secondary infection has occurred. In the early stages (hyperemia and edema), cystoscopy may not be helpful, but the changes associated with schistosomiasis later become obvious. Again, the finding of eggs in the urine or on cystoscopic biopsy establishes the diagnosis.

Vesical neoplasm may be differentiated by proper urinalysis (eggs) and cystoscopic biopsy. It must be remembered, however, that the incidence of squamous cell carcinoma is high in schistosomiasis.

Complications

Complications of schistosomiasis may include vesical fibrosis and contracture, bladder neck obstruction, perineal or suprapubic fistulas, vesical calculus, squamous cell carcinoma of the bladder, ureteral obstruction with hydronephrosis, vesicoureteral reflux, secondary infection with perivesical abscess, pyelonephritis, and general sepsis.

Treatment

Treatment is quite satisfactory if the diagnosis is made before complications develop.

A. Specific Measures:

1. Stibocaptate (Astiban) is the drug of choice. It is less toxic than tartar emetic and is given intramuscularly rather than intravenously. The total dose is 50 mg/kg divided into 5 equal injections given over a period of 1 week for 5 weeks.

2. Other useful drugs include niridazole (Ambilhar) and antimony potassium or sodium tartrate (tartar emetic).

B. General Measures: Secondary infection can be combated with the sulfonamides and antibiotics. Supportive treatment may be indicated (eg, transfusions for anemia).

C. Treatment of Complications: If vesical fibrosis is of such a degree that urinary frequency is a problem, colocystoplasty or ileocystoplasty is indicated. Urethral fistulas or strictures will require plastic repair. Vesicoureteral obstruction (or reflux) indicates the need for ureterovesical reimplantation.

Control

Sanitary measures can do a great deal to reduce the incidence of schistosomiasis in endemic areas. Attempts at control have been made by draining ponds and canals, thus decreasing the population of freshwater snails. Little, however, has been accomplished. Chemicals may be added to water to minimize snail infestation. Intensive chemotherapy of infected persons has so far failed to decrease the incidence of the disease.

Prognosis

If the diagnosis is made early (at the time of initial vesical symptoms), medical treatment is almost always curative. Reinfection may occur in endemic areas.

In the later stages of the disease (fibrosis, secondary infection), the prognosis is only fair. Specific therapy, even if it eradicates the fluke and kills the eggs, cannot reverse the disabling secondary changes. In many endemic areas, schistosomiasis ranks high on the list of fatal diseases.

FILARIASIS

Filariasis is endemic in the countries bordering the Mediterranean, in South China and Japan, the West Indies, and the South Pacific islands, particularly Samoa. Limited infection, as seen in American soldiers during World War II, gives an entirely different clinical picture than the frequent reinfections usually encountered among the native population.

Etiology

Wuchereria bancrofti is a threadlike nematode about 0.5 cm or more in length which lives in the human lymphatics. In the lymphatics the female gives off microfilariae, which are found, particularly at night, in the peripheral blood. The intermediate host (usually a mosquito), biting an infected person, becomes infested with microfilariae which develop into larvae. These are in turn transferred to another human being, in whom they reach maturity. Mating occurs, and microfilariae are again produced. *Brugia malayi,* a nematode, acts in a similar fashion.

Pathogenesis & Pathology

The adult nematode in the human host invades and obstructs the lymphatics; this leads to lymphangitis and lymphadenitis. In long-standing cases, the lymphatic vessels become thickened and fibrous; there is a marked reticuloendothelial reaction.

Clinical Findings

A. Symptoms: In mild cases (few exposures), the patient suffers recurrent lymphadenitis and lymphangitis with fever and malaise. Not infrequently, inflammation of the epididymis, testis, scrotum, and spermatic cord occurs. These structures then become edematous, boggy, and at times tender. Hydrocele is common. In advanced cases (many exposures), obstruction of major lymph channels may cause chyluria and elephantiasis.

B. Signs: Varying degrees of painless elephantiasis of the scrotum and extremities develop as obstruction to lymphatics progresses.

C. Laboratory Findings: Chylous urine may look normal if minimal amounts of fat are present, but, in an advanced case or following a fatty meal, it is milky. On standing, the urine layers: the top layer is fatty, the middle layer is pinkish, and the lower layer is clear. In the presence of chyluria, large amounts of protein are to be expected. Hypoproteinemia is found, and the albumin:globulin ratio is reversed. Both white and red cells are found. The fat will be dissolved by chloroform; the urine will therefore become clear.

Marked eosinophilia is the rule in the early stages. Microfilariae may be demonstrated in the blood, which should preferably be drawn at night. The adult worm may be found by biopsy. Skin and complement fixation tests are highly successful in diagnosis.

D. X-Ray Findings: Retrograde urography and lymphangiography may reveal the renolymphatic connections in patients with chyluria.

Prevention

In endemic areas, mosquito abatement programs must be intensively pursued.

Treatment

A. Specific Measures: Diethylcarbamazine (Hetrazan) is the drug of choice. The dose is 3 mg/kg orally 3 times daily for 21 days. This drug kills the microfilariae but not the adult worms. Several courses of the drug may be necessary.

B. General Measures: Prompt removal of recently infected patients from the endemic area almost always results in regression of the symptoms and signs in early cases.

C. Surgical Measures: Elephantiasis of the scrotum may require surgical excision.

D. Treatment of Chyluria: Mild cases require no therapy. If nutrition is impaired, the lymphatic channels may be sealed off by irrigating the renal pelvis with 2% silver nitrate solution. Should this fail, renal decapsulation and resection of the renal lymphatics should be performed.

Prognosis

If exposure has been limited, resolution of the disease is spontaneous and the prognosis is excellent. Frequent reinfection may lead to elephantiasis of the scrotum or chyluria.

ECHINOCOCCOSIS
(Hydatid Disease)

Involvement of the urogenital organs by hydatid disease is relatively rare in the USA. It is common in Australia, New Zealand, South America, Africa, Asia, and Europe, especially where sheep are raised.

Etiology

The adult tapeworm *(Echinococcus granulosus)* inhabits the intestinal tracts of carnivorous animals, especially dogs. Their eggs pass out with the feces and may be ingested by such animals as sheep, cattle, pigs, and occasionally men. Larvae from these eggs pass through the intestinal wall of the various intermediate hosts and are disseminated throughout the body. In man, the liver is principally involved, but about 3% of infected humans develop echinococcosis of the kidney.

If a cyst of the liver should rupture into the peritoneal cavity, the scoleces (tapeworm heads) may directly invade the retrovesical tissues, thus leading to the development of cysts in this area.

Clinical Findings

If renal hydatid disease is closed (not communicating with the pelvis), there may be no symptoms until a mass is found. If communicating, there may be symptoms of cystitis, and renal colic may occur as cysts are passed from the kidney. Eosinophilia is the rule. X-ray films may show calcification in the wall of the cyst (Fig 13–4), and urograms often reveal changes typical of a space-occupying lesion. Angiography reveals lucent masses. Needle aspiration will reveal chocolate-colored fluid containing scoleces and hooklets. The finding of scoleces and hooklets in the urine is

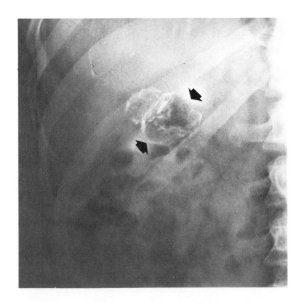

Figure 13–4. Hydatid disease, right kidney. Plain film showing 2 calcified hydatid cysts.

pathognomonic. A positive skin sensitivity test (Casoni) is suggestive. Complement fixation tests are positive in 90% of cases.

Retroperitoneal (perivesical) cysts may cause symptoms of cystitis, or acute urinary retention may develop secondary to pressure. The presence of a suprapubic mass may be the only finding. It may rupture into the bladder and cause hydatiduria, which establishes the diagnosis.

Treatment

Nephrectomy is generally the treatment of choice

of renal hydatid disease, although aspiration and marsupialization have also been recommended. Retroperitoneal cysts are best treated by marsupialization and curettage.

Prognosis

Echinococcosis of the kidney usually has a good prognosis. The problem presented by perivesical cysts is more troublesome. After surgical intervention, drainage may be prolonged. It must be remembered, too, that involvement of other organs, especially the liver, is usually present.

● ● ●

References

Tuberculosis

Bjørn-Hansen R, Aakhus T: Angiography in renal tuberculosis. Acta radiol (diag) 11:167, 1971.

Bloom S, Wechsler H, Lattimer JK: Results of a long-term study of non-functioning tuberculous kidneys. J Urol 104:654, 1970.

Bowersox DW & others: Isoniazid dosage in patients with renal failure. New England J Med 289:84, 1973.

Christensen WI: Genitourinary tuberculosis: Review of 102 cases. Medicine 53:377, 1974.

Citron KM: Tuberculosis. Brit MJ 2:296, 1973.

Cooper HG, Robinson EG: Treatment of genitourinary tuberculosis: Report after 24 years. J Urol 108:136, 1972.

Ehrlich RM, Lattimer JK: Urogenital tuberculosis in children. J Urol 105:461, 1971.

Kollins SA & others: Roentgenographic findings in urinary tract tuberculosis: A 10-year review. Am J Roentgenol 121:487, 1974.

Küss R & others: Indications and early and late results of intestino-cystoplasty: A review of 185 cases. J Urol 103:53, 1970.

Lattimer JK, Reilly RJ, Segawa A: The significance of the isolated positive urine culture in genitourinary tuberculosis. J Urol 102:610, 1969.

Mangelson NL, Saunders JC, Brosman SA: Urogenital tuberculosis. J Urol 104:309, 1970.

Report: Controlled clinical trial of four short-course (6-months) regimens of chemotherapy for treatment of pulmonary tuberculosis. Lancet 1:1331, 1973.

Riley HD: Current concepts in therapy: Rifampin. South MJ 66:273, 1973.

Roylance J & others: Radiology in the management of urinary tract tuberculosis. Brit J Urol 42:679, 1970.

Symes JM, Blandy JP: Tuberculosis of the male urethra. Brit J Urol 45:432, 1973.

Wolinsky E: New antituberculosis drugs and concepts of prophylaxis. M Clin North America 58:697, 1974.

Amicrobic (Abacterial) Cystitis

Hewitt CB, Stewart BH, Kiser WS: Abacterial pyuria. J Urol 109:86, 1973.

Moore T, Parker C, Edwards EC: Sterile non-tuberculous pyuria. Brit J Urol 43:47, 1971.

Numazaki Y & others: Acute hemorrhagic cystitis in children. Isolation of adenovirus type II. New England J Med 278:700, 1968.

Candidiasis

Béland G, Piette Y: Urinary tract candidiasis: Report of a case with bilateral ureteral obstruction. Canad MAJ 108:472, 1973.

Boldus RA, Brown RC, Culp DA: Fungus balls in the renal pelvis. Radiology 102:555, 1972.

Sales JL, Mundy HB: Renal candidiasis: Diagnosis and management. Canad J Surg 16:139, 1973.

Schönebeck J: Studies on Candida infection of the urinary tract and on the antimycotic drug 5-fluorocytosine. Scandinav J Urol Nephrol (Suppl 11), 1972.

Schönebeck J, Segerbrand E: *Candida albicans* septicaemia during first half of pregnancy successfully treated with 5-fluorocytosine. Brit MJ 4:337, 1973.

Wise GJ & others: Candidal cystitis management by continuous bladder irrigation with amphotericin B. JAMA 224:1636, 1973.

Actinomycosis

Anhalt M, Scott R Jr: Primary unilateral actinomycosis: Case report. J Urol 103:126, 1970.

Fass RJ & others: Clindamycin in the treatment of serious anaerobic infections. Ann Int Med 78:853, 1973.

Grobert MJ, Bischoff AJ: Actinomycosis of the testicle: Case report. J Urol 87:567, 1962.

McPartland N, Grove JS, Chomet B: Actinomycosis of penis. J Urol 86:95, 1961.

Trichomoniasis in the Male

Davidson F: Short-term high-dose metronidazole for vaginal trichomoniasis. J Obst Gynec Brit Common 80:368, 1973.

Keighley EE: Trichomoniasis in a closed community: Efficacy of metronidazole. Brit MJ 1:207, 1971.

Lumsden WHR, Robertson DHH, McNeillage GJC: Isolation, cultivation, low temperature preservation, and infectivity titration of *Trichomonas vaginalis*. Brit J Ven Dis 42:145, 1966.

McClean AN: Nitrimidazine (Naxogin) compared with metronidazole (Flagyl) in the treatment of trichomonal vaginitis. Brit J Ven Dis 48:69, 1972.

Pereyra AJ, Nelson RM, Ludders DJ: Flunidazole: A new drug for systemic treatment of urogenital trichomoniasis. Am J Obst Gynec 112:963, 1972.

Summers JL, Ford ML: The Papanicolaou smear as a diagnostic tool in male trichomoniasis. J Urol 107:840, 1972.

Schistosomiasis (Bilharziasis)

Al-Ghorab MM, El-Badawi AA, Effat H: Vesico-ureteric reflux in urinary bilharziasis: A clinico-radiological study. Clin Radiol 17:41, 1966.

Farid Z & others: Symptomatic, radiological, and functional improvement following treatment of urinary schistosomiasis. Lancet 2:1110, 1967.

Farid Z & others: Urinary schistosomiasis treated with sodium antimony tartrate: A quantitative evaluation. Brit MJ 3:713, 1968.

Forsyth DM, Rashid C: Treatment of urinary schistosomiasis. Lancet 1:130, 1967.

Ghoneim MA, Ashamallah A, Khalik MA: Bilharzial strictures of the ureter presenting with anuria. Brit J Urol 43:439, 1971.

Khafagy MM, El-Bolkainy MN, Mansour MA: Carcinoma of the bilharzial urinary bladder. Cancer 30:150, 1972.

Koraitim M: A new concept of bilharzial bladder neck obstruction: The triple mechanism. J Urol 109:393, 1973.

Filariasis

Akisada M, Tani S: Filarial chyluria in Japan: Lymphangiography, etiology and treatment in 30 cases. Radiology 90:311, 1968.

Cahill KM: Filarial chyluria: A biochemical and radiologic study of five patients. J Trop Med 68:27, 1965.

Campbell BL, Wilson JD, Scott PJ: Studies of the anatomy, physiology and clinical variability of chyluria. Australasian Ann Med 15:336, 1966.

Chang C-Y, Lue YB, Lapides J: Surgical treatment for chyluria. J Urol 109:299, 1973.

Lang EK, Redetzki JE, Brown RL: Lymphangiographic demonstration of lymphaticocalyceal fistulas causing chyluria (filariasis). J Urol 108:321, 1972.

Echinococcosis (Hydatid Disease)

Baltaxe HA, Fleming RJ: The angiographic appearance of hydatid disease. Radiology 97:599, 1970.

Birkhoff JD, McClennan BL: Echinococcal disease of the pelvis: Urologic complication, diagnosis and treatment. J Urol 109:473, 1973.

Deliveliotis A, Kehayas P, Varkarakis M: The diagnostic problem of the hydatid disease of the kidney. J Urol 99:139, 1968.

Kirkland K: Urological aspects of hydatid disease. Brit J Urol 38:241, 1966.

Silber SJ, Moyad RA: Renal echinococcus. J Urol 108:669, 1972.

14 . . .
Urologic Aspects of Venereal Diseases in the Male

GONORRHEA

Gonorrhea is primarily a urethral infection. If untreated it is a self-limiting disease, the bacteria dying out as a rule within 6 months. Infection does not confer immunity against reinfection.

Antibiotics have diminished the incidence of gonorrhea, but it is still the most common reportable infectious disease in the USA. Fortunately, disabling complications (prostatitis, epididymitis, urethral stricture, endocarditis, and arthritis) are now relatively rare.

Neisseria gonorrhoeae is almost without exception transmitted through sexual contact. The organisms are kidney-shaped and arranged as diplococci with their relatively flat surfaces apposed. They are gram-negative and are typically located within the neutrophils, although they are frequently found extracellularly as well. Other pyogenic cocci (eg, staphylococci) are also located intracellularly at times, but these can usually be differentiated morphologically from gonococci.

The pathologic findings consist mainly of diffuse infiltration of the tissues by neutrophils, lymphocytes, and plasma cells.

Clinical Findings

A. Symptoms: The first symptom of gonorrhea is a purulent urethral discharge, which usually appears 4–10 days after sexual exposure. There is usually some burning on urination, and urethral itching is common. Frequency, urgency, and nocturia do not occur unless the posterior urethra and prostate become involved (rare with antibiotic therapy).

B. Signs: The purulent urethral discharge is yellow or brown. The meatus is red and edematous, and its lips are everted. The urethra may be thickened and tender. The inflammation is mucosal and submucosal.

Prostatic massage and urethral instrumentation are contraindicated during the acute phase of the disease. If severe urinary symptoms are present and urinary obstruction supervenes, palpation of the prostate may show it to be swollen, hot, and tender (acute prostatitis).

C. Laboratory Findings: The urethral discharge should first be examined, unstained and in saline, for trichomonads. Examination of smears stained with Gram's stain and methylene blue should be done in order to establish a bacteriologic diagnosis. If microscopic study reveals the typical intracellular gram-negative diplococci, cultures are not necessary. If discharge is unobtainable, the first part of the urine should be centrifuged and the sediment treated as urethral discharge.

When the infection is limited to the anterior urethra, only the first portion of the urine is cloudy. If posterior urethritis develops, the entire stream becomes purulent. Gonococci are then found in the stained sediment of the midstream specimen.

In equivocal cases, cultures of the purulent discharge are necessary. This is particularly true in the diagnosis of pharyngeal and rectal involvement. Because gonococci die rapidly on drying, specimens must be cultured promptly on special media (chocolate blood agar) in an atmosphere of 10% CO_2.

Asymptomatic gonorrhea is common in men who have had sexual contact with women with proved infection. Such men should have cultures made. This is best done by urethral swab or urethral scrapings with a loop. Culture of the first 10 ml of urine passed is also a rewarding diagnostic procedure.

Differential Diagnosis

Nonspecific and trichomonal urethritis causes the same symptoms as gonorrhea, although the discharge in the latter is usually more purulent and profuse. Study of the discharge, both fresh and stained, demonstrates the etiologic organisms.

Complications

Most complications are local (periurethral) and prostatic. They are rare, but may still occur if the diagnosis is missed or if improper treatment (without antibiotics) is instituted. Periurethritis may develop and may lead to abscess formation; in the healing process, periurethral fibrosis will cause stricture. Posterior urethritis and prostatitis occur if the disease process extends beyond the external sphincter. Symptoms of cystitis may occur at this stage, and all of the urine passed is purulent. The infection may then descend to the epididymis, causing a very painful swelling of that organ.

Gonorrheal arthritis is occasionally observed as a

complication of bacteremia, which may be manifested by typical cutaneous lesions. Acute polyarthritis may develop, and monarticular disease with effusion may be seen. These usually respond promptly with definitive antibiotic therapy. Meningitis and endocarditis are quite rare. Of more importance is involvement of the rectum and pharynx in homosexual men. Gonococcal ophthalmia neonatorum is on the increase.

Prevention

A single and almost foolproof method of prevention of gonorrhea is the proper use of antibiotics in the first few hours before or after exposure (does not prevent syphilis): (1) penicillin, 1 million units orally or 300,000 units IM; (2) chlortetracycline, chloramphenicol, oxytetracycline, tetracycline, or erythromycin, 1 g orally as one dose; or (3) streptomycin, 1 g IM.

It has been shown that doxycycline, 300 mg by mouth, kanamycin, 2 g IM, and spectinomycin, 2 g IM, each given as a single dose, are also quite efficacious. Sulfamethoxazole-trimethoprim (co-trimoxazole), 4 tablets orally every 12 hours for 2 days, is particularly effective.

Treatment

The gonococcus is very sensitive to most antibiotics, although there is some evidence that it is becoming increasingly resistant to penicillin. At least 90% of patients respond promptly to the proper drug given in adequate dosage. The discharge usually disappears in 12 hours, and complications seldom develop. In about 10–15% of patients, a scanty, thin discharge will remain following treatment. This usually disappears within a few days, particularly when treated with tetracycline.

Proof of cure rests on the absence of gonococci in whatever discharge remains or in the washings from the urethra (the first portion of the voided urine). If gonococci are absent, culture of the first portion of a urine specimen should then be done. If this is negative for gonococci, cure has been established. If the infective bacteria have not been eradicated by one antibiotic, another drug or combination of drugs should be used. Since syphilis may also have been contracted simultaneously, serologic tests for syphilis must be done in 3 weeks and then after 3, 6, 12, and 24 months.

A. Specific Measures: Repository penicillin, 4.8 million units IM, cures over 90% of cases. This effect may be enhanced by giving 2.5 g of probenecid one-half hour before the injection. Oral penicillins are also effective. A single dose of ampicillin, 3.5 g orally, preceded by probenecid, also results in a high cure rate. The tetracyclines also cure 90% of infected persons. It has recently been reported that the gonococci in the Far East are showing increasing resistance to penicillin whereas they are quite sensitive to the tetracyclines. Since we can expect this strain in other parts of the world, the combination of penicillin and a tetracycline seems indicated. A total of 10 g can be administered in doses of 0.5 g every 6 hours.

B. General Measures: Response to the antibiotics is so prompt that general measures are not necessary. Sexual intercourse should be avoided until cure has been established.

C. Treatment of Complications: Complications are exceedingly rare. If any of the following develops, more extensive antibiotic therapy is indicated: acute prostatitis, acute epididymitis, periurethral abscess, cystitis, and arthritis. Urethral stricture requires urethral dilatations.

Prognosis

The prognosis is excellent if gonorrhea is diagnosed early and treated properly.

THE PRIMARY PENILE LESION OF SYPHILIS

Syphilis is caused by infection with *Treponema pallidum,* a distinctive spirochete. It makes its appearance about 2–4 weeks after sexual exposure. A painless papule or pustule develops on the glans, corona, foreskin, shaft, or even the pubic area or on the scrotum, and breaks down to form an indurated, punched-out ulcer. The lesion may be so small and transient that it may be missed.

Microscopically, the tissues are heavily infiltrated with small round cells and plasma cells. Some proliferation of the intimal linings of the blood vessels develops. Neutrophils may be numerous if secondary infection occurs.

Clinical Findings

A. Symptoms and Signs: The patient usually presents himself because of the appearance of a painless penile sore 2–4 weeks after sexual contact. The ulcer is relatively deep, has indurated edges, a clean base, and is not painful on pressure. If untreated, spontaneous healing is slow. Discrete, enlarged inguinal lymph nodes may be palpable. They are not tender unless the primary lesion has become infected by pyogenic organisms, which occurs very rarely.

B. Laboratory Findings: The diagnosis is made by finding the pathogenic spirochetes in the serous discharge from the ulcer on dark-field examination. Serologic tests for syphilis may remain negative for 1–3 weeks or longer after the appearance of the chancre.

Differential Diagnosis (Table 14–1)

The primary penile lesions of chancroid, lymphogranuloma venereum, granuloma inguinale, gangrenous and erosive balanitis, and herpes simplex may resemble the chancre of syphilis. All penile ulcers must be considered syphilitic until proved otherwise. *Borrelia refringens* may be present and is most difficult to distinguish from *T pallidum* in the dark field.

Erythroplasia of Queyrat (see p 286) may resemble a chancre. Dark-field examination and biopsy will clarify the diagnosis.

Complications

Urologic complications of syphilis are rare. They include gummas of the testis and neurogenic bladder due to neurosyphilis.

Prevention

Give benzathine penicillin G, 2.4 million units IM in one dose.

Treatment

Give 2.4 million units of procaine penicillin G with 2% aluminum monostearate into the buttocks and then 1.2 million units IM every other day for a total dose of 4.8 million units. Other satisfactory regimens include (1) benzathine penicillin G, 1.2 million units in each gluteal muscle, or (2) procaine penicillin G, 600,000 units IM daily for 8 days.

Prognosis

The prognosis is excellent. Relapse is rare and requires more intensive penicillin therapy. The blood serology of the patient should, however, be rechecked every 6 months for 3 years after treatment. The spinal fluid should be examined to rule out CNS syphilis, which requires more intensive treatment.

The patient should be cautioned not to have sexual intercourse until cure has been obtained.

CHANCROID
(Soft Chancre)

Chancroid is a common venereal disease whose primary ulcer may simulate the chancre of syphilis or lymphogranuloma venereum. It is usually accompanied by inguinal adenitis. The highest incidence occurs in men with long foreskins who practice poor hygiene.

The infecting organism is *Haemophilus ducreyi,* a short, nonmotile, gram-negative streptobacillus which usually occurs in chains. It is found with difficulty on stained smear; cultures are more successful. The incubation period is 1–5 days.

Macroscopically, one or several small penile ulcers are present. Biopsy of chancroid shows endothelial proliferation without much fibroplasia in the midzone; the deeper tissues are diffusely infiltrated with small round cells and plasma cells. These findings are considered to be diagnostic.

Inguinal adenitis, usually unilateral, develops in about 50% of cases. Progression is rapid, although the lesion may resolve spontaneously or go on to suppuration and spontaneous evacuation.

Clinical Findings

A. Symptoms: A few days after sexual exposure, one or more painful, dirty-appearing ulcers may be noted. They enlarge gradually. In 2 or 3 weeks, large, tender inguinal lymph nodes appear. These may suppu-

rate and drain spontaneously. About 50% of patients have fever to 39 °C (102.2 °F), malaise, and headache.

B. Signs: The ulcer is rarely more than 1–2 cm in diameter. It is usually shallow and has irregular edges. The base is friable and bleeds easily. On occasion it may become very extensive and destructive.

C. Laboratory Findings: Diligent search of a smear stained with Gram's stain shows *H ducreyi* in 50% of cases. Culture, if available, is more successful. Skin tests (Ducrey test) are positive in about 75% of cases. Biopsy is diagnostic in all cases. Tests for other venereal ulcers should be done to establish or rule out the possibility of double infections: (1) dark-field examination for spirochetes (syphilis and erosive balanitis), (2) complement fixation or Frei test (lymphogranuloma venereum), (3) search for "Donovan bodies" (granuloma inguinale), and (4) serologic tests for syphilis.

Differential Diagnosis (Table 14–1)

Chancroid must be differentiated from other ulcerative lesions of the external genitalia.

Complications

Secondary infection with *Borrelia refringens* and fusiform bacilli may cause marked destruction of tissue, but this is not common. Phimosis or paraphimosis may develop during the healing stage.

Prevention

Thorough washing of the genitalia with soap and water after sexual intercourse, or any of the antibiotics which are useful in treatment, will prevent the disease.

Treatment

A. Specific Measures: Even in the bubo stage, response to the tetracyclines is excellent. The optimum dose is 0.5 g every 6 hours for 7 days. The sulfonamides, 4 g/day for 10 days, are only slightly less effective. For those that are resistant to this treatment, give kanamycin, 500 mg IM twice a day for 7–14 days, depending on the response. Penicillin is without effect.

B. General Measures: Cleanliness is of the greatest importance. The parts should be washed regularly with bland soap and water. Oils and greases are contraindicated.

C. Treatment of Complications: If the symbiotic infection of fusiform bacilli and spirochetes complicates the picture, penicillin should be used in addition, although the antibiotics which are administered for the chancroidal infection will probably overcome these infections also. If phimosis or paraphimosis develops, surgical correction may be necessary. During the acute stage, only a dorsal slit is indicated. Later, circumcision can be done. Aspiration of fluctuant inguinal nodes may be necessary.

Prognosis

With proper antibiotic therapy, the prognosis for immediate cure is excellent.

LYMPHOGRANULOMA VENEREUM
(Lymphopathia Venereum)

Lymphogranuloma venereum is an infectious venereal disease caused by a specific bacterial organism of the psittacosis-LGV-trachoma (Chlamydia) group. The disease is characterized by a transient genital lesion followed by lymphadenitis and at times, in the female, rectal stricture. In men, because of the anatomy of the lymphatics, the inguinal and subinguinal nodes become matted, and, although many resolve, the majority undergo suppuration and form multiple sinuses.

Microscopically, the lesion shows acute and subacute inflammation. There is nothing specific or diagnostic in its appearance. The lymph nodes show abscesses and heavy infiltration with neutrophils. Hyperplasia of lymphoid elements then takes place and plasma cells appear. In the late stages, the capsular areas become fibrotic; the centers are necrotic.

Clinical Findings

A. Symptoms and Signs: The penile lesion develops 30–60 days after sexual exposure; it heals spontaneously and rapidly and thus is often not seen. This lesion may be papular or vesicular, although only a superficial erosion may occur. A few days or weeks later, painful enlargement of inguinal nodes develops; because the primary lesion is so often missed, this may be the initial symptom. Later, the matted nodes usually break down, whereupon multiple sinuses develop. At the stage of bubo formation, constitutional symptoms are present. These include chills, fever, headache, generalized joint pains, and nausea and vomiting. Skin rashes are frequent.

Rectal stricture is a late manifestation of the disease in females. If present, it can usually be palpated. It tends to be annular in type and may almost close the lumen. When this has developed, a change in bowel habits is evident.

B. Laboratory Findings: The white blood cell count may reach 20,000/μl during the stage of lymph node invasion. Anemia may also develop. The sedimentation rate is accelerated. Serum proteins (globulin) are increased. The Frei test (intradermal) is positive in about two-thirds of persons who have or have had the disease. Complement fixation tests, if positive, are almost pathognomonic for present or past lymphogranuloma venereum. These tests cannot differentiate reliably between infection caused by any member of the chlamydia group of organisms. The serologic test for syphilis may give a weak false-positive reaction. This is usually transient, however.

Differential Diagnosis (Table 14–1)

All penile ulcers should be regarded as of syphilitic origin until proved otherwise; dark-field examinations for *T pallidum* and serologic studies are essential. Lymphogranuloma venereum must be suspected in any rectal stricture in a female.

Complications

Untreated or late cases may develop multiple sinuses from involved lymph nodes. Elephantiasis of the genitalia can occur if lymphatic drainage is severely obstructed. Occasionally in women (rarely in men), proctitis and rectal stricture may occur. Stricture sometimes becomes manifest years after the initial infection.

Prevention

Washing the genitals with soap and water immediately after sexual exposure is a successful preventive measure. One of the tetracycline group of antibiotics given for 1–2 days immediately after exposure may be a useful means of prophylaxis.

Treatment

A. Specific Measures: Chloramphenicol and the tetracyclines are effective even in the stage of bubo formation. The usual dose for each is 0.5–1 g every 6 hours for a total dose of 15–30 g. These antibiotics are also reported to be moderately effective in relieving the anorectal stricture. They do not affect the fibrous tissue, however; their value probably lies in controlling viral activity and suppressing secondary infection, thus reducing edema associated with the inflammation.

Sulfonamides, 4 g/day for 3–4 weeks, although they probably have little effect upon the causative agent, control secondary infection.

Streptomycin and penicillin are not effective.

B. Treatment of Complications: Aspiration of fluctuant inguinal nodes is indicated. Draining sinuses may have to be excised. Rectal stenosis may require surgical measures.

Prognosis

The prognosis is excellent. Only the late complications seen in old cases present difficulties (genital elephantiasis and rectal stricture).

GRANULOMA INGUINALE

Granuloma inguinale is a chronic venereal infection of the skin and subcutaneous tissues of the genitalia, perineum, or inguinal regions. The incubation period is 2–3 months.

The infective agent is *Calymmatobacterium granulomatis,* a bacterium related to *Klebsiella pneumoniae* (Friedländer's bacillus). It grows with difficulty on artificial media containing egg yolk or in the yolk sac of the chick embryo.

The ulcer does not excite a constitutional reaction and does not involve the lymph nodes or lymphatics.

The microscopic picture shows nonspecific infection, with necrosis of the skin and small abscesses. In the deeper portions there is an infiltration of plasma cells, giant cells, neutrophils, and large monocytes; the cytoplasm of the monocytes contains numerous "Donovan bodies," the intracellular stage of the etiologic organism.

Clinical Findings

A. Symptoms and Signs: The first sign of the disease is an elevation on the skin of the genitals or adjacent skin (commonly the groin), which finally breaks down. This moderately painful superficial ulcer gradually spreads and can become quite extensive. The base of the ulcer is covered by pink granulation tissue which bleeds easily. There is a more or less purulent discharge, particularly if secondary infection develops.

B. Laboratory Findings: Identification of the "Donovan body" in large monocytes on a stained smear makes the diagnosis. Scrapings from the base of the lesion are placed on a slide, fixed in air, and stained. Wright's and Giemsa's staining technics are both adequate.

In case of doubt, biopsy may be done. The bacteria take up hematoxylin as well as silver salts.

Complement fixation and skin sensitivity tests are not dependable and not readily available.

Differential Diagnosis

See Table 14—1.

Complications

Secondary infection may cause deep ulceration and tissue destruction. Sinuses may result. Marked phimosis may occur in advanced cases, even to the point of urinary obstruction. Other venereal diseases may be present at the same time.

Prevention

The use of a condom does not prevent perigenital inoculation. Thorough washing with soap immediately after contact will often prevent infection. Tetracycline antibiotics given for several days following contact may afford protection.

Treatment

A. Specific Measures: The tetracyclines and chloramphenicol have proved curative in a high percentage of cases. Dosage is 1 g/day in divided doses for 7—14 days.

Streptomycin is also effective. The dose is 1 g/day IM for 10 days.

B. Treatment of Complications: Secondary infection is effectively combated in most instances by the drug used to cure the primary disease. If fusiform bacilli and spirochetes *(Borrelia refringens)* are present, penicillin may be used also.

Prognosis

There are no serious complications, and antibiotics are quite efficient in treatment. The prognosis is excellent.

EROSIVE & GANGRENOUS BALANITIS

This is one of the less common penile lesions, presumably of venereal origin. A long foreskin is almost a necessary prerequisite to the development of the lesion since the infecting organisms are anaerobic. Poor local hygiene also contributes to the establishment of the disease. The lesion ulcerates progressively and proceeds to gangrene of the glans and at times even of the shaft of the penis. The incubation period is 3—7 days.

The infecting organisms are a spirochete *(Borellia refringens)* and a gram-positive bacillus (vibrio) acting in symbiosis. Both organisms are stained by the common dyes.

Microscopic examination of a biopsy specimen shows nothing specific; the picture is one of acute inflammation. Neutrophilic and small round cell infiltration is extensive.

Clinical Findings

A. Symptoms: The patient complains of local pain, a profuse, foul discharge, and, if the foreskin can be retracted, a progressive ulcerative lesion of the glans, foreskin, or shaft of the penis. In acute cases, chills, fever, and marked malaise may develop. Burning on urination is common and is caused by the inflammatory reaction in and about the urinary meatus.

B. Signs: The ulceration usually starts in the region of the corona under a tight, unclean prepuce. The ulcer gradually spreads and produces a foul, often profuse discharge. The accompanying edema may prevent retraction of the foreskin; a dorsal slit may be necessary before the lesion can be observed. As the disease progresses, the invasion of the penile tissue goes deeper, and, if it is not treated by appropriate means, portions of the penis may become gangrenous. In extreme cases the entire penis and even the scrotum may be destroyed.

C. Laboratory Findings: The finding of many spirochetes and fusiform bacilli in a smear is strongly suggestive, but it must be remembered that other ulcerative venereal lesions can be secondarily invaded by these organisms.

Differential Diagnosis

See Table 14—1.

Complications

If the disease is untreated, severe damage may occur to the penis and adjacent structures. If the infection is mild or is aborted by appropriate means, some fibrosis of the foreskin may occur. Contracture of this tissue leads to phimosis.

In elderly men, the fulminating form of this disease is to be feared, as overwhelming sepsis is often rapidly fatal.

Prevention

Proper hygienic care of the redundant foreskin

Table 14–1. Differential diagnosis of genital ulcers.

	Syphilitic Chancre	Chancroid	Lymphogranuloma Venereum	Granuloma Inguinale	Erosive and Gangrenous Balanitis	Herpes Progenitalis	Epithelioma
Etiology	*T pallidum*	*H ducreyi* (Ducrey's bacillus)	Chlamydia bacterium	*Calymmatobacterium granulomatis*	Vibrio and spirochete *(Borrelia refringens)*	Herpesvirus type 2	. . .
Incubation time	2–4 weeks	3–10 days	3–21 days	2–3 months	3–7 days	Unknown (often recurrent)	. . .
Early lesion	Enlarging papule which finally ulcerates	Macule → papule, then formation of ulcer	Transient, usually not seen. Papule or macule heals rapidly.	Superficial ulcer of skin	Single or multiple ulcerations which fuse and spread	Multiple superficial vesicles on the foreskin or glans	May appear as small ulcer
Advanced local lesion	Ulcer becomes deep and edges indurated. Heals spontaneously.	Ulcer gradually spreads. May become extensive. Multiple lesions.	None	Becomes serpiginous and may spread widely	Ulcers become deep and painful. May spread rapidly. Profuse foul discharge.	Vesicles may coalesce and form superficial ulcer which heals spontaneously	May become large and destructive
Local pain	Absent unless secondarily infected	Very painful	None	Little	Very painful	Slight local burning or itching	None unless secondarily infected
Involvement of inguinal lymph nodes	Discrete, rubbery, nontender	In 50% of cases, nodes are enlarged and tender. May suppurate.	In almost all cases in 2–8 weeks after primary sore. Matted, tend to break down. Multiple sinuses.	None	Discrete, only mildly tender	None	Metastases usually unilateral. Painless.
Definitive diagnosis	*T pallidum* on dark-field examination. Serology.	Skin test, stained smear or culture, biopsy	Frei test, complement fixation test	Stained organisms in scrapings from ulcer or biopsy	Spirochetes and fusiform bacilli on dark-field examination or stained smear	Isolation of virus	Biopsy

will prevent the disease, but circumcision is definitive. This is a disease of filth and neglect.

Treatment

A. Specific Measures: Penicillin is the drug of choice; 0.6–1.2 million units/day for 5–7 days usually suffice. The tetracyclines are also effective; the dosage is 2 g/day in divided doses for 5–7 days.

B. General Measures: If response to antibiotics is not prompt, dorsal slit of the prepuce may be indicated for purposes of hygiene and because aerobic conditions discourage the organisms. Mild soap and water or hydrogen peroxide soaks are helpful and will combat the malodorous discharge.

C. Treatment of Complications: Plastic procedures on a badly damaged organ may be necessary. Circumcision is indicated if phimosis develops.

Prognosis

If diagnosed and treated early, the prognosis is excellent. Superficial loss of skin is replaced spontaneously with surprisingly little scar. Neglected patients may, however, suffer severe local tissue destruction.

•   •   •

References

General

Symposium on venereal diseases. M Clin North America 56:1057, 1972.

Wisdom A: *Color Atlas of Venereology.* Year Book, 1973.

Gonorrhea

Barrett-Connor E: Gonorrhea and the pediatrician. Am J Dis Child 125:233, 1973.

Baynel & others: Oral amoxicillin in acute uncomplicated gonorrhea. Canadian MAJ 111:685, 1974.

Corman LC & others: The high frequency of pharyngeal gonococcal infection in a prenatal clinic population. JAMA 230:568, 1974.

Handsfield HH, Hodson WA, Holmes KK: Neonatal gonococcal infection. 1. Orogastric contamination with *Neisseria gonorrhoeae.* JAMA 225:697, 1973.

Handsfield HH & others: Asymptomatic gonorrhea in men. New England J Med 290:117, 1974.

Harris JRW, McCann JS, Mahony JDH: Gonococcal arthritis: A common rarity. Brit J Ven Dis 49:42, 1973.

Judson FN, Allaman J, Dans PE: Treatment of gonorrhea: Comparison of penicillin G, procaine, doxycycline, spectinomycin and ampicillin. JAMA 230:705, 1974.

Kilpatrick ZM: Gonorrheal proctitis. New England J Med 287:967, 1972.

Kohen DP: Neonatal gonococcal arthritis: Three cases and review of literature. Pediatrics 53:436, 1974.

Lightfoot RW Jr, Gotschlich EC: Gonococcal disease. Am J Med 56:347, 1974.

Moffett M & others: Doxycycline HCl (Vibramycin) as a single dose oral treatment of gonorrhoea in women. Brit J Ven Dis 48:126, 1972.

Moore G & others: Gonorrhea detection by urine sediment culture. JAMA 224:1499, 1973.

Owen RL, Hill JL: Rectal and pharyngeal gonorrhea in homosexual men. JAMA 220:1315, 1972.

Pederson AHB & others: Spectinomycin and penicillin G in the treatment of gonorrhea. JAMA 220:205, 1972.

Sayeed ZA & others: Gonococcal meningitis. JAMA 219:1730, 1972.

Snowe RJ, Wilfert CM: Epidemic reappearance of gonococcal ophthalmia neonatorum. Pediatrics 51:110, 1973.

Svindland HB: Treatment of gonorrhoea with sulfamethoxazole-trimethoprim: Lack of effect on concomitant syphilis. Brit J Ven Dis 49:50, 1973.

Tanowitz HB, Adler JJ, Chirito E: Gonococcal endocarditis. New York J Med 72:2782, 1972.

Thompson TR, Swanson RE, Wiesner PJ: Gonococcal ophthalmia neonatorum: Relationship of time of infection to relevant control measures. JAMA 228:186, 1974.

Wiesner PJ & others: Clinical spectrum of pharyngeal gonococcal infection. New England J Med 288:181, 1973.

Wheeler JK, Heffron WA, Williams RC Jr: Migratory arthralgias and cutaneous lesions as confusing initial manifestations of gonorrhea. Am J Med Sc 260:150, 1970.

Primary Penile Lesion of Syphilis

Desmond FB: The diagnosis of infectious syphilis. New Zealand MJ 73:135, 1971.

Fluker JL: Syphilis. Practitioner 209:605, 1972.

Nicolis G, Loucopoulos A: Cephalothin in the treatment of syphilis. Brit J Ven Dis 50:270, 1974.

Penicillin in the treatment of syphilis. (Editorial.) Brit MJ 2:259, 1973.

Schroeter AL & others: Treatment for early syphilis and reactivity of serologic tests. JAMA 221:471, 1972.

Youmans JB: Syphilis and other venereal diseases. M Clin North America 48:573, 1964.

Chancroid

Alergant CD: Chancroid. Practitioner 209:624, 1972.

Marmar JL: The management of resistant chancroid in Vietnam. J Urol 107:807, 1972.

Granuloma Inguinale

Davis CM: Granuloma inguinale. JAMA 211:632, 1970.

Lal S, Nicholas C: Epidemiological and clinical features in 165 cases of granuloma inguinale. Brit J Ven Dis 46:461, 1970.

Ribeiro J: Granuloma inguinale. Practitioner 209:628, 1972.

15 . . .
Urinary Stones

Urinary lithiasis is one of the most common diseases of the urinary tract. It occurs more frequently in men than in women but is rare in children and in blacks; a familial predisposition is often encountered.

If a stone is not obstructive, it is not apt to cause injury or symptoms. If it blocks a urinary passage (eg, the ureteropelvic junction), it leads to severe symptoms and renal damage. Since stones tend to recur, a patient with a nonobstructive stone may later form a stone which will cause obstruction; for this reason, investigation of the cause of the first stone is of importance in the prevention of later renal injury.

RENAL STONE*

Etiology

All the causes of renal stone formation are not known, but in most cases multiple factors are involved. An adequate stone analysis is the key to an understanding of the pathogenetic mechanisms involved. In the USA, two-thirds of all renal stones are composed of either calcium oxalate or mixtures of calcium oxalate with calcium phosphate in the form of hydroxyapatite. Pure apatite or brushite (calcium hydrogen phosphate dihydrate) stones are very rare. Magnesium ammonium phosphate (struvite) accounts for 15% of all stones and occurs almost exclusively in patients with urinary tract infections with urea-splitting organisms and persistently alkaline urine. Uric acid and cystine stones account for about 10%. Miscellaneous stones are composed of xanthine, silicates, or matrix and occasionally of artifacts brought in by patients as "kidney stones."

The following factors are known to influence the formation and growth of uroliths:

A. Hyperexcretion of Relatively Insoluble Urinary Constituents:

*Portions of the section on renal stone are contributed by Felix O. Kolb, MD, Clinical Professor of Medicine, Research Physician and Associate Director, Metabolic Research Unit, University of California School of Medicine (San Francisco); Chairman, Division of Endocrinology and Metabolism, Mount Zion Hospital (San Francisco).

1. Calcium—(Normal urinary excretion of calcium on a low-calcium diet [no milk or cheese for 4 days] is 100–175 mg/24 hours.) On regular diets, normal females excrete less than 250 mg/24 hours and males less than 300 mg/24 hours. The major calcium foods are milk and cheese. Hypercalciuria may be seen in some adults who drink a quart or more of milk per day. It has been shown that the lactose in milk and dietary protein causes increased absorption of calcium from the gut.

Prolonged immobilization (spinal cord injury, fractures, poliomyelitis) and certain bone diseases (eg, metastatic cancer, myeloma, Paget's disease) cause hypercalciuria. Under these circumstances, calcium excretion may reach 450 mg/day or more.

Primary hyperparathyroidism causes hypercalciuria and hyperphosphaturia as well as hypercalcemia and hypophosphatemia. Two-thirds of these patients have renal stones.

Idiopathic hypercalciuria occurs most commonly in males. Serum calcium is normal and serum phosphorus is decreased. Even on a low-calcium intake, these patients may excrete as much as 500 mg of calcium in 24 hours. This may reflect increased absorption of calcium from the gut.

Hypervitaminosis D may so increase absorption of calcium from the intestine that urinary excretion of this ion may reach pathologically high levels.

Renal tubular acidosis causes hyperexcretion of calcium since the formation of ammonia and titratable acidity is defective.

2. Oxalate—Although oxalate is the major component of two-thirds of all renal stones, hyperoxaluria as a cause of lithiasis is relatively rare. Cabbage, rhubarb, spinach, tomatoes, celery, black tea, and cocoa contain large amounts of oxalate, but limitation of these foods usually has little effect in prevention because the major source of oxalate is endogenous and dietary oxalate is usually poorly absorbed.

Primary hyperoxaluria is a rare, often lethal genetic disorder affecting the metabolism of glyoxylic acid, which forms oxalate rather than glycine. It is an important cause of nephrolithiasis and nephrocalcinosis in children. Acquired forms of hyperoxaluria include pyridoxine deficiency, ethylene glycol poisoning, methoxyflurane anesthesia, and small bowel disease with hyperabsorption of dietary oxalate.

3. Cystine—Cystinuria is a hereditary disease. It is somewhat uncommon, except in infants and children, and only a small percentage of patients form stones. Other amino acids (ornithine, lysine, and arginine) are also lost simultaneously; however, these are quite soluble and do not form stones. The loss of these amino acids is due to a defect in renal tubular reabsorption.

4. Uric acid—Uric acid stones may form when there is rapid tissue breakdown, eg, in the chemotherapeutic treatment of leukemia, polycythemia, and carcinoma; for this reason, it is important to maintain an alkaline dilute urine when treating these diseases. The administration of allopurinol (Zyloprim) should also be considered. Many uric acid stone formers have normal serum uric acid levels but show a consistently low urinary pH. This may be caused by decreased tubular formation of ammonia. Many of these patients are Italians or Jews. Patients with chronic diarrheal states or with ileostomies also have strongly acid urines and may form uric acid stones. Elevated serum uric acid is often observed secondary to thiazide diuretic therapy, but this can be controlled by giving allopurinol. Many patients with gout form uric acid calculi, particularly when under treatment for their arthritis; most of these patients have elevated blood uric acid levels and increased urinary uric acid excretion. Gout is not a necessary condition for the formation of uric acid stones, however.

5. Xanthine—A rare cause of renal stone is associated with lack of xanthine oxidase and very low uric acid levels. Recently, a few cases have been observed after the use of allopurinol in the hyperuricemia of leukemia or Lesch-Nyhan syndrome.

6. Silicon dioxide—Long-term use of magnesium trisilicate in the treatment of peptic ulcer may rarely lead to the formation of radiopaque silicon stones.

B. Physical Changes Which Occur in the Urine:

1. Increased concentration of salts and organic compounds—This may be due to low fluid intake; excessive water losses in febrile diseases, in hot climates, or in occupations causing excessive perspiration; or excessive water losses due to vomiting and diarrhea.

2. Urinary magnesium/calcium ratio—This appears to have some influence on stone formation. Acetazolamide (Diamox) causes a decrease in the ratio and is related to an increased incidence of stone formation. The thiazides, which appear to help prevent recurrences of stone, cause an increase in the ratio.

3. Urinary pH—The mean urinary pH is 5.85. It is influenced by diet, by ingestion of acid or alkaline medications (eg, treatment of peptic ulcer), and by acetazolamide in the treatment of glaucoma. The latter causes an increase in urinary pH. Urea-splitting bacteria—usually *Proteus mirabilis*—make the urine strongly alkaline (pH 7.5+) by liberating ammonia. The inorganic salts are less soluble in an alkaline medium (calcium phosphate forms at a pH of 6.6 or higher, and magnesium ammonium phosphate precipitates at pH of 7.2 or higher). Organic substances (eg, cystine, uric acid) are least soluble at a pH below 7.0 (maximum insolubility, pH 5.5).

4. Colloid content—It has long been claimed that the colloids in the urine allow the inorganic salts to be held in a supersaturated state. Recent work has tended to negate this theory.

5. "Good" and "evil" urine—Howard finds that some types of urine promote while others prevent stone formation. When rachitic rat cartilage is placed in "good" urine, calcification does not occur. In "evil" urine, the cartilage becomes calcified. "Evil" urine, however, becomes "good" urine following the oral administration of 3–6 g/day of phosphate with enhanced urinary excretion of pyrophosphate and polyphosphates. The use of aluminum hydroxide gels which absorb phosphate in the gut is therefore probably contraindicated if an attempt is being made to prevent calcium stone formation.

C. A Nidus (Core or "Nucleus") Upon Which Precipitation Occurs: Randall observed that calcific plaques ("Randall's plaques") are commonly seen on the renal papillae. He believed that they develop as a result of injury to cells of the collecting tubule secondary to infection elsewhere. Randall postulated that when the overlying mucosa finally ulcerates, the calcification acts as a nidus to which the insoluble substances in the urine can adhere. Vermeulen has recently verified this observation.

Some investigators believe that most stones develop by precipitation of crystals (eg, calcium oxalate) on an organic matrix formed of amino acids and carbohydrates, but support for the primary role of matrix in initiating stone disease is lacking. Other masses that can act as nidi include blood clots, clumps of epithelial or pus cells, or even bacteria.

Necrotic ischemic tissue and foreign bodies may encourage the precipitation of relatively insoluble substances. Tissues of this sort may be caused by neoplasms, retained necrotic papillae, or ulceration of mucous membranes by infection.

D. Structural Anomalies, Including Calicectasis and Medullary Sponge Kidney: These disorders may be complicated by stones which form secondary to stasis or infection of urine in the dilated collecting tubules.

Pathology

The size and position of the stone govern the development of secondary pathologic changes in the urinary tract. The obstruction caused by a small stone lodged in the ureteropelvic junction or in the ureter may slowly destroy a kidney (Fig 10–4), whereas a relatively large stone may be so placed as to cause little renal damage.

Infection is a common complication of an obstructing renal stone because of the stasis which it causes. The very presence of such a foreign body seems to decrease the local resistance to hematogenous infection. The parenchymal ischemia caused by local pressure from an enlarging staghorn stone may progressively damage a kidney, but the major cause of progressive renal damage is the renal infection that caused the stone to form.

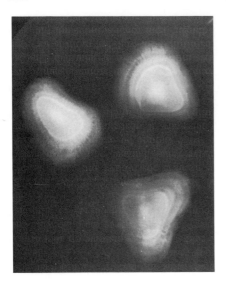 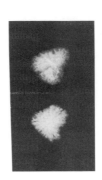 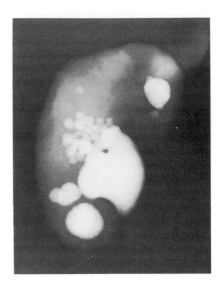

Figure 15–1. X-ray appearance of stones. ***Left:*** Calcium phosphate, laminated. ***Center:*** Calcium oxalate, spiculated. ***Right:*** Cystine, homogeneous. (Reproduced, with permission, from Albright & Reifenstein: *Parathyroid Glands and Metabolic Bone Disease.* Williams & Wilkins, 1948.)

The Physical Characteristics of Urinary Calculi (Fig 15–1)

(1) Calcium phosphate stones (often mixed with magnesium ammonium phosphate) may be soft or hard; they are usually yellow or brown (sometimes dark), often form staghorn masses, and are frequently laminated. They are readily seen on x-ray films; the lamination, if present, is clearly visible.

(2) Magnesium ammonium phosphate stones are usually yellow and somewhat friable. Staghorn formation is common. On radiograms, their density lies between that of calcium oxalate and cystine. Lamination may be noted if calcium oxalate or phosphate is also present.

(3) Calcium oxalate stones ("jackstones," "mulberry stones") are usually small, rough, and hard. Staghorn formation is rare. Spicules radiating from a central core can often be seen on x-rays.

(4) Cystine stones are smooth and light yellow or yellow-brown. They have a "waxy" appearance and are usually multiple and bilateral. They may enlarge quite rapidly, sometimes coalescing to form staghorn calculi. Although their density is relatively low, they can be identified on a roentgenogram as homogeneous, slightly opaque, smoothly rounded bodies (Fig 15–2). On occasion they contain some calcium salts, in which

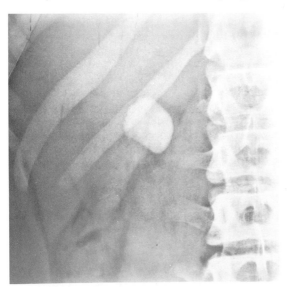 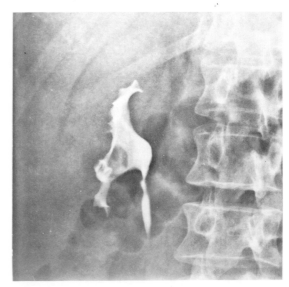

Figure 15–2. Cystine and uric acid stones. ***Left:*** Plain film showing homogeneous, mildly opaque stone, typically cystine. ***Right:*** Excretory urogram showing uric acid stone as "negative" shadow because radiopaque medium is more dense than the stone.

case the stone may show some lamination.

(5) Uric acid crystals can precipitate in the renal parenchyma. The stones formed from these crystals in the renal pelvis are usually small and hard, varying in color from yellow to reddish-brown. They may be multiple. If they are composed of pure uric acid crystals, they cannot be seen on plain x-ray films. On excretory urograms, they are present as "negative" shadows (Fig 15–2).

Radiopacity

Radiopacity is directly related to the density of the stone compared to that of water (Table 15–1).

Clinical Findings

A. Symptoms: The history should include a survey of fluid intake, diet (amount of milk, cheese), drugs (alkalies, analgesics, acetazolamide, vitamin D), periods of immobilization, previous passage of stones, and the presence of gout. There may be a family history of stone formation due to hereditary hyperoxaluria, cystinuria, hyperuricemia, or renal acidosis.

If the stone is still submucosal (Randall's plaque) or adherent to the parenchyma, there are no symptoms. The same is usually true of a small stone trapped in a minor calyx.

If the stone is free and obstructs a calyx or the ureteropelvic junction, there will be dull flank pain due to parenchymal and capsular distention and colic due to hyperperistalsis and smooth muscle spasm of calyces and pelvis; total hematuria; nausea and vomiting; and abdominal distention from paralytic ileus. Chills, high fever, and vesical irritability are due to infection.

Staghorn calculus may be asymptomatic even if infection is present. Symptoms which occur are most apt to be gastrointestinal and simulate gallbladder disease, peptic ulcer, or less specific enteric syndromes. Urologic symptoms may include mild back or flank pain, hematuria, and those due to infection (chills, fever, increased renal pain, and symptoms of cystitis).

B. Signs: Tenderness in the costovertebral angle or over the kidney may or may not be present. Acute renal infection may cause more definite findings. If marked hydronephrotic atrophy has occurred as a result of prolonged ureteral obstruction, a mass in the flank may be seen, felt, or percussed. Some muscle rigidity over the kidney may be found, and rebound

Table 15–1. Stone density as related to degree of radiopacity.

	Density	Degree of Radiopacity
Calcium phosphate	22.0	Very opaque
Calcium oxalate	10.8	Opaque
Magnesium ammonium phosphate	4.1	Moderately opaque
Cystine	3.7	Slightly opaque
Uric acid	1.4	Nonopaque
Xanthine	1.4	Nonopaque

tenderness may be elicited, particularly if acute infection is present. Abdominal distention and diminished peristalsis usually accompany acute renal colic.

C. Laboratory Findings:

1. Blood count–The white blood count may be increased as a result of complicating infection. If renal function is not adequate, anemia may be found.

2. Urinalysis–Protein may be noted because of the presence of hematuria. Pus cells and bacteria may be seen. Oxalate bodies are often observed in hyperparathyroidism, renal tubular acidosis, and hyperoxaluria. Calcium phosphate casts suggest hypercalciuria.

If the pH of the urine is higher than 7.6, urea-splitting organisms must be present, for the kidneys cannot produce urine in this range of alkalinity. Such a finding strongly suggests that the stones are composed of magnesium ammonium phosphate. Fixation of the pH at 6.0–6.5 is compatible with renal tubular acidosis. Consistently low pH is a common cause of the formation of uric acid calculi.

A search should be made for crystals in the sediment; the type may afford a clue to the type of stone (Fig 5–1). Cystine and uric acid crystals may be precipitated by adding a few drops of glacial acetic acid (which lowers the pH to about 4.0) to a test tube of urine which is then refrigerated. Cystine crystals resemble benzene rings; uric acid crystals are typically amber-brown.

A simple chemical screening test for cystine is as follows: To 5 ml of urine made alkaline with ammonium hydroxide, add 2 ml of 5% sodium cyanide and let stand for 5 minutes. Add a few drops of fresh 5% sodium nitroprusside. A deep purplish-red color means hypercystinuria. The definitive diagnosis and proper treatment rest upon quantitative estimation of the amount of alpha-aminonitrogen and of cystine (and cysteine) excreted in 24 hours. Normal people excrete about 1 mg/lb (up to 150 mg/24 hours) of alpha-aminonitrogen and 50–180 mg of cystine (and cysteine) in a like period. Mild cystinurics excrete 200–400 mg of cystine (and cysteine); moderate cystinurics excrete 400–1000 mg; and those with a severe tubular defect, up to 3000 mg/day.

The Sulkowitch test should be done, in conjunction with specific gravity determination, on all patients with urinary stone. If strongly positive (especially if the urine is dilute), hypercalciuria is present. A positive test should be repeated after milk and cheese have been withdrawn for 4 days. If the test is still strongly positive, blood chemistry studies should be done (see below) since hyperparathyroidism may be the cause.

After 4 days on a diet free of milk and cheese, the amount of calcium excreted in the urine in 24 hours should be determined. More than 175 mg of calcium per 24 hours suggests hyperparathyroidism or idiopathic hypercalciuria unless some obvious cause for calcium excess is found (eg, immobilization). The finding of hyperphosphaturia is compatible with a renal phosphate leak and strongly suggests hyperparathyroidism when hypercalcemia and hypercalciuria are found.

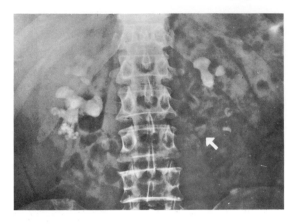 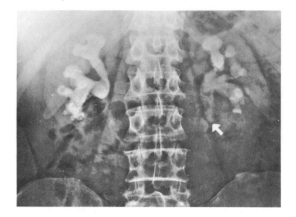

Figure 15–3. Bilateral staghorn calculi and left upper ureteral stone. *Left:* Plain film. Arrow points to ureteral stone. *Right:* Excretory urogram showing bilateral impaired function.

A 24-hour urine specimen should be subjected to a quantitative test for oxalate. The upper limit of normal is 50 mg. Levels as high as 200–300 mg/24 hours may be encountered in primary hyperoxaluria. The normal uric acid excretion is 300–600 mg/24 hours.

A test for the presence of urea-splitting bacteria may be performed by incubating noninfected acid urine overnight with a few drops of the infected urine. If the pH increases, urea-splitting organisms are present.

3. Renal function tests—The PSP may be normal even in the presence of bilateral staghorn stones or in chronic unilateral obstruction due to stone. Acute obstruction at the ureteropelvic junction may suddenly depress the PSP to two-thirds of normal. The complication of renal infection may also interfere with renal function.

A serum creatinine or urea nitrogen determination is indicated if the PSP is less than 30% in one-half hour. Unless the patient is dehydrated, elevation of any one of these indicates decreased renal function.

4. Blood chemistry studies—Fasting serum calcium and phosphorus should be determined on 3 occasions. Serum proteins should also be estimated, since almost half of the calcium is normally un-ionized and bound to protein. If serum proteins are decreased but total calcium is normal, an increase in ionized calcium is indicated (Fig 15–4, left). Hypercalcemia with hypophosphatemia strongly suggests primary hyperparathyroidism, but normal serum phosphate is found in 60% of these patients. Estimation of serum chloride concentration may prove helpful in the differential diagnosis of hypercalcemia. It is above 102 mEq/liter in hyperparathyroidism and below this figure in other conditions (eg, cancer of the breast).

Hypercalcemia is most commonly seen in association with osteolytic or disseminated malignant disease, especially cancers of the breast and lung, multiple myeloma, leukemia, and sarcoidosis, but serum phosphate is usually normal.

Determination of the tubular reabsorption of phosphate (TRP) may prove helpful in the diagnosis of hyperparathyroidism when minimal hypercalcemia and normal blood phosphate levels are obtained. The normal range of tubular reabsorption of phosphate is about 90–95% with low phosphate intake and 75–85% with high phosphate intake. In hyperparathyroidism the values range from 40–80%, demonstrating the typical phosphate leak. Radioimmunoassay of parathyroid hormone is becoming increasingly available. If elevated with serum calcium levels to above 10.7 mg/100 ml, the diagnosis of hyperparathyroidism is strongly suggested.

Serum alkaline phosphatase (normal is 2–4.5 Bodansky units) is increased in hyperparathyroidism only if bone disease (eg, osteitis fibrosa cystica) is present.

Elevated serum uric acid (normal is 2–6 mg/100 ml) is found in 50% of uric acid stone formers.

If CO_2 combining power of the plasma or serum is decreased, acidosis is present. Such a finding might be the clue to the cause of hypercalciuria and stone formation, because when renal tubular damage is advanced, calcium is excreted as fixed base rather than sodium and ammonium. Low CO_2 combining power in the presence of high serum chloride is compatible with renal tubular acidosis or severe chronic renal insufficiency. An ammonium chloride load test will bring out latent cases of renal tubular acidosis. Electrophoretic analysis of the serum will point to sarcoidosis or myeloma as the cause of hypercalcemia.

D. X-Ray Findings: At least 90% of renal stones are radiopaque and are readily visible on a plain film of the abdomen unless they are small or overlie bone. It is necessary to differentiate renal stone from calcified mesenteric lymph nodes, calcium in rib cartilage, gallstones, and solid medication (pills) present in the intestinal tract. Because the plain film is 2-dimensional, it has only presumptive value except in the case of a staghorn stone, which is never confused with other findings (Fig 15–3).

The morphology of the stone may give a clue to

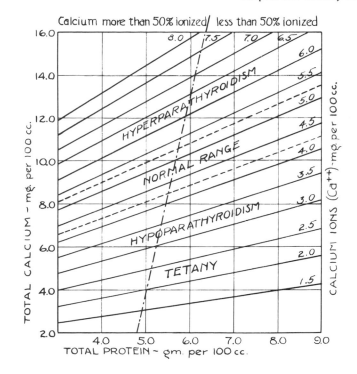

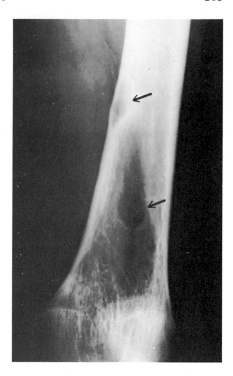

Figure 15–4. *Left:* Nomogram showing relation of calcium level to total proteins. (Reproduced, with permission, from McLean & Hastings: Am J Med Sc 189:601, 1935.) *Right:* Osteitis fibrosa cystica with hyperparathyroidism. Note cystic changes in femur (arrows).

its chemical nature (Fig 15–1).

Bone disease may be discovered in the hands, ribs, spine, pelvis, or femoral heads. This may afford a clue to the cause of hypercalciuria (eg, hyperparathyroidism, metastatic carcinoma, Paget's disease). X-rays of the long bones and skull may also show changes typical of these disorders (Fig 15–4, right). The pathognomonic sign of hyperparathyroidism is cortical subperiosteal resorption in the phalanges.

Excretory urograms are necessary because they accurately localize the calcific shadow unless the kidney is without function or unless it is acutely blocked by a stone (Fig 15–3). Oblique views may also be helpful. If a urogram is not obtained but the kidney shadow becomes dense (nephrogram, Fig 15–9), acute obstruction of a good kidney has probably occurred. If the stone is nonopaque, the films will demonstrate obstruction (dilatation), and the stone may appear as a darker area ("negative" shadow) in the renal pelvis (Fig 15–2). Excretory urograms also measure renal function, which is helpful in judging definitive treatment.

If function is poor, retrograde urograms may be needed.

E. Renal Scan: If the excretory urograms imply poor renal function, isotope studies may prove helpful in further assessing this factor (see Chapter 8). If the damage is irreversible, the [203]Hg scan will show little uptake by the tubules while the scintillations afforded by ^{131}I will be minimal. [99m]Tc will reveal poor vascularity. Such findings might indicate the need for

nephrectomy rather than nephrolithotomy.

F. Instrumental Examination: Cystoscopy for diagnostic purposes is seldom necessary if the excretory urograms are satisfactory. Ureteral catheterization may prove helpful in localizing infection and measuring renal function. Such studies in conjunction with retrograde urograms may be the deciding factor in the choice of treatment (pyelolithotomy vs nephrectomy).

G. Examination of Stone: Examination of previously passed stones and chemical examination of stones removed or passed is useful in establishing the cause of stone formation, especially in differentiating "primary" (metabolic) stones from "secondary" stones (eg, stones formed due to infection).

Differential Diagnosis

Acute pyelonephritis may start with acute and severe renal pain, thus mimicking a renal stone lodged at the ureteropelvic junction. Pus and bacteria are found in the urine, although it must be remembered that infection may be a complication of renal stone. Urograms will decide the issue. Chronic infection may be associated with little or no back pain and few if any vesical symptoms. Urinalysis and radiographic study will settle the diagnosis.

Renal tumor may sometimes simulate stone, particularly if a blood clot causes obstruction (pain, hematuria). Urography will establish the diagnosis.

A tumor of the renal pelvis or calyx can cause renal colic and hematuria. The urogram, showing a space-occupying lesion, may be confused with a non-opaque stone (Figs 15–2 and 18–7). Cytologic examination of the urine sediment is helpful in differential diagnosis, but at times the diagnosis is made at the operating table.

Renal tuberculosis may be painful and, if associated with bleeding, may mimic renal stone. A plain abdominal x-ray may show calcium deposits in the renal shadow. Stone complicates tuberculosis in 10% of cases. A "sterile" pyuria and a suspicion of tuberculosis on urography suggest the diagnosis. Demonstration of acid-fast bacilli is diagnostic.

Papillary necrosis may be confused with renal stone because if sloughed papillae are not passed they tend to undergo peripheral calcification, thus giving the radiographic appearance of a uric acid stone containing an outer shell of calcium. The history, diminished renal function, pyuria, and the typical radiographic appearance of papillitis should make the diagnosis (Fig 12–4).

Infarction of the kidney, commonly secondary to a cardiac lesion, usually occurs without pain or gross hematuria; if the infarction is massive, however, renal pain and microscopic or even gross hematuria may be produced. Evidence of a cardiac lesion (eg, subacute bacterial endocarditis, atrial fibrillation) should suggest the possibility of infarction. Excretory urograms will show lack of secretion, and angiography will reveal arterial occlusion.

Complications

The presence of a stone lowers resistance to bacterial invasion. This is particularly true if the stone is obstructive. Calculi complicated by infection may cause pyonephrosis and ultimate complete destruction of the kidney, which becomes a cavity containing stones and purulent material only.

Obstruction of the ureter at the ureteropelvic junction leads to hydronephrosis. If this progresses, the parenchyma of the kidney is ultimately destroyed. Obstruction of a calyx causes hydrocalycosis and focal renal damage. Complicating infection contributes to further injury.

While an enlarging staghorn stone may cause some renal damage as a result of the pressure it exerts on the parenchyma, the major effect on kidney function is caused by pyelonephritis.

The rare epidermoid carcinoma of the renal pelvis is almost always associated with an infected kidney containing a stone.

Prevention

Patients who have formed stones should be managed prophylactically in an attempt to prevent recurrences. The measures indicated depend upon the type of stone formed in the past. If a stone is not available for chemical analysis, its composition may be surmised from the following data: (1) x-ray density and morphology of stones in the urinary tract, (2) types of crystals in the urine, (3) positive test for urinary alpha-aminonitrogen and cystine, and (4) abnormalities in blood chemistry (calcium, phosphorus, uric acid).

A. General Measures: Stone-formers must maintain a high urine volume to keep solutes well diluted. Fluids should be taken at bedtime so that nocturia will occur; on waking, more water should be taken. This will prevent relative nocturnal dehydration. Combat infection by use of appropriate antibiotics. Eliminate obstruction and stasis by surgical means. Avoid recumbency.

Ask the patient if he is a "vitamin addict." He may be taking vitamin D, as well as mineral preparations which may include considerable calcium. Calcium stone formers should maintain an acid urine and should be asked about overuse of alkalies for gastric distress.

B. Specific Measures: Prophylactic treatment specific for the various types of stones is as follows:

1. Calcium and magnesium ammonium phosphate stones—If caused by primary hyperparathyroidism, the parathyroid glands should be explored.

a. Diet—Eliminate milk and cheese (dairy products) if hypercalciuria is discovered. A low carbohydrate intake may be of value.

b. Urinary pH—Calcium phosphate and magnesium ammonium phosphate stones form most readily in neutral or alkaline urine. The pH of the urine should be kept below 6.0. It may be tested by the patient with Nitrazine paper. Cranberry juice, 200 ml 4 times a day; ascorbic acid, 1 g 4 times a day; and sodium or potassium acid phosphate are the most efficient acidifiers. In renal tubular acidosis, alkali should be given in the form of sodium and potassium citrate; this will dramatically reduce the output of urinary calcium.

c. Converting stone-forming urine to nonstone-forming urine—According to Howard, stone formers manufacture "evil" urine. This effect can be negated by the administration of 2.5 g of neutral sodium (or potassium) phosphate (Na_2HPO_4) daily in divided doses. Sodium (or potassium) acid phosphate, 4–6 g/day, is also effective. The potassium salts are preferable. Neutra-Phos and K-Phos Neutra are commercially available preparations. Give enough to furnish 1–2 g of phosphate. Attempt to increase urinary phosphate excretion to 1500–2000 mg/24 hours. Cellulose phosphate may be of value in the treatment of hypercalciuric patients who absorb calcium excessively. This is an expensive drug and not generally available (see Pak & others, 1974).

d. Diuretics—Yendt (1973) has observed that the administration of a benzothiadiazine diuretic (eg, hydrochlorothiazide [HydroDiuril], 50 mg twice a day) decreases the amount of calcium in the urine by half in patients with idiopathic hypercalciuria. Potassium supplements must be given. There have, however, been a few reports of hypercalcemia and increased stone formation following this regimen.

2. Oxalate stones (calcium oxalate)—Prescribe phosphate and limit calcium intake (see above). There is no entirely effective method for decreasing the amount of oxalate in the urine even in hyperoxaluria.

Foods high in oxalate should be deleted from the diet, especially in patients with ileitis or shunts. Pyridoxine in large doses may be helpful.

The administration of magnesium oxide, 150 mg 3 times a day, may control recurrence of oxalate stones. It does not diminish the level of urinary excretion; the magnesium may combine with oxalate, thus forming a more soluble complex. Marked restriction of calcium is contraindicated.

3. Metabolic stones (uric acid, cystine)—Keep the pH at 7.0 or higher, thereby increasing the solubility of these substances (up to 100%). This can sometimes be done with an alkaline-ash diet (high in vegetable and fruit content, low in protein), but added alkalies are usually needed (give 50% sodium citrate solution, 1–2 tsp 4 times daily or oftener as needed, or a mixture of sodium and potassium bicarbonate). The patient can follow his urine pH with paper indicators. A low-purine diet (one weekly serving of meat, poultry, or fish) should be prescribed for the uric acid stone-former. Allopurinol (Zyloprim), a xanthine oxidase inhibitor, by decreasing the endogenous production of uric acid, has proved very effective in preventing recurrence of uric acid calculi. The dose is 300–600 mg/24 hours.

In severe cystinurics (over 1200 mg/24 hours), a low-methionine diet may be necessary in order to decrease the amount of endogenous cystine, but this diet is not very palatable. If the above measures fail to decrease the urinary cystine to safe levels, penicillamine (Cuprimine) should be added to the regimen. This preparation (30 mg/kg/day in divided doses) usually reduces the amount of cystine in the urine to 100 mg or less per day. Pyridoxine, 50 mg/day, should also be given. Stone formation ceases; some stones may dissolve. Skin rashes are not uncommon but can be controlled by corticosteroids, which are given for a few weeks and then withdrawn. The nephrotic syndrome has been observed as a complication of the drug. It subsides when the drug is stopped.

4. Urease inhibitors—Recently, use of urease inhibitors such as acetohydroxamic acid has been proposed as a potentially effective means of treatment of magnesium ammonium phosphate stone formers.

5. Methylene blue—Methylene blue has not proved an effective measure for treatment or prevention of renal calculi.

6. Aluminum hydroxide—Although aluminum hydroxide gels had been advocated for the prevention of phosphate calculi, long-term studies have shown that hypercalciuria and osteomalacia are produced and that the low phosphate content of urine may promote calcium oxalate and calcium phosphate stone formation.

C. Mixed Stones: If the patient forms more than one type of stone and the prophylactic regimens interfere with each other, it is best to determine which is the primary stone and direct prophylactic measures against that type of stone in an effort to prevent recurrence.

Treatment

A. Conservative Measures:

1. No surgery is necessary in the following cases—

a. Randall's plaque requires no treatment as long as it remains submucosal. Later, however, it may become free and pass down the ureter and cause obstruction.

b. A small stone trapped in a minor calyx and causing few if any symptoms and no renal damage is best ignored.

c. In the elderly poor-risk patient, a coralline stone is best left alone unless it causes significant symptoms. In younger individuals, removal of such stones should be considered since their primary cause (urea-splitting organisms) cannot be eradicated as long as the stone (containing embedded bacteria) remains. After nephrolithotomy, the renal infection can usually be treated successfully (Nemoy & Stamey, 1971).

d. Stones due to renal tubular acidosis should be treated conservatively even if multiple since they may pass spontaneously with adequate medical treatment (alkalies).

2. Combat infection—This is of particular importance if the bacteria are urea-splitting, for they encourage the progression of calcium phosphate or magnesium stone formation. Unfortunately, this is often not successful unless the stone is removed.

3. Attempts at dissolution—Chemical dissolution of renal stones requires indwelling ureteral catheters for constant "through-and-through" irrigation with G (or M) solution and is usually mechanically impracticable. Sand and stone fragments occlude the catheters and cause acute obstruction. This may lead to exacerbation of pyelonephritis, and bacteremia and renal cortical abscesses may result.

Some uric acid stones may dissolve on allopurinol (Zyloprim) therapy. Cystine stones may likewise disappear when penicillamine (Cuprimine) is administered.

B. Surgical Measures: Removal of the stone is indicated if the stone is obstructive and causes undue pain or progressive renal damage or if the infection complicating a stone cannot be eradicated. Nephrectomy may be necessary if obstruction and infection have markedly impaired renal function.

Prognosis

The recurrence rate of renal stone is significant, and the prognosis must therefore be guarded. The patient must be carefully followed for months or even years. The real danger from renal stone is not the pain but the kidney destruction caused by obstruction and infection.

NEPHROCALCINOSIS*

Nephrocalcinosis is a precipitation of calcium in the tubules, parenchyma, and, occasionally, in the glomeruli of the kidney. The presence of nephrocalcinosis often signifies that primary or secondary impairment of renal function has occurred. It is therefore a more serious disease than calculus. Nephrocalcinosis and calculus formation may exist together.

Etiology & Pathogenesis

A common cause of nephrocalcinosis with hypercalcemia is hyperparathyroidism. Hypercalciuria with hypercalcemia may be due to hyperparathyroidism; hypervitaminosis D, particularly when accompanied by a high calcium intake; acute osteoporosis due to immobilization, especially in children; metastatic malignancy involving bone; or hyperthyroidism.

Hypercalciuria without hypercalcemia may be caused by chronic renal insufficiency, particularly that due to chronic pyelonephritis, glomerulonephritis, or polycystic kidney disease, all of which are sometimes accompanied by calcific deposits in the kidneys. Hyperchloremic acidosis (eg, renal tubular acidosis) resulting from loss of the power of the tubules to elaborate ammonia leads to excretion of calcium as well as potassium and sodium. The hypercalciuria contributes to the precipitation of calcium salts.

Nephrocalcinosis without hypercalciuria is most commonly due to excessive intake of milk and soluble alkalies, particularly in the treatment of peptic ulcer. It is also observed in hyperoxaluria and in association with structural anomalies, eg, medullary sponge kidney.

Pathology

The kidneys may be grossly normal or there may be obvious changes suggesting advanced renal disease (eg, hydronephrosis, chronic pyelonephritis). Calcific deposits in the tubules are seen microscopically. Primary tubular or glomerular lesions may also be noted.

Metastatic calcification is not uncommonly found in many other organs, including the skin, lungs, stomach, spleen, pancreas, cornea, thyroid, and around the joints.

Clinical Findings

A. Symptoms: There are no symptoms which suggest nephrocalcinosis, although these patients at times pass stones and sand. The complaints are those of the primary disease (eg, primary hyperparathyroidism or renal insufficiency). In childhood, there may be lack of normal growth and bone changes suggestive of rickets.

B. Signs: The physical examination is usually negative. Signs of the primary cause may be found, as follows: (1) parathyroid adenoma or hyperplasia, (2) metastatic calcifications around the joints or in the

---

*The section on nephrocalcinosis is contributed in part by Felix O. Kolb, MD. (See p 200, *Note.*)

cornea ("band keratopathy") as viewed with a slit-lamp, (3) punched-out lesions in the fingertips (sarcoidosis), (4) pseudofractures (osteomalacia), (5) bilateral renal masses (polycystic kidneys), (6) dwarfism, or (7) renal osteodystrophy.

C. Laboratory Findings: Anemia may be noted in advanced renal disease. The urinary pH is fixed between 6.0–6.5 in renal tubular acidosis. Pus and bacteria will be found in the urine in association with chronic renal infection. Casts and protein are constant findings in glomerulonephritis. Calcium phosphate casts may be seen. The Sulkowitch test is positive in states of hypercalciuria; it may be positive with secondary parathyroid hyperplasia as well. In advanced renal disease, hypocalciuria may be seen.

Renal function tests will demonstrate some impairment of function whether the primary cause of the calcification is renal or not. Nitrogen retention is common.

Hypercalcemia and hypophosphatemia are to be expected in primary hyperparathyroidism. In chronic renal disease (with secondary hyperparathyroidism), the serum calcium may be low or normal and the phosphate normal or elevated.

Hyperchloremic acidosis (low blood pH) and hypokalemia accompany renal tubular acidosis.

Serum alkaline phosphatase will be elevated if nephrocalcinosis is accompanied by bone disease (osteitis, osteomalacia, etc).

D. X-Ray Findings: A plain film of the abdomen

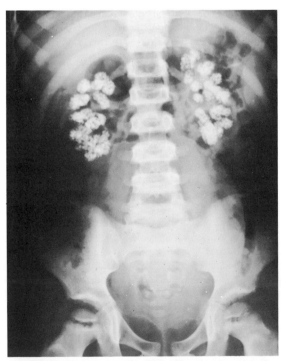

Figure 15–5. Nephrocalcinosis. Plain film showing parenchymal calcification in both kidneys. Large globular soft tissue shadow (greatly distended bladder) in midline extending from pelvis to level of lower poles of kidneys. It has displaced the bowel to the flanks.

will show the pathognomonic parenchymal calcifications (Fig 15–5). These consist of minute calcific densities with a linear arrangement in the region of the renal papillae and radiating outward from the calyces. If renal function is not seriously impaired, excretory urograms will show that the calcium is in the renal parenchyma and not in the calyces although true stones may be present as well. These films may reveal changes compatible with atrophic pyelonephritis or hydronephrosis. X-rays of bones may show osteitis fibrosa generalisata and a soft tissue calcification of "renal rickets" (renal osteodystrophy).

Differential Diagnosis

Renal stones are usually discrete and lie in the calyces or pelvis.

In renal tuberculosis, renal calcification is also parenchymal but tends to be related to the pericalyceal zones. Furthermore, the calcification is punctate rather than striated. Pus cells and tubercle bacilli are present, and excretory urograms will usually show the mucosal ulcerations or abscess cavities of tuberculosis.

Medullary sponge kidneys may develop multiple small calculi in their dilated cystic collecting tubules. Renal function is usually normal. Metabolic defects may coexist (Stella & others, 1973). Excretory urograms help in the differentiation.

Complications

Calcification secondary to extrarenal disease (eg, hyperparathyroidism) often causes minimal impairment of renal function. The calcium deposits secondary to preexisting renal disease cause more damage. If stones form and cause obstruction—particularly if secondary infection ensues—further renal injury occurs.

Treatment

A. Specific Measures: Treat the primary cause of the disease (eg, remove the parathyroid adenoma, relieve obstruction, and treat urologic infection).

B. General Measures: Discontinue vitamin D and give a low-calcium diet (delete dairy products, especially milk and cheese), encourage mobilization, and force fluids. If osteomalacia is present, vitamin D and calcium may have to be given in spite of nephrocalcinosis.

If renal function is reasonably good and hyperchloremic (renal tubular) acidosis exists, replace base to decrease hypercalciuria: Give a 50% solution of sodium or potassium citrate (or a combination of both), 4–8 ml 4 times daily. Sodium bicarbonate, 4 g 4 times daily, can be given in orange juice or water. The goal is alkalinization (pH of 7.0–7.5) of the urine. Additional potassium is also indicated. At times the degree of nephrocalcinosis decreases with alkali treatment of renal tubular acidosis.

Prognosis

If the nephrocalcinosis is secondary to primary renal disease, the prognosis is poor although life can be prolonged significantly with adequate treatment. If the

renal calcification has developed because of extrarenal disease and if renal function is fairly good, correction of the underlying disease may terminate the progression of kidney damage. Frequently, however, the outlook is poor even in these instances.

URETERAL STONE

Ureteral stones originate in the kidney. Gravity and peristalsis both contribute to spontaneous passage into and down the ureter.

Ureteral stones are seldom completely obstructive; they are usually spiculated, so that urine can flow around them. Occasionally, a stone will remain lodged in a ureter for many months without harming the kidney. Partial obstruction is usually present, however, and causes dilatation of the ureter and renal pelvis proximal to the stone. In the early phase, this dilatation is due more to distention than to "hydronephro-

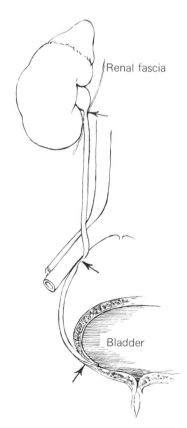

Figure 15–6. Points of ureteral narrowing. The ureter is narrow at 3 points: (1) at the ureteropelvic junction, (2) at the point where the ureter crosses over the iliac vessels, and (3) in the ureterovesical zone. A stone which passes the ureteropelvic junction has an excellent chance, therefore, of continuing the whole distance. If it becomes arrested, it is usually in the lower 5 cm of the ureter.

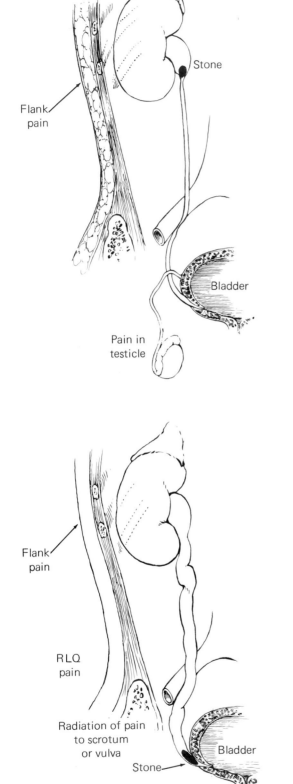

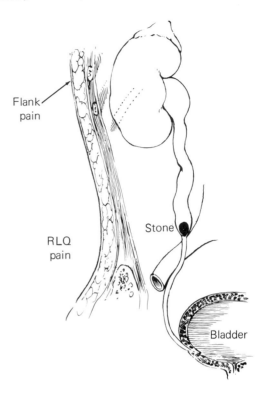

Figure 15—7. Radiation of pain with various types of ureteral stone. ***Above left:*** Ureteropelvic stone. Severe costovertebral angle pain from capsular and pelvic distention; acute renal and ureteral pain from hyperperistalsis of smooth muscle of calyces, pelvis, and ureter, with pain radiating along the course of the ureter (and into the testicle, since the nerve supply to the kidney and testis is the same). The testis is hypersensitive. ***Above right:*** Midureteral stone. Same as above but with more pain in the lower abdominal quadrant. ***Left:*** Low ureteral stone. Same as above with pain radiating into bladder, vulva, or scrotum. The scrotal wall is hyperesthetic. Testicular sensitivity is absent. When the stone approaches the bladder, urgency and frequency with burning on urination develop as a result of inflammation of the bladder wall around the ureteral orifice.

sis," which implies definite renal damage. If the stone passes within a few days, no evidence of renal injury can be shown. However, if the stone is definitely obstructive and is allowed to remain for weeks or months, irreparable damage to the renal parenchyma can occur (Fig 7–4). A stone is apt to be arrested at the narrowest points in the ureter (Fig 15–6). If infection complicates the urinary stasis, further renal damage results.

Clinical Findings

A. Symptoms: Pain is usually abrupt in onset and becomes severe within minutes (Fig 15–7). There are 2 types of pain: (1) radiating, colicky, agonizing pain (from hyperperistalsis of the smooth muscle of the calyces, pelvis, and ureter); and (2) the rather constant ache in the costovertebral area and flank (from obstruction and capsular tension). The radiation of pain at times suggests the position of the stone. If the stone is high in the ureter, the colic may radiate to the testicle. As the stone nears the bladder, the pain may spread to the scrotum or appear in the vulva. This is due to the common innervation of these organs and the lower ureter. At times the pain comes on more slowly and may be felt more anteriorly. It may occasionally be quite mild. In these instances, the diagnosis may not at first be obvious.

Gastrointestinal symptoms are commonly associated with stone in the ureter. Nausea and vomiting almost always occur, and abdominal distention due to paralytic ileus is always present. These symptoms may be so severe that the renal and ureteral pain may be overshadowed and an intraperitoneal lesion sought (eg, bowel obstruction, ruptured peptic ulcer, cholelithiasis, or acute appendicitis).

Gross hematuria is observed in about one-third of cases; small clots may be passed.

Even in the absence of infection, symptoms of urgency and frequency may develop when the stone approaches the bladder.

Existing chronic renal infection may be exacerbated by the ureteral obstruction. Chills and fever with increased back pain may be noted. It is not common for stone to be complicated by acute (new) infection unless it is introduced by instrumentation. If this does occur, chills, fever, and sepsis are to be expected.

B. Signs: The patient is usually in agony, pacing the floor rather than lying quietly in bed (as a patient with peritoneal irritation is apt to do). Nothing he does affords relief. His skin may be cold and clammy, and he may exhibit other signs of mild shock. There is marked tenderness in the costovertebral angle and flank. Fist percussion posteriorly causes severe pain. Spasm of the abdominal muscles on the affected side is to be expected.

Fever indicates that infection is a complicating feature. The abdomen is distended, tympanitic, and quiet on auscultation. The ipsilateral testis may be hypersensitive if the stone is in the upper ureter. It may be retracted. The scrotal skin may be hyperesthetic if the stone lies low. A juxtavesical ureteral stone may at times be felt vaginally.

C. Laboratory Findings: They are the same as for renal stone (see p 200).

D. X-Ray Findings: A plain film of the abdomen may show a calcific body in the region of the ureter. This constitutes merely presumptive grounds for the diagnosis, however, for the shadow may be a phlebolith or some other intra-abdominal calcification.

Excretory urograms are invaluable (Fig 15–8). The ureterogram places the calcification in the ureter and usually demonstrates dilatation of the ureter above the stone. It also reveals what is happening to the kidney (degree of obstruction). On occasion, no "dye" may enter the renal pelvis or ureter because of the obstruction but a marked density of the renal shadow occurs (nephrogram effect) (Fig 15–9). This is evidence of good kidney function and acute ureteral obstruction. The acute ureteral obstruction may cause extravasation of the radiopaque fluid in the region of the renal hilum. This finding in itself is rarely of consequence.

In the case of a nonopaque stone, a "negative" gray or black shadow is seen within the white area of the ureter. This may be difficult to differentiate from ureteral tumor or blood clot.

The diagnosis of ureteral stone may be established by demonstrating that the suspicious shadow hugs the cystoscopically placed ureteral catheter in both the anteroposterior and oblique views. This would only be necessary if the excretory urograms failed to visualize the ureter.

E. Instrumental Examination: Cystoscopy and ureteral catheterization are seldom needed for the diagnosis of ureteral stone. Instrumental examination should be avoided unless a proper conclusion cannot be drawn otherwise. No matter how careful one is, instrumentation always carries bacteria from the urethra into the urinary tract. Infection introduced in this way unnecessarily complicates the problem.

Differential Diagnosis

Passage of crystals down the ureter may occur during treatment or an exacerbation of gout or in oxaluria after excessive ingestion of foods high in oxalate content. Symptoms and signs are the same as those seen in stone, and hematuria is just as common. X-ray examination is usually normal. The presence of many crystals in the urine may explain the colic.

A tumor of the kidney or renal pelvis may bleed, and a clot or piece of necrotic tumor tissue may pass down the ureter. This will simulate ureteral stone perfectly. Excretory urograms should demonstrate a space-occupying lesion in the kidney and a "negative" shadow in the ureter. Retrograde urograms may then be indicated for more definitive diagnosis.

Ureteral tumor is often obstructive and may cause colic. Hematuria is common. X-ray visualization of the urinary tract should make the diagnosis.

Obstructive chronic lesions of the ureter may cause severe recurrent pain. These include congenital ureteral stenosis and extraureteral obstructions such as

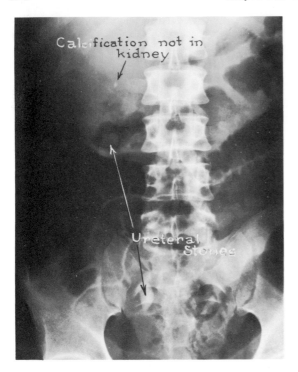

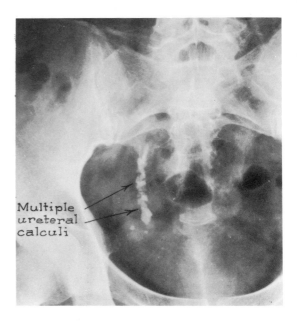

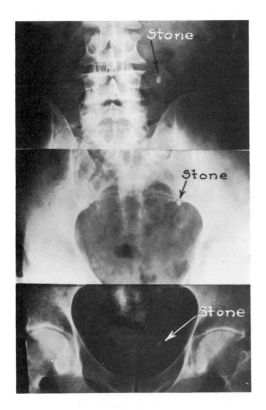

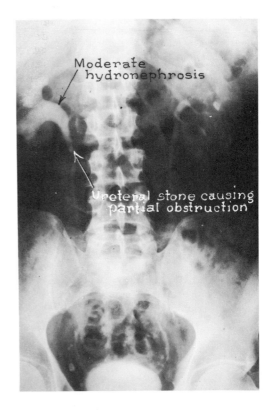

Figure 15—8. Radiograms showing ureteral stones. *Above left:* Two stones in right ureter, mildly radiopaque: cystine. *Above right:* Multiple stones, right ureter. *Below left:* Plain films showing progress of stone down ureter. *Below right:* Stone in upper right ureter causing moderate obstruction.

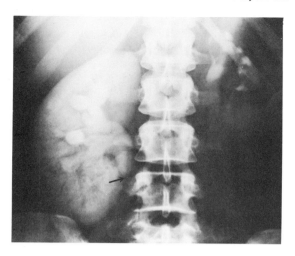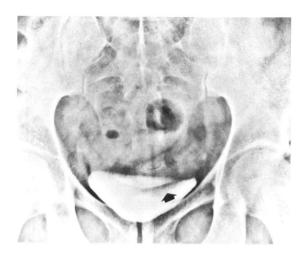

Figure 15—9. Ureteral stone. *Left:* "Nephrogram" caused by acute ureteral obstruction. Marked density of renal parenchyma with moderate hydronephrosis. Arrow points to nonopaque (uric acid) stone. Left kidney is contracted and scarred from previous infections. *Right:* Patient has just passed left ureteral calculus. Note secondary edema of left intravesical ureter as depicted by arrow and a second stone in the left ureter just above the bladder.

may be caused by lymph nodes containing cancer. A careful history and physical examination and excretory urograms should lead to the correct diagnosis.

Acute pyelonephritis may start so abruptly and the pain may be so acute as to suggest stone. The finding of pyuria and bacteriuria with normal urograms should establish the diagnosis.

Acute gallbladder disease (stone or infection) may be confused with ureteral stone if severe pain is referred to the back. A history of dyspepsia or jaundice is helpful. It is true, however, that renal and ureteral stones also cause gastrointestinal symptoms. Red cells in the urine suggest urinary stone. Cholecystograms and urography should settle the matter.

An aneurysm of the abdominal aorta may cause pain suggestive of left renal colic. Palpation of the aneurysm, absence of hematuria, and normal excretory urograms will differentiate the two. Aortography is definitive.

A sloughed papilla passing down the ureter may simulate ureteral stone. Urinalysis shows evidence of infection. Excretory urograms will reveal the typical changes of papillary necrosis.

Complications

The major complication of ureteral stone is obstruction, usually only partial. Permanent renal damage is rare except in the case which remains undiagnosed or is inadequately treated. Bilateral ureteral calculi may cause anuria, in which case drainage of the kidney by ureteral catheters or removal of the stones must then be accomplished.

Infection may gain a foothold in the presence of the obstruction, but it is usually introduced by the cystoscopist in his attempts to remove the stone. Drainage either by catheter or surgical attack is indicated in addition to appropriate antibiotic therapy.

Prevention

See p 206.

Treatment

A. Specific Measures: About 80% of stones which reach the ureter can pass spontaneously and should always be allowed to do so as long as complications do not develop. Antispasmodics may be helpful. Physical activity should be encouraged and adequate fluid intake maintained to increase ureteral peristalsis. A stone small enough to pass down the ureter will have no difficulty traversing the urethra.

Cystoscopic manipulation, electronic lithotripsy, or operation (ureterolithotomy) is necessary if the stone is too large to pass spontaneously. Stones up to 0.5 cm in diameter and even a few up to 1 cm in diameter may pass without surgical or cystoscopic assistance. The onset of infection may require removal of the obstructing agent before sepsis can be controlled. If periodic excretory urograms show progressive hydronephrosis or if pain remains intense and incapacitating, removal of the stone is indicated.

B. General Measures: Morphine or a similar opiate given intravenously is necessary to control pain. Morphine sulfate, 8 mg IV, or a comparable drug in the same relative strength, should be given immediately and repeated in 5 minutes if relief has not been obtained. Pain can usually be controlled thereafter by subcutaneous injection. Initial subcutaneous morphine, even in doses of 30 mg, is not adequate for relief of pain of this degree.

Atropine, 0.8 mg subcut, is the antispasmodic of choice. Methantheline bromide (Banthine), 0.1 g IV, will usually relieve the pain; unfortunately, it may paralyze bladder action for some hours as well. Other antispasmodics can be given by mouth, but their efficacy is questionable.

Heat to the flank or a hot bath is often helpful as an adjunct to drug analgesia.

Prognosis

About 80% of stones which enter the ureter will pass spontaneously in a few days or weeks. If the effect of the stone upon the kidney is evaluated at intervals with excretory urograms, the physician will be able to intervene as necessary in order to prevent kidney damage.

VESICAL STONE

Primary vesical stones are rare in the USA but occur commonly in northwest India, the Middle East, and parts of China. The cause is not known, but a dietary cause is assumed. Vitamin B_6 deficiency may play a role. Once they are removed, primary vesical stones rarely recur.

Secondary vesical stone develops as a complication of other urologic disease; 95% occur in men. The most common cause of secondary vesical stone is infection of residual urine with urea-splitting organisms (eg, proteus). This partial urinary retention may be due to prostatic or bladder neck obstruction, cystocele, or neurogenic bladder. Stagnation is particularly marked in vesical diverticula; stones are often found when diverticula are present (Fig 15—11).

A stone that passes through the ureter into the bladder usually passes on through the urethra. If obstruction or urinary stasis is present, the stone may remain in the bladder and act as a nidus for precipitation of more urinary salts.

A markedly inflamed or ulcerated bladder may predispose to stone formation. This is seen in vesical schistosomiasis and following irradiation of the bladder.

Foreign bodies occasionally are introduced into the bladder, particularly in women (see Chapter 26). These include nonabsorbable sutures, candles, nail files, chewing gum, and even crochet hooks. They may act as nidi for the precipitation of calcific deposits (Fig 15—10). Infection complicates the picture and hastens calculus formation, particularly if the bacteria are urea-splitters.

Prolonged use of an indwelling catheter may permit the formation of calcium encrustations which may become dislodged when the catheter is removed.

Pathology

Vesical stones may be single or multiple. If single, they are ovoid; if multiple, they often are faceted (Fig 15—11). In addition to the infection which is uniformly present with secondary stones, their presence further increases the inflammation of the bladder.

Most vesical stones are radiopaque (calcium phosphate, calcium oxalate, or ammonium magnesium phosphate), but some are radiolucent (uric acid). Even calcium stones are at times invisible on a plain film. This may be due to the presence of large amounts of matrix.

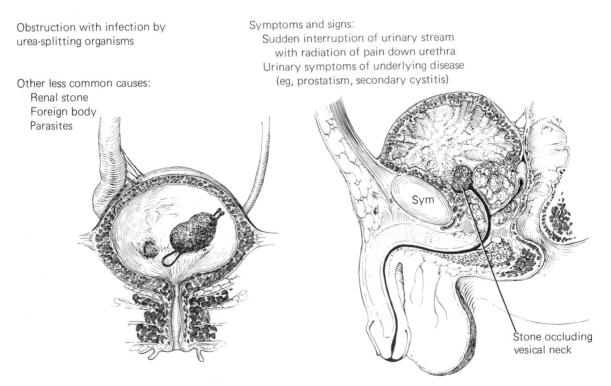

Obstruction with infection by urea-splitting organisms

Other less common causes:
  Renal stone
  Foreign body
  Parasites

Symptoms and signs:
  Sudden interruption of urinary stream
    with radiation of pain down urethra
  Urinary symptoms of underlying disease
    (eg, prostatism, secondary cystitis)

Sym

Stone occluding vesical neck

Figure 15—10. Genesis and symptoms and signs of vesical calculus.

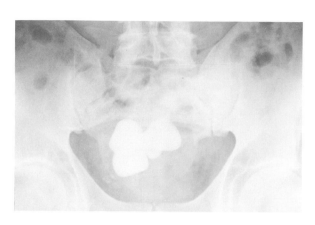

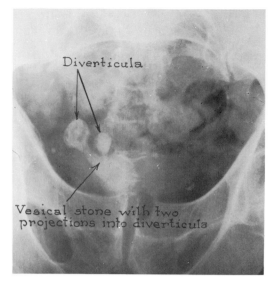

Figure 15—11. Vesical stones. *Left:* Plain film showing multiple-faceted stones. *Right:* Plain film showing dumbbell-shaped stone in bladder with projections into diverticula.

Clinical Findings

A. Symptoms: Symptoms of chronic urinary tract obstruction or stasis and infection occur in most cases, for these are the common causes of vesical stone. There may be a history of introduction of a foreign body into the bladder or prolonged vesical catheter drainage. The male patient may complain of sudden interruption of the urinary stream associated with pain radiating down the penis when the stone rolls over the bladder neck. He may be unable to void except in certain positions which cause the stone to move off the bladder neck. Considerable hematuria may be noted, although this can occur also with pure obstruction or infection.

B. Signs: Only giant calculi can be felt suprapubically. The bladder may be visible, palpable, or percussible if there is a great deal of residual urine. Palpation of the urethra may reveal a thickening compatible with stricture. Rectal examination may demonstrate a relaxed anal sphincter (neurogenic bladder) or an enlarged or hard (cancerous) prostate. Cystocele may be noted.

C. Laboratory Findings: The urine is almost always infected. Blood cells are commonly found. Excretion of PSP may be depressed because of chronic obstruction. A flattened curve (first and second half-hour specimens about equal in amount) suggests residual urine.

D. X-Ray Findings: Vesical stones are usually visible on a plain film (Fig 15—11). They must be differentiated from calcified ovaries and fibroids. Oblique films are usually helpful. Excretory urograms may show back pressure changes in the kidneys, and a film taken after voiding may reveal residual urine. Diverticula may be noted. Stones will be localized in the excretory or retrograde cystograms.

E. Instrumental Examination: The attempt to pass a catheter or sound may lead to the diagnosis of urethral stricture. Successful passage of a catheter after urination allows estimation of the degree of obstruction and stasis by recovering residual urine. The positive diagnostic step of "sounding" for stone may be accomplished by passing a sound into the bladder. The definitive "click" of the instrument on the stone can readily be heard or felt. Cystoscopy usually visualizes the stone or stones and the obstructive lesion with its secondary vesical changes (Fig 10—1).

Differential Diagnosis

A pedunculated tumor of the bladder can suddenly occlude the vesical orifice, thereby simulating vesical stone. Cystoscopy will make the differentiation.

Extravesical calcifications on x-rays of the vesical region may appear to be in the bladder but are actually in the veins, omental fat pads, ovaries, or fibroids of the uterus. Cystoscopy will help in differentiating these.

Complications

A primary stone will lead eventually to infection. If infection is present, it will be worsened by the presence of the calculus, which in turn will defeat attempts to sterilize the urine.

Vesicoureteral reflux is commonly associated with vesical calculi. Removal of the calculi may cause spontaneous cessation of the reflux.

A small vesical concretion may pass down the urethra and become lodged there (Amin, 1973). This may cause complete urinary obstruction.

Prevention

Stasis and infection, whether primary or secondary, must be eradicated.

Treatment

A. Specific Measures:

1. Cystoscopy and surgical removal—

a. Transurethral route—Small stones can be removed by cystoscopic manipulation; large ones can be crushed (litholapaxy) and the fragments washed out. If the patient has an obstructing prostate which can be removed by transurethral resection, both procedures may be undertaken at the same time.

Stones may be cracked by an instrument called an electrohydraulic lithotrite. This instrument is passed transurethrally into the bladder, filled with water, and its tip pressed against the stone. An electric charge is delivered, breaking up the stone.

b. Suprapubic route—This route must be used for removal of stones which are too large for transurethral removal or crushing. Suprapubic prostatectomy may also be done.

2. Chemical dissolution—This is usually successful, but it fails to treat the cause of the stone formation. It may be indicated if the patient is considered to be an unwarranted surgical risk or if he refuses surgery or cystoscopic removal.

In the dissolution of calcium and magnesium ammonium phosphate calculi, excellent results are obtained with hemiacidrin (Renacidin). Thirty ml of 10% solution are instilled, and the catheter is clamped for 30—60 minutes. This is repeated 4—6 times a day. A continuous drip through a 3-way Foley catheter may also be used.

Calcium salts and magnesium ammonium phosphate are highly soluble in citric acid. Suby and Albright have evolved buffered solutions of this compound:

"Solution G" (pH 4.0)

Citric acid (monohydrated)	32.25
Magnesium oxide (anhydrous)	3.84
Sodium carbonate (anhydrous)	4.37
Water, qs ad	1000.0

If this solution proves irritating, the amount of sodium carbonate can be increased to 8.74 g ("solution M," which has a pH of 4.5).

In order to dissolve organic matrix, 0.05% pepsin should be added to the solution. The resulting mixture can be sterilized by passing it through a millipore filter.

Through an indwelling catheter, 60—100 ml of solution G (or M) are introduced into the bladder. The fluid is retained for one-half hour, and the bladder is then drained. This procedure is repeated several times at intervals of 1—2 hours.

These solutions may fail with markedly radiopaque (hard) stones. They have no effect on uric acid or cystine stones.

In order to prevent precipitation of calcium salts on an indwelling catheter, Rollins & Finlayson (1973)

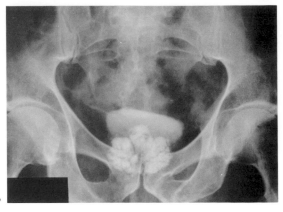

Figure 15—12. Prostatic calculi seen in typical locations behind the symphysis pubis.

recommend the use of 65 mg of methylene blue 4 times a day by mouth.

B. General Measures: Analgesics for pain and antibiotics for control of infection are used for relief of distressing symptoms until the stone can be removed and its cause eliminated.

C. Treatment of Complications: Infection cannot be eradicated until the stone and the cause of the obstruction are removed. Urethral stone may be extracted transurethrally or pushed back into the bladder and then extracted or crushed.

Prognosis

The rate of recurrence of vesical stone is low if the primary cause (obstruction) is successfully treated.

PROSTATIC CALCULI

Prostatic calculi are seldom of clinical importance. They are commonly seen in association with benign prostatic hyperplasia, although in rare cases in younger persons they may be secondary to an advanced but healing tuberculous prostatitis.

Prostatic calculi are formed of desquamated epithelial cells which finally acquire a shell of calcium. They average about 1—2 mm in diameter and are brown to black in color. They are situated between the hypertrophied adenoma and the surgical capsule. Therefore, on enucleation of the enlarged prostate or complete transurethral prostatectomy, they tend to be extruded.

On a plain film they are situated in the region of the pubic symphysis (Fig 15—12).

The importance of prostatic calculi lies in the fact that they cause indurated areas in the prostate which may be mistaken for carcinomas.

•   •   •

References

Renal Stone

Barzilay BI, Kedar SS: Surgical treatment of staghorn calculus by lower partial nephrectomy and pyelocalicolithotomy. J Urol 108:689, 1972.

Bender RA, Hansen H: Hypercalcemia in bronchogenic carcinoma: A prospective study of 200 patients. Ann Int Med 80:205, 1974.

Bissada NK, Meacham KR, Redman JF: Nephrostoscopy with removal of renal pelvic calculi. J Urol 112:414, 1974.

Blacklock NJ, Macleod MA: Calcium-47 absorption in urolithiasis. Brit J Urol 46:377, 1974.

Blacklock NJ, Macleod MA: The effect of cellulose phosphate on intestinal absorption and urinary excretion of calcium: Some experience in its use in the treatment of calcium stone formation. Brit J Urol 46:385, 1974.

Boyce WH, Elkins IB: Reconstructive renal surgery following anatrophic nephrolithotomy: Follow-up of 100 consecutive cases. J Urol 111:307, 1974.

Coe FL, Raisen L: Allopurinol treatment of uric-acid disorders in calcium-stone formers. Lancet 1:129, 1973.

Dunegan LJ & others: Primary hyperparathyroidism: Pre-operative evaluation and correlation with surgical findings. Am J Surg 128:471, 1974.

Earnest DL & others: Excessive absorption of oxalate contributes to hyperoxaluria in patients with ileal disease. Gastroenterology 64:723, 1973.

Elliott JS: Calcium stones: The difference between oxalate and phosphate types. J Urol 100:687, 1968.

Ekburg M, Jeppsson J-O, Denneberg T: Penicillamine treatment of cystinuria. Acta med scandinav 195:415, 1974.

Ettinger B, Kolb FO: Factors involved in crystal formation in cystinuria: In vivo and in vitro crystallization dynamics and a simple, quantitative colorimetric assay for cystine. J Urol 106:106, 1971.

Ettinger B, Kolb FO: Inorganic phosphate treatment of nephrolithiasis. Am J Med 55:32, 1973.

Farrell RM, Marshall VF: Urolithiasis in children. Urology 4:51, 1974.

Freed SZ: The alternating use of an alkalizing salt and acetazolamide in the management of cystine and uric acid stones. J Urol 113:96, 1975.

Gellman AC, Malament M: Partial nephrectomy in renal calculus disease. Urology 1:355, 1973.

GibbonsRP: Use of water-pik and nephroscope. Urology 4:605, 1974.

Goldman L, Gordan GS, Roof BS: The parathyroids: Progress, problems and practice. Curr Probl Surg 1:64, 1971.

Herrin JT: The child with urolithiasis: Practical considerations in diagnosis and management. Clin Pediat 10:306, 1971.

Howard JE: Tried, true, and new ways to treat and prevent kidney stones. Res Staff 16:67, 1970.

Joekes AM, Rose, GA, Sutor J: Multiple renal silica stones. Brit MJ 1:46, 1973.

Knisley RE: Hypercalcemia associated with leukemia. Arch Int Med 118:14, 1966.

Kolb FO: General approach to the treatment of patients with renal stones. Mod Treat 4:464, 1967.

Lavengood RW Jr, Marshall VF: The prevention of renal phosphatic calculi in the presence of infection by the Shorr regimen. J Urol 108:368, 1972.

Lund HT: Primary hyperparathyroidism in childhood. Acta paediat Scandinav 62:317, 1973.

Mahmood P, Morales PA: Extended pyelolithotomy (Gil Vernet's pyelotomy). J Urol 109:772, 1973,

Mallette LE & others: Primary hyperparathyroidism: Clinical and biochemical features. Medicine 53:127, 1974.

Nemoy NJ, Stamey TA: Surgical, bacteriological, and biochemical management of "infection stones." JAMA 215:1470, 1971.

Ofstad J, Nordahl EH, Gjersvik T: Renal function in patients with unilateral staghorn calculi. Acta med scandinav 194:65, 1973.

Oreopoulos DG, Soyanno MAO, McGeown MG: Magnesium/calcium ratio in urine of patients with renal stones. Lancet 2:420, 1968.

Ozog LS, Tomskey GC: Diagnosis and treatment of cystinuria. Urology 3:197, 1974.

Pak CYC, Delea CS, Bartter FC: Successful treatment of recurrent nephrolithiasis (calcium stones) with cellulose phosphate. New England J Med 290:175, 1974.

Palmer FJ, Nelson JC, Bacchus H: The chloride-phosphate ratio in hypercalcemia. Ann Int Med 80:200, 1974.

Patel VJ: The coagulum pyelolithotomy. Brit J Surg 60:230, 1973.

Paulson DF & others: Pediatric urolithiasis. J Urol 108:811, 1972.

Powell D & others: Primary hyperparathyroidism. New England J Med 286:1169, 1972.

Prien EL Sr, Gershoff SF: Magnesium oxide-pyridoxene therapy for recurrent calcium oxalate calculi. J Urol 112:509, 1974.

Raisz LG: The diagnosis of hyperparathyroidism (or what to do until the immunoassay comes). New England J Med 285:1006, 1971.

Rasmussen K: Observations during treatment of cystinuria with D-penicillamine. Acta med scandinav 189:367, 1971.

Rose GA, Harrison AR: The incidence, investigation and treatment of idiopathic hypercalciuria. Brit J Urol 46:261, 1974.

Scholten HG, Bakker NJ, Cornil C: Urolithiasis in childhood. J Urol 109:744, 1973.

Silver S, Brendler H: Use of magnesium oxide in management of familial hyperoxaluria. J Urol 106:274, 1971.

Singh M, Tressider GC, Blandy J: The fate of the unoperated staghorn calculus. Brit J Urol 45:581, 1973.

Smith LH: The diagnosis and treatment of metabolic stone disease. M Clin North America 56:977, 1972.

Smith LH, Fromm H, Hoffmann AF: Acquired hyperoxaluria nephrolithiasis and intestinal disease. New England J Med 286:1371, 1972.

Smith MJV: Concretions and methylene blue. J Urol 107:164, 1972.

Smith MJV & others: Uricemia and urolithiasis. J Urol 101:637, 1969.

Stauffer JQ, Humphreys MH, Weir GJ: Acquired hyperoxaluria with regional enteritis after ileal resection: Role of dietary oxalate. Ann Int Med 79:383, 1973.

Stein J, Smythe HA: Nephrotic syndrome induced by penicillamine. Canad MAJ 98:505, 1968.

Stuart AE: Operative nephroscopy using bronchofiberscope. J Urol 111:9, 1974.

Symposium on urinary stone. Am J Med 45:654, 1968.

Thompson RB, Stamey TA: Bacteriology of infected stones. Urology 2:627, 1973.

Ts'ai-Fan Y, Gutman AB: Uric acid nephrolithiasis in gout. Ann Int Med 67:1133, 1967.

Uhlir K: The peroral dissolution of renal calculi. J Urol 104:239, 1970.

Valman HB, Oberholzer VG, Palmer T: Hyperoxaluria after resection of ileum in childhood. Arch Dis Childhood 49:171, 1974.

Vermeulen CW, Ellis JE, Hsu T-C: Experimental observations on the pathogenesis of urinary calculi. J Urol 95:681, 1966.

Vermeulen CW, Fried FA: Observations on dissolution of uric acid calculi. J Urol 94:293, 1965.

Vermeulen CW & others: The renal papilla and calculogenesis. J Urol 97:573, 1967.

Wallace MR, MacDiarmid J, Reeder J: Exacerbation of nephrolithiasis by a carbonic anhydrase inhibitor. New Zealand MJ 79:687, 1974.

Weber AL: Primary hyperoxaluria. Am J Roentgenol 100:155, 1967.

Williams HE: Nephrolithiasis. New England J Med 290:33, 1974.

Yendt ER: Renal calculi. Canad MAJ 102:479, 1970.

Yendt ER: Thiazide prophylaxis for calcium stones. Med World News, Urol/1973, p 33.

Yendt ER, Gagne RJA: Detection of primary hyperparathyroidism, with special reference to its occurrence in hypercalciuric females with "normal" or borderline serum calcium. Canad MAJ 98:331, 1968.

Nephrocalcinosis

Buckalew VM & others: Hereditary renal tubular acidosis: Report of 64 member kindred with variable clinical expression including idiopathic hypercalciuria. Medicine 53:229, 1974.

Courey WR, Pfister RC: The radiographic findings in renal tubular acidosis: Analysis of 21 cases. Radiology 105:497, 1972.

Farrell RM, Horwith M, Muecke EC: Renal tubular acidosis and nephrocalcinosis: Diagnosis and clinical management. J Urol 111:429, 1974.

Fletcher RF, Jones JH, Morgan DB: Bone disease in chronic renal failure. Quart J Med 32:321, 1963.

Nash MA & others: Renal tubular acidosis in infants and children: Clinical course, response to treatment, and prognosis. J Pediat 80:738, 1972.

Punsar S, Somer T: The milk-alkali syndrome. Acta med scandinav 173:435, 1963.

Scholz DA & others: Diagnostic considerations in hypercalcemic syndromes. M Clin North America 56:941, 1972.

Stanbury SW, Lumb GA: Parathyroid function in chronic renal failure: A statistical survey of the plasma biochemistry in azotemic renal osteodystrophy. Quart J Med 35:1, 1966.

Stella FJ & others: Medullary sponge kidney associated with parathyroid adenoma: A report of 2 cases. Nephron 10:332, 1973.

Vazquez AM: Nephrocalcinosis and hypertension in juvenile primary hyperparathyroidism. Am J Dis Child 125:104, 1973.

Young JD Jr, Martin LG: Urinary calculi associated with incomplete renal tubular acidosis. J Urol 107:170, 1972.

Ureteral Stone

Arnaldsson Ö, Holmlund D: Defects in the urographic contrast medium above and below a ureteric calculus. Acta radiol diag 11:26, 1971.

Bowers L: Loop catheter delivery of ureteral calculi. J Urol 110:178, 1973.

Constantian HM: Use of the Davis nylon loop extractor for removal of low ureteral calculi. J Urol 97:248, 1967.

Kettlewell M & others: Spontaneous extravasation of urine secondary to ureteric obstruction. Brit J Urol 45:8, 1973.

Mahon FB Jr, Waters RF: A critical review of stone manipulation: A 5-year study. J Urol 110:387, 1973.

Nagel R, Marquardt H, Grull S: Treatment of ureteral calculi with the Zeiss loop. Internat Urol Nephrol 4:215, 1972.

Olsson O: Frequency of backflow in acute and renal colic. Acta radiol diag 12:469, 1972.

Reuter HJ, Kern E: Electronic lithotripsy of ureteral calculi. J Urol 110:181, 1973.

Skolnick AM, Lome LG, Presman D: Spontaneous urinary extravasation secondary to acute ureteral obstruction. J Urol 110:391, 1973.

Smulewicz JJ & others: Spontaneous rupture of the collecting system of the kidney: An evaluation. J Urol 104:507, 1970.

Walsh A: An aggressive approach to stones in the lower ureter. Brit J Urol 46:11, 1974.

Wisoff CP, Parsavand R: Edema of the interureteric ridge: A useful Roentgen sign. Am J Roentgenol 86:1123, 1961.

Vesical Stones

Alfthan O, Murtomaa M: Experiences with the clinical and experimental use of Urat-I lithotriptor. Scandinav J Urol Nephrol 6:23, 1972.

Amin SA: Urethral calculi. Brit J Urol 45:192, 1973.

Andersen DA: The nutritional significance of primary bladder stones. Brit J Urol 34:160, 1962.

Angeloff A: Hydro electrolithotripsy. J Urol 108:867, 1972.

Aurora AL, Taneja OP, Gupta DN: Bladder stone disease of childhood. 1. An epidemiological study. 2. A clinico-pathological study. Acta paediat scandinav 59:177, 385, 1970.

Mulvaney WP, Henning DC: Solvent treatment of urinary calculi: Refinements in technique. J Urol 88:145, 1962.

Raney AM: Electrohydraulic lithotripsy: Experimental study and case reports with the stone disintegration. J Urol 113:345, 1975.

Reuter HJ, Jones LW: Trocar lithotripsy: A new perspective. J Urol 110:197, 1973.

Rollins R, Finlayson B: Mechanism of prevention of calcium oxalate encrustation by methylene blue and demonstration of the concentration dependence of its action. J Urol 110:459, 1973.

Prostatic Calculi

Eykyn S & others: Prostatic calculi as a source of recurrent bacteriuria in the male. Brit J Urol 46:527, 1974.

Fox M: The natural history and significance of stone formation in prostate gland. J Urol 89:716, 1963.

Gawande AS, Kamat MH, Seebode JJ: Giant prostatic calculi. Urology 4:319, 1974.

Meares EM Jr: Infection stones of prostate gland: Laboratory diagnosis and clinical management. Urology 4:560, 1974.

Sutor DJ, Wooley SE: The crystalline composition of prostatic calculi. Brit J Urol 46:533, 1974. 7

16...
Injuries to the
Genitourinary Tract

EMERGENCY MANAGEMENT

Orkin has evolved a method of examining the severely injured patient from the urologic point of view. These steps are never contraindicated and contribute greatly to the early diagnosis of urologic injuries, thus materially decreasing the mortality and morbidity rates.

If possible, after shock and hemorrhage have been treated, a complete description of the accident should be obtained from the patient or from an observer. The site of injury and the principal location of the pain should be ascertained. Hematuria, oliguria, or anuria requires careful attention. Blood from the urethra, unassociated with urination, suggests urethral injury distal to the external urinary sphincter.

Evidence of trauma to the kidneys, ureters, bladder, or urethra must be sought. Significant signs of injury include ecchymoses over the various organs, local tenderness, masses (from bleeding or urinary extravasation), blood from the urethra, and the passage of bloody urine. Injuries to the external genitalia should be obvious. Abdominal paracentesis should be performed if intraperitoneal hemorrhage is suspected. Frequent careful examinations are essential to discover rapidly enlarging masses, which may represent profuse bleeding (as from a lacerated kidney).

Rectal examination must be made and repeated. It may reveal upward displacement of the prostate if the gland has been torn from the membranous urethra. Swelling and bogginess of the tissues about the urethra suggest extravasation.

X-rays should be made when the patient can be moved. A plain film of the abdomen is invaluable. A fractured pelvis is often associated with urethral or vesical injury; fracture of the lower ribs or transverse processes of the upper lumbar vertebrae is often seen with injury to the kidney. Extravasation of blood or urine from an injured kidney will be revealed by a large area of grayness in the vicinity of the kidney and obliteration of the renal and psoas shadows.

Special Examinations

Instrumental examination should be made as symptoms indicate and the patient's condition warrants. No inflexible rules can be made about when these should be performed; the physician must carefully evaluate each patient.

A. Catheterization and X-Ray Examinations: The following steps should be performed in the sequence given.

1. Catheterization—An attempt should be made to confirm the continuity of the urethra by passing a urethral catheter. Microscopic blood found in the urine is of no significance (catheter trauma), but grossly bloody urine means injury to the urinary tract. If the catheter cannot be passed into the bladder, urethrograms should be made.

2. Excretory urograms—The catheter should then be clamped and excretory urograms taken unless significant hypotension is present, in which case renal blood flow is impaired and visualization of the kidneys poor or absent. Infusion urography (the technic of choice) may reveal lack of excretion by one kidney, extravasation of opaque fluid from a tear in any of the urinary organs, or blood clots if there is hemorrhage into the hollow excretory passages.

3. Retrograde cystograms—Retrograde filling of the bladder should then be done by instilling at least 350 ml of radiopaque fluid through the catheter. An x-ray film of the bladder area is then taken. The catheter is opened and the fluid allowed to drain. Films taken at this time will reveal extravasation posterior to the bladder.

4. Urethrograms—The catheter should then be withdrawn into the urethra and 20–30 ml of opaque material again instilled. It should not contain lubricating jelly, for its extravasation will cause increased fibrosis with healing. Appropriate x-ray films may reveal periurethral extravasation or a collection of fluid about the prostate or anterior to the bladder. If a catheter cannot be successfully passed, a urethrogram should be made as the catheter is withdrawn from the point of obstruction.

B. Cystoscopy and Retrograde Urography: These examinations are seldom needed but should be done when more information is needed and if the condition of the patient warrants it.

C. Indwelling Catheter: An indwelling catheter should be left in the bladder. A small tear in the urethra or bladder, if missed on the above examinations, may heal without complications. It is essential for monitoring renal perfusion if the patient is in shock.

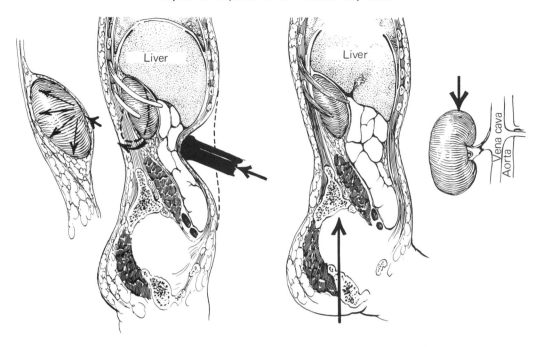

Figure 16—1. Mechanisms of renal injury. *Left:* Direct blow to abdomen. Smaller drawing shows force of blow radiating from the renal hilum. *Right:* Falling on buttocks from a height (contrecoup of kidney). Smaller drawing shows direction of force exerted upon the kidney from above. Tear of renal pedicle.

INJURIES TO THE KIDNEY

Traumatic injuries to the kidney are not common, but they are potentially serious and may be complicated by injuries to other organs or structures (eg, liver, spleen). They occur most commonly during athletic activities or in industrial or traffic accidents. Ninety percent occur in men. Mild trauma may rupture an abnormal kidney (eg, hydronephrosis, Wilms's tumor), especially in children.

Etiology (Fig 16—1)

The most common mode of injury is direct trauma to the abdomen, flank, or back. Indirect ("contrecoup") injury, caused by falling from a height and landing on the feet or buttocks, is less common, as are injuries caused by bullets or knives. On rare occasion, acute abdominal muscle contractions have caused a hydronephrotic kidney to burst.

Pathogenesis

The mechanics of renal lacerations are explained by the fact that the kidney contains a large amount of fluid, ie, urine and blood. The force of a sudden blow to the kidney is therefore transmitted equally throughout its tissues. The fibrous capsule which surrounds the kidney does to some extent protect the parenchyma from splitting.

The relative rarity of serious renal injury is due to the fact that the kidneys are protected by the rib cage and by the heavy muscles of the back. Furthermore, the kidneys are mobile in their adipose beds and are thus able to absorb the shock of a blow.

Pathology & Classification (Fig 16—2)

A. Early Pathologic Findings: Lacerations usually occur transverse to the long axis of the kidney or tend to radiate from the hilus. Renal injuries are classified pathologically as follows:

1. Simple bruising and ecchymosis—Contusion or bruising of the renal parenchyma is the most common lesion.

2. Hematoma—If, in association with contusion, the renal capsule is ruptured, a small perirenal hematoma may form.

3. Fissures—Incomplete fissures of the parenchyma may occur. If they involve the renal pelvis only, hematuria without perinephric hematoma occurs. If the renal capsule is torn, a large perirenal hematoma may develop. Hematuria is usually microscopic.

4. Lacerations—If the laceration extends through capsule and pelvis, extravasation of both blood and urine occurs. Hematuria may be marked. Tears in the renal pelvis or ureter lead to urinary extravasation with only slight bleeding. This is rare as an isolated lesion.

5. Rupture of the renal vascular pedicle—This causes massive bleeding which may prove rapidly fatal. Traumatic thrombosis of the renal artery has been reported.

6. Other pathologic lesions associated with renal lacerations include peritoneal tears with intraperitoneal bleeding, other visceral injuries, and fractures of the spine or ribs.

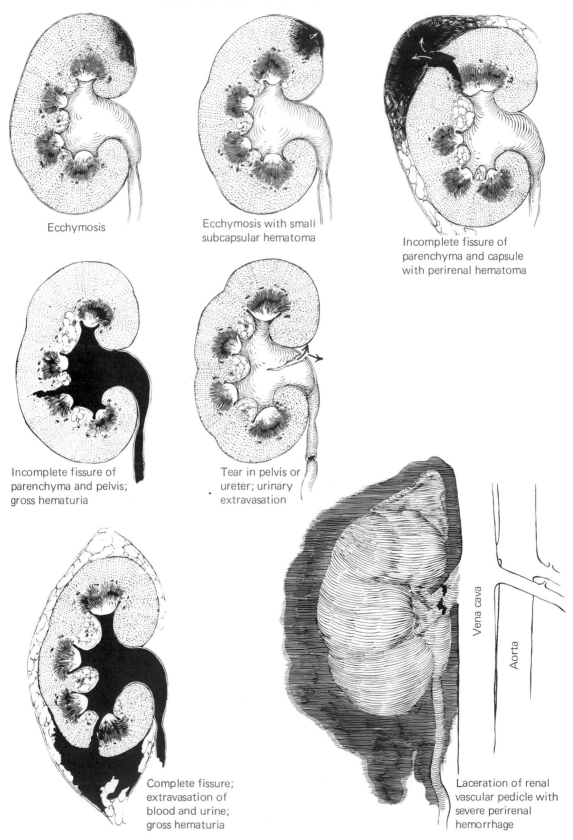

Ecchymosis

Ecchymosis with small subcapsular hematoma

Incomplete fissure of parenchyma and capsule with perirenal hematoma

Incomplete fissure of parenchyma and pelvis; gross hematuria

Tear in pelvis or ureter; urinary extravasation

Complete fissure; extravasation of blood and urine; gross hematuria

Vena cava

Aorta

Laceration of renal vascular pedicle with severe perirenal hemorrhage

Figure 16—2. Types and degrees of renal injury.

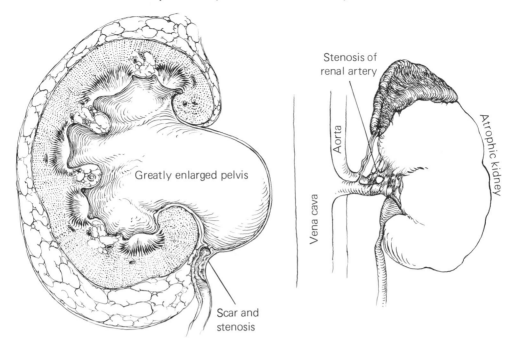

Figure 16—3. Late pathology. *Left:* Ureteropelvic stenosis with hydronephrosis secondary to fibrosis from extravasation of blood and urine. *Right:* Atrophy of kidney caused by injury (stenosis) of arterial blood supply.

B. Late Pathologic Findings: (Fig 16–3)

1. Hydronephrosis and infection—At times the perirenal tissues will undergo fibrosis following extravasation of blood or urine, and ureteral obstruction may develop; this leads to hydronephrosis. Renal infection may then follow.

2. Atrophy or fibrosis—If the blood supply to the organ is impaired (rupture, thrombosis), atrophy is to be expected. Renovascular hypertension may develop. Renal lacerations heal by fibrosis; scar formation may be extensive if vascular damage was great or bleeding extensive.

3. A few cases of renal arteriovenous fistula have been reported.

C. Spontaneous Cessation of Bleeding: If bleeding stops spontaneously, the hematoma may absorb, become infected, or liquefy. The blood in the latter case is then absorbed and a collection of clear amber fluid remains (ie, perirenal cyst).

Clinical Findings

Gross hematuria following any injury means trauma to the urinary tract. Signs and symptoms localized to one flank and the finding of impaired function of that kidney are strongly suggestive. Extravasation of opaque medium, as shown on x-ray films, is diagnostic.

A. Symptoms: A history or evidence of physical injury is usually present. Pain in the renal area may be obscured by the severity of other injuries (eg, fractures or injury to other viscera). Gross hematuria, not necessarily proportionate to the severity of the injury, is usually noted with the first voiding. It may be intermittent or continuous. Nausea, vomiting, and abdom-

inal distention due to intestinal ileus are common in the presence of retroperitoneal bleeding. Urinary retention may occur from clots in the bladder. There may be symptoms of injuries to other organs.

B. Signs: Shock or signs of hemorrhage may be found with severe renal injury or in the presence of multiple injuries. Ecchymosis may be noted over the flank or back. Local tenderness is present. A mass in the flank may be caused by extravasation of blood or urine, but if the overlying peritoneum has been torn these fluids may leak into the peritoneal cavity; hence, no flank mass develops. If local tenderness precludes careful palpation, percussion is invaluable. Rigidity of the abdominal muscles on the affected side and rebound tenderness are common. Abdominal distention and hypoperistalsis are to be expected. The ipsilateral testicle may be hypersensitive. The possibility of injuries to organs of the chest or of the abdomen should be explored. Fracture of the pelvis should cause one to suspect injury to the bladder or urethra. Oliguria may accompany the hypotensive phase of shock.

C. Laboratory Findings: The hematocrit, especially when followed serially, is of the greatest importance; progressive anemia means progressive hemorrhage which may require heroic surgical intervention. Hematuria is present in almost all cases. It is usually marked at first. Infection may be found later if ureteral obstruction develops.

D. X-Ray Findings: A plain film of the abdomen may prove quite helpful. It may show increased grayness of the renal area, loss of renal and psoas shadows, scoliosis of the spine with concavity on the affected side; fractures of the transverse processes, spine, lower ribs, or pelvis; and changes in the bowel pattern compatible with paralytic ileus.

An upright film, if it can be taken, may reveal gas under the diaphragm because of rupture of the intestinal tract.

In the face of hypotension, infusion urography is the method of choice for visualizing the upper urinary tract. These should be obtained as soon as practicable (Fig 16–4). They may show a normal kidney on the opposite side (on more than one occasion a solitary kidney has been removed because of injury); normal function and configuration, if injury is minimal; delayed visualization, if injury (or hypotension) is present; deformed renal pelvis or calyces, if lacerations (or blood clots) have occurred; extravasation of dye within the renal shadow or into the perirenal space; and displacement or deformity of the pelvis or ureter from extrarenal extravasation of blood or urine. Nonvisualization does not necessarily mean severe damage. Lack of function may be secondary to shock or reflex in origin, even though damage is minimal.

Retrograde urograms delineate the degree of injury quite clearly, but they are seldom needed. In case of doubt about the degree of injury, particularly of the major renal arteries, angiography should be done. Greater detail is gained if the selective technic is used. If splenic or hepatic injury is suspected, a selective angiogram of the celiac axis will reveal it.

E. Renal Scanning: Rectilinear scanning of the kidneys with ^{203}Hg has proved helpful in judging renal blood flow and tubular function. Lack of uptake implies injury or laceration of the renal artery. Areas of decreased activity are compatible with renal contusion. Absence of uptake in one renal pole suggests its amputation. The gamma camera affords more information, however. In addition to the changes observed with mercury, the hippurate shows areas of decreased or absent function as well as perirenal extravasation of the radioactive urine. Technetium study reveals absence of perfusion of blood into the kidney with injury to the renal artery or localized absence of activity if the kidney is fragmented (Fig 8–7).

F. Instrumental Examination: Cystoscopy and ureteral catheterization may be necessary. If excretory urography shows the contralateral kidney to be normal, there is no need to catheterize that side.

Differential Diagnosis

Trauma to the lumbar muscles or fractures of ribs, spine, or transverse processes may cause local symptoms suggesting renal injury. Hematuria is absent and urograms normal.

Complications

A. Early: The immediate complication of importance is perirenal hemorrhage, which may cause rapid exsanguination. The patient with an injured kidney must be observed closely. Blood pressure, pulse, and hematocrit should be taken frequently. Evidence of an enlarging mass must be sought. It is often helpful to outline a mass with ink on the skin so its progress can

be followed. It must be remembered, however, that serious renal trauma may be accompanied by a peritoneal tear which may allow the escape of blood and urine into the peritoneal cavity. Hence, the expected mass will not develop. In 70–80% of cases, bleeding will stop spontaneously. If the kidney has been badly fractured, the degree of bleeding will warrant early surgery. Secondary bleeding and its accompanying shock may develop as late as 1–2 weeks following the injury.

Even though the extravasation of urine and the bleeding cease, secondary perirenal infection may supervene. Perirenal blood will cause fever to 37.5–38.5 °C (99.5–101.3 °F). Higher temperatures suggest infection. Increased pain and tenderness are to be expected. Abdominal muscle rigidity may become marked; rebound tenderness may develop. Edema of the skin over the back may be observed.

B. Later: The patient should be reexamined (including excretory urograms) after an interval of 3–6 months to determine the presence of progressive hydronephrosis from periureteral fibrosis, which may occur in the healing process; renal atrophy, if the blood supply has been impaired; and perirenal cyst, if complete absorption of the hematoma (or urinary extravasation) does not occur.

If thrombosis of the renal artery develops, hypertension secondary to the renal ischemia may supervene.

Treatment

A. Emergency Measures: Treat shock and hemorrhage.

B. Surgical Measures: Since two-thirds of injured kidneys are merely contused, bleeding will cease spontaneously. Even some of the ruptured organs will heal without surgical care (Fig 16–4). Ten to 20% of cases may require early surgical intervention because of alarming hemorrhage. Drainage of the perirenal space, suture of the renal laceration, or partial or total nephrectomy may be necessary.

C. General Measures: Opiates for pain should be withheld until the completion of the diagnostic steps; they may mask accompanying intra-abdominal or pulmonary lesions. Bed rest is indicated until hematuria has ceased and local signs of injury have largely subsided.

D. Treatment of Complications: Perinephric infection requires surgical drainage. Late complications may require nephrectomy or repair of secondary ureteral obstruction.

Prognosis

In contusions of the kidney, the prognosis is excellent; they heal spontaneously and leave no demonstrable renal lesion. When rupture occurs, serious complications may supervene. It is important to follow these cases by periodic urography and blood pressure determinations for many months.

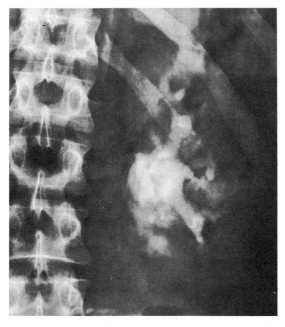 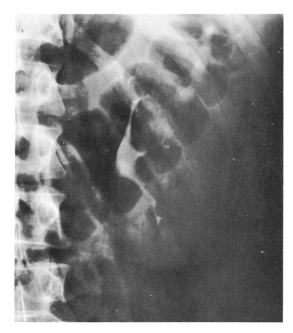

Figure 16—4. Renal injury. *Left:* Excretory urogram showing extravasation of radiopaque fluid. Conservative treatment. *Right:* Excretory urogram, same patient, 10 days later; normal urogram.

INJURIES TO THE URETER

Injuries to the ureter from external violence or penetrating wounds are relatively rare. They usually occur accidentally during difficult and extensive gynecologic operations or during abdominoperineal resection of the rectum. They may also occur from cystoscopic ureteral manipulation.

Etiology

A large pelvic tumor may displace a ureter far from its usual site. In this instance the surgeon may inadvertently cut it. Marked inflammatory adhesions may make the ureter hard to identify, in which case it may be easily injured during surgery. If a ureter is invaded by tumor of the rectum, colon, or ovary, it may have to be resected with the tumor. Extensive lymph node dissection or x-ray therapy to the area may impair ureteral blood supply, and necrosis may follow.

A ureter may be injured by blunt trauma or a penetrating object (eg, a bullet), causing urinary extravasation. Injury to neighboring viscera must be sought. The ureter may be perforated by the cystoscopist, particularly if the ureteral wall is diseased. This occurs most commonly in association with manipulation of a ureteral stone.

Pathogenesis & Pathology

If the ureter is completely or partially divided during surgery but the surgeon is unaware of the accident, urinary extravasation will occur. Extravasation may be intraperitoneal or extraperitoneal. A urinary fistula may form between the severed ureter and the surgical wound or the vagina, or an enlarging collection of urine at the site of the injury will become evident. If the urine becomes infected, signs of peritonitis or cellulitis will develop. If uninfected, urine in the free peritoneal cavity may cause few symptoms other than gradual abdominal distention from the urine itself. Some degree of ureteral compression or stenosis is to be expected with ureteral injury; this leads to hydronephrosis.

Should the ureter be inadvertently sutured or ligated, progressive hydronephrosis will develop. Renal infection may then occur. Because of ischemia, the ureter may slough at the site of ligation. Delayed extravasation or fistula formation may then be observed.

Clinical Findings

A. Symptoms: If the accident is not recognized at the time of surgery, the patient usually complains of pain in the flank and lower abdominal quadrant. Vomiting may be severe. Paralytic ileus is often marked. The patient will become quite ill if pyelonephritis or peritonitis complicates the picture. Urine may suddenly begin to drain through the abdominal or perirenal wound or through the vagina, which may relieve all the foregoing symptoms. Anuria following pelvic surgery suggests bilateral ureteral injury or occlusion.

B. Signs: Abdominal distention and lack of peristalsis are evident if ileus is marked. Signs of peritonitis (rebound tenderness) may be noted if there is leakage of urine into the free peritoneal cavity. Urine may be seen draining from the surgical wound or vagina. If

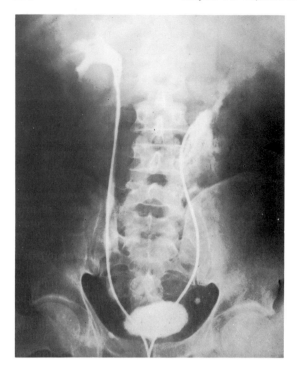 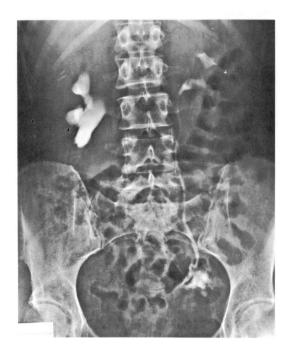

Figure 16—5. Ureteral injury. *Left:* Perforation of left upper ureter by catheter. *Right:* Carcinoma of cervix; preoperative irradiation therapy and Wertheim operation. Partial ureteral obstruction on right (hydronephrosis), ureterovaginal fistula on left. Site of ureteral fistula demonstrated.

there is any question about whether the fluid is actually urine, the patient can be given 0.2 g of methylene blue by mouth or 5 ml of indigo carmine IV. The injection of the latter causes transient hypertension. Both are excreted by the kidney and stain the urine. Vaginal examination may reveal the site of the urinary fistula.

C. Laboratory Findings: Blood count and urinalysis contribute little to the diagnosis. The PSP may be slightly depressed if one ureter is occluded. The serum creatinine will rise quickly if bilateral ureteral obstruction is present.

D. X-Ray Findings: A plain film of the abdomen may reveal a large area of increased density in the region of the injured ureter due to a large collection of extravasated urine.

Excretory urograms may demonstrate extravasation of the radiopaque fluid at the site of injury (Fig 16—5). When the injury is near the bladder, however, it may be confused with a vesicovaginal fistula. Ureteral injuries are usually associated with some degree of ureteral obstruction; thus, hydronephrosis and hydroureter down to the point of trauma are to be expected.

If the ureter is completely occluded as a result of recent injury, no radiopaque material will collect in the renal pelvis, but progressive increase in density of the renal parenchyma may be observed on the later films.

Retrograde ureterograms will show the site and degree of the injury.

E. Isotope Scanning: (See Chapter 8.) If one

ureter has been ligated, the radioisotope renogram will show a further increase of counts, rather than a drop-off after the secretory phase due to accumulation of urine in the renal pelvis (Fig 8—8). The scintillation camera, using ^{131}I, will show slow transport of the isotope to the pelvis where the photon activity will become intense because of stasis.

F. Instrumental Examination: Cystoscopy and ureteral catheterization demonstrate patency or obstruction and afford ureterograms and urograms (Fig 16—5).

Differential Diagnosis

Postoperative peritonitis may be mimicked by ureteral injury if there is leakage of infected urine into the peritoneal cavity. Ureteral catheterization or excretory urograms should make the differentiation clear.

Oliguria may be due to dehydration or bilateral but incomplete ureteral injury. A survey of fluid and electrolyte intake and output (urinary, gastrointestinal, and invisible losses), body weight, PSP test, hematocrit, and the urinary specific gravity should establish the diagnosis with regard to dehydration. Immediate total anuria means bilateral obstruction. The isotope renogram or the camera scan should contribute useful information.

Acute renal failure, due to shock or transfusion with incompatible blood, also causes oliguria. It may be differentiated from surgical ureteral injury by finding no more than a trace of PSP excretion in 1 hour, and fixation of the urinary chloride concentration at 30–40 mEq/liter. In case of doubt, ureteral catheterization will be definitive. Isotope studies are also helpful.

Evisceration may be confused with ureteral injury since the early sign of eventration is the onset of profuse drainage of clear, odorless transudate from the wound which may be mistaken for urine. In case of doubt, the skin should be opened widely and the peritoneal rent sought.

Complications

Complications of ureteral injury include urinary fistula, ureteral stenosis with hydronephrosis, renal infection; peritonitis, if urine drains into the peritoneal cavity; and uremia, if the injury is bilateral.

Treatment

Reparative surgery should be undertaken as soon as the injury is recognized. In simple perforation from a ureteral catheter or other instrument, surgical drainage is usually not necessary. The ureteral wall will heal spontaneously.

A. Immediate: The ureter should not be tied off. The ureteral tip usually undergoes necrosis, and fistula results. If the tie holds, progressive hydronephrosis is inevitable.

The following surgical methods are available if the injury is recognized when it occurs:

1. Anastomosis of the 2 ends over a catheter or "T" tube.

2. Implantation of the proximal end of the ureter into the bladder (ureteroneocystostomy), or into a tube formed from a bladder flap if a segment of the ureter has been resected. The injured ureter can also be anastomosed into the side of the contralateral ureter.

3. If a bladder flap tube cannot be made long enough, the defect can be replaced with an isolated section of ileum.

4. Temporary ureterostomy or nephrostomy, if the patient's condition does not permit primary anastomosis, preserves kidney function and permits elective repair later.

B. Late: If the injury is discovered during the postoperative period, early intervention is indicated before the inflammatory reaction becomes severe or fibrosis occurs. If delayed ureteral repair is attempted, the methods available are end-to-end anastomosis, implantation of the ureter into the bladder or into a bladder flap, transureteroureterostomy, and replacement of the damaged ureter with an isolated ileal segment. Autotransplantation of the kidney into the iliac fossa has been accomplished for high ureteral injury. Nephrectomy may be indicated if the other kidney is normal.

Prevention

The surgeon must be careful to identify the ureters when extensive pelvic surgery is done. In case of doubt, the surgeon should perform a high longitudinal ureterotomy and pass a catheter down the ureter. This area should be drained extraperitoneally. In difficult cases, preliminary to surgery, indwelling ureteral catheters should be placed so that the ureters may be easily felt. The insignificant risks in such a maneuver are greatly outweighed by the advantages.

Prognosis

Prognosis is best in those injuries repaired at the time they are sustained. Patients operated upon within the first week following injury usually achieve good ureteral repair. After marked fibrosis has developed, the results are not very good; nephrectomy may be required.

INJURIES TO THE BLADDER

The urinary bladder may be injured by external forces; during surgery, including accidental incision in pelvic surgery or in the repair of hernia; and in transurethral manipulations.

Rupture of the bladder caused by a direct blow presupposes a bladder distended with urine. It can also be perforated by bony spicules from a fractured pelvis.

Pathogenesis & Pathology

A sudden blow to the full bladder causes a sharp rise in intravesical pressure; this may either contuse the wall or split it (Fig 16–6). With such an injury, the extravasation of urine is usually intraperitoneal. If the vesical contents are infected, death from peritonitis will occur unless the laceration is closed surgically or seals itself spontaneously. If the urine is sterile, few symptoms may develop immediately although anuria with uremia becomes obvious and "ascites" develops as the urine progressively fills the peritoneal cavity. If this urine becomes infected (following catheterization or cystoscopy or from bacteria carried there by the blood stream), true peritonitis supervenes. A few cases of spontaneous rupture have been reported. This presupposes obstruction distal to the bladder.

Vesical lacerations secondary to fracture of the pelvis cause extraperitoneal extravasation of urine. If this urine is infected or later becomes so, a spreading cellulitis develops and death occurs unless adequate drainage is afforded. Rupture and perforation of the bladder, then, are fatal injuries unless treated promptly. The most common cause of death in this instance is hemorrhage secondary to the pelvic fracture.

Clinical Findings

A history of an injury or blow to the lower abdomen followed by low abdominal pain and hematuria is strongly suggestive of vesical injury. Fracture of the pelvis is commonly accompanied by injury to the bladder. The finding of suprapubic tenderness or a mass is suggestive; signs of peritonitis may be elicited. Cystography is the most dependable test. If, however, clinical judgment suggests the presence of vesical

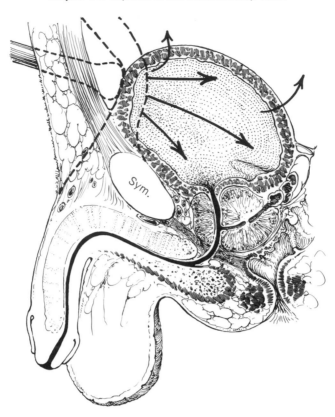

Figure 16—6. Mechanism of vesical injury. A direct blow over the full bladder causes increased intravesical pressure. If the bladder ruptures, it will usually rupture into the peritoneal cavity.

trauma, even a normal cystogram should be ignored.

A. Symptoms: There is usually a history of injury. If the patient can urinate, hematuria is to be expected, but he may not be able to urinate at all. Pain is present low in the abdomen. Pain in the shoulder may be noted if there is urine in the peritoneal cavity. High fever suggests infection.

B. Signs: Shock may be profound, especially if multiple injuries have been suffered. There may be evidence of local trauma such as a bullet or knife wound or ecchymosis. Marked tenderness in the suprapubic area is to be expected. There may be rebound tenderness if the laceration involves the peritoneum. Spasm of the muscles of the lower abdomen occurs even though the extravasation is perivesical. A board-like abdomen suggests intraperitoneal rupture. The skin over the symphysis commonly becomes quite cool immediately after extraperitoneal rupture occurs. A large suprapubic mass may be felt or percussed as the perivesical collection of fluid develops. This will contain blood, urine, and sometimes pus. Rectal examination may reveal a large boggy mass obliterating the normal landmarks. Evidence of other injuries is usually present.

C. Laboratory Findings: The hematocrit may demonstrate anemia from loss of blood or hemoconcentration from shock. The white blood count and neutrophils are increased. Urinalysis reveals hematuria,

either gross or microscopic. The presence of bacteria means infection, either preexisting or new. If a significant amount of urine escapes into the peritoneal cavity, the serum BUN:creatinine ratio is significantly increased.

D. X-Ray Findings: A plain film may reveal fractures of the pelvic bones. About 15% of patients with a fractured pelvis will have a vesical injury (Fig 16—7). Increased grayness from a perivesical collection of urine and blood may be seen. Excretory urograms will be helpful in surveying the kidneys for damage. Extravasation of the opaque material may be noted in the perivesical tissues. The bladder may be displaced or compressed by extravesical blood or urine.

A cystogram is the most dependable test for vesical injury (Fig 16—7). Instill 350—400 ml of radiopaque fluid and take anteroposterior and oblique films. Then drain the vesical contents and take another film. This may reveal small amounts of extravasated fluid lying behind the bladder or in the cul-de-sac.

E. Instrumental Examination: The passage of a catheter will detect possible injury to the urethra. If an injured person cannot void, he should be catheterized. The presence of bloody urine must be investigated.

If 350—500 ml of sterile solution is instilled into the bladder and the full amount is recovered, the bladder is probably intact. On occasion, however, this may afford erroneous information; omentum or blood

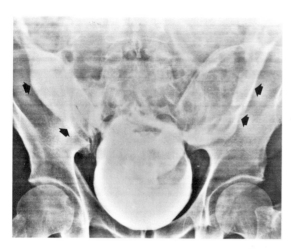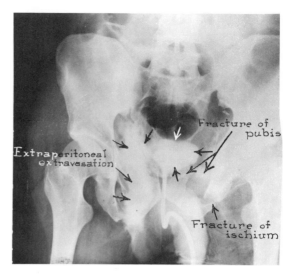

Figure 16—7. Vesical injuries. *Left:* Retrograde cystogram showing intraperitoneal extravasation. Note radiopaque material in both lumbar gutters. *Right:* Retrograde cystogram showing extraperitoneal rupture of the bladder secondary to fracture of the pelvis.

clot may temporarily plug the laceration.

Cystoscopy is usually not very helpful. Bleeding and clots may obscure vision, and a laceration may be missed.

Differential Diagnosis

Hematuria and signs of injury to abdominal organs can also arise from an injured kidney. A mass and tenderness in the flank and evidence of fractures in the renal area are suggestive of renal injury. Changes on a plain film of the abdomen or on excretory urograms should establish the diagnosis. A normal cystogram will relieve any lingering doubt.

Urethral injury may accompany fractures of the pelvis. Exploration of the urethra with a catheter is helpful, and a urethrogram will show extravasation through the injured wall.

Complications

In extraperitoneal rupture, the extravasation of large amounts of blood and urine is often complicated by infection. If untreated, a necrotizing phlegmon ensues; the mortality rate in this instance is high. Abdominal or peritoneal fistulas may develop.

In intraperitoneal rupture, if the urine becomes infected generalized peritonitis occurs. If this is untreated, death is to be expected.

Treatment

A. Emergency Measures: Treat shock and hemorrhage.

B. Specific Measures:

1. **Extraperitoneal rupture**—If the rupture is extraperitoneal, the site of the injury should be drained surgically. Urologists as a rule favor suprapubic cystostomy as a more reliable method than catheterization for keeping the bladder empty and at rest. The perito-

neum should be opened and intraperitoneal organs explored for associated injury.

2. **Intraperitoneal rupture**—When the tear is intraperitoneal, it should be closed transperitoneally. If the point of rupture is inaccessible, suprapubic cystostomy permits healing without complications. Extravasated fluid in the peritoneal cavity should be aspirated. Injury to other organs should be sought.

3. **Fractured pelvis**—If there is evidence of a fractured pelvis and massive hemorrhage, a transfemoral iliac angiogram should be done to seek the site of bleeding. The catheter can then be passed into the bleeding artery and occluded by injecting clotted autogenous blood into the catheter.

Prognosis

If the diagnosis is made and proper treatment instituted within 6—12 hours after the injury, morbidity and mortality will be minimal. If treatment is delayed for a few days, perivesical infection or peritonitis may develop and may not be controllable; the number of deaths under these circumstances will be significant.

INJURIES TO THE URETHRA

The various parts of the urethra can be contused, lacerated, or avulsed. Injuries to the deep urethra are the most serious and are often associated with fracture of the pelvis. Urethral stricture is a common complication.

Because treatment and sequelae vary with the nature and site of the trauma, these injuries are discussed as injuries to the membranous urethra, the bulbous urethra, and the pendulous urethra.

1. INJURIES TO
THE MEMBRANOUS URETHRA

Etiology

The urogenital diaphragm (ie, triangular ligament) encloses the membranous urethra, Cowper's glands, and most of the external urinary sphincter. It is firmly attached to the pubic bone. In pelvic fractures, this fascia may be torn, shearing off the prostate from the membranous urethra. Bony spicules may perforate the urethra, and the bladder also may be lacerated.

Pathogenesis & Pathology (Fig 16–8)

These injuries usually occur in association with trauma to other organs or structures. They occur just above the urogenital diaphragm. This causes extravasation of blood and urine into the periprostatic and perivesical tissues. Only if the triangular ligament is badly damaged will the extravasation present in the perineum. The extravasated urine leads to a necrotizing phlegmon which may become infected. If this is not properly treated, early death may ensue from sepsis.

Clinical Findings

A. **Symptoms**: Urethral bleeding may be noted. A history of injury, usually severe, is always obtained. Pain is present in the perineum or low in the abdomen. The patient may be unable to void.

B. **Signs**: Urethral bleeding or hematuria is present. There may be a mass in the suprapubic area. The area may be dull to percussion. Suprapubic tenderness may be marked. This may be due to extravasation or to a fracture of the pelvis with associated hematoma. Rectal examination may reveal a large boggy mass of extravasated blood and urine. The prostate may be dislodged upward if it has been avulsed from the membranous urethra (Fig 16–8).

C. **Laboratory Findings**: There may be anemia from hemorrhage or hemoconcentration from shock. The white blood count is elevated, especially if infection has supervened. The urine usually is grossly bloody. In the case of minor contusions, hematuria may be only microscopic.

D. **X-Ray Findings**: A fracture of the pelvis may be shown on a plain film. Radiopaque fluid (20–30 ml) should be instilled into the catheter passed to the point of arrest. An x-ray will show the site of extravasation (Fig 16–9). If the catheter passes to the bladder, a cystogram will demonstrate vesical injury.

E. **Instrumental Examination**: If a catheter can be passed to the bladder, the urethral lesion is minor. In more extensive injuries, the catheter may be arrested at the site of injury.

Differential Diagnosis

Vesical and urethral injuries often occur following severe trauma and fracture of the pelvis. Rectal examination may reveal that the prostate is riding free from the membranous urethra. In the latter instance, a catheter will not pass. X-rays following instillation of radiopaque fluid will reveal the true site of injury.

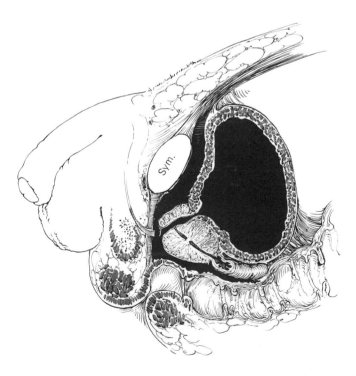

Figure 16–8. Injury to the membranous urethra. The prostate has been avulsed from the membranous urethra secondary to fracture of the pelvis. Extravasation occurs above the triangular ligament and is periprostatic and perivesical.

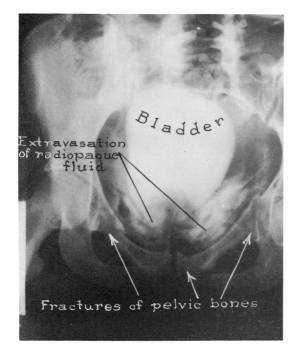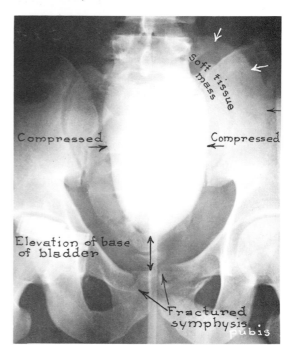

Figure 16—9. Injury to the membranous urethra. *Left:* Retrograde cystogram showing periprostatic extravasation; laceration of membranous urethra with fracture of pelvis. *Right:* Retrograde cystogram showing elevation and lateral compression of bladder due to periprostatic and perivesical extravasation of blood and urine; laceration of membranous urethra from fracture of pelvis.

In injury to the bulbous urethra there is perineal swelling due to blood, urine, or both. A urethrogram is diagnostic.

Complications

Hemorrhage about the prostate and bladder may be marked in the early stages. It usually emanates from the fractured pelvis. Urinary extravasation may occur if the patient is unable to urinate. This may lead to severe sepsis if diagnosis is late.

Urethral stricture is a common late complication, particularly if proper treatment is not instituted early. Sexual impotence (loss of erection) develops in one-third of men, probably as a result of nerve injury, though Gibson (1970) believes it is caused by thrombosis of the arterioles to the corpora cavernosa. Impaired control of urination occasionally results. This may be due to direct injury to the external sphincter or may be secondary to nerve damage.

Treatment

A. Emergency Measures: Treat shock and hemorrhage.

B. Specific Measures: If a urethral catheter of adequate size (22—24F) can be passed to the bladder, it should be left in place for 14—21 days. Simple lacerations usually heal well with only this simple splinting. If a catheter cannot be passed to the bladder, surgical intervention is imperative. There is no unanimity of opinion about definitive treatment. Each of the follow-

ing methods of management has its proponents:

1. Suture the injured urethra and place a splinting urethral catheter in the bladder (Fig 16—10). Place a cystostomy tube. The urethral catheter should be left in for 3 weeks (Pierce).

2. If repair by suture cannot be done, an indwelling Foley catheter should be placed through the urethra into the bladder; 0.5 kg of traction upon the external end of the catheter will bring about apposition of the ruptured urethra (Fig 16—10). Drainage by cystostomy tube is essential. The urethral catheter should be left in place for 3 weeks (Gibson, 1974; Meyers & DeWeerd, 1972). An alternative is to place sutures in the prostatic tissue lateral to the apex and pass them out through the perineum with the catheter in place. Traction is exerted by the pull of rubber bands taped to the thighs.

3. Morehouse, Belitsky, & MacKinnon (1972) recommend immediate cystostomy only with reconstruction of the urethra later. They feel that complications (impotence, incontinence, and stricture) occur less often and are less severe with this technic.

4. The retropubic area must be drained.

C. General Measures: If treatment has been instituted late and sepsis is already present, broad-spectrum antibiotics should be used as a lifesaving measure as well as to minimize fibrous reaction. Analgesics and sedation should be used as indicated.

D. Treatment of Complications: It must be assumed that all patients suffering from deep urethral

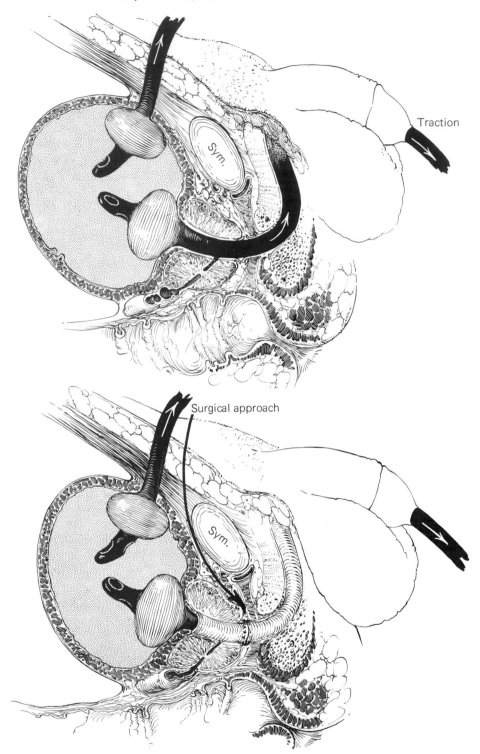

Figure 16—10. Methods of repair of injuries of the membranous urethra. ***Above:*** Retropubic exposure and suture of membranous urethra over an indwelling catheter; suprapubic cystostomy. ***Below:*** If suture of the urethra is not feasible, a Foley (self-retaining) catheter should be placed and traction exerted on the catheter in order to appose the ends of the divided urethra. Tying the ends of the 2 catheters together with braided silk will guard against dislodgment of the urethral catheter should its bag deflate.

injuries will develop strictures until proved otherwise. It is therefore necessary to get urethrograms or pass urethral sounds periodically for as long as 6–12 months in order to discover the development of a stricture. If stricture does occur, definitive treatment is required.

There is no treatment that will correct loss of erections. The implantation of a Silastic penile prosthesis should be considered (see under Impotence, Chapter 31). Little can be done for the patient with impaired sphincteric function. A condom collecting device may be necessary.

Prognosis

Unless other serious injuries have been sustained, the mortality rate for injury to the membranous urethra is quite low; this is true even though perivesical phlegmon has developed because of delayed treatment. The antibiotics are successful in combating this.

The most troublesome complication is urethral stricture, which may require the periodic passage of a sound for the rest of the patient's life. Surgical correction of the stricture may be necessary. If this is not done, chronic infection of the bladder and even of the kidneys may develop; vesical and renal stones may form because of stasis and complicating infection.

2. INJURIES TO THE BULBOUS URETHRA

Etiology

Injuries to the bulbous urethra, which lies just inferior to the urogenital diaphragm, may result from instrumentation but are most commonly caused by forcibly falling astride an object. The urethra is apt to be contused or lacerated (Fig 16–11).

Pathogenesis & Pathology

A. Contusion: If the urethra is only contused, some evidence of perineal hematoma may be noted. In all probability, this will resolve without sequelae. A large hematoma might require drainage. Mild stricture, caused by healing, may result from the fibrosis.

B. If laceration occurs, blood and urine extravasate into the perineum; if extravasation is extensive, it spreads to the scrotum and penis, then up the abdominal wall. It is limited by Colles' fascia (Figs 1–9 and 16–11). Serious infection ensues if diagnosis is late. If the laceration is untreated, stricture formation is inevitable.

Clinical Findings

A. Symptoms: A history of perineal injury, either external or by a urethral instrument, can usually be obtained. There is local pain and some bleeding from the external meatus. If a urethral tear is present, an attempt at urination may cause sudden perineal swelling from extravasation. If the patient is seen a few days after the accident, there may be symptoms of severe sepsis (eg, fever, prostration).

B. Signs: Some urethral bleeding may be seen. Its degree is not necessarily a measure of the severity of the injury. Local tenderness is present in the perineum. A large mass may be found locally. This may represent blood, urine, or both. If seen late, swelling and discoloration of the skin of the scrotum, penis, and lower abdominal wall may be noted. This represents extensive extravasation and at times inflammation.

C. Laboratory Findings: Anemia is not common, for blood loss is usually not excessive. The white count may be markedly elevated, particularly if secondary infection of the perineum, genitalia, and abdominal wall has developed. Blood is present in the urine if the patient is able to void.

D. X-Ray Findings: The instillation of 20–30 ml of radiopaque fluid into the urethra will demonstrate the site and degree of the injury (Fig 16–12).

E. Instrumental Examination: A catheter may pass to the bladder if the urethra is merely contused or lacerated on one side. If the catheter is arrested, the injury is more serious.

Differential Diagnosis

Laceration or avulsion of the membranous urethra often accompanies fracture of the pelvis. The extravasation of blood and urine in this type is almost always above the urogenital diaphragm, whereas that from the bulb is into the perineum and external genitalia. A urethrogram will answer the question.

Complications

Considerable bleeding from injury to the corpus spongiosum may occur early. If the urethra is ruptured, urinary extravasation occurs when the patient attempts to urinate.

Stricture at the site of trauma is a common late complication, particularly in the more severe injuries.

Treatment

A. Specific Measures:

1. Nonobstructed urethra—If the patient can void well and the perineal hematoma is not extensive, the injury should be left alone. The blood will almost surely be absorbed, and the contused urethra will heal. If the hematoma becomes infected, it should be drained. Later, urethral sounds must be passed or urethrograms done to be sure that stricture does not develop. If stricture should occur, periodic dilation or even surgical repair will be required (see Chapter 27).

2. Severe injuries—If there is urinary extravasation, or if urination is impossible, an attempt should be made to pass a catheter to the bladder. If this is successful, the catheter should be left in place for 3 weeks. If it is not successful (due to more severe urethral injury), surgical exploration and repair are required. A splinting catheter should be left in the urethra for 3 weeks.

3. Extensive extravasation—If urinary extravasation is extensive, these areas (perineum, scrotum, lower

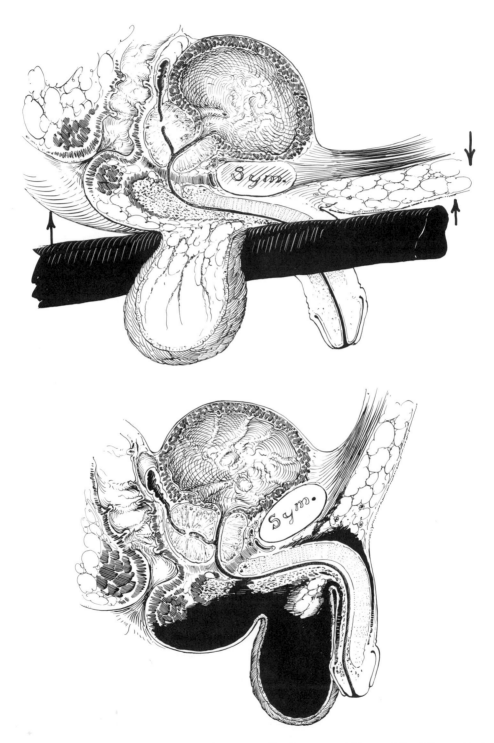

Figure 16–11. Injury to the bulbous urethra. *Above:* Mechanism: Usually a perineal blow or fall astride an object; crushing of urethra against inferior edge of symphysis pubis. *Below:* Extravasation of blood and urine enclosed within Colles' fascia (Fig 1–9).

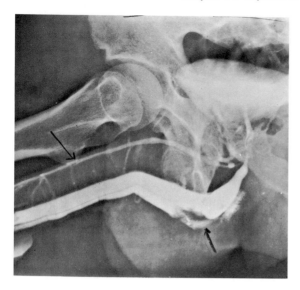

Figure 16–12. Urethral injury. Oblique urethrogram showing extravasation in region of bulbous urethra. Pressure injection caused radiopaque solution to enter venous system. (This is the mechanism for emboli if oily lubricants are injected into the urethra.)

abdominal wall) must also be drained. It is questionable, however, whether the radical drainage formerly prescribed is still necessary now that potent antibiotics are available.

The caliber of the urinary stream must be observed during the next few months. If stenosis develops, the stricture must be treated.

4. Very severe injuries—If the patient has been badly hurt, suprapubic cystostomy and drainage of the perineum may be all that can be accomplished initially; later it may be necessary to resect the stenotic portion of the urethra and anastomose its healthy ends. Postoperative stricture must be sought and, if present, treated.

B. General Measures: When the urethral injury is adjudged minor and no specific treatment is indicated, antimicrobial drugs are not warranted. If urinary extravasation has occurred, antimicrobials should be administered.

Prognosis

Mortality is low unless there are more severe injuries to other structures. Antibiotics and surgical drainage will almost always save the patient with urinary extravasation, even if it has been initially neglected.

Urethral stricture is the only serious complication. If this is not treated, urinary tract infection and its complications (stone, renal damage) may ensue.

3. INJURIES TO THE PENDULOUS URETHRA

Etiology

Injuries to the penile urethra from direct blows are not common since the penis, except during erection, tends to "ride" with a blow. The erect organ may, however, be fractured (rupture of the corpora cavernosa) and the urethra become torn.

The urethra is most often injured by injudicious instrumentation. The most common injury of this sort is the perforating injury that may result when a metal sound of small caliber is being passed to dilate a stricture. The pendulous urethra may also sustain injury from penetrating wounds.

Pathogenesis & Pathology

These injuries are usually mild and little more than contusions. Some periurethral bleeding may develop, but this is usually quickly absorbed. The urethra may be injured by the passage of the relatively large resectoscope (size 28F) used for transurethral prostatectomy. Postoperative stricture may ensue.

Clinical Findings

A. Symptoms and Signs: Some urethral bleeding is to be expected. Swelling of the pendulous portion of the penis is common.

B. Laboratory Findings: If the patient can urinate, red cells are found in the urine.

C. X-Ray Findings: A urethrogram may reveal the site of injury, although extravasation is rare with these injuries (Fig 16–13).

D. Instrumental Examination: Attempts to pass a catheter may fail if the laceration is extensive.

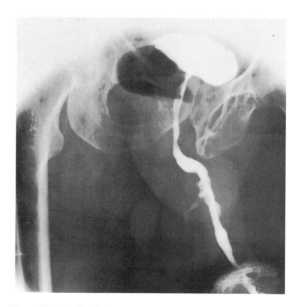

Figure 16–13. Urethral injury. Urethrogram showing extravasation of the radiopaque material from lacerated pendulous urethra at penoscrotal junction.

Differential Diagnosis

Swellings from lesions of the bulb are in the perineum; swellings from injuries to the distal urethra are local. In case of doubt, a urethrogram will demonstrate the site of the injury.

Complications

Large hematomas and urinary extravasation are not common unless the urethra has been badly torn. Urethral stenosis may develop as the urethra heals.

Treatment

A. Specific Measures: If urination proceeds normally, an indwelling catheter is not needed. Small hematomas will be absorbed. Large ones may require drainage. If bleeding is profuse, a catheter can be passed and the penis then tightly bandaged to prevent further bleeding. If a small amount of urine should pass into the tissues, it will be absorbed; if it is extensive, surgical drainage is indicated. When extravasation of urine occurs, a catheter should be passed to the bladder and left in place for 10 days. If the injury is severe and if passage of a catheter is unsuccessful, surgical repair of the injured urethra is indicated. A splinting catheter should be left in place for 14 days.

B. General Measures: Antibacterial drugs are not needed unless infection has occurred.

Prognosis

These injuries are usually not serious. The only sequel of note is urethral stricture, the complications of which can be serious. These include chronic infection of the urinary tract and urolithiasis.

INJURIES TO THE PENIS

The penis may be injured by a penetrating object (eg, knife, bullet) or by a blow when the organ is erect. The placement of a constricting band about the shaft (eg, metal washer, string, rubber band) can also cause injury from ischemia which may lead to gangrene. Self-emasculation is occasionally seen.

The skin may be lacerated or even avulsed if caught in machinery. One or more of the corpora can be ruptured, in which case profuse bleeding may occur beneath Colles' fascia; this may spread over the scrotum, perineum, and up over the lower abdomen. Pressure from swelling may lead to gangrene. Associated urethral injury is not uncommon.

The history of injury is usually obtainable. The skin may be lacerated or avulsed. Great swelling from bleeding may be evident. Edema distal to a constricting band may be marked. The bleeding from laceration or contusion will usually cease spontaneously. Large hematomas may require evacuation.

Constricting bodies must of course be removed. Immediate or late urethral injury should be sought. Extensive loss of skin will require skin grafting.

INJURIES TO THE SCROTUM

Local injuries or blows may cause ecchymosis or hematoma. They are not serious and heal spontaneously. Lacerations may need suture; avulsion will require skin grafts.

INJURIES TO THE TESTIS

Because of their mobility, the testes are seldom injured. If traumatized, the patient experiences severe pain. Nausea and vomiting are common, and shock may result. The injury may be a mild contusion or the testis may be lacerated, in which case bleeding into the tunica vaginalis (hematocele) may be profuse. Only in the latter case is surgical intervention required; suture of the tear is imperative.

On rare occasion, a severe local injury may dislocate the testicle into the abdomen, penis, perineum, or adjacent areas. Replacement in the scrotum requires surgical intervention.

Even mild wounds may result in thrombosis of blood vessels which leads to atrophy of the testis. Penetrating wounds will require closure of the scrotal and testicular incisions.

OBSTETRIC INJURIES TO THE URETHRA & BLADDER

If there is disproportion between the circumference of the baby's head and the mother's pelvis and if labor is therefore prolonged, urethral ischemia may occur. Necrosis may cause a urethrovaginal (or vesicovaginal) fistula. Improperly placed forceps may tear these urologic structures. Surgical repair is required.

Because of attenuation of supporting tissues of the urethra and base of the bladder during delivery, weakness of these structures develops. Thus the urethra and bladder sag into the vagina (urethrocele, cystocele), and stress incontinence may result. Operations to improve the support of the urethra and vesical base or to elevate and fix the bladder neck usually relieve this distressing symptom (see Chapter 26).

References

Emergency Management

Baker WNW, Mackie DB, Newcombe JF: Diagnostic paracentesis in the acute abdomen. Brit MJ 3:146, 1967.

Kaufman JJ, Brosman SA: Blunt injuries of the genitourinary tract. S Clin North America 52:747, 1972.

Lucey DT, Smith MJV: Initial diagnosis and management of urinary tract injuries. Clin Med 80:17, 1973.

Orkin LA: The diagnosis of urological trauma in the presence of other injuries. S Clin North America 33:1473, 1953.

Richter MW & others: Radiology of genitourinary trauma. Radiol Clin North America 11:593, 1973.

Injuries to the Kidney

Cass AS, Ireland GW: Renal injuries in children. J Trauma 14:719, 1974.

Champion H & others: Indications for early haemodialysis in multiple trauma. Lancet 1:1125, 1974.

Cosgrove MD, Mendez R, Morrow JW: Traumatic renal arteriovenous fistula: Report of 12 cases. J Urol 110:627, 1973.

Del Villar RG, Ireland GW, Cass AS: Management of renal injury in conjunction with the immediate surgical treatment of the acute severe trauma patient. J Urol 107:208, 1972.

Esho JO, Ireland GW, Cass AS: Renal trauma and pre-existing lesions of the kidney. Urology 1:134, 1973.

Jameson RM: Transient hypertension associated with closed renal injury. Brit J Urol 45:482, 1973.

Joachim GR, Becker EL: Spontaneous rupture of the kidney. Arch Int Med 115:176, 1965.

Kalish M & others: Traumatic renal hemorrhage: Treatment by arterial embolization. J Urol 112:138, 1974.

Koehler PR & others: Association of subcapsular hematomas with the nonfunctioning kidney. Radiology 106:537, 1973.

Krahn HP, Axenrod H: The management of severe renal lacerations. J Urol 109:11, 1973.

Marks LS & others: Arterography in penetrating renal trauma. Urology 3:18, 1974.

Peterson NE, Kiracofe LH: Renal trauma: When to operate. Urology 3:537, 1974.

Peterson NE, Norton LW: Injuries associated with renal trauma. J Urol 109:766, 1973.

Scott R Jr, Carlton CE Jr, Goldman M: Penetrating injuries of the kidney: An analysis of 181 patients. J Urol 101:247, 1969.

Skinner DG: Traumatic renal artery thrombosis: A successful thrombectomy and revascularization. Ann Surg 177:264, 1973.

Slade N: Management of closed renal injuries. Brit J Urol 43:639, 1971.

Toguri AG & others: Traumatic bilateral renal artery thrombosis. J Urol 112:430, 1974.

Vermillion CD, McLaughlin AP, Pfister RC: Management of blunt renal trauma. J Urol 106:478, 1971.

Injuries to the Ureter

Beckly DE, Waters EA: Avulsion of the pelvi-ureteric junction: A rare consequence of non-penetrating trauma. Brit J Radiol 45:423, 1972.

Calame RJ, Nelson JH Jr: Ureterovaginal fistula as a complication of radical pelvic surgery. Arch Surg 94:876, 1967.

Carlton CE Jr, Scott R Jr, Guthrie AG: The initial management of ureteral injuries: A report of 78 cases. J Urol 105:335, 1971.

Goldstein AG, Conger KB: Perforation of the ureter during retrograde pyelography. J Urol 94:658, 1965.

Gross M, Peng B, Waterhouse K: Use of the mobilized bladder to replace the pelvic ureter. J Urol 101:40, 1969.

Hardy JD: High ureteral injuries: Management by autotransplantation of the kidney. JAMA 184:97, 1963.

Herman G, Guerrier K, Persky L: Delayed ureteral deligation. J Urol 107:723, 1972.

Hulse CA & others: Conservative management of ureterovaginal fistula. J Urol 99:42, 1968.

Lankford R, Block NL, Politano VA: Gunshot wounds of the ureter: A review of 10 cases. J Trauma 14:848, 1974.

Lee RA, Symmonds RE: Ureterovaginal fistula. Am J Obst Gynec 109:1032, 1971.

Reznichek RC, Brosman SA, Rhodes DB: Ureteral avulsion from blunt trauma. J Urol 109:812, 1973.

Thompson IM, Ross G Jr: Long-term results of bladder flap repair of ureteral injuries. J Urol 111:483, 1974.

Thompson JD, Benigno BB: Vaginal repair of ureteral injuries. Am J Obst Gynec 111:601, 1971.

Wesolowsky S: Bilateral ureteral injuries in gynecology. Brit J Urol 41:666, 1969.

Injuries to the Bladder

Brosman SA, Fay R: Diagnosis and management of bladder trauma. J Trauma 13:687, 1973.

Carswell JW: Intraperitoneal rupture of the bladder. Brit J Urol 46:425, 1974.

Cass AS, Ireland GW: Bladder trauma associated with pelvic fractures in severely injured patients. J Trauma 13:205, 1973.

Del Villar RG, Ireland GW, Cass AS: Management of bladder and urethral injury in conjunction with the immediate surgical treatment of the acute severe trauma patient. J Urol 108:581, 1972.

Dhall GI, Dhall K, Pathak IC: Massive hematuria after obstructed labor. Obst Gynec 28:360, 1966.

Graber EA, O'Rourke JJ, McElrath T: Iatrogenic bladder injury during hysterectomy. Obst Gynec 23:267, 1964.

Kamat MH, Corgan FJ, Seebode JJ: Spontaneous rupture of the bladder. Arch Surg 100:735, 1970.

Kerr WS Jr & others: Arteriography in pelvic fractures with massive hemorrhage. J Urol 109:479, 1973.

Van Nagell JR Jr & others: Bladder or rectal injury following radiation therapy for cervical cancer. Am J Obst Gynec 119:727, 1974.

Injuries to the Membranous Urethra

Allison RC: Urethrography in pelvic trauma. J Urol 111:778, 1974.

Clark SS, Prudencio RF: Lower urinary tract injuries associated with pelvic fractures: Diagnosis and management. S Clin North America 52:183, 1972.

Gibson GR: Impotence following fractured pelvis and ruptured urethra. Brit J Urol 42:86, 1970.

Gibson GR: Urological management and complications of

fractured pelvis and ruptured urethra. J Urol 111:353, 1974.

Morehouse DD, Belitsky P, MacKinnon K: Rupture of the posterior urethra. J Urol 107:255, 1972.

Myers RP, Deweerd JH: Incidence of stricture following primary realignment of the disrupted proximal urethra. J Urol 107:265, 1972.

Pierce JM Jr: Management of dismemberment of the prostatic membranous urethra and ensuing stricture disease. J Urol 107:259, 1972.

Ragde H, McInnes GF: Transpubic repair of severed prostatomembranous urethra. J Urol 101:335, 1969.

Injuries to the Bulbous Urethra

Ezell WW & others: Mechanical traumatic injury to the genitalia in children. J Urol 102:788, 1969.

Injuries to the Pendulous Urethra

Blumberg N: Anterior urethral injuries. J Urol 102:210, 1969.

Injuries to the Penis

Engelman ER & others: Traumatic amputation of the penis. J Urol 112:774, 1974.

Fleming JP: Reconstruction of the penis. J Urol 104:213, 1970.

Kendall AR, Karafin L: Repair of the denuded penis. J

Urol 98:484, 1967.

Mears EM Jr: Traumatic rupture of the corpus cavernosum. J Urol 105:407, 1971.

Mendez R, Kiely WF, Morrow JW: Self-emasculation. J Urol 107:981, 1972.

Shiraki IW, Trichel BE: Traumatic dislocation of the penis. J Urol 101:186, 1969.

Stuppler SA & others: Incarceration of penis by foreign body. Urology 2:308, 1973.

Tuerk M, Weir WH Jr: Successful replantation of a traumatically amputated glans penis. Plast Reconstr Surg 48:499, 1971.

Injuries to the Scrotum

Millard R Jr: Scrotal construction and reconstruction. Plast Reconstr Surg 33:10, 1966.

Injuries to the Testis

Merricks JW, Papierniak FB: Traumatic rupture of the testicle. J Urol 103:77, 1970.

Schulman CC: Traumatic rupture of the testicle: An underestimated pathology. Urol Internat 29:31, 1974.

Sethi RS, Singh W: Traumatic dislocation of testes. J Urol 98:501, 1967.

Talarico RD, Clark JC: Nonpenitrating testicular rupture. Urology 1:365, 1973.

17 . . .
Immunology of Genitourinary Tumors

J. Vivian Wells, MD, & H. Hugh Fudenberg, MD

The classical therapeutic approaches to cancer have been surgery, radiotherapy, and chemotherapy. In addition, for about the last 50 years, there have been sporadic attempts to influence the outcome of tumors in individual patients by influencing immunologic mechanisms. The rapid expansion of knowledge in the field of immunology in the past 15 years has been accompanied by a corresponding increase in interest in the role of immunology in the development and progress of malignancy. The intention of this chapter is to briefly outline immunologic concepts as they relate to etiology, diagnosis, therapy, and prognosis of genitourinary tumors.

IMMUNOLOGIC CONCEPTS OF ONCOGENESIS

The hypothesis of "immunologic surveillance" against cancer was proposed independently by Burnet and Thomas in the early 1960s. They proposed that an important function of the normal immune system is to recognize mutant or aberrant patterns in the body—such as malignant cells—and eliminate them. This implied the existence of foreign antigenic determinants on tumor cells, their recognition by the immune system of the host, and the development of effector mechanisms to destroy or neutralize these cells. A considerable body of evidence has accumulated to support this hypothesis.

Tumor-Associated Antigens (TAAs)

Tumor-associated antigens (TAAs) have been demonstrated in a wide variety of tumors in experimental animals, both those arising spontaneously and those induced by viral, chemical, or physical carcinogens. The term tumor-specific transplantation antigens was used in studies in inbred strains of animals with tumors induced by chemical carcinogens, eg, methylcholanthrene (MCA). The tumor in each animal

J Vivian Wells is Senior Staff Specialist in Clinical Immunology, Kolling Institute of Medical Research, Sydney. H Hugh Fudenberg is Professor of Medicine, University of California School of Medicine, San Francisco, and Professor of Immunology, University of California, Berkeley.

Abreviations Used in This Chapter

AFP	Alpha-1-fetoprotein
BCG	Bacillus Calmette-Guérin
CEA	Carcinoembryonic antigen
DHSR	Delayed hypersensitivity reaction
DNCB	Dinitrochlorobenzene
HL-A	Human leukocyte-antigen
MCA	Methylcholanthrene
MER	Methanol-extractable residue
MIF	Migration inhibition factor
PBL	Peripheral blood lymphocytes
PHA	Phytohemagglutinin
PPD	Purified protein derivative
RNA	Ribonucleic acid
TAA	Tumor-associated antigen
TF	Transfer factor
UCEA	Urinary carcinoembryonic antigen

appeared to have individually unique or specific antigens. More recently, studies in these animals suggest that they also contain TAAs with weak cross-reactivity between different animals. MCA-induced bladder tumors show weakly cross-reacting TAAs in both rats and mice. Furthermore, MCA-induced rat bladder papillomas and carcinomas share TAAs. By comparison, animals with virus-induced tumors show easily detectable cross-reacting TAAs.

TAAs have been clearly demonstrated in a variety of human tumors, including neuroblastoma, melanoma, osteogenic sarcoma, leukemia and lymphoma, cerebral tumors (eg, meningioma), hepatoma, nasopharyngeal carcinoma, ovarian carcinoma, breast carcinoma, lung carcinoma, genitourinary tumors, etc. The genitourinary tumors include renal adenocarcinoma, nephroblastoma, transitional cell carcinoma of the genitourinary tract—including carcinoma of the bladder—and carcinoma of the prostate. Comparisons with studies of TAAs in animal models led to proposals that human genitourinary tumors such as nephroblastoma are of viral etiology while bladder carcinoma is chemically induced. Renal adenocarcinoma can be induced in animals by chemical, viral, or physical agents, but the cause in man is still unknown. This is unfortunate, since malignant renal tumors comprise 1.2% of all human malignancies excluding skin malignancies, and adenocarcinoma is clearly the most frequent malignant renal tumor (89%).

TAAs have not yet been isolated in pure form and characterized for the great majority of tumors studied. They appear mainly on the membrane of affected cells; attempts at purification are complicated by the presence of various normal membrane components. Hence, the detection of TAAs has classically been based on their elicitation of immune responses in the tumor-bearing host.

Immune Responses to TAAs

TAAs elicit immunologic responses from both components of the immune system: humoral and cellular. Humoral immunity is mediated by circulating antibodies or immunoglobulins secreted by plasma cells which develop from B cells (bursa- or bone marrow-derived lymphocytes). Cellular immunity is mediated by T cells (thymic-derived). Humoral responses to TAAs are therefore detected by a variety of methods for antitumor antibodies. Cellular responses to TAAs are detected by appropriate tests for cell-mediated immunity. These are discussed below in the section on immunologic diagnosis of tumors. It should be emphasized here, however, that in an individual patient with a tumor the 2 components of humoral and cellular immunity have varying degrees of importance and interrelationships during different stages of the tumor in that patient.

IMMUNOLOGIC METHODS IN TUMOR DIAGNOSIS

General Diagnostic Considerations

Although many of the procedures outlined below require sophisticated laboratory technics and considerable experience with them, evaluation of histologic sections of tumor tissue is of great help in estimating the prognosis. Such approaches have shown that, for example, infiltration of breast tumor tissue by immunologically competent cells is associated with a much better prognosis, both in terms of life span in untreated patients (in the prechemotherapy days) and in terms of chances of response to chemotherapy. Personal experience with urologic tumors, limited mainly to embryonal cell carcinoma of the testis, indicates that, regardless of clinical stage, patients whose tumors are heavily infiltrated with plasma cells, lymphocytes, and eosinophils survive much longer than the average. It is, therefore, highly recommended that these simple histologic evaluations be performed in any tumors removed.

In addition to the standard investigations to diagnose a tumor in a patient—eg, x-rays, radionuclide scanning, and biopsy—a general assessment of the patient's immunologic status should be made:

A. Humoral Immunity: Commonly used technics such as electrophoresis of serum proteins and measurement of serum immunoglobulin levels are usually not helpful unless the patient has an associated monoclonal gammopathy, but a test of the patient's antibody response to primary immunization may be of value. One study measured the antibody response to immunization with monomeric flagellin antigen from *Salmonella adelaide;* the response was depressed significantly in patients with active cancer compared with sick but not cancerous control patients. A significant correlation was found between the degree of depression and overall survival. Antibody responses in patients with clinically cured cancer were significantly greater than those in both hospital controls and patients with active cancer but still were less than those in healthy subjects.

B. Cellular Immunity: There are 4 main methods of measuring cellular immunity in patients: (1) delayed skin hypersensitivity reactions (DHSR), (2) in vitro transformation of peripheral blood lymphocytes (PBL), (3) elaboration of MIF and other cellular mediators, and (4) measurement of "active" and total T cells in peripheral blood.

The first 3 tests are performed with standard specific antigens, eg, PPD, mumps antigen, and streptokinase-streptodornase. Significant abnormalities in individual cases usually are found in more advanced malignancies where the diagnosis is already obvious and the abnormalities are an indication of the altered general immunologic status of the patient.

Peripheral blood T cells spontaneously bind sheep red blood cells to form a rosette; approximately 70–80% of normal human PBLs are rosette-forming T cells. "Active" T cells, measured by a different rosetting technic, are 28 ±6.8% in persons. A reduced "active" T rosette cell count may be found in some patients with tumors before metastases develop. Viral infections also lower the "active" T rosette cell count. It should be emphasized that this test does not indicate the type or site of the postulated tumor.

Specific Diagnosis

These methods detect immune responses in patients to the specific TAA.

A. Humoral Responses: These tests include immunofluorescence, complement fixation, immune cytolysis, and immunodiffusion.

Immunofluorescence has been widely used to demonstrate serum antibodies in patients with tumors. The specificities of the antibodies determine whether they react only with the autologous tumor, the autologous tumor and metastases from the primary tumor, tumors of the same histologic type in other patients, or long-term cultures of malignant cells of the same histologic type. Immunofluorescent methods have also been used to label antisera prepared in animals against TAAs, eg, human nephroblastoma.

B. Cellular Responses: The methods consist of lymphocyte-mediated cytotoxicity, in vitro stimulation of PBL by TAA, release of mediators from PBL, and DHSR to TAA.

The latter 3 methods refer to responses to the specific TAA for a particular type of tumor and not to general immune responses. They require the preparation of TAA from the tumor under study.

In cytotoxicity studies, PBL from the patient are tested for their ability to inactivate or kill labeled tumor cells in vitro. This method has been used in several laboratories to study renal carcinoma, nephroblastoma, and, more recently, transitional cell carcinoma of the bladder. In each case, cell-mediated immunity was demonstrable, but in bladder carcinoma some studies have demonstrated non-T-cell-mediated cytotoxicity.

Oncofetal Antigens

TAAs, by definition, are not found in normal tissues. However, another group of antigens is found in certain malignancies which can be detected in very small amounts in normal tissues or in diseased but nonmalignant tissues. Since these antigens can be found in significant amounts in fetal tissues, they have been called oncofetal antigens. Some workers include in this group abnormal hormones and enzymes, and antigens which have not been fully studied. We will discuss the 2 best-known examples: carcinoembryonic antigen (CEA) and alpha-1-fetoprotein (AFP).

A. Carcinoembryonic Antigen (CEA): Gold and his colleagues in Montreal in the mid 1960s extracted a glycoprotein substance from human colonic carcinomas and prepared antisera against this glycoprotein. They found material with the same antigenic characteristics in fetal tissues, and it was therefore called CEA. The initial impression that CEA was associated with gastrointestinal malignancy has been fully confirmed, but extensive studies have shown CEA to be associated with a variety of malignancies (including genitourinary tumors) and nonmalignant diseases. Many different technics have been employed to measure CEA, but those most frequently used show a plasma level of less than 2.5 ng/ml in over 98% of normal subjects. Slight to moderate increases in CEA are found with a variety of inflammatory diseases—pancreatitis, ulcerative colitis, etc—and malignancies. Markedly increased levels (> 40 ng/ml) are very likely to be associated with malignancy, especially carcinoma of the colon, pancreas, breast, or lung. Table 17–1 lists some published data on the incidence of CEA in various conditions.

The height of the plasma CEA is related to the mass of the tumor rather than its histologic type or parent tissue. The routine CEA test is not specific for any one tumor and is therefore not suitable for use as a screening test. Its principal current applications are in monitoring therapy and indicating prognosis. In a patient with a tumor and a markedly elevated plasma CEA level, complete removal of the tumor leads to a fall to normal CEA levels, generally within 14 days. A fall to an intermediate but still increased CEA level indicates residual primary tumor tissue or the presence of secondary deposits. Patients with full removal of the tumor and a fall to normal CEA levels can then be

Table 17–1. Plasma CEA levels.
(Normal: < 2.5 ng/ml)

Diseases	% Increase (> 2.5 ng/ml)
Gastrointestinal	
Carcinoma of colon, rectum	72–95
Carcinoma of pancreas	63
Colorectal polyposis	9–19
Diverticulitis	21
Respiratory	
Carcinoma of lung	72–76
Chronic bronchitis and emphysema	25–35
Carcinoma of breast	47–67
Genitourinary	
Carcinoma of kidney	35
Carcinoma of bladder	33
Carcinoma of prostate	40
Carcinoma of cervix	42
Carcinoma of ovary	35
Testicular tumors	33

monitored at regular intervals of 3–6 months. An increasing plasma CEA level in such a patient under observation suggests local recurrence of the tumor, growth of secondary deposits, or, what is more unlikely, the development of a separate CEA-secreting tumor.

CEA has the following properties:

Molecular weight: 200,000
Sedimentation rate: 7S–8S
Carbohydrate/protein ratio: 6:1 to 1:1
Sialic acid content: Markedly variable
N-Acetylglucosamine content: High
N-Acetylgalactosamine content: Trace
Polydispersion on gel electrophoresis.

Studies in the past 5 years have demonstrated molecules in trace amounts in normal and neoplastic tissues which show cross-reactivity with CEA, indicating sharing of antigenic determinants. It appears likely that there are several similar molecules or a family of CEA molecules with slight antigenic and structural differences.

Urinary CEA. Measurement of CEA levels in the urine in male subjects showed that 95% had less than 35 ng of CEA per ml of urine. A survey of patients with urothelial tumors of all stages showed 52% had increased urinary CEA levels. The elevated urinary CEA levels are specific to urothelial carcinomas if infection is excluded since urinary CEA levels are normal in malignancies such as prostatic cancer and carcinoma of the colorectal region even if plasma levels are raised with the latter tumors. Only if the latter tumors directly invade the urinary tract do they show elevated urinary CEA levels. The urinary CEA level is influenced by the tumor mass and not by the histologic type or degree of differentiation of the tumor.

The incidence of positive tests and the amount of urinary CEA show an increase with increasing tumor mass and therefore with the tumor stage. Thus, urinary CEA levels were increased in 33% of stage T1 tumors and 79% of stage T4 tumors. Successful surgery for bladder carcinoma leads to a fall to normal levels of urinary CEA; a return of increased levels indicates local recurrence, the development of metastases, or a new tumor.

Further research suggests that the component studied in urine has slight but definite antigenic and structural differences from CEA prepared from colon cancer tissue and has therefore been designated urinary carcinoembryonic antigen (UCEA). A test specific for UCEA has not yet been devised.

Combined measurements of both plasma and urinary CEA are therefore of value in estimating the effects of treatment of urothelial tumors and in detecting local or distant recurrences.

B. Alpha-1-Fetoprotein (AFP): Serum levels of AFP are high in the fetus but low in adult animals and humans. High levels are also found with certain tumors such as hepatoma (72–95%) and embryonic tumors (13–75%). Serum AFP levels are increased in teratocarcinoma or embryonal cell carcinoma of the gonad (45–75%) and in choriocarcinoma (13%). The serum AFP level is normal in seminoma, other gonadal tumors, nephroblastoma, etc. More sensitive technics now detect slightly increased levels of serum AFP in a small proportion of patients with nonmalignant conditions, eg, infectious hepatitis.

Measurement of serum AFP levels is therefore helpful only in a small proportion of patients with genitourinary tumors, ie, patients with teratocarcinoma.

IMMUNOLOGIC FACTORS IN PROGNOSIS

There are many examples in both animals and man which confirm the view that changes in general immunologic status influence both the development and course of malignancies. Analysis of cases reported to the Immunodeficiency Cancer Registry shows that patients with primary immunodeficiency have a far greater risk of developing malignancies (2–10%) than normal subjects. This is most significant when their short life spans are considered. Patients receiving immunosuppressive therapy after renal allotransplantation have a significantly higher risk of developing malignancies, especially of unusual types. Malignancy in patients with severe impairment of their immune system generally carries a poorer prognosis.

An important point is that some forms of treatment of malignancy can be severely immunosuppressive, eg, radiotherapy and chemotherapy. This effect can of course be counterproductive in terms of the main aim of curing the malignancy.

Specific Immune Responses & Clinical Stages

Specific responses to TAAs occur during the life of a tumor in a host, as outlined above. The relative balance between cellular and humoral responses is probably the major factor in determining the overall outcome of a tumor in immunologic terms.

Lymphocytes from patients with actively growing in vivo tumors were shown by means of in vitro tests to be cytotoxic for the patient's own tumor or a tumor of the same type from other patients. This disparity between in vivo and in vitro findings was postulated to be due to factors which "blocked" in vivo the cytotoxic effect of lymphocytes against tumor cells. Blocking of this sort can occur for 2 main reasons:

(1) Blocking factor: IgG antibody-antigen complexes (probably in antigen excess) have now been detected in such patients which bind to the tumor cells (apparently without damaging them) and prevent the cytotoxic lymphocytes from attaching to the tumor cells via the TAAs.

(2) Circulating TAAs: The second mechanism which might occur with large tumor masses is that membrane-bound TAAs are released into the circulation as soluble glycoproteins. These are subsequently bound to the surface of specific lymphocytes, and the cells can no longer bind to TAAs on tumor cells in the main tumor mass.

The result of these mechanisms is in vivo growth of the tumor since the specific cellular response to the tumor is blocked by the serum blocking factors.

The degree of lymphocyte cytotoxicity in bladder cancer varies with the course of the disease. A strong response generally indicates a good prognosis, especially after radiotherapy. The absence of cytotoxicity may have 2 entirely different interpretations: (1) at least temporary cure of tumor, or (2) extensive tumor growth, metastases, and a very bad prognosis.

The second major point is that serum from some patients with tumors has the opposite effect and reverses the "blocking" activity of serum found in patients with growing tumors. This "deblocking" activity due to "deblocking factors" is usually seen with regressing tumors. It was proposed that this deblocking activity was due to the elimination of antigen-antibody complexes by additional antibody.

The serum from one patient with a transitional cell carcinoma of the bladder contained an IgG antibody which induced lymphocyte cytotoxicity against the tumor and did not require complement for this activity. The IgG antibody induced cytotoxicity in the lymphocytes from patients with or without bladder cancer, and the cytotoxicity was tumor-specific. It acted against transitional cell carcinoma but not against normal adult cells, normal embryonal cells, nor nephroblastoma cells. The IgG antibody and TAA had first to make contact before one could show this antibody-induced, noncomplement-dependent lymphocyte cytotoxicity for tumor cells.

Tests with TAAs for lymphocyte transformation and DHSR have also been performed in patients with various stages of malignant disease. Skin tests generally were positive in remission and negative in relapse. A remission with treatment was accompanied by a return of a positive DHSR. This is not due simply to DHSR to antigens in general but is tumor-specific. Stimulation of lymphocytes by TAAs was found to be positive in equal numbers in patients in remission or in relapse. This lack of correlation between in vivo and in vitro tests of specific responses to TAAs has not yet been explained.

These various opposing mechanisms resulting in tumor growth or tumor destruction may therefore operate to different degrees in a single patient during the history of his tumor. This fact must be taken into consideration with the effects of therapy on the patient's immune system and the form of immunotherapy which might be employed.

GENERAL IMMUNOLOGIC CONSIDERATIONS IN TUMOR THERAPY

The greater the number of tumor cells of a given tumor injected into experimental animals, the shorter the survival of the host. This correlation between size of tumor and survival is apparently true with tumors in man. Unfortunately, in most patients at the time of diagnosis, the tumor load is already great. The aim of therapy is therefore rapid elimination of the tumor. This is accomplished if possible by surgical removal or radiotherapy. Chemotherapy is the method of choice with disseminated tumors. Cytotoxic drugs used for this purpose can be divided into 3 classes: (1) Agents killing cells in all phases of the cell cycle irrespective of proliferative capacity (mechlorethamine, carmustine [BCNU], gamma irradiation). (2) Agents killing cells in only one phase of the cell cycle (vinblastine, methotrexate). (3) Agents killing cells in all phases of the cell cycle but closely correlated with the fraction of cells in the proliferative phase (fluorouracil, dactinomycin, cyclophosphamide).

Combination regimens of drugs have been used to achieve killing of maximal numbers of tumor cells. The use of surgery, radiotherapy, and chemotherapy is an important first stage in treatment since the immune system is best suited to the elimination of small numbers of tumor cells rather than a large tumor mass. The latter indicates a failure in immunologic mechanisms.

An important corollary to combination drug regimens is the suppressive effect they have on bone marrow cells and other rapidly dividing cells such as those of the gastrointestinal tract. They also have an immunosuppressive effect on lymphoid cells, and this further prompted study of agents which stimulate the immune system of the patient.

IMMUNOTHERAPY

The methods used to stimulate the immune responses of patients with tumor are discussed under the 3 main headings of active, passive, and nonspecific immunotherapy.

Active Immunotherapy

Attempts are made to stimulate the patient's own immunity by one or more of the methods listed in Table 17–2. Numerous animal experiments have confirmed the efficacy of many of these measures. Living tumor cells can be administered intradermally in small numbers which will not cause progressive tumor growth but will stimulate immunity. For obvious reasons, including ethical ones, living fresh tumor cells are generally not used in man. Instead, tumor cells are administered after inactivation or, in many cases, modification. The various methods for modifying the tumor cells are directed toward increasing their immunogenicity, frequently by causing changes in membrane structure.

Another approach is to prepare subcellular components from the tumor cells and inject these into tumor-bearing subjects. These can be crude extracts of TAAs purified from membranes.

Finally, active immunity can be stimulated by the use of an adjuvant such as BCG. In man, the available adjuvants are limited compared with the number that can be used in experimental animals.

The applications of these methods in man have thus far been limited mainly to leukemias, malignant melanoma, and sarcomas. Remission maintenance in chronic granulocytic leukemia can be accomplished by the injection of inactivated tumor cells. They have not yet been sufficiently well studied in carcinomas and genitourinary tumors.

Table 17–2. Active immunotherapy.

Whole tumor cell vaccines
Living tumor cells
Autologous
Allogeneic
Inactivated tumor cells
Irradiation
Mitomycin C
Freezing and thawing
Heat
Modified tumor cells
Carrier protein
Chemical (iodoacetate)
Neuraminidase
Concanavalin A
Vaccines to subcellular components
Crude cell extracts
Isolated cell membranes
Purified cell surface TAAs
Immune adjuvants
Freund's adjuvant
BCG
MER (methanol-extractable residue)
Corynebacterium parvum
Levamisole

Passive Immunotherapy

This includes the administration of antitumor antisera, lymphocytes, or lymphocyte fractions to passively transfer immunity to tumor-bearing patients from normal subjects or subjects cured of cancer (Table 17–3).

A. Antitumor Antisera: Antisera prepared in animal species against various human tumors have generally yielded disappointing results when tested in tumor-bearing patients. They do not appear to be suitable for the elimination of a large tumor mass. The patient also tends to become sensitized to the foreign proteins in the antiserum, and this limits the treatment schedule.

Human plasma from 2 sources can be used to treat tumors. Normal subjects may be immunized with tumor extracts or TAAs and their plasma subsequently collected. Ethical considerations generally preclude widespread use of this approach. The other approach is to use plasma from patients who are in long-term remission or clinically "cured" (with or without treatment). Obviously, the plasma must be ABO compatible and negative for the serum hepatitis antigen (hepatitis B antigen). Careful serial monitoring of clinical and laboratory parameters is needed to make certain that the treatment produces tumor destruction and not enhancement of tumor growth by blocking antibodies. A plasma donor must be selected who has an IgG "deblocking" antibody specific for the patient's tumor. If suitable donors are available, this type of therapy will undoubtedly be used more frequently in selected patients with genitourinary tumors.

B. Lymphocytes: Lymphocytes from many sources have been administered to cancer patients to transfer passive immunity. This could circumvent the patient's own immunologic defects. Several studies have reported improvement in small numbers of selected patients with widespread disease.

1. Xenogeneic lymphocytes–The procedure is to immunize a selected animal against a particular tumor, harvest lymphocytes from the animal after sensitiza-

tion, and inject these lymphocytes into the arterial blood supply of the patient's tumor. The pig has been selected as a suitable donor because it is easy to handle, is free of infection, and has a long continuous mesenteric lymph node chain. This approach was used in one study of 16 patients with advanced (stage T4) carcinoma of the bladder. Seven patients received significant benefit. The main disadvantages are that the foreign lymphocytes do not survive very long in the recipient and that readministration might cause serious anaphylactoid reactions.

2. Nonactivated lymphocytes–The donors of the lymphocytes may be other patients with the same or some other type of cancer, preferably in long-term remission. The main problem limiting the efficacy of this treatment is histoincompatibility. Genetic differences exist between lymphocytes of different subjects, and these lead to interactions between them and subsequent elimination of the foreign cells. HL-A typing is performed with serologic methods to detect one system of genetic cellular markers. To avoid this rejection phenomenon, one can use lymphocytes from the genetically identical normal twin of a patient. Most patients do not have an identical twin, and a sibling is sought with the same HL-A type. Even if such a match is obtained, sensitization to the donor's cells usually occurs as a result of other genetic differences. The final method is to take the patient's own lymphocytes, grow them in vitro in short-term cultures, and then reinfuse them into the patient. The aim is to increase the cytotoxicity of the cells, eg, by the removal of blocking factor. The results obtained to date have been largely disappointing.

3. Activated lymphocytes–An alternative way of overcoming the problem of the short survival of the infused lymphocytes is to make them more effective in their active period by prior in vitro activation. Lymphocytes from any of the donors listed above can be stimulated in vitro by PHA or TAAs. The TAAs are usually provided by monolayers of long-term cultures of the specific tumor cells. After exposure, the lymphocytes are collected and infused into the patient.

4. Cross-transplantation of tumors–This complicated approach has certain problems, including ethical considerations. Patients with tumors are matched for tumor type and ABO and Rh groups. Tumor samples are exchanged between the patients and placed subcutaneously. After a period of time has elapsed to allow for "sensitization," plasma and leukocytes are exchanged between the patients. Reports of studies with small numbers of patients with advanced cancer have claimed complete regression in 3–5% and partial regression in 15–20%. The contributions of anti-HL-A reactions and anti-TAA reactions to these results have yet to be analyzed.

C. Extracts of Sensitized Lymphoid Cells: A persistent problem in long-term treatment with infusions of whole lymphocytes has been incompatibility from HL-A and other antigens. Studies were therefore undertaken to eliminate tumors with lymphoid cell extracts which do not have HL-A specificity.

Table 17–3. Passive immunotherapy.

Antitumor antisera
   Xenogeneic
   Allogeneic
Lymphocytes
   Xenogeneic
   Nonactivated lymphocytes
      Allogeneic cancer patients
      Normal identical twins or HL-A matched sibling
      Autologous lymphocytes grown in vitro
   Lymphocytes activated in vitro
      PHA
      TAAs
   Lymphocytes sensitized by cross transplantation
      of tumors
Extracts of sensitized cells
   Transfer factor
   Immune RNA

---

1. Transfer factor (TF)—TF is an extract of lymphocytes which transfers DHSR and other parameters of cellular immunity from one subject to a recipient. The mechanisms of this transfer are not yet clear. TF is a small dialyzable molecule of approximately 7000 molecular weight. It is stable against repeated freezing and thawing, lyophilization, storage for over 5 years, and the action of DNase, RNase, and trypsin. It does not contain immunoglobulin or HL-A antigens.

Administration of TF to a subject transfers DHSR in 1–7 days, and this may last up to 1 year. It also transfers the production of mediators of cellular immunity, eg, MIF. It does not lead to transfer of antigen-induced lymphocyte transformation. It has been used with success in the clinical management of selected patients with defects in cellular immunity.

Trials are currently proceeding to assess the role of TF in certain types of malignancy—osteogenic sarcoma, malignant melanoma, carcinoma of the breast, etc. A major problem is the supply of donors, since TF must be obtained from the lymphocytes of human donors with proved cellular immunity against the specific type of tumor. Suitable donors are restricted to close household contacts who have demonstrable cellular immunity to the tumor, as "nonspecific" transfer factor is of no value and might even be deleterious. "Recovered" (5-year-disease-free) patients almost always lack such immunity.

2. Immune RNA—The alternative approach is to prepare RNA extracts from lymphoid cells. This immune RNA can be prepared in animals as it is not species-specific. One theoretical risk is the possibility of transferring RNA from oncogenic viruses in the immune RNA. Immune RNA has not yet been sufficiently tested in preliminary trials to ascertain whether it will have clinical applications.

NONSPECIFIC IMMUNOTHERAPY

This refers to the use of the immune adjuvants listed in Table 17–2. The rationale appears to be a general stimulation of the patient's immune system which will result in control or eradication of a growing tumor. Animal studies have clearly confirmed the efficacy of some of these adjuvants under selected experimental conditions.

BCG

BCG can be administered to skin lesions such as metastatic nodules by direct injection or into non-involved areas by scarification. Multiple BCG treatments are preferred for maximal effect. The progress of the anergic patient is followed by noting clinical progress, the acquisition of DHSR to the chemical DNCB (dinitrochlorobenzene), and laboratory parameters such as tumor-specific lymphocyte cytotoxicity. Studies in malignant melanoma and other tumors showed the immunopotentiating effect of BCG, and its clinical benefits were enhanced by simultaneous chemotherapy appropriate for disseminated solid tumors. One such study administered 6×10^8 viable units of fresh liquid Pasteur strain BCG by scarification on days 7, 12, and 17 of a course of chemotherapy. The regimen was repeated every 21 days if the patient's blood counts were acceptable. The appropriate chemoimmunotherapy courses for disseminated renal and bladder cancers have yet to be determined.

Levamisole

This drug is widely used in the treatment of roundworms and hookworms and is now known to stimulate a wide spectrum of immunologic functions. The administration of 150 mg levamisole per day for 3 days to anergic patients with cancer restored DSHR. Patients were tested for DHSR to DNCB and PPD. Trials are now in progress to see if levamisole, alone or in combination with antitumor chemotherapy, has any effect on the clinical course of disseminated malignant disease. To date, the results have been disappointing.

Interferon

This protein, a product of activated T cells (and perhaps other cells as well), inhibits viral replication. Preliminary trials with interferon preparations in human osteosarcoma (which is presumably a virally induced tumor) have proved promising and clearly warrant further investigation.

CONCLUSION

There is considerable evidence that a defect in immune surveillance permits the development of cancers or at least hampers their eradication. It is clear that various facets of a subject's immune response to a developing tumor play crucial roles in determining the outcome of that tumor. It is another clear example of a "seed and soil" relationship.

The aim of immunotherapy is to stimulate the immune system to eliminate an established tumor, prevent a recurrence, and prevent the development of a new tumor. Unfortunately, we still cannot predict with certainty the effects of specific immunization in an individual patient with a tumor. Both humoral and cellular immunity may be stimulated by a particular regimen and lead to enhancement of tumor growth by blocking antibodies rather than tumor destruction by cytotoxicity and the production of deblocking antibodies rather than blocking antibodies. Studies with active immunization and passive transfer for genitourinary tumors are necessary to achieve this aim. In the meantime, disseminated tumors are being studied with a combination of chemotherapy and immunotherapy with adjuvants (BCG or levamisole). If suitable donors were to become available, future therapy might involve plasma infusions with tumor-specific deblocking antibody and injection of tumor-specific TF. At present, these procedures remain experimental ones and are not generally available.

• • •

References

Baker MA, Taub RN: Immunotherapy of human cancer. Progr Allergy 17:227, 1973.

Burnet FM: Implications of cancer immunity. Australian New Zealand J Med 3:71, 1973.

DeVita VT, Schein PS: The use of drugs in combination for the treatment of cancer: Rationale and results. New England J Med 288:998, 1973.

Fudenberg HH & others: The therapeutic uses of transfer factor. Hosp Practice 9:95, Jan 1974.

Golub SH, O'Connell TX, Morton DL: Correlation of in vivo and in vitro assays of immunocompetence in cancer patients. Cancer Res 34:1833, 1974.

Hakala TR & others: Antibody-induced lymphocyte cytotoxicity. New England J Med 291:637, 1974.

Hellstrom KE, Hellstrom I: The role of cell-mediated immunity in control and growth of tumors. Page 233 in: *Clinical Immunobiology*. Vol 2. Bach FH, Good RA (editors). Academic Press, 1974.

Kersey JH, Spector BD, Good RA: Primary immunodeficiency disease and cancer: The Immunodeficiency-Cancer Registry. Internat J Cancer 12:333, 1973.

Laurence DJR, Neville AM: Foetal antigens and their role in the diagnosis and clinical management of human neoplasms: A review. Brit J Cancer 26:335, 1972.

Morton DL: Immunotherapy of cancer: Present status and future potential. Cancer 30:1647, 1972.

Neville AM & others: Aspects of the structure and clinical role of the carcinoembryonic antigen (CEA) and related macromolecules with particular reference to urothelial carcinoma. Brit J Cancer 28 (Suppl I):198, 1973.

Perlman P, O'Toole C, Unsgaard B: Cell-mediated immune mechanisms of tumor cell destruction. Fed Proc 32:153, 1973.

Prehn RT: Immunological surveillance: Pro and con. Page 191 in: *Clinical Immunobiology*. Vol 2. Bach FH, Good RA (editors). Academic Press, 1974.

Prehn RT: Immunosurveillance, regeneration and oncogenesis. Progr Exp Tumor Res 14:1, 1971.

Reynoso C & others: Carcinoembryonic antigen in patients with tumors of the urogenital tract. Cancer 30:1, 1972.

Stjernswärd J & others: Tumour-distinctive cellular immunity to renal carcinoma. Clin Exper Immunol 6:963, 1970.

Symes MO & others: The treatment of advanced bladder cancer with sensitized pig lymphocytes. Brit J Cancer 28 (Suppl I):276, 1973.

Tanaka T, Cooper EH, Anderson CK: Lymphocyte infiltration in bladder carcinoma. Rev Europ Etud Clin Biol 15:1084, 1970.

Wahren B, Edsmyr F: Fetal proteins occurring in testicular teratomas. Internat J Cancer 14:207, 1974.

18 . . .
Tumors of the Genitourinary Tract

Neoplasms of the prostate gland, bladder, and kidney are among the most common abnormal growths which afflict the human body. They are often silent, so that diagnosis may not be possible until quite late. Tumors of the testis are highly malignant and afflict young men. Neoplasms of the ureter, urethra, penis, scrotum, epididymis, and seminal vesicle are rare.

Adrenal tumors are discussed in Chapter 20.

MANIFESTATIONS OF UROGENITAL TRACT NEOPLASMS

Hematuria

Gross or microscopic hematuria is common when ulceration of a vesical, ureteral, or renal pelvic neoplasm occurs or when a renal parenchymal tumor breaks through the pelvic lining. It is seen often with benign prostatic hypertrophy, in which case bleeding is usually from dilated veins in the region of the bladder neck. Symptoms of prostatism plus hematuria do not, therefore, necessarily mean prostatic cancer; in fact, bleeding from the malignant prostate does not occur until the tumor grows through the mucosa of the bladder or urethra.

Pain

A. Renal Pain: Renal carcinoma can incite pain in the costovertebral angle (from renal capsular distention) if the tumor bleeds into its own substance. Renal and ureteral colic may occur if a blood clot or a mass of cells passes down the ureter. This type of pain is due to hyperperistalsis of the pelvis or ureter.

B. Ureteral Pain: Ureteral tumors (rare) usually cause ureteral obstruction and occasionally colic.

C. Vesical Pain: Ulceration of a vesical tumor predisposes to midtract (bladder) infection, which causes painful urination. With extravesical extension, constant suprapubic pain which increases with urination may be experienced.

D. Low Back Pain: Pain low in the back with radiation down one or both legs in an elderly man strongly suggests metastases to the pelvis and lumbar spine from cancer of the prostate. Local (perineal) pain is seldom a symptom of neoplasia of the prostate.

E. Testicular Pain: Testicular neoplasm typically causes little or no pain, but if spontaneous bleeding occurs into the tumor it can mimic painful lesions (eg, torsion of the spermatic cord, acute epididymitis).

Dysuria

Hesitancy, impaired caliber and force of the urinary stream, and terminal dribbling are most commonly caused by benign prostatic hypertrophy, but cancer of the prostate produces the same difficulties. A tumor of the bladder on or near the internal vesical orifice may cause similar symptoms. Cystoscopy is therefore necessary in all cases of bladder neck obstruction.

Tumor of the urethra causes progressive diminution of the urinary stream. A palpable urethral mass suggests tumor or stricture. Biopsy may be needed for positive differentiation.

Skin Lesions

Tumors or ulcers of the penile and scrotal skin may be benign or malignant but can be caused by infection. If there is the slightest doubt, a specimen should be obtained for pathologic study.

Palpable Mass

A. Renal Mass: Renal tumors frequently present no symptoms other than the discovery of a tumor mass by the patient or the doctor. Neoplasms can be confused with simple renal cysts, polycystic kidney, hydronephrosis, cyst of the pancreas, or an enlarged spleen.

B. Abdominal Mass: An intra-abdominal mass near the umbilical region should suggest metastases to the preaortic lymph nodes from tumor of the testis. A suprapubic midline mass may represent a dilated (obstructed) bladder or may be caused by gastrointestinal or gynecologic tumor. It is not common for a vesical neoplasm to be palpable suprapubically except on bimanual (abdominorectal or abdominovaginal) examination under anesthesia.

C. Prostatic Mass: When the prostate is diffusely stony-hard and fixed it is almost certainly cancerous, but a hard area in the gland may pose a problem in differential diagnosis. The possibilities include early cancer, fibrosis from chronic infection, prostatic calculi, granulomatous prostatitis, and tuberculosis. At

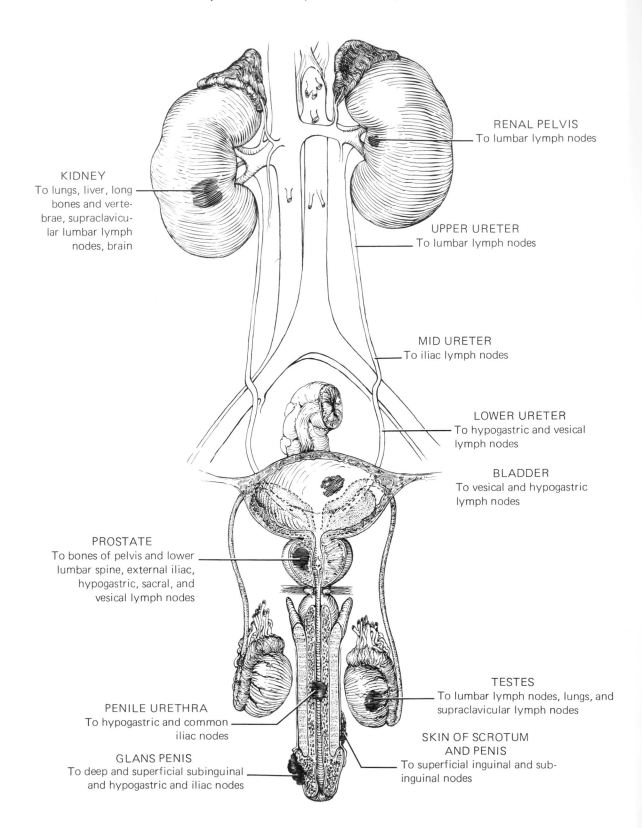

RENAL PELVIS
To lumbar lymph nodes

KIDNEY
To lungs, liver, long
bones and verte-
brae, supraclavicu-
lar lumbar lymph
nodes, brain

UPPER URETER
To lumbar lymph nodes

MID URETER
To iliac lymph nodes

LOWER URETER
To hypogastric and vesical
lymph nodes

BLADDER
To vesical and hypogastric
lymph nodes

PROSTATE
To bones of pelvis and lower
lumbar spine, external iliac,
hypogastric, sacral, and
vesical lymph nodes

TESTES
To lumbar lymph nodes, lungs, and
supraclavicular lymph nodes

PENILE URETHRA
To hypogastric and common
iliac nodes

SKIN OF SCROTUM
AND PENIS
To superficial inguinal and sub-
inguinal nodes

GLANS PENIS
To deep and superficial subinguinal
and hypogastric and iliac nodes

Figure 18–1. Sites of origin and metastases in the male.

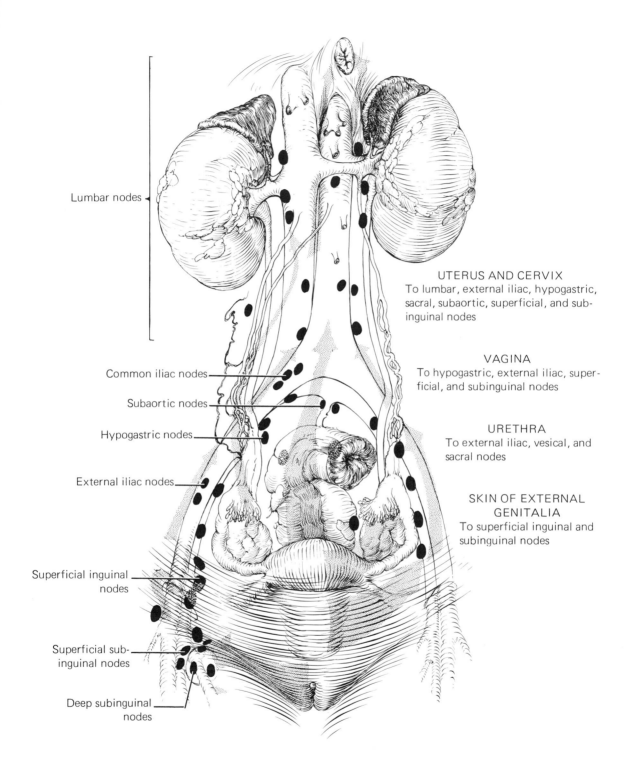

Figure 18–2. Sites and routes of metastases in the female.

times the differentiation can only be made by biopsy.

D. Testicular Mass: A painless, firm testis should be regarded as neoplastic until proved otherwise. Gummas may cause induration, but they are rare; serology will be helpful in differentiation.

Fever

Tumors of the kidney may excite no symptoms other than fever. Tumors of the urinary organs may also cause obstruction and be complicated by sepsis.

Hypertension

Hypertension is noted in about half of patients with Wilms's tumor, in some with renal adenocarcinoma, and in patients with juxtaglomerular adenomas.

Anemia

With advanced cancer in any urologic organ, anemia is to be expected even in the absence of blood loss. This is particularly true with prostatic malignancy, when bone marrow is extensively involved.

Erythrocytosis

Erythrocytosis occurs in association with 4% of renal cancers, including Wilms's tumor. It may also be noted with certain benign renal lesions.

Urinalysis

In most individuals with vesical neoplasms and transitional cell tumors of the ureter or renal pelvis, the urinary sediment stained with methylene blue will reveal round (transitional) epithelial cells; therefore, the presence of these cells should always arouse suspicion of tumor. Cytologic examination of urine sediment using Papanicolaou technics is discussed in Chapter 5.

SYMPTOMS & SIGNS OF METASTASES

Tumors of the genitourinary tract often cause no local symptoms or definite signs. Clinical manifestations may arise only from metastases.

Central nervous system. Tumors of the kidney or prostate may metastasize to the central nervous system. The first symptoms may therefore be neurologic.

Lungs. Tumors of the kidney, prostate, and testis often spread to the lungs. Pleuritic pain may suggest secondary pleural involvement.

Liver. Renal tumors frequently metastasize to the liver, which then becomes enlarged and nodular. If compression of the common duct occurs, jaundice will be noted.

Lymph nodes. Enlargement of the left supraclavicular lymph nodes may be the only finding in cancer of the kidney or testis. Palpable para-aortic abdominal masses in a young man may mean tumor of the testis. Edema of one or both legs may develop from compression of the iliac vessels by masses of lymph nodes

containing tumor cells from cancer of the prostate or bladder (Figs 18–1 and 18–2).

Bones. Metastasis to the skeletal system is most common from cancer of the prostate and kidney. This may cause pain in the bone, spontaneous fracture, or neurologic manifestations due to metastasis to the spine.

TUMORS OF THE RENAL PARENCHYMA

BENIGN TUMORS

From the clinical standpoint, benign tumors of the kidney are rare. However, small adenomas are often seen at autopsy. Their cells resemble those of the adult renal tubule. There is evidence that these adenomas are the source of the carcinomas of the renal parenchyma which are seen quite frequently in the adult.

Benign tumors of the renal parenchyma include adenomas, hemangiomas, fibromas, endometriosis, lipomas, myomas, and neurofibromas. Most of these are small, little more than 1–2 cm in diameter.

Large tumors of this type do occur and present signs and symptoms similar to those described under carcinoma; it is almost impossible to differentiate these from the malignant variety by urographic means. The kidney must, therefore, be removed.

Angiomyolipoma (Hamartoma)

This tumor appears in 3 forms: (1) unilateral single tumor without stigmas of tuberous sclerosis; (2) multiple and bilateral hamartomas in patients showing widespread connective tissue defects; and (3) so-called fetal hamartoma or mesoblastic nephroma.

A. Angiomyolipoma, Single and Unilateral: These benign tumors are made up of fat, smooth muscle, and blood vessels. Grossly, the tumor resembles adenocarcinoma of the kidney, from which it must be differentiated. Most occur in women between the ages of 40–60 years. The first symptoms are due to sudden spontaneous perirenal hemorrhage. The patient usually develops severe flank pain, an enlarging flank mass, and, in many cases, gross hematuria. Shock due to exsanguination is common.

On the plain abdominal film, areas of lucency may be noted in the tumor, which displaces and distorts calyces. Evidence of a large perinephric mass (blood) may be noted. Infusion urography shows increased vascularity, yet with areas of lucency in the tumor if the content of fat is significant. These films ordinarily are suggestive of hamartoma but not diagnostic. Selective renal angiography shows multiple small aneurysms, and in the early phase a fine network of tortuous vessels. Areas of lucency are seen. The vessels fail to undergo spasm after the infusion of epinephrine. In this way, they mimic adenocarcinoma; on late films, little venous and sinusoidal vascularity is noted. This is in contradistinction to the findings with cancer. Whorls of contrast material similar to those seen in uterine myomas are observed.

In the absence of signs of bilateral disease and the stigmas of tuberous sclerosis, immediate nephrectomy should be performed as a lifesaving procedure.

B. Tuberous Sclerosis: This syndrome is characterized by the presence of multiple and bilateral renal hamartomas, miscellaneous cutaneous lesions including "adenoma sebaceum," mental retardation, epilepsy, tumorlike swellings of the retina, and various mixed tumors in the brain, heart, and lungs.

There are usually no symptoms directly related to the kidneys. The presence of other signs of tuberous sclerosis may lead to excretory urography or infusion nephrotomography, which reveals large kidneys containing many lucent areas, thus mimicking polycystic renal disease. Angiography will, however, reveal the vascular nature of these lesions.

Surgical treatment should be conservative. If spontaneous bleeding occurs, watchful waiting and blood replacement may be the treatment of choice in the hope that the hemorrhage will cease. If it does not, partial nephrectomy should be done if feasible.

With the involvement of so many organ systems the prognosis is guarded. Progression of growth of the renal lesions may lead to renal insufficiency.

C. Renal Fetal Hamartoma, Mesoblastic Nephroma: These benign tumors are seen in the first few weeks or months of life. Until recently, they were diagnosed as Wilms's tumors. The mass consists of fetal mesenchymal tissue, largely hamartomatous and leiomyomatous elements. They have also, therefore, been considered fibrosarcomas and leiomyomas.

The tumor presents as a mass in the flank. Excretory urograms show changes typical of a space-occupying lesion. Angiography may fail to differentiate them from Wilms's tumors, although areas of lucency due to fat may be noted. Some neovascularity may be seen.

Since Wilms's tumor is very rarely present at birth, fetal hamartoma should be considered in this age group. Preoperative radiotherapy should not be given without a positive biopsy diagnosis. Treatment for these benign tumors consists of nephrectomy only.

Juxtaglomerular Cell Adenoma (Hemangiopericytoma)

These relatively rare, small, benign tumors secrete renin and therefore cause severe hypertension. Urinary aldosterone levels are elevated; plasma renin, particularly from the renal vein of the involved kidney, is elevated and hypokalemia is found. The lesion may be depicted on selective renal angiograms. The effect of nephrectomy is dramatic.

ADENOCARCINOMA
(Grawitz' Tumor; Hypernephroma)

About four-fifths of renal neoplasms are adenocarcinomas, and two-thirds of these occur in men. More than 150 cases have been reported in children. Because adenocarcinomas produce symptoms relatively late, the prognosis is only fair.

Etiology

There has been considerable disagreement over the origin of adenocarcinomas. Grawitz thought they arose from intrarenal adrenal rests, and the term "hypernephroma" was coined to describe them. The leading opinion now, however, is that they arise from cells of the renal tubules or from the benign adenomas. This theory is based on the histologic findings. Some of these tumors secrete hormones. Among those reported are parathyroidlike hormone, gonadotropins, ACTH, erythropoietin, and prostaglandin A, an antihypertensive.

Pathogenesis & Pathology

Adenocarcinoma usually arises in one of the renal poles. As the neoplasm expands, it compresses adjacent renal tissue and displaces calyces, blood vessels, and the pelvis, which then become distorted and tend to surround the mass. It is this characteristic which leads to urographic diagnosis. Multiple adenocarcinomas are often found in patients suffering from Lindau's disease (see Chapter 21).

The renal veins and even the vena cava are frequently invaded. This may be associated with the nephrotic syndrome or hepatic dysfunction. At times a column of tumor extends into the right heart. Occlusion of the renal vein may cause marked dilatation of the perirenal vessels and varicocele. As enlargement increases, intraperitoneal organs may be displaced (eg, stomach, intestines, spleen) or the diaphragm elevated. The tumor may invade adjacent muscle or organs (eg, duodenum, diaphragm).

Adenocarcinoma usually has a well-defined fibrous capsule. On section, the tumor is yellow and often contains zones of hemorrhage or necrosis. It produces a definite expansion of the kidney. Calcification may develop and may be visible on x-ray film.

Microscopically, varying patterns of cells may be seen even in the same tumor. In general, the cells resemble renal tubule cells and have small eccentric nuclei and an abundant clear cytoplasm. At times the cytoplasm may be more opaque and granular. A papillary or even anaplastic pattern may be seen. Tumors with well-differentiated clear cells seem to offer the best prognosis.

Most visceral metastases occur by way of the blood stream. The liver, lungs, and long bones (and occasionally the brain and adrenal glands) may be affected. Lumbar lymph nodes about the renal pedicle may become involved, and enlarged left supraclavicular nodes are occasionally seen. The kidney is involved

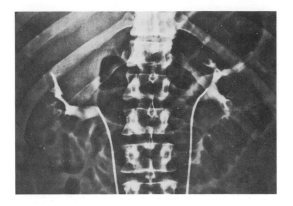
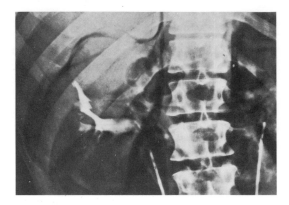
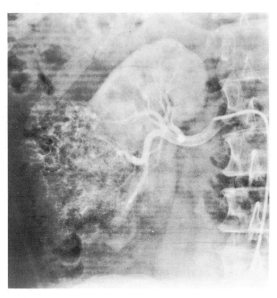
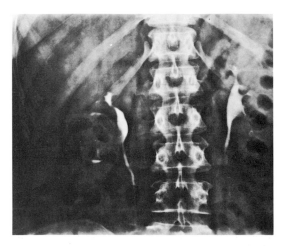

Figure 18–3. Adenocarcinoma of the kidney. *Above left:* Retrograde urogram showing lateral displacement of upper pole of right kidney and elongation and distortion of upper calyces (carcinoma). Left urogram normal. *Above right:* Same patient. Retrograde urogram combined with pneumogram shows extent of mass and its relation to calyces. Normal right adrenal. *Below left:* Selective renal angiogram showing marked vascularity of mass in lower portion of right kidney typical of malignant tumor. *Below right:* Excretory urogram. Distortion of the pelvis, middle and lower calyces of right kidney. Space-occupying lesion (adenocarcinoma). The left kidney is normal.

secondarily by metastases from other organs in 7.6% of cases. The bronchus is the most common primary site.

Clinical Findings

A. Symptoms: Gross total hematuria is the most common symptom and is usually not accompanied by pain. It occurs in two-thirds of patients. Pain may be the initial symptom but is usually a late manifestation. It may be of the dull type felt in the back, resulting from back pressure from ureteral compression, perirenal extension, or hemorrhage into the substance of the kidney; or it may be colicky if a clot or mass of tumor cells passes down the ureter.

Occasionally a patient may discover a mass in the flank in the absence of other symptoms. Gastrointestinal complaints resembling the syndromes of peptic ulcer or gallbladder disease may be the only subjective manifestations. These are caused by reflex action or by

displacement or invasion of intraperitoneal organs. Unexplained low-grade fever may be the only symptom.

Symptoms from metastases may also occur as the first manifestations of renal tumor. These include unexplained loss of weight, increasing weakness, and anemia. Bone pain, spontaneous fracture, pulmonary difficulties, or a mass in the left side of the neck (Virchow's nodes) may be the presenting complaint.

B. Signs: A mass is often discovered in the flank. It must be pointed out, however, that the kidneys lie rather high, particularly on the left side. In an obese or muscular person, considerable enlargement can be present and still defy detection. Fixation may mean local invasion. Involvement of the vena cava by tumor or thrombosis may cause the development of dilated veins on the abdominal wall. An acute hydrocele or varicocele may develop as a rare and late sign if the

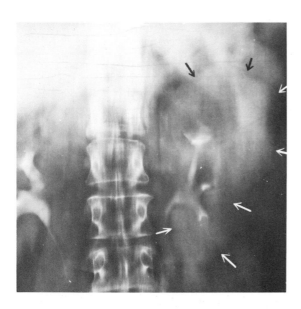

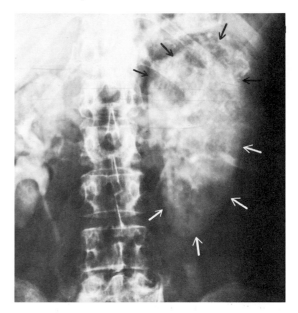

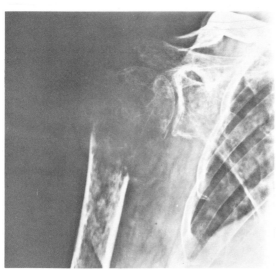

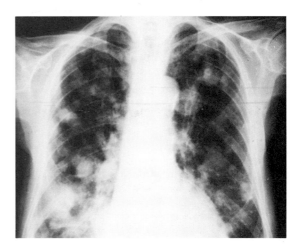

Figure 18–4. Adenocarcinoma of the kidney. *Above left:* Excretory urogram with tomography showing marked expansion of upper pole and elongated upper calyx, left kidney. *Above right:* Infusion urogram, same patient, showing pooling of radiopaque fluid in cancer of upper pole, left kidney. *Below left:* Osteolytic metastases to humerus. *Below right:* Metastases to lung. Note typical "cannonball" lesions.

spermatic vein is occluded. This is most apt to occur on the left side because this vein drains into the left renal vein.

Arteriovenous fistulas are occasionally observed in association with renal adenocarcinoma. This is suggested in the presence of cardiomegaly, diastolic hypertension, and a systolic murmur and bruit over the mass. The diagnosis is made on angiography.

Metastatic signs are varied and may be the presenting manifestations of the illness. A palpable mass in the left supraclavicular region may mean metastases to lymph nodes. Physical examination of the lung fields may reveal no pathologic changes even though

metastases are present. Tenderness or even a palpable mass may be found over bone involved by tumor. Edema of the legs may be secondary to neoplastic involvement of the vena cava. The liver is a common site of metastases, in which case it may be enlarged and nodular. Ascites may be found. Loss of weight may be marked.

C. Laboratory Findings: Gross or microscopic hematuria is the cardinal finding, and even a few red cells must be explained. Erythrocytosis with an increased plasma erythropoietin level occurs in 3–4% of patients. Anemia may be present in advanced disease. Total renal function is usually not impaired, for even the involved kidney retains some function and bilateral renal cancer is rare. The sedimentation rate is usually accelerated. Hypercalcemia with secondary effects on muscle, heart, and brain may be noted; a parathyroid-like hormone can be extracted from the tumor in these patients. A few tumors have been found that secrete ACTH. This has led to a cushingoid appearance. Elaboration of gonadotropins causes gynecomastia in the male. One tumor was found to elaborate prostoglandin A. Only after the tumor was removed did hypertension develop.

The presence of a hypernephroma may cause hepatic insufficiency as shown by tests of liver function. Removal of the tumor causes the test results to return to normal.

D. X-Ray Findings (Simple Technics): A plain film of the abdomen often shows an enlarged kidney; a definite bulge of its contour is significant. The incidence of cystic or curvilinear calcification is 7%. The psoas margin may be obscured if a solid tumor overlies the muscle. If the tumor is a cyst, the psoas margin may be visible through it (Fig 6–12). The renal shadow may be displaced in any direction, depending upon the location of the tumor. A low left kidney in particular must not be ignored. Osteolytic metastases may be noted on bone x-rays.

Excretory urograms usually show a filling defect caused by a space-occupying lesion (Fig 18–3). Calcyes are bent, elongated, or otherwise distorted by the enlarging tumor. On rare occasion the ureter may be compressed, and hydronephrosis may develop. If considerable renal tissue is destoryed by tumor, visualization may be poor. If the renal vein is involved, no excretion of dye may be seen; this is a bad prognostic sign.

Infusion angionephrotomograms may show the renal capsule separated from the parenchyma. This might represent bleeding from a small cortical tumor. Selective angiography will be definitive.

If excretory urograms do not afford the necessary information for diagnosis, ureteral catheterization and retrograde urograms must be done (Fig 18–3). Oblique and lateral views should also be taken in order to depict minor deformities of the calyces and pelvis.

A chest film may show the typical nodular metastases, usually multiple (Fig 18–4). A gastrointestinal series or barium enema will show displacement of the stomach or bowel if the renal mass is large. Roentgenologic bone surgery may reveal osteolytic metastases. Pathologic fracture may be observed.

E. Ultrasonography: B-scan ultrasound differentiates between cyst and tumor in 90% of cases (see Chapter 8).

F. Special Radiographic Studies: Nephrotomography almost always reveals increased opacification of a tumor because of its increased vascularity (Fig 18–4). Renal angiography, particularly the selective type, produces a dense renal shadow (due to the presence of contrast material in the renal vessels and tubules) and may thereby reveal a bulge of the renal outline, indicating a tumor. Furthermore, because of

the great vascularity of the tumor (Fig 18–3), pooling of the opaque material will occur within it on the late films (5 seconds after injection). A cyst will cast no shadow at all.

Some tumors are relatively avascular, and the diagnosis may be in doubt. The infusion of epinephrine just before the radiopaque fluid is instilled will show marked spasm of the arterioles of normal renal tissue but not of the vessels in a tumor.

In some cases, numerous arteriovenous aneurysms are seen. Early opacification of the renal vein is therefore noted. This readily accounts for diastolic hypertension and an audible bruit heard over the kidney.

Venacavagraphy or selective renal phlebography may reveal the presence of tumor in the renal vein or vena cava.

G. Isotope Scanning: A rectilinear scan, using ^{203}Hg, will reveal a "cold" area because functioning parenchyma has been displaced by the tumor. The scan will be similar to that seen with simple renal cyst (Fig 21–4). The gamma camera will show a negative shadow with both ^{203}Hg and ^{131}I; but with ^{99m}Tc, which reveals the vasculature of the kidney, the tumor area will show normal or increased perfusion (Fig 8–3). A cyst shows none. A bone scan may reveal evidence of osseous metastases (Chapter 8).

H. Special Examinations: If the special radiologic studies fail to differentiate between cyst and tumor, a needle can be passed into the mass. The recovery of blood will suggest tumor.

I. Instrumental Examination: If the patient has gross hematuria when seen, immediate cystoscopy will demonstrate its source. Postponing cystoscopy almost guarantees that this valuable information will be lost, for renal tumors bleed intermittently.

J. Cytology: The Papanicolaou technic has been applied to the urinary sediment but rarely proves helpful.

K. Plasma or Urinary Carcinoembryonic Antigen (CEA): Chu & others (1974) note that about half of patients with adenocarcinoma reveal significant elevation of CEA levels. Following nephrectomy, the amount of this antigen decreases. In those who have demonstrable metastasis, more than 85% will have elevations of CEA.

Differential Diagnosis

Hydronephrotic kidney may be accompanied by pain, tumor, and hematuria. Gross bleeding, however, is rare. Urography will establish the diagnosis.

Polycystic kidney disease may also present with hematuria and a renal mass, but total renal function is usually impaired even though only one kidney is large enough to be felt. Hypertension is common with polycystic disease. Renal angiography or a technetium scan should differentiate the 2 lesions.

Simple cyst of the kidney may cause flank pain and may be palpable, but gross or even microscopic hematuria is unusual. Tumors are often associated with an increased sedimentation rate; cysts are not. Tumor and cyst both occupy space in the kidney, and so urograms of both may be similar. Cysts tend to be more extrinsic; solid tumors are prone to occupy the deeper renal tissues. If the renal mass overlies the psoas, the muscle is apt to be obliterated by a solid tumor but may be visible through a cyst (Fig 6–12). Infusion nephrotomograms (Fig 6–5) or angiograms (Fig 18–3) will usually make the differentiation: A cyst fails to opacify; a tumor becomes unusually dense.

If the radiographic diagnosis is cyst, this can be further confirmed by passing a needle into the mass. The fluid recovered should be analyzed for fat, whose absence confirms the diagnosis of cyst, and subjected to cytologic examination. Radiopaque fluid is then introduced and appropriate films taken (Fig 21–5). Differentiation may be possible only at surgery.

Renal tuberculosis can cause renal pain, a palpable mass, and gross hematuria, but symptoms of vesical irritability and pyuria are usually present. Acid-fast bacteria can almost always be demonstrated by culture. Cystoscopy may reveal tuberculous cystitis, and urograms should make an unequivocal differentiation.

A stone in the kidney or ureter can cause renal pain and hematuria, but the pain is often more acute. Roentgenograms should differentiate between stone and tumor.

Ureteral or renal pelvic tumor may mimic renal tumor, causing renal pain and often a palpable hydronephrotic kidney. Gross hematuria may also be present. Urography will clearly differentiate the two.

Adrenal or other extrarenal tumor (pancreatic pseudocyst) may present a palpable mass (either the tumor or a displaced kidney), but hematuria and pain are unusual. Most adrenal tumors are functional and cause definite signs and symptoms (eg, hirsutism, amenorrhea, obesity). Pheochromocytoma and neuroblastoma elaborate increased amounts of vanilmandelic acid in the urine. Urography and other studies will show a mass displacing the kidney whose calyces are normal.

Chronic pyelonephritis often causes renal pain and hematuria, but such kidneys are not enlarged. Symptoms of cystitis are often noted. The finding of pus and bacteria in the urine is suggestive. Urography should establish the diagnosis.

The xanthogranulomatous pyelonephritic kidney usually does not show function on excretory urograms, but retrograde urograms reveal a distorted calyceal system not unlike that seen with tumor. The differentiation is often made only at surgery, but angiography may prove helpful.

Tumors of the bladder usually cause hematuria. Excretory urograms will reveal an absence of calyceal distortion, although hydronephrosis may be present if a ureteral orifice is partially occluded. The cystogram may reveal a defect consistent with tumor (Fig 18–9). Cystoscopy will reveal the growth.

A kidney deformed by scarring due to infarction or multiple attacks of acute pyelonephritis may develop focal areas of renal compensatory hypertrophy which, with expansion, may deform the calyces, thus

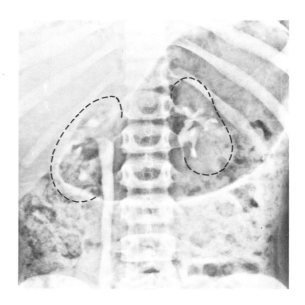

Figure 18–5. Renal pseudotumor. Bilateral healed pyelonephritis secondary to vesicoureteral reflux. Localized compensatory hypertrophy in lower pole of left kidney displaces calyces suggesting presence of space-occupying lesion.

simulating tumor (Fig 18–5). A similar picture may be caused by a very large column of Bertin which may resemble a tumor on excretory urography. An infusion nephrotomogram using abdominal compression will show the mass to be more dense than the surrounding parenchyma. It extends to the capsule and is seen between the upper and middle calyces. Angiography will fail to show the neovascularity of cancer.

Renal lymphoma or Hodgkin's disease may lead to deformity of the calyces. The tumors are usually bilateral and multiple. Evidence of lymphoma elsewhere is helpful in differential diagnosis. Angiography may be helpful, but Hodgkin's tumor may be very vascular.

Complications

The complications of adenocarcinomas are largely related to local invasion or distant metastases. A few patients develop hydronephrosis from ureteral compression, hypertension from interference with the blood supply to the organ, or arteriovenous fistula. Occlusion of the renal vein by tumor may cause findings compatible with the nephrotic syndrome. Rarely, hematuria may be severe enough to threaten to cause death from exsanguination.

Treatment

A. Radical Nephrectomy: If there are no demonstrable metastases, radical nephrectomy, including removal of the perinephric fat, should be performed. If hemorrhage is intractable, nephrectomy may be necessary even though metastases are demonstrated. Erythrocytosis, if present, subsides after nephrectomy. Tests implying impaired liver function will return to normal.

Hypercalcemia will react in kind. The red cell count and serum calcium may rise again if metastases occur. In a few patients, pulmonary metastases may regress following nephrectomy. Most, however, again become obvious in a few months. Almgard & others (1973) suggest that, should the tumor mass be very large, autologous muscle suspension can be injected into the renal artery in conjunction with selective renal angiography. The resulting partial thrombosis causes the kidney to shrink, making nephrectomy easier. Brandstetter & Schwentker (1973) recommend the injection of isobutyl-2-cyanoacrylate to accomplish the same purpose.

Partial nephrectomy for cancer in a solitary kidney should be considered.

B. X-Ray Therapy: Adenocarcinomas of the kidney and their metastases are usually radioresistant. Most authorities feel that x-ray therapy is therefore not indicated either preoperatively or postoperatively, but a few authors disagree.

C. Chemotherapy: Chemotherapy has been disappointing. The administration of medroxyprogesterone or testosterone has had some palliative effect in a few cases.

D. Follow-Up Care: This includes abdominal palpation for tumor in the renal bed or enlarging nodular liver and a chest film. Angiography may reveal the hypervascularity of local recurrence.

Prognosis

About 35% of patients suffering from cancer of the kidney are alive 5 years after nephrectomy. The outlook is poor if the renal vein or vena cava has been invaded by tumor. Metastases may develop even 10–15 years after removal of the primary growth. The percentage of cures can only be increased by subjecting all patients suffering from hematuria—microscopic or gross; persistent, transient, or intermittent—to complete urologic study. The prognosis in children is more promising.

EMBRYOMA
(Wilms's Tumor;
Adenomyosarcoma, Nephroblastoma)

Embryoma of the kidney is a highly malignant mixed tumor. It is almost exclusively a disease of children under the age of 6 years; in this age group it is second in incidence only to leukemia and is the most common abdominal neoplasm in children. Ten percent are bilateral. The incidence is 1:10,000.

Etiology

Wilms's tumor is considered by most investigators to be congenital and to arise from embryonal cells trapped in the kidney. About 6% are clinically present at birth, and these, if large, may cause dystocia.

Pathogenesis & Pathology

Wilms's tumor may arise in any portion of the kidney. It usually becomes quite large before it is discovered. Pain is not common. Hematuria is rare and late, for this tumor seldom breaks through the renal pelvis.

The tumor is usually large, pale, and lobulated. The surface of the kidney is usually covered by large, thin-walled veins. Little viable renal tissue may be left. On cut section, the tissue is usually yellow or white and heterogeneous; hemorrhagic and cystic areas are often found. Microscopically the major tissues are of connective tissue origin: muscle, cartilage, and myxomatous or lipomatous tissue. The epithelial structures may be undifferentiated or may resemble renal tubules or even glomeruli. The term "adenomyosarcoma" has therefore been used to describe these tumors. Possibly half of them will show abnormal chromosome sets.

If preoperative x-ray treatment has been given, the tumor may be small; in fact, the kidney may be only slightly enlarged. The entire tumor may be necrotic and hemorrhagic, although viable sarcoma and carcinoma cells are usually found microscopically. These primitive cells are quite radiosensitive.

The usual route of metastasis is through the bloodstream; the lungs, liver, and brain are most commonly involved. Regional lumbar lymph nodes may be affected.

Clinical Findings

A. Symptoms: The most common symptom is a palpable mass in the flank, usually discovered by the child's parents. Rarely, pain may be experienced from local invasion or ureteral compression (hydronephrosis). Other symptoms include loss of weight, anorexia or vomiting from displacement or invasion of the enteric tract, and hematuria (unusual).

B. Signs: A palpable mass in the flank of a child under age 6 must be regarded as Wilms's tumor (or neuroblastoma of the adrenal) until proved otherwise. The mass does not transilluminate. An enlarged nodular liver strongly suggests that metastasis from the renal tumor has occurred. The lungs usually reveal no abnormal physical signs even though they contain metastases. Hypertension is common in children with embryoma of the kidney. There is evidence to suggest that these tumors secrete renin (Ganguly, 1973). The hypertension is usually relieved by removal of the involved organ. Weight loss is a prominent feature of the late stage of the disease. In 1–2% of cases, congenital aniridia has been observed. This is often associated with microcephaly, cataracts, glaucoma, and mental retardation. Hemihypertrophy is occasionally seen.

C. Laboratory Findings: Anemia may be present. Urinalysis is usually normal; the finding of red cells is unusual. Tests of total renal function are usually normal, for even the involved kidney usually retains some function.

D. X-Ray Findings:

1. Simple technics—A greatly enlarged renal

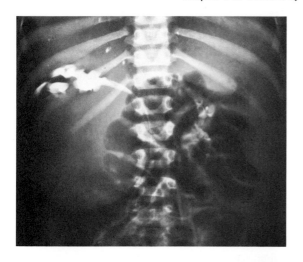

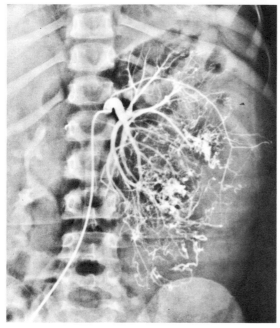

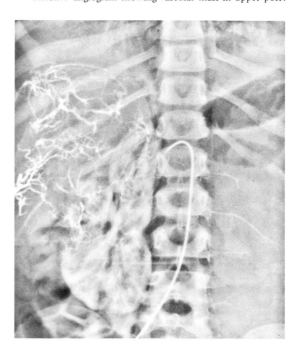

Figure 18–6. Wilms's tumor. *Left:* Exeretory urogram showing large globular mass in right upper quadrant with displacement and distortion of calyces. Upper right ureter displaced over spine. *Below:* Bilateral embryomas as shown on angiography. *Left:* Early phase of left selective angiogram showing arcing of major renal arteries, vascular pooling, and typical tumor vessels. *Right:* Late phase of right selective angiogram showing vascular mass in upper pole.

shadow is usually evident on a plain film of the abdomen. There may be a rim of calcification around the periphery of the tumor. The bowel, as demonstrated by the gas pattern, may be displaced. There may be evidence of enlargement of the liver.

Excretory urograms usually show great distortion of the pelvis and clayces on the involved side (Fig 18–6), although lack of excretion may occur. Retrograde urograms may then be necessary.

A chest film may disclose metastases to the lungs.

2. **Special radiographic studies**—Renal angiography will show the enlarged renal mass (Fig 18–6). Unlike adenocarcinoma, vascularity is sparse; zigzag arterioles are seen. There is no pooling of opaque medium, nor are arteriovenous fistulas observed. The midstream study may show metastatic deposits in the liver.

E. Instrumental Examination: Cystoscopy and

ureteral catheterization are indicated for the purpose of obtaining retrograde urograms if excretory urograms are inadequate, but this is rare.

F. Cytologic Examination: Papanicolaou studies will seldom be of help for the tumor rarely breaks through the pelvic lining.

Differential Diagnosis

Neuroblastoma of the adrenal medulla is an exceedingly malignant tumor which, for the most part, afflicts children under age 3. It usually presents as a mass in the flank, but since it metastasizes early and widely and by both lymphatics and blood vessels, the first symptoms may be caused by metastases. Neuroblastoma tends to invade the muscles of the back; it may therefore present a visible bulge in the costovertebral angle. Urography, either excretory or retrograde, should permit differentiation. Neuroblastoma tends to displace the kidney; Wilms's tumors are intrinsic renal lesions and therefore distort the calcyes. Neuroblastomas frequently contain stippled calcification on the plain film. The osseous metastases are frequently bilateral and almost symmetrical, involving many bones. The urinary vanilmandelic acid level is increased with neuroblastoma but is normal with Wilms's tumor.

Fetal hamartoma (congenital mesoblastic nephroma) is a benign tumor discovered during the first few months of life. On infusion urography and angiography, lucent areas representing fat are seen. The vascular changes are typical of hamartoma.

Hydronephrosis may also cause a mass in the flank. It is usually softer than a tumor. It may transilluminate. If secondarily infected, pyuria will be found. Urography is diagnostic.

Multicystic kidney seen in the newborn presents as a nodular mass in one flank and may, therefore, be confused with Wilms's tumor. This cystic kidney fails to secrete radiopaque material. The ureter is usually not connected to the mass; therefore retrograde urography will not afford a urogram. Angiography may be required to settle the matter, but the diagnosis may be made only at the operating table.

Polycystic kidney disease may cause a palpable mass, although enlargement is usually bilateral. Renal function tests are depressed, and urograms show bilateral calcyeal distortion. It must be remembered, however, that 10% of Wilms's tumors are bilateral. Renal angiography may be needed in case of doubt.

Treatment

A. Specific Measures:

1. Radiation therapy—Only if it is judged that the tumor is too large to allow nephrectomy readily should preoperative irradiation be administered. If the diagnosis is accurate, dramatic shrinkage of the mass should be observed. Following nephrectomy, radiotherapy to the tumor bed should be given. In patients under 1 year of age, there is some danger of damaging the vertebrae, leading to kyphosis or scoliosis.

2. Nephrectomy—The kidney should be removed through a transperitoneal incision as soon as the diagnosis is made. In the face of bilateral renal involvement, some cures have been obtained by removal of one kidney and partial removal of the other. Bilateral nephrectomy followed by renal transplantation has its advocates.

3. Chemotherapy—This tumor has proved to be quite sensitive to dactinomycin, which should be started a few days before surgery and continued daily for 1 week and then at weekly intervals. Other dosage schedules have also been suggested. Other useful chemotherapeutic drugs include vincristine and adriamycin. Multiple courses of dactinomycin should be given to control subsequent pulmonary metastases.

B. Palliative Measures: If metastases are widespread—and particularly if they are discovered in bone or the brain—the prognosis appears to be hopeless, though radiotherapy and chemotherapy should not be withheld. Vincristine has been found useful under these circumstances. Instances have been reported in which resection of pulmonary and even hepatic metastases has led to cure.

C. Follow—Up Care: The patient should undergo palpation of the flank for evidence of local recurrence. Serial chest films are essential because pulmonary metastases are common.

Prognosis

In the absence of demonstrable metastases, about 80–90% of these children will be cured by nephrectomy, radiation therapy and chemotherapy. Even in the presence of pulmonary lesions, combined therapy offers cure in about 50% of cases. The younger the child, the better the outlook. Since it seems probable that the tumor has its inception at the time of conception, cure may be assumed if the child lives for a period equal to nine months plus its age at the time of surgery. Thus, a patient operated upon at the age of 20 months may be considered cured if he is free of disease 29 months after surgical intervention (Collins). The prognosis is improved if the capsule has not been invaded.

SARCOMA

Sarcomas of the kidney are rare. They may be made up of smooth or striated muscle, fibroplastic tissue, or fat. They may become quite large and fill the flank. Spread is usually by way of the blood stream; the lungs and bones are commonly involved.

The signs and symptoms are usually the presence of a mass and local pain. Hematuria is not common. Spontaneous perirenal hemorrhage may cause the first symptoms (pain, shock).

The diagnosis rests on urographic evidence of a space-occupying lesion. Preoperative differentiation from all other types of renal tumor is difficult.

In the absence of metastases, nephrectomy is indicated unless lymphoblastoma is suspected, in which case radiation therapy should be used. The prognosis is quite poor for the entire group. The incidence of distant metastases and local recurrence after surgical extirpation is high.

TUMORS OF THE
RENAL PELVIS & URETER

Histologically, the epithelial tumors of the renal pelvis and ureter resemble the tumors of the bladder. They may be benign or malignant.

Although malignant tumors of the ureter arising

from mesenchymal tissues have been described, they are rare and will therefore not be discussed here. Suffice it to say that clinically they mimic the more common epithelial growths and benign polyps.

TUMORS OF THE RENAL PELVIS

Most tumors arising from the calyceal or pelvic mucosa are papillary in type. They comprise about 10% of tumors of the kidney. Hematuria is usually the earliest symptom. Eighty percent are transitional cell tumors, and most of these occur in men. Squamous cell carcinoma has an incidence of about 15%, and the majority occur in women. Adenocarcinomas and sarcomas are rare.

Etiology

The cause of the papillary growths is not known. Their tendency to "seed" in the ureter and bladder suggests that the mucosa generally is susceptible to such change. The rare epidermoid carcinoma is usually associated with chronic infection or stone; chronic inflammation may therefore play a part in its genesis.

The metabolites of tryptophan (alpha-aminophenols) are suspect as carcinogenic agents. For a discussion of this subject, see section on etiology of tumors of the bladder, p 262.

Reports from Yugoslavia and Scandinavia incriminate phenacetin abuse as a cause of transitional cell tumors. This is associated with interstitial nephritis—even papillary necrosis. Renal insufficiency is noted in half of these patients. In 10% of these cases, the lesion is bilateral.

Pathogenesis & Pathology

These tumors may cause obstruction to calyces or even the ureteropelvic junction, thereby causing renal pain and the changes associated with back pressure. The more malignant types tend to invade the parenchyma. Hematuria occurs earlier than in adenocarcinomas of the parenchyma. Similar tumors may also be found in the ureter and bladder, particularly in the region of the ipsilateral ureteral orifice. It is therefore necessary to remove the kidney, ureter, and adjacent bladder wall when dealing with these growths. Most papillary tumors of the renal pelvis are malignant. Metastases are usually not widespread. The regional lumbar nodes may be involved.

Microscopically, these tumors show a central core of connective tissue which is covered by transitional epithelium. Invasion of the supporting stroma or mucosa or the finding of many cells in mitosis is evidence of malignancy, but at times it is difficult to draw the line between the malignant and benign types. Epidermoid cancers are invasive and highly malignant, and survival is rare. They are usually associated with severe chronic infection or lithiasis. They also spread to the regional lymphatics. Microscopic examination reveals the typical picture presented by squamous cell tumors seen elsewhere in the body.

Clinical Findings

A. Symptoms: Gross painless hematuria is the most common complaint of patients with renal pelvic tumor. Bleeding is at times quite profuse. Flank pain may be due to ureteral obstruction from the tumor; there may be ureteral colic from passage of clots.

B. Signs: Tenderness may be found over the kidney, particularly if ureteral obstruction has occurred or if infection has supervened. A palpably enlarged kidney is not common.

C. Laboratory Findings: Anemia can be marked if bleeding is profuse. Gross or microscopic hematuria is to be expected, but at intervals the urine may be free of red cells. Renal infection can result from obstruction or can be primary with epidermoid tumors, in which case pus and bacteria will be found in the urine. Renal function tests will be of little help; although the kidney may be gradually destroyed by the tumor, the other kidney will assume the lost function.

D. X-Ray Findings: A plain film of the abdomen will probably not be of much value, for the kidney is ordinarily not grossly enlarged. Excretory urograms, if good filling occurs, will show a space-occupying lesion in the pelvis (Fig 18–7) or a calyx. A chest film should be taken routinely, although metastases to the lungs are not common.

Retrograde urography should reveal the filling defect. Secondary ureteral growths may also be demonstrated. Selective renal angiography usually reveals an enlarged pelviureteric artery, fine neovascularity, and often a tumor blush.

E. Instrumental Examination: Cystoscopy must be done immediately if and when gross bleeding is present; blood may be seen spurting from one ureteral orifice. During cystoscopy, search must be made for "satellite" tumors on the bladder wall.

F. Cytologic Examination: The Papanicolaou technic or methylene blue smear of the urinary sediment is usually positive. The chances for a positive test are enhanced if the pelvis is irrigated with saline and the washings submitted for study.

G. Plasma or Urinary Carcinoembryonic Antigen (CEA): It has been reported that possibly two-thirds of these patients will have elevated levels of CEA.

Differential Diagnosis

Adenocarcinoma of the kidney will cause hematuria. Such a tumor is apt to be palpable or may be visible on a plain film of the abdomen as an expansion of a portion of the kidney. Urograms will show the intrarenal nature of the growth. However, blood clots in the renal pelvis can mimic pelvic tumor.

A nonopaque renal stone may cause hematuria and renal pain. A mass may be palpable if hydronephrosis develops. Urograms will show a space-occupying lesion of the pelvis, but the outline of the negative (black) shadow (representing the stone) tends to be smoothly round or oval with stone and irregular (papil-

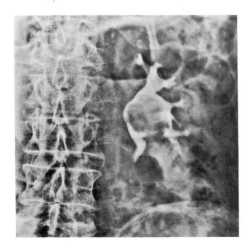

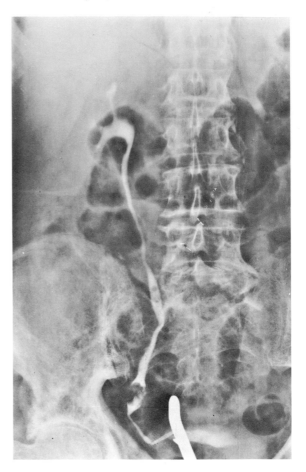

Figure 18—7. *Left:* Excretory urogram showing space occupying lesion of left renal pelvis. Transitional cell carcinoma. *Right:* Retrograde urogram showing "negative" shadow caused by transitional cell carcinoma of the lower right ureter without evidence of obstruction.

lary) with tumor (Fig 15—2). With tumor, cytology is usually positive.

An opaque renal stone may be associated with an epidermoid carcinoma of the renal pelvis. Diagnosis under these circumstances may be difficult and may be possible only at the time of surgical exploration for the treatment of the calculus.

Renal tuberculosis may mimic pelvic neoplasm. The urogram may show irregularity of the pelvic outline due to ulceration. This might suggest tumor. The patient with urinary tract tuberculosis usually complains of vesical irritability and has a "sterile" pyuria. Acid-fast organisms can be demonstrated in the urine.

Cholesteatoma of the renal pelvis comprises a mass of keratinized squamous cells. Urography shows an intrapelvic mass. The urine is loaded with squamous cells. Angiography reveals no evidence of tumor.

An ectopic or aberrant renal papilla projecting into the renal pelvis will show on urography as a space-occupying lesion. Selective angiography is definitive.

Hemangioma, an occasional cause of hematuria involving the renal pelvis or submucosal parenchyma, is usually too small to be seen on a urogram. A large

hematoma will present on the urogram as a space-occupying lesion of the pelvis. Renal angiography makes the diagnosis (Fig 18—8).

Complications

On rare occasion, hemorrhage may be so severe that emergency nephrectomy is necessary.

Hydronephrosis or hydrocalycosis may arise from progressive obstruction. Secondary infection may then develop.

Treatment

A. Specific Measures: Once the diagnosis has been made and evidence of metastasis ruled out, the kidney, ureter, and the periureteral portion of the bladder must be removed. This radical procedure is necessary because secondary ureteral and vesical tumors may be present or may develop later in the ureteral stump or bladder.

B. Palliative Measures: Even though metastases are demonstrated it may be advisable to remove the affected kidney if pain or infection from obstruction is severe or if bleeding is profuse.

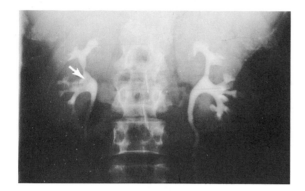
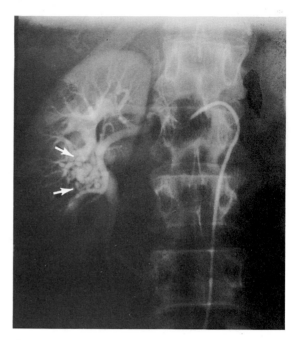

Figure 18–8. Renal hemangioma. *Left:* Excretory urogram showing filling defect in right renal pelvis. *Right:* Selective renal angiogram. Note multiple tortuous vessels.

Tumors of the renal pelvis are radioresistant. Little can be expected from radiotherapy.

C. Follow-Up Care: The patient should be seen periodically and examined by abdominal palpation to search for local recurrence and enlargement or nodulation of the liver. Serial chest films are indicated. Since vesical or contralateral pelvic tumors may develop, urinary cytology should be ordered.

Prognosis

The prognosis for the patient suffering from benign tumor is excellent. With low-grade malignancies the outlook is good (75% are alive after 5 years); it is fair to poor if the papillary tumor is undifferentiated (25% are alive after 5 years). Epidermoid carcinoma is almost always fatal within 1 year.

TUMORS OF THE URETER

Tumors of the ureter are rare; the majority are malignant and papillary in type. About two-thirds of them occur in men, and most are seen in the lower ureter.

Etiology

Although the cause of these tumors is not known, there is increasing evidence that carcinogens are involved (see section on etiology of tumors of the bladder, p 262). The incidence of this lesion is higher than normal in persons who habitually take large doses of phenacetin.

Pathogenesis & Pathology

Ureteral tumors may be primary or may be associated with similar tumors of the renal pelvis or bladder. Although they usually bleed, many of the symptoms are caused by ureteral obstruction (eg, renal and ureteral pain).

These neoplasms are similar in all respects to those of the renal pelvis and bladder. Most are papillary; a few are sessile. Squamous cell carcinoma is rare. Benign fibrous polyps are occasionally seen. Endometriosis has been reported.

Transitional cell carcinomas range from a low to a high grade of malignancy. The most malignant show invasion of the stroma and ureteral wall by pleomorphic cells which have a marked tendency to metastasize to regional lymph nodes, lungs, and liver.

Metastatic tumors from other sources are occasionally seen. The primary sites include the uterus, colon, breast, and prostate.

Clinical Findings

A. Symptoms: The most common symptom is hematuria, usually intermittent and sometimes quite profuse. There may be a dull pain over the kidney, caused by ureteral obstruction. Acute renal colic can occur from the passage of clots down the ureter. There may be symptoms of urinary tract infection (secondary to obstruction). These include fever, back pain, and vesical irritability.

B. Signs: Physical findings are usually absent. If the kidney has become hydronephrotic from ureteral obstruction, it may be palpable. If it is infected, it may be tender. An enlarged liver or a mass of lymph nodes (metastatic involvement) may be felt.

C. Laboratory Findings: Anemia may be found if bleeding is prolonged or severe. Gross or microscopic hematuria is usually present. Evidence of infection may be found on urinalysis. Renal function will ordinarily not be impaired unless the other kidney is also diseased.

D. X-Ray Findings: A plain film of the abdomen may show an enlarged renal shadow (hydronephrosis) secondary to ureteral obstruction. Excretory urograms will usually make the diagnosis (Fig 18–7). There is often dilatation of the urinary passages proximal to the obstructive tumor, and an intraureteral space-occupying lesion may be noted as the cause for the obstruction. An x-ray of the chest should be taken as soon as the diagnosis of ureteral tumor is made since metastases may be found in the lungs.

A ureteral catheter passed up the ureter for urography often forms a loop at the site of the tumor. A retrograde urogram will demonstrate the lesion. Oblique views are often helpful.

E. Instrumental Examination: Cystoscopy should be done immediately if the patient is actively bleeding in order to locate the source of the hemorrhage. It must be done also to observe for "seeding" of secondary growths on the bladder wall. Occasionally the tumor can be seen protruding from the ureteral orifice.

Ureteral catheterization may cause considerable blood to drain from the catheter when it passes by the tumor. When its tip reaches the renal pelvis, the urine becomes clear; this may therefore be of diagnostic significance.

F. Cytologic Examination: Papanicolaou studies or a methylene blue smear of the urinary sediment will usually reveal abnormal transitional cells.

Differential Diagnosis

Ureteral calculus, if it is radiolucent, may cause the same symptoms and signs as ureteral tumor. The urogram in each case will show a "negative" or black shadow in the ureter with dilatation of the tract above it. Stone is suggested if a "grating" feeling is noted as a catheter is passed by it. The correct diagnosis may be possible only at surgery.

Ureteral stenosis, often secondary to compression by masses of lymph nodes involved by cancer (eg, cervix), can mimic ureteral tumor. The discovery of a primary tumor will make the diagnosis.

A blood clot from a renal stone, adenocarcinoma, or pelvic tumor will also show as a "negative" shadow within the ureter. The urograms should make the differentiation. Air bubbles introduced through a ureteral catheter may cause some confusion.

Complications

Hydronephrosis is often found with ureteral tumor.

Because obstruction is usually present, infection may develop. The bacteriuria usually fails to clear despite appropriate medication; this should indicate the need for urography, which will demonstrate the tumor.

Treatment

A. Specific Measures: In the absence of demonstrable metastases, ureteronephrectomy and the resection of the periureteral bladder wall are necessary. When dealing with transitional cell tumors, if the lower ureter is left in, there is a 10–15% chance of recurrence of tumor in this segment. For benign or very low grade tumors, sleeve resection of the involved ureteral segment with end-to-end anastomosis should be considered.

B. Palliative Measures: Little can be accomplished if metastases are present, since these tumors are usually radioresistant. Ureteronephrectomy may be necessary to relieve pain due to the obstruction or to control otherwise intractable bleeding. It may also be indicated because of severe and persistent infection of the kidney. Chemotherapy has not been effective.

C. Follow-Up Care: Evidence of recurrence in the retroperitoneum and metastasis to the liver and lungs should be sought. Periodic urine cytologic examination must be done to search for clues to the development of new transitional tumors in the other kidney or bladder.

Prognosis

The prognosis in the benign type is excellent; with the malignant transitional cell carcinomas, it is only fair, particularly if they are invasive. The higher the grade, the poorer the outlook. Patients with squamous cell tumors or tumors which have involved the ureteral muscle and regional lymph nodes are rarely cured.

TUMORS OF THE BLADDER

Tumors of the bladder are the second most common of all genitourinary neoplasms. (Only prostatic tumors occur more frequently.) Seventy-five percent are found in men. Most are seen after age 50. Papillomatous growths submit readily to transurethral treatment if diagnosed early. Infiltrating (transitional cell) types constitute one of the most difficult of all urologic problems.

Etiology

It has long been established that prolonged exposure to certain industrial aromatic amines (eg, 2-naphthylamine, benzidine, 4-aminodiphenyl) may be associated with a high incidence of vesical neoplasm. Recent work suggests that the multiple transitional cell tumors involving the urinary tract (eg, renal pelvis, ureter, bladder) probably are caused by carcinogens, particularly tryptophan. This substance and the industrial amines listed above are metabolized to ortho-aminophenols by the liver, conjugated with sulfate or glucuronic acid, and excreted through the kidneys. These materials are attacked by hydrolytic enzymes (betaglucuronides), thus liberating orthophenols, some of which have been proved to be carcinogenic in dogs and mice. These carcinogens are found in increased concentration in the urines of those patients harboring vesical tumors (Boyland, 1963). It is thought that many years of exposure to these carcinogens are necessary to stimulate the growth of these tumors.

There is evidence that the activity of urinary beta-glucuronidase is increased merely by forcing fluids and by the presence of vesical infection, even schistosomiasis. This substance is also found in increased amounts in the presence of other cancers, benign enlargement of the prostate, renal infection, renal cyst, and urolithiasis. Kallet and Lapcol claim that this enzyme is elaborated by urologic epithelial cells which have been damaged; therefore, increases in urinary levels of beta-glucuronidase are of no diagnostic significance.

Smoking has been cited as a cause of the increased incidence of vesical neoplasm. It has recently been shown that smokers experience a 50% increase in carcinogenic metabolites of tryptophan excreted in the urine. On cessation of smoking, the levels return to normal. Rose & Wallace (1973) studied urinary chemiluminescence in both smokers and nonsmokers as well as patients with vesical cancer. The latter showed the highest levels; smokers had next highest levels; and nonsmokers had low levels. They found that ascorbic acid decreased this activity both in those who smoked and in those who did not. The high incidence of cancer of the bladder in patients with severe vesical schistosomiasis is well known.

Pathogenesis & Pathology

It is customary to judge transitional cell vesical carcinomas in 2 ways: (1) The degree of differentiation of the cells, and (2) the depth of penetration of the tumor into the vesical wall or beyond (Fig 18–9).

A. The Grade and Stage of the Tumor:

1. Grade–The degree of cell differentiation.

Grade I tumors are quite well differentiated. The lamina propria is usually not involved. Most are relatively small, are papillary in type, and have a narrow base. These are curable by transurethral means but are radio-resistant.

Grade II tumors are papillary in type, show less differentiation of their cells, and are apt to invade the lamina propria if not the detrusor muscle itself. They tend to be larger than the grade I tumors and have a wider connection with the bladder wall. They are often curable by transurethral resection. They do not respond too well to radiotherapy.

Grade III and IV neoplasms are poorly differentiated, even anaplastic. They tend to be nodular rather than papillary, and as a rule are quite invasive. They respond poorly to transurethral removal as well as cystectomy but are sensitive to radiotherapy.

2. Stage–The degree of invasion. Two methods of staging vesical tumors are in vogue: The Jewett method, which is commonly used in the USA, and the international (UICC) system. The former uses letters

O, A, B_1, B_2, C, D; while the latter utilizes "T" numbers.

Stage O (T1S) represents a papillary tumor which has not invaded the lamina propria.

Stage A (T1) tumors have invaded the lamina propria but not the muscle of the vesical wall.

Stage B_1 (T2) neoplasms have extended into the superficial half of the detrusor muscle.

Stage B_2 (T2) tumors are found in the deep muscle layers.

Stage C (T3) tumors have extended into the perivesical fat or have involved overlying peritoneum.

Stage D (T4) tumors have demonstrable metastases (eg, lymph nodes, liver).

B. Type and Location: Since 80% of vesical tumors arise on the base of the bladder, they may involve one or both ureteral orifices or the vesical neck. Hydroureteronephrosis and pyelonephritis are common complications. When tumors ulcerate, they bleed and often become infected.

Most growths are papillary in type and are malignant. They may be single or multiple; generalized papillomatosis is not uncommon. Generally speaking, the larger the tumor and the broader its base, the more malignant it is, and nodular tumors are more malignant than the papillary types.

In the male, secondary tumors may develop in the urethra.

Lamb (1967) has noted that aberrations in chromosome count and structural abnormality are apt to be seen in the undifferentiated tumors.

After successful treatment of even the grade I and II types that are superficial (stages O [T1S] and A [T1]), there is a definite tendency for new tumors to develop elsewhere in the bladder. This suggests that the appearance of these tumors is in some way related to a generally increased susceptibility of the mucosa to neoplastic proliferation, perhaps in response to carcinogens. This is true also of the renal pelvic and ureteral transitional cell tumors.

Vesical neoplasms most commonly metastasize to the vesical, hypogastric, common iliac, and lumbar nodes. The bones, liver, and lungs are at times affected.

Rarely, other types of vesical neoplasms may be encountered:

(1) Epidermoid carcinoma: About 5% of vesical neoplasms are of the squamous cell variety. These are ordinarily highly malignant (anaplastic), deeply invasive, and metastasize early. With a few exceptions, they are incurable.

(2) Adenocarcinoma is very rare. It often arises in a urachal remnant.

(3) Rhabdomyosarcomas and leiomyosarcomas are quite rare. They occur most frequently in male children and adolescents. They infiltrate widely, metastasize early, and are usually fatal.

(4) Primary malignant lymphomas, carcinosarcomas, neurofibromas, hemangiomas, and pheochromocytomas are rare. The latter may be associated with attacks of hypertension during voiding.

(5) Cancers of the skin (melanoma), stomach,

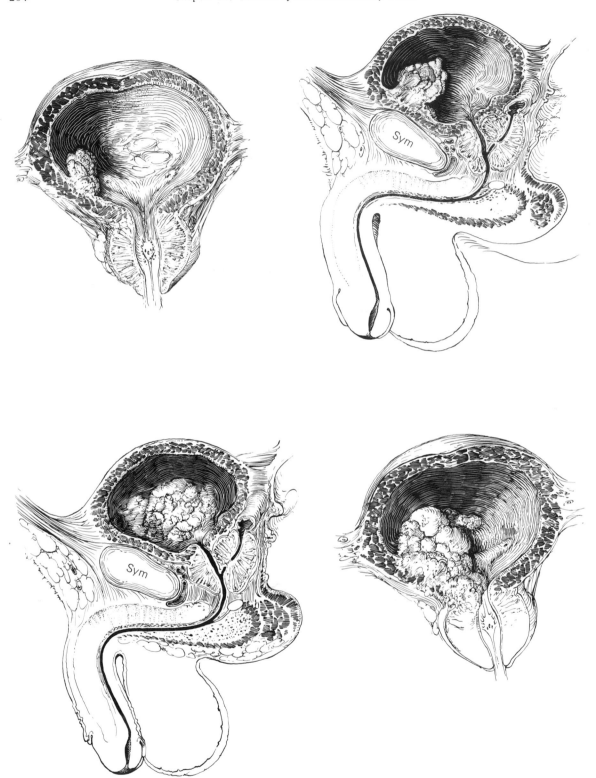

Figure 18–9. Transitional cell carcinomas of the bladder. ***Above left:*** Transitional cell (papillary) carcinoma with minimal invasion of the bladder wall. This is compatible with a grade II, stage A (T1) tumor. ***Above right:*** Larger, more invasive transitional cell carcinoma, probably grade II–III, stage B$_1$ (T2). ***Below left:*** More extensive transitional cell carcinoma involving the right ureteral orifice, compatible with grade III, stage B$_2$ (T3). ***Below right:*** Advanced large, invasive carcinoma of the bladder; occlusion of right ureteral orifice with extension into the bladder neck and prostate (grade IV, stage C [T3]).

lung, and breast may metastasize to the bladder. Vesical invasion by endometriosis may occur.

Clinical Findings

A. Symptoms: Gross hematuria is the most common symptom. As with all tumors of the urinary tract, hematuria is usually intermittent. All bleeding, severe or mild, prolonged or transient, must be accounted for. If infection supervenes, symptoms of cystitis will usually be present. These include burning on urination, urgency, frequency, and nocturia. Symptoms of bladder neck obstruction may develop if the tumor encroaches on the internal orifice. These include hesitancy and decrease in force and caliber of the urinary stream. If there is perivesical extension, suprapubic pain may be constant and severe. Pain in the flank may be noted if the growth obstructs a ureteral orifice and produces hydronephrosis. This may be complicated by renal infection, which may cause increased pain and high fever. If metastases are present, if infection is severe, if both ureteral orifices become occluded, or if anemia has developed, the patient may complain of weakness and loss of weight.

B. Signs: In most cases nothing abnormal can be found on physical examination. Renal tenderness or enlargement may be present due to ureteral obstruction and infection. A suprapubic mass may be noted on rare occasion. This might be due either to a large cancer or to urinary retention caused by clots or inva-sion of the bladder neck by tumor. On vaginal examination a mass at the base of the bladder may be noted. Less often, rectal examination may reveal an invasive mass in the trigonal area. Bimanual palpation (abdominorectal or abdominovaginal) is of the greatest importance in feeling and estimating the size and extent of the growth. This is best done under anesthesia. Signs of metastases may be noted. These include palpable abdominal masses (involved lymph nodes along the iliac vessels) and edema of one or both legs from occlusion of the iliacs.

C. Laboratory Findings: Anemia is not uncommon and may be from loss of blood, severe infection, or uremia caused by occlusion of both ureteral orifices by the growth. The urine may be very bloody, but between bouts of bleeding few if any red cells may be found. Pus and bacteria may also be noted. Renal function tests are usually normal unless there is bladder neck obstruction with residual urine or obstruction of both ureteral orifices.

D. X-Ray Findings: Excretory urograms are essential. While they are usually normal, they may show the tumor itself (Fig 18–10), evidence of ureteral obstruction, or a primary tumor of the renal pelvis or ureter as a cause of the "primary" vesical growth. Retrograde cystograms may show the tumor if it is large enough. A "fractionated" cystogram may afford evidence of invasion of the tumor into the vesical wall. First, the vesical capacity is determined. This amount of diluted

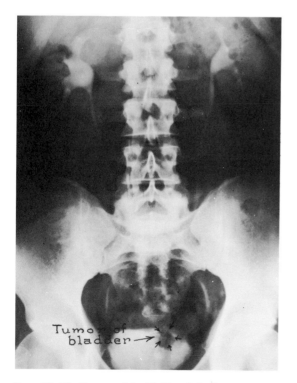 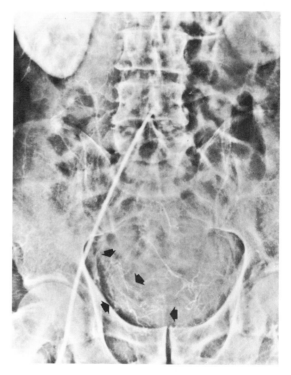

Figure 18–10. Tumors of the bladder. *Left:* Excretory urogram showing space-occupying lesion (transitional cell carcinoma) on the left side of the bladder; the upper tracts are normal. *Right:* Vesical angiogram, delayed film, showing increased vascularity of a deeply invasive transitional carcinoma grade IV, stage C, right vesical wall. Some of these vessels are presumed to be typical of tumor.

radiopaque medium is then prepared. One-fourth of this amount is then instilled into the bladder and an x-ray exposure made. The other three-fourths are successively instilled, and an x-ray exposure is then made on the same film. If the tumor is superficial, the vesical wall will fill symmetrically; in the presence of invasion, that portion of the wall will not expand. Vesical angiography may afford information concerning depth of infiltration of the tumor. It is quite accurate in revealing stage C (T3) and stage D (T4) tumors (Fig 18–10). Lymphangiography will reveal evidence of lymph node metastases.

E. **Instrumental Examination:** Cystoscopy almost always reveals the tumor. Biopsy of the lesion should be routine. A few tumors may be missed by this means, but these can be visualized if the patient is given tetracycline for a few days before cystoscopy, using ultraviolet illumination. The tetracycline causes fluorescence of the tumor.

Carcinoma in situ is often difficult to diagnose. The mucosa shows some erythema and has a granular and velvety appearance. This lesion leads to vesical contraction. In case of doubt, multiple biopsies are indicated.

F. **Cytologic Examination:** Papanicolaou preparations or the simpler methylene blue stain of fresh urinary sediment will almost always reveal transitional cells shed from the tumor. Well-differentiated tumors shed round cells of rather uniform size with large nuclei. When anaplastic tumors are present the urinary sediment usually reveals large epithelial cells (often in clumps) with very large dark staining nuclei.

Trott & Edwards (1973) have suggested the following technic: 50 ml of normal saline are instilled into the bladder via the cystoscope or catheter. The solution is washed back and forth 3 times and then fixed for cytologic examination. They have found this method significantly superior to a similar study of the voided urine.

This procedure is also useful in the follow-up of these patients and as a screening test for those exposed to chemical carcinogens. Suspicious cells (carcinoma in situ) may be noted months before a tumor can be discovered cystoscopically.

G. **Plasma or Urinary Carcinoembryonic Antigen (CEA):** Studies have shown that 60–70% of these patients have increased levels of CEA. Following definitive therapy, increasing amounts of CEA suggest recurrence or metastasis.

Differential Diagnosis

Renal or ureteral tumors also cause hematuria. Urograms will demonstrate the renal or ureteral lesion. Palpation or a plain abdominal film may reveal an enlarged kidney. It must be remembered that tumors of the renal pelvis or ureter may "seed" to the bladder wall, and the "primary" vesical neoplasm may really be "secondary."

Endometriosis occasionally involves the bladder. Bleeding and vesical irritability may be most marked at the time of the menses. Cystoscopically, the lesion is bluish in color and looks like a vascular tumor. Pelvic examination usually reveals evidence of other sites of involvement.

Acute nonspecific infections of the bladder or prostate may cause hematuria, but bleeding is usually terminal and associated with symptoms of cystitis. A tumor often becomes infected, however. Differentiation depends upon cystoscopy.

Benign prostatic hypertrophy commonly causes hematuria, often initial or terminal. Cystoscopy is necessary in the differential diagnosis.

Tuberculosis of the urinary tract often causes bleeding. A "sterile" pyuria is usually found, and tubercle bacilli can be demonstrated by special technics. Excretory urograms will be negative for tumor but may show evidence of calyceal ulceration. Again, cystoscopy will establish the diagnosis.

Renal, ureteral, or vesical stones may mimic tumor, but a plain film or excretory urogram will usually demonstrate them.

Acute hemorrhagic nephritis in an adult may require differentiation from tumor. The urinary findings (casts), hypertension, and edema should lead to the proper diagnosis. In case of doubt, cystoscopy is indicated.

Tumors of the cervix or bowel may invade the bladder. Demonstration of the primary tumor and a biopsy of the vesical lesion should settle the diagnosis.

Complications

Secondary infection of the bladder is common when the tumor ulcerates. It may be severe. Renal infection is not uncommon when ureteral obstruction ensues. Urinary retention may develop if the tumor invades the bladder neck.

Hydronephrosis due to ureteral occlusion is common. If bilateral, uremia supervenes. This is the most common cause of death.

Hemorrhage may become a problem. If it is intractable, instill 10% (some authors suggest 4%) formalin solution, via catheter, to capacity. Drain the bladder after 15 minutes and then irrigate with normal saline or with 10% alcohol followed by saline. Catheter drainage is maintained for the next few days. This procedure is highly successful, though occasionally it must be repeated. A cystogram must be done before instituting treatment. If vesicoureteral reflux is demonstrated, the use of formalin is contraindicated (Kalish & others, 1973).

Prevention

Employment in aniline dye factories should be restricted to 3 years, during which time periodic urinary Papanicolaou studies and cystoscopy are indicated. The clinical significance of endogenous carcinogenic agents has not been established. Schlegel & others (1970) have adduced evidence that the administration of ascorbic acid, 0.5 g 3 times a day, may prevent the formation of vesical tumors through neutralization of urinary carcinogens. Rose (1972) has found that giving large doses of pyridoxine decreases tryptophan metabolites in the urine. It seems worthwhile, therefore, to prescribe these drugs for those patients in whom the diagnosis has been made.

Treatment

There is still considerable disagreement about the proper treatment of vesical neoplasms. Certainly the low-grade superficial tumors lend themselves well to transurethral resection. For the more malignant and invasive tumors, the physician must choose between radiotherapy and radical surgery or a combination thereof.

A. Surgical Measures: Most single or multiple papillomas are best treated by transurethral resection, care being taken to "saucerize" deeply into the wall of the bladder in order to remove the base of the tumor completely. This procedure will cure many of the papillary carcinomas (eg, stage O, A, B_1 [T1S, T1, T2], grade I, II). However, if the tumor has invaded deeply into the vesical muscle (stage B_2, C [T3]), this method will usually fail.

Partial (segmental) cystectomy is feasible if the malignant tumor does not lie on the base of the bladder, for in this case one or both ureteral orifices might have to be sacrificed. Unfortunately, fewer than 20% of vesical tumors are restricted to areas far removed from the trigone.

Total cystectomy (with removal of the prostate) is often practiced for the treatment of papillomatosis and many of the more undifferentiated invasive tumors. Diversion of the urinary stream presents a problem. Ureterosigmoidostomy results in urinary continence but frequently causes ureteral obstruction or reflux with hydronephrosis and renal infection. Many of these patients die of renal insufficiency rather than of cancer. A few will develop symptomatic hyperchloremic acidosis from absorption of the chloride ions in the urine. Hypokalemia may occur. The administration of potassium citrate will usually correct these electrolytic defects. The most popular method of urinary diversion today is anastomosis of the ureters to an isolated loop of ileum (or sigmoid) with one end of this loop brought to the skin to act as a conduit. Renal complications and electrolyte problems are minimized.

Some urologists advocate radical pelvic node dissection in conjunction with the cystectomy. Since similar tumors may develop in the urethra in both men and women, urethrectomy—particularly in the male— should be done.

B. Radiation Therapy: In general, the more undifferentiated the tumor the more radiosensitive it is. It is therefore most useful in the grade III–IV, stage B_2 (T3) and C (T3) lesions. There is mounting evidence that radiotherapy in this type of neoplasm offers at least as good a control rate as radical surgery without the mortality associated with the latter. The optimal dose is 6000 rads given over a period of 6 weeks or more. This is compatible with the maintenance of good vesical function. If, after irradiation, viable tumor is still demonstrable, cystectomy can still be considered. There has been recent enthusiasm for use of radiother-

apy (4500 rads) followed by planned cystectomy 1–2 months later. It has been observed that 20–30% of these bladders are found to be free of tumor. This seems to reflect the significant value of modern radiation therapy. Blackard (1972), however, compared the control rate of patients treated solely by radiation, by cystectomy alone, and by preoperative irradiation followed by cystectomy. The result with all 3 modalities of treatment was the same.

Hewitt & others (1972) advocate the use of intracavitary radium for treatment of superficial low grade tumors and carcinoma in situ. They report better than 50% control of these lesions at 5 years.

C. Chemotherapy: Palliation of advanced high grade vesical neoplasms with parenteral anticancer drugs has been reported. These include 5-fluorouracil, mitomycin C, bleomycin, methotrexate, adriamycin, and hydroxurea. Ogata & others (1973) have infused mitomycin C via the internal iliac artery. They were encouraged by their results. By and large, however, the effects of chemotherapy have not been dramatic. The instillation by catheter of 60 mg of thiotepa dissolved in 30–60 ml of normal saline has been suggested by Veenema & others (1969) in the treatment of superficial lowgrade papillomas. Four to 6 weekly treatments should be given. This should be followed by instillations every month for 6–10 months. Success is judged by urinary cytology and cystoscopy. Similar therapy is indicated if new tumors appear following transurethral resection of a low-grade superficial neoplasm. This may change the nature of the mucosa; the appearance of new tumors may cease. Before each instillation, a white cell and platelet count should be obtained. Should the white count be less than 4000 or the platelets below 100,000 cu mm, treatment should be deferred until the hemogram improves.

British urologists have had considerable experience with instillations of triethylene glycol diglyceridyl ether (Epodyl). Since it is poorly absorbed through the vesical wall, blood dyscrasia has not been observed. Inject 100–200 ml of a 1% solution (in distilled water) via catheter. Remove the catheter and instruct the patient to retain the drug for at least an hour. This instillation is repeated every week for 12 weeks, then every month for a year, and then every 3 months. If the response is poor, a 2% solution should be used.

D. Miscellaneous: Helmstein (1972) advocates the utilization of a hydrostatic technic in the treatment of the more malignant tumors, though England & others (1973) found that only the stage A (T1) tumors responded. Under anesthesia, a balloon is placed in the bladder transurethrally and filled with water until the intravesical pressure approaches the systolic blood pressure. This pressure is maintained for 5½–7 hours. A catheter is left in place for a few days. Tumor necrosis is caused by the ischemic effect of the balloon pressing on the tumor. It is too early to accurately judge its efficacy.

Reuter (1972) claims good results with transurethral freezing (cryosurgery) of vesical tumors.

E. Rhabdomyosarcoma: Triple therapy is preferred: (1) prostatocystectomy with resection of the pelvic lymph nodes; (2) postoperative irradiation; and (3) chemotherapy (dactinomycin and vincristine).

F. Treatment of Complications: Infection can usually be controlled with antibiotics. It cannot be completely eradicated, however, as long as ulceration (either spontaneous or following electrosurgery) is present. Radiotherapy may control excessive bleeding. An infected hydronephrotic kidney, secondarily obstructed by the growth, may have to be removed.

Follow-Up Care & Prognosis

The superficial, well-differentiated tumors may recur, or new papillomas may appear. Constant vigilance, with periodic cystoscopy and urinary cytologic examination, is therefore necessary for at least 3 years. New tumors may also be well controlled by transurethral means, but if they tend to recur they are apt to become progressively invasive and of higher grade. Cystectomy or radiation therapy must then be considered.

Prognosis with any vesical tumor varies, in general, with the stage (invasion) and grade (differentiation). The best results are obtained by transurethral resection of the grade I–II, stage O (T1S), A (T1), and B₁ (T2) tumors. Cystectomy cures about 15–25% of grade III–IV, stage B₂ and C (T3) lesions with an accompanying mortality from the operation of 5–15%. Radiotherapy for the same serious neoplasms offers about 15–25% control at 5 years.

Few if any cures of rhabdomyosarcoma are achieved during the first year of life. Possibly 30–40% can be controlled in those that develop in childhood. Leiomyosarcomas offer a somewhat better outlook.

TUMORS OF
THE PROSTATE GLAND

The prostate is the urologic organ most often affected by benign or malignant neoplasm. Cancer of this organ is almost as common as malignancy of the lung or gastrointestinal tract.

The danger from adenomatous hypertrophy is not from the lesion per se but from the effects of obstruction: hydronephrosis and renal infection. The same is true, to a large extent, of prostatic cancer, although metastases may contribute to the death of the patient.

BENIGN PROSTATIC
HYPERPLASIA (OR HYPERTROPHY)

There is some debate about the cause of the prostatic enlargement. One group believes that the obstructing tissue represents hyperplasia of the periurethral glands with compression of the true prostatic tissue peripherally to form the "surgical capsule." Thus, "prostatectomy" is not prostatectomy at all. The hyperplastic periurethral glandular tissue is removed; the prostate is not. Others believe that the prostatic lobes lying proximal to the verumontanum (the 2 lateral and subcervical lobes) undergo hyperplasia but in addition are invaded by the periurethral glands, thus giving the fibromuscular tissue its often striking glandular component. If this be true, then prostatectomy is accomplished. The latter theory is favored (Hutch & Rambo, 1970).

Benign prostatic hyperplasia causes progressive obstruction to the flow of urine and, in the later stages, causes back pressure in the kidneys (hydronephrosis) and contributes to the establishment of infection in the urinary tract.

Etiology

Some enlargement begins to develop in most men by age 50. The majority have palpable evidence of hyperplasia by age 60. Not all have symptoms of obstruction, however, nor is the hyperplasia necessarily progressive.

The cause of this disease is not entirely clear, although its relationship to hormonal activity is borne out by much experimental and clinical evidence. Animal investigation reveals that prostatic obstruction is common in aging male dogs, but this does not develop if the animal has been previously castrated. Orchiectomy causes atrophy of the gland and therefore terminates the elaboration of prostatic fluid. Dogs with Sertoli cell (estrogen) tumors of the testis do not develop prostatic hyperplasia.

Previous castration also seems to prevent prostatic hypertrophy in men. However, administration of estrogens or even castration has little if any effect upon the gross size of the enlarged gland, although microscopically some atrophy of the epithelial structures may be noted. The administration of estrogens or androgens has little effect upon the amount of acid phosphatase elaborated by the gland.

Certainly androgens per se cannot be blamed for this hyperplasia, for the disease occurs at a time when the androgenic activity of the organism is decreasing. Therefore, an imbalance between androgens and estrogens may be the causative factor. It is not clear why hyperplasia of the prostate develops in some men and not in others and affects different individuals in varying degrees.

Pathogenesis
(See Chapter 10.)

The enlarged gland produces its harmful effects by obstructing the bladder neck and by upsetting the mechanisms which force open and funnel the vesical orifice.

A. Changes in the Bladder:

1. **Early**—As the degree of obstruction increases, the vesical detrusor undergoes compensatory hyper-

trophy in order to overcome the increasing urethral resistance. The muscle wall may become more than 2 cm thick. This power of compensation varies. One patient with a markedly obstructive gland may have few symptoms, whereas another may have great difficulty with a milder obstruction. There is therefore little relationship between the size of the gland and the severity of symptoms.

As compensatory hypertrophy develops, the following take place:

a. Trabeculation of the bladder wall—Taut, intertwined hypertrophic muscle bundles lift up the mucosa.

b. Hypertrophy of the trigone and interureteric ridge.

c. Diverticula—As the intravesical voiding pressure rises (as it must to overcome increased urethral resistance), the mucosal layer may be forced between the muscle fibers and finally balloon into the perivesical fat. It may then grow to large size. The diverticulum has no muscular wall and therefore cannot empty itself; the urine it contains easily becomes infected.

2. Late—In many men the power for further vesical compensation becomes exhausted when the muscle can no longer hypertrophy, and decompensation occurs. Urine is then retained in the bladder in increasing amounts, and symptoms may become severe. With chronic urinary retention, the hitherto thickened bladder wall may become markedly attenuated and atonic.

B. Changes in the Ureter and Kidney: With secondary hypertrophy of the trigonal-ureteral complex, there is increased downward traction on the intramural ureteral segments, thus increasing resistance to urine flow. This is further aggravated when there is significant residual urine which causes further stretching and, therefore, pull on the intramural ureter. This leads to progressive proximal dilatation and is the common cause of ureterohydronephrosis and its accompanying impaired renal function. Significant residual urine leading to chronic vesical distention may cause a vesicorenal reflex which is manifested by diminution of renal urinary secretion. In either case, catheter drainage or prostatectomy, by relieving trigonal stretch and allowing resolution of the trigonal hypertrophy, causes the hydroureteronephrosis to recede (Fig 18–11).

In a few advanced cases of prostatic enlargement, the ureterovesical "valves" may become incompetent. This not only hurts the kidney hydrodynamically but encourages the development and perpetuation of pyelonephritis.

C. Infection: In the presence of vesical residual urine or urethrovesical reflux, the urologic defense against infection is defeated. Some such patients develop cystitis which is, in all probability, secondary to a preexisting prostatitis. It is possible, however, that impaired urethral washout secondary to the obstruction may allow abnormal ascent of urethral flora.

If the organisms split urea (eg, proteus), vesical stones may form. If vesicoureteral reflux develops, pyelonephritis ensues. The renal lesion is the important complication of prostatic obstruction.

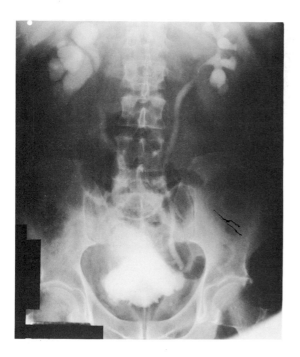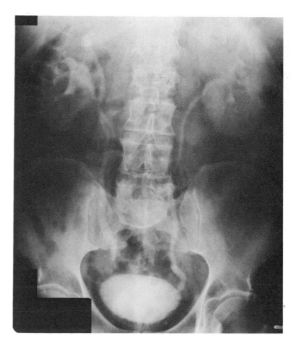

Figure 18–11. Benign prostatic hypertrophy. *Left:* Preoperative 1-hour excretory urogram showing bilateral hydronephrosis and a heavily trabeculated bladder. *Right:* Postoperative excretory urogram revealing regression of hydronephrosis. Bladder now of normal contour.

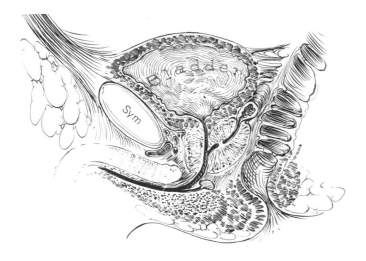

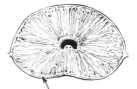

Normal adult prostate

Apple-peel-thin anatomic capsule

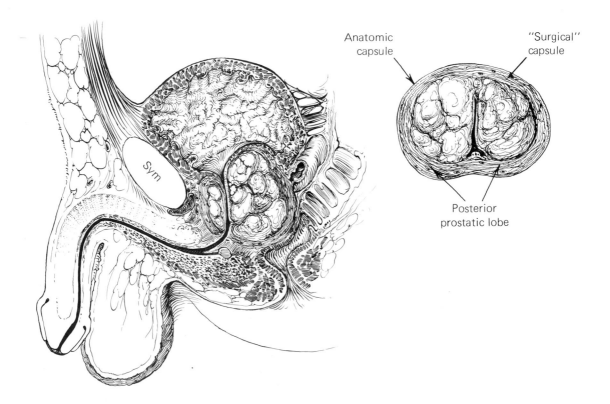

Anatomic capsule

"Surgical" capsule

Posterior prostatic lobe

Figure 18–12. Pathogenesis of benign prostatic hyperplasia. *Above:* Normal bladder and prostate. Inset shows normal prostate (containing prostatic urethra) and thin fibrous anatomic capsule. *Below:* Enlarged prostate enclosed by relatively thick "surgical" capsule which is composed of the posterior prostatic lobe.

Pathology (Fig 11–12)

The prostate in the young adult may be compared to an apple; its true capsule is thin and intimately attached to the underlying secretory tissue. For this reason, intracapsular enucleation of the young man's prostate is impossible. The enlarged gland, on the other hand, is more like an orange. It has a thick "surgical" capsule (the peripherally compressed extraurethral prostate) which is poorly connected to the central obstructing tissue; this permits easy "shelling out" of the hyperplastic prostatic lobes, leaving the "surgical" capsule behind. It should be noted that the posterior prostatic lobe is left as part of this surgical capsule. Since it is in this lobe that carcinoma develops, intracapsular prostatectomy is not prophylactic against cancer developing later.

There are 3 lobes which commonly undergo hyperplasia: the 2 lateral lobes and the subcervical lobe. At times only the lateral lobes enlarge. Again, a fairly pure subcervical lobe hyperplasia is seen. In this instance the rectal examination may reveal a prostate of normal size, for this lobe cannot be felt. Very commonly, all 3 enlarge together. The gland becomes elongated and the lobes tend to herniate through the bladder neck; intravesical protrusion may be marked. Under these circumstances the true size of the gland, as judged by rectal palpation, will not be revealed.

On section the adenomatous pattern is usually obvious; multiple nodules are noted. The "surgical" capsule is composed of atrophic true extraurethral (posterior lobe) prostatic tissue which has been compressed and displaced to the periphery. It may be 2–5 mm in thickness. This capsule is poorly connected to the hyperplastic lobes, which therefore may be easily enucleated.

Microscopically, the hyperplasia affects glandular, muscular, and fibrous tissue in varying degrees. The epithelial cells are of the tall columnar type. They may pile up into a papillary pattern. There are no mitoses.

Clinical Findings

Benign prostatic enlargement seldom causes significant symptoms before age 50. The complaints are referable to the obstruction and may be increased by infection. Rectal examination may or may not reveal prostatic enlargement. Urinary infection may be present. The PSP may be depressed because of incomplete emptying of the bladder (residual urine); back pressure on the kidneys will cause true impairment of renal function. Cystoscopy will reveal hypertrophy of the prostate and secondary changes in the bladder wall.

A. Symptoms: (The physiologic explanation for the obstructive symptoms is discussed in Chapter 10.) In the early stages, the patient may notice that if the bladder becomes too full there is a little hesitation in starting the stream and some loss of force and caliber of the stream. Later, the symptoms are more persistent and severe.

1. Bladder symptoms—Hesitancy in starting the stream may be marked. Considerable straining may be necessary. Because of the increased urethral resistance,

decrease in caliber of the bladder neck, and derangement of the normal mechanisms which open the bladder neck, the stream is small and lacks force. This will be worse if the urge to urinate must be put off, for the smooth muscle of the bladder becomes overstretched and loses tone. Toward the end of urination the stream tends to diminish gradually and may end as a mere dribble. Frequency (both day and night) develops, depending on the degree of irritability of the bladder and the amount of residual urine; the greater this amount is, the smaller is the working capacity of the organ. If infection complicates the picture, all of the above symptoms are increased. The inflammatory edema of the prostate or bladder neck will increase the degree of obstruction and will cause more residual urine, thereby further increasing frequency. Infection diminishes vesical capacity, thus further increasing the degree of frequency. Hematuria is not uncommon. It may be due to rupture of dilated veins at the bladder neck which are apt to develop with straining. Acute urinary retention may develop suddenly in a patient who has had few premonitory symptoms. At other times it occurs after some months or years of increasing symptoms of prostatism. The patient then experiences marked suprapubic pain and marked urgency; he is miserable until relieved by catheterization.

2. Renal symptoms—The hydronephrosis secondary to prostatic obstruction is usually painless unless it becomes infected. In a few men with vesicoureteral reflux, renal pain may be experienced during the act of voiding. In the advanced stage of the disease, symptoms of uremia may be noted: somnolence, vomiting, diarrhea, and loss of weight.

B. Signs: A visible mass low in the midline of the abdomen may be seen, felt, or percussed. In acute retention, it is quite tender. In chronic urinary retention, the bladder may be so flabby that only percussion will reveal it. On rectal examination the prostate may or may not be enlarged. One lobe may be larger than the other. The surface is usually smooth; it may be firm (fibromuscular) or unduly soft and boggy (adenomatous). Areas of induration should be sought (suggesting cancer).

It should be mentioned that the degree of obstruction is measured not by rectal examination but by the severity of the symptoms and the amount of residual urine.

Unless acute urinary infection is present or the patient is verging on complete urinary retention, the gland should be massaged. If pus is found in the secretion or if the gland is found to be overful of secretion, conservative treatment may afford some relief from obstructive symptoms. Tenderness over a kidney may indicate renal infection. The maximum intravesical voiding pressure is significantly increased; voiding flow rate is reduced. Hypertension may be found. It may be caused by renal back pressure (ischemia).

C. Laboratory Findings: Urinalysis may reveal an otherwise completely silent complicating infection (pus, bacteria). Renal function as measured by PSP is a very important step in examination. It also indirectly estimates the presence or absence of residual urine. If the PSP is 50% or more at 30 minutes after injection and the urine volume is small, total renal function is normal and there can be no significant residual urine. If it is only 25%, either residual urine is present or renal function is depressed. Determine the serum creatinine. If it is normal, then the man's kidneys must have excreted 60% of the dye. The residual urine would therefore have to be about equal to the volume of urine passed at one-half hour (see p 46). The passage of a catheter immediately after voiding will accurately measure the degree of retention.

D. X-Ray Findings: A plain film of the abdomen and excretory urograms may show complicating calculi. Often, ureterohydronephrosis is portrayed (Fig 18–11). This is usually caused by hypertrophy and chronic stretch of the trigone which applies increased occlusive pull on the intravesical ureteral segments. Intravesical encroachment of the prostate and even ureteral reflux may be revealed on urethrography and cystography (Fig 18–13). The bladder may be raised well above the upper edge of the symphysis if the gland is significantly elongated.

E. Instrumental Examination: The amount of urine retained after voiding is a measure of the degree of decompensation of the bladder. This is ascertained by passing a catheter to the bladder immediately after voiding or its estimation by means of the PSP test.

Cystoscopy or panendoscopy will show the degree of enlargement of the prostatic lobes and the secondary changes in the bladder wall (eg, trabeculation, diverticula, infection). It will also reveal complications such as vesical stone or incidental neoplasm.

F. Sonography: Transrectal sonograms of the prostate will reveal its size most accurately (Watanabe & others, 1971).

Differential Diagnosis

The neurogenic bladder also causes difficulty with urination and a low maximum voiding flow rate. There is often a history of spinal cord or peripheral nerve injury. Diabetic neuropathy may be present. Tranquilizers (eg, diazepam) lead to vesical atony. Neurologic examination may reveal definite abnormality (particularly perianal anesthesia), and the anal sphincter may be found to be atonic (relaxed). A cystometrogram is helpful. The bethanechol supersensitivity test (originally described by Lapides) is definitive (Melzer, 1972). With 100 ml of water in the bladder, intravesical pressure is estimated. A subcutaneous injection of 2.5 mg of bethanechol chloride (Urecholine) is given. If, after 30 minutes, the intravesical pressure has risen 15 cm of water or more, the test is positive for vesical atonicity. Cystoscopy may show little in the way of obstruction. A positive serologic test for syphilis of blood or spinal fluid may be suggestive. Herpes zoster involving the sacral spinal ganglia has caused urinary retention in a few patients.

Ganglionic blocking agents and parasympatholytic drugs in the treatment of peptic ulcer and hypertension, as well as tranquilizers, weaken the power of detrusor contraction, thus causing symptoms simulating vesical neck obstruction. In a man with moderate prostatism, such drugs may cause urinary retention.

Contracture of the vesical neck caused by chronic prostatitis (rare) mimics the symptoms of benign enlargement perfectly. A fibrous or nodular prostate is to be expected, and its secretion will contain pus. Cystoscopy will settle the diagnosis.

Cancer of the prostate will be suggested by the finding of a hard gland. Besides the obstructive symptoms, lumbosacral backache with pain radiating

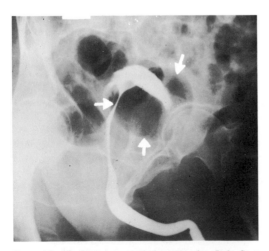
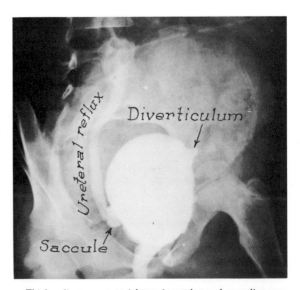

Figure 18–13. Benign prostatic hypertrophy. *Left:* Cystourethrogram. Thick radiopaque material seen in urethra and spreading over superior surface of greatly enlarged intravesical prostate. Arrows outline bladder filled with air. *Right:* Lateral voiding cystourethrogram showing diverticulum of the bladder ("Hutch" saccule; see Fig 11–4) and vesicoureteral reflux. Postoperative prostatectomy.

down one or both legs suggests metastases to the bony pelvis or extension along the perineural lymphatics. If the disease is extensive, the serum acid phosphatase is increased. Serum alkaline phosphatase is elevated when the tumor has metastasized to bone. Osteoblastic metastases to the pelvic bones usually mean prostatic cancer. Biopsy of the prostate is definitive.

Acute prostatitis will cause obstructive symptoms, but this disease is acute, is associated with marked febrile response, and often occurs in young individuals. Pyuria is always found. Rectal examination will reveal a prostate which is enlarged, but it is hot, exquisitely tender, and often fluctuant (abscess).

Urethral stricture also causes obstruction to urinary flow. A history of complicated gonorrhea (now rare) or perineal trauma should suggest the possibility. Urethral discharge, pyuria, and pus in the prostatic secretion usually accompany this abnormality. Urethral exploration with catheter or sound makes the diagnosis.

Sarcoma of the prostate is rare and affects younger men and boys. Symptoms are those of obstruction. A large, soft, or firm mass is felt in the prostatic area.

Vesical stone will be suggested by sudden interruption of the urinary stream accompanied by pain radiating down the penis. It will be revealed by radiography or cystoscopy.

Complications

Obstruction may lead to infection. This may involve the bladder, kidneys, and the prostate itself. From the latter, epididymitis may develop. Stones may form in the bladder.

The obstruction may cause vesical diverticula. Hydronephrosis may occur from hypertrophy of the trigone or when a ureterovesical "valve" gives way. At times, hematuria may be brisk.

Treatment

Since benign prostatic hyperplasia is not necessarily a progressive disease, conservative therapy should be used where applicable. The problem is to decide which patients can be treated in this manner and which require surgery. Criteria for operation vary, but the following seem feasible: (1) Impaired renal function due to the obstruction corroborated by excretory urography. (This indication is hardly debatable.) (2) A degree of symptoms which so upsets the patient that he requests relief. This will vary, since one man may be distressed at urinating 3 times during the night, whereas another may not be particularly inconvenienced by nocturia of 6 times.

A. Conservative Measures: Regular intercourse is the best means of combating prostatic congestion. If necessary, this may be replaced or augmented by 3 or 4 prostatic massages given at intervals of 14 days. At times improvement is striking.

Prostatitis should be treated with antimicrobials (effects will not be dramatic), prostatitic massage (not oftener than once a week), and sitz baths.

If pyuria is present, antibiotics or sulfonamides may afford considerable relief. The choice of drug will depend upon the organism found. If there is a great deal of residual urine, drug therapy will probably not be successful.

To protect vesical tone, the patient should be conditioned to avoid excessive intake of fluids in a short period of time. Rapid distention of the bladder may cause the hypertrophic muscle to lose its tone and lead to sudden exacerbation of symptoms or even acute retention. The patient should be cautioned about the diuretic effect of alcohol (Richmond, 1974), which, combined with the volume of fluid taken, may lead to retention despite the fact that his symptoms up to that time had been moderate. In fact, such an episode is the most common cause of acute urinary retention. For the same reason, the patient should void as soon as he feels the urge to do so, thus preventing the bladder from becoming overdistended.

The use of antiandrogen therapy (estrogens or orchiectomy) may have some beneficial effect upon benign prostatic hypertrophy, but the cost to the patient (impotence) is too high.

Men who are given testosterone for other reasons may notice improvement in their obstructive symptoms from increased vesical tone. Care should be taken that the patient does not have cancer of the gland, because androgen therapy will hasten its growth. The administration of cyproterone acetate has afforded some encouragement in the treatment of benign enlargement. Its use is still experimental.

Catheterization is mandatory for acute retention. If the patient is still unable to void spontaneously, and particularly if there have been few antecedent symptoms, a catheter should be left indwelling for 2–4 days. Thus, prostatic congestion is relieved, vesical tone is reestablished, and fairly normal voiding may return. If catheterization by any means is impossible, cystostomy must be performed. After a few days, the power of spontaneous urination may be restored. A permanent indwelling catheter (or cystostomy) may occasionally be indicated in the debilitated patient.

B. Surgery: There are 4 operations in vogue at present, but it is impossible to state the indications for each. The choice of operation is a personal matter for the surgeon.

Transurethral prostatectomy is most often used. In some hands only a small amount of tissue is removed; in others, this procedure is essentially a complete intracapsular removal. The latter method is to be preferred, since only this can compete with the results afforded by open surgery. The mortality is about 1–2%, and the urinary result is good in most instances. Potency is maintained, and hospitalization is relatively short.

Suprapubic transvesical prostatectomy is still the most popular open method of removal of the hypertrophied tissue. Its mortality rate is 1–3%. The urinary result is excellent, probably more consistently so than with the transurethral method. Potency is maintained.

Retropubic extravesical prostatectomy has a

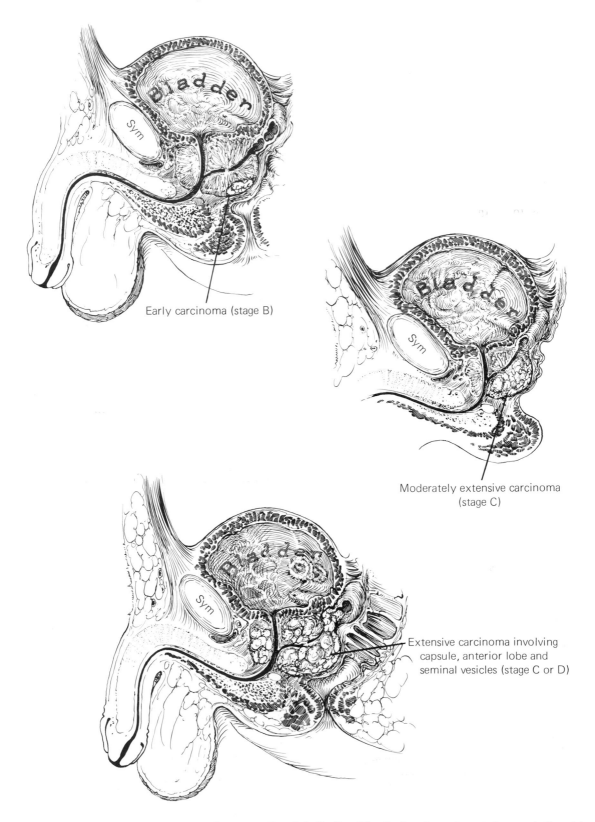

Figure 18—14. Pathogenesis of carcinoma of prostate. *Above left:* Small, well-localized carcinoma in posterior aspect of prostate, easily felt on rectal examination. *Above right:* Extension of carcinoma into posterior half of prostate. *Below:* Advanced carcinoma of prostate; trabeculation of bladder wall.

mortality rate of 1–2%. The urinary result is excellent. Potency is maintained.

Perineal prostatectomy involves little risk (1–2%), but impotence may occur, there is often some delay in regaining perfect urinary control, and on occasion some degree of stress incontinence persists. Rectourethral fistual has a definite incidence (1–5%), and is most distressing.

Cryosurgery. Some enthusiasm for this method of treatment is being evinced for the poor-risk patient. The instrument is passed down the urethra with the freezing unit placed in the prostatic urethra. Liquid nitrogen is circulated through the probe until the temperature in the prostatic capsule reaches 0–10 °C. This leads to death and slough of the obstructing tissue. Blood loss is usually minimal. The result in possibly 10% of patients is less than optimal. Further evaluation of this method is awaited.

C. Follow-Up Care: Periodic urinalysis with stained smear or culture should be done postoperatively. Healing should be complete after 2 months, at which time an appropriate antibiotic should clear any residual infection.

Prognosis

Most patients can be given considerable relief by conservative means. If on follow-up their symptoms increase or renal function, as measured by the PSP test, begins to diminish, surgical intervention is indicated.

CARCINOMA OF THE PROSTATE

Carcinoma of the prostate is rare before age 60 and increases in frequency thereafter, probably afflicting 25% of men in the eighth decade. The disease is rare in Orientals but more common in blacks, in Maoris and in white New Zealanders, and in Scandinavians. There is a significant familial incidence, which suggests a genetic component. Multiple cancers are common in these patients. It metastasizes principally to the bones of the pelvis and the pelvic lymph nodes. Ureteral obstruction, with secondary renal injury, may develop from direct extension, compression by pelvic nodes, intramural metastases, or hypertrophy of the trigone secondary to the vesical neck obstruction.

Three instances of the elaboration of adrenocorticotropin have been reported. These patients presented with hypokalemic acidosis, diabetes, psychosis, and hypertension.

Etiology

The true cause of prostatic carcinoma is not known, but it is quite clear that its growth is strikingly influenced by sex hormones. The adult prostate is the major site of elaboration of acid phosphatase. In advanced prostatic cancer, particularly when it has metastasized to bone, three-fourths of patients will have markedly increased amounts of this enzyme in the blood.

The administration of androgens usually increases the rate of growth of this tumor and increases the acid phosphatase level in the serum. Estrogen therapy (or orchiectomy) slows the growth of these tumors and maintains the amount of acid phosphatase in the blood at a normal level. Determination of the amount of acid phosphatase in the serum is therefore an index of the extent of the tumor; it also indicates the degree of success of antiandrogen therapy.

Pathogenesis & Pathology (Fig 18–14)

Cancer of the prostate is usually associated coincidentally with benign prostatic hyperplasia but does not develop from it. Most malignancies originate in the posterior lobe in the surgical capsule (compressed peripheral prostatic tissue), although a few may be found within the hyperplastic benign prostatic lobes. These latter tumors are usually very small ("occult" or "academic" cancers, stage A) and apparently are often completely removed by intracapsular enucleation of the enlarged gland.

The initial lesion is usually a firm area on the posterolateral surface. It gradually spreads in the capsule (posterior lobe) and involves the hyperplastic tissue as well. The seminal vesicles then become involved. Later, the tumor may extend through the urethral mucosa or bladder wall; the external sphincter may be invaded. The rectal wall is singularly immune; only rarely does the tumor invade Denonvilliers' fascia.

The cancer spreads in the perineural lymphatics. The vesical, sacral, external iliac, and lumbar lymph nodes then become involved. The left supraclavicular node is occasionally affected. When the seminal vesicles are involved, 80% of patients will have invasion of the pelvic nodes.

Metastases also occur by way of the veins, particularly through the vertebrals. This mechanism accounts for the predilection of this tumor for the bones of the pelvis, heads of the femurs, and the lower lumbar spine. Other bones, including the skull, are occasionally involved. Spread to the skin and viscera (eg, lungs, liver) is also seen. Infiltration of the bone marrow is particularly common.

Grossly, cancers of the prostate are white or yellow. They may be quite hard, if fibrous; or merely firm, if more cellular. Multiple zones of cancer are not uncommon. Rarely, a tumor may be medullary and so soft as to simulate abscess.

On microscopic study, the tissue may be largely epithelial or may be scirrhous. The epithelial elements may assume a papillary pattern or may be anaplastic. Invasion of the stroma is usually obvious. Mitoses are common. Invasion of perineural sheaths is an outstanding feature but is not necessarily of prognostic importance.

After antiandrogen therapy, retrogressive changes may be marked. The gland becomes smaller and assumes a more normal consistency. This change may be marked within 3 months after therapy is instituted. Obstructive symptoms regress to some extent. Microscopically, the malignant cells have become smaller and stain more darkly. The cytoplasm becomes scanty. The number of these cells is markedly diminished. Similar changes occur in metastatic tumors.

A few transitional cell carcinomas arising from the epithelium of the ducts have been reported. They are highly malignant, cause osteolytic metastases, respond poorly to irradiation, and so require radical cystoprostatectomy. Lymphomatous infiltration is occasionally seen.

Adenocarcinoma of the prostate is staged as follows:

Stage A: Rectal examination normal. The tumor is found incidentally in tissue removed in the treatment of benign enlargement or at autopsy.

Stage B: There is a localized induration in the prostate which is confined within the capsule. The serum acid phosphatase is normal. Such a lesion lends itself to radical prostatectomy.

Stage C: There is extracapsular extension of the tumor. Serum acid phosphatase may be elevated. Surgical cure is unlikely.

Stage D: There are distant metastases (eg, lymph nodes, bone).

Clinical Findings

A. Symptoms: The presenting symptoms in 95% of men with prostatic malignancy are from obstruction to the flow of urine, infection, or both. They are similar to those described in the discussion of benign prostatic enlargement.

1. Bladder symptoms—Hesitancy and straining to initiate the stream, loss of force and caliber of the stream, terminal dribbling, frequency with nocturia, symptoms of infection of the bladder, and urinary retention. Localized tumors unassociated with benign hyperplasia provoke no symptoms at all.

2. Symptoms due to metastases—One out of 20 patients have their first symptoms from metastases. Metastatic spread causes the following: pain in the lumbosacral region, which may radiate into the hips or down the legs; a mass in the right upper abdominal quadrant (ie, liver involvement), supraclavicular mass (ie, sentinel node metastasis), anemia and loss of weight, and hematuria late in the course of the disease when the bladder or urethra is invaded. Symptoms of renal insufficiency may be due to obstruction of the ureteral orifices by the primary tumor or by hypertrophy of the trigonal muscle; or to compression of the ureters by masses of iliac lymph nodes involved by metastatic cancer.

B. Signs: Rectal examination is the most important step in the diagnosis of cancer of the prostate. The early lesion is difficult to differentiate from certain benign conditions which cause areas of induration. A cancerous nodule is usually not raised above the surface of the gland. There is a sudden change in consistency between it and surrounding tissue (Fig 4–2). Diagnosis may not be possible without biopsy.

The more advanced lesion is usually stony hard, and the gland is fixed. It may be nodular. The seminal vesicles may be indurated. Occlusion of the rectum by surrounding growth is very rare.

Other signs of prostatic cancer include an enlarged, nodular liver, pathologic fracture from metastasis (including sudden paraplegia from collapse of a vertebral body), and an enlarged, hard left supraclavicular node.

C. Laboratory Findings: Anemia may be extreme in the later stages, when bone marrow is replaced by tumor; hemorrhage and infection will also contribute to this. Urinalysis may or may not show infection. Red cells may be present.

In the early stages of obstruction, renal function is unimpaired. Later, if the ureters are occluded or if obstruction is so marked that renal back pressure develops, the PSP may be depressed because of renal impairment, residual urine, or both; serum creatinine or BUN may be increased.

Serum phosphatase determinations are important in the diagnosis of prostatic cancer. The normal serum acid phosphatase in men is 1–5 King-Armstrong units (or 0.5–2 Bodansky or Gutman units). When the cancer extends outside the prostatic capsule and metastases are present, 75% of patients will have elevations to above 10 units. This is pathognomonic of advanced prostate carcinoma, whether metastases can be demonstrated or not. With antiandrogen therapy these abnormal levels tend to revert to normal.

The serum alkaline phosphatase (normally 5–13 King-Armstrong units, 2–4.5 Bodansky units, 3–10 Gutman units) will be elevated if there are bony metastases. This is a nonspecific reaction and merely reflects the amount of osteogenic activity in the body. After an initial further rise, it too tends to return to normal levels when hormonal treatment is instituted.

Raskin & others (1973), found hypocalcemia (below 8.6 mg/100 ml) in 16% and hypercalcemia in 9% of their patients.

D. X-Ray Findings: A chest film may show evidence of metastases to the hilar nodes, lungs, or ribs. A plain film of the abdomen may reveal the typical osteoblastic metastases from prostatic tumor (Fig 18–15). The common sites include the pelvic bones, the lumbar spine, and the femoral heads. Excretory urograms may show hydronephrosis from bladder neck or ureteral obstruction (Fig 18–16).

E. Scanning Technics: Although ^{85}Sr and ^{18}F bone scans have been widely used, ^{99m}Tc polyphosphate is probably the method of choice for it has a relatively short half-life (see Chapter 8). The scan is much more sensitive than osteography in demonstrating metastases.

F. Instrumental Examination: Passage of a catheter immediately after voiding will measure the amount of residual urine. Cystoscopy will usually show nonspecific vesical changes from obstruction (eg, trabeculation, diverticula, infection). Only very late will invasion of the bladder be seen. Obstruction of the prostatic urethra will be evident. The gland may be found to be relatively fixed on movement of the instrument.

G. Cytologic Examination: Papanicolaou technics

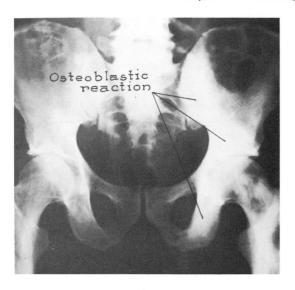

Figure 18—15. Metastases to bone from carcinoma of the prostate. Plain film of pelvis showing osteoblastic metastases to the lumbar vertebrae, ilium, ischium, and left femur.

are of no value in the early cases. By the time malignant cells can be demonstrated in prostatic secretion, the diagnosis is usually quite evident clinically.

H. Biopsy: If the lesion is extensive, a positive diagnosis can be made on pathologic studies of tissue removed by transurethral resection. In early cases (limited to the capsule), this method fails. Needle biopsy through the perineum, or transrectally, is a very useful procedure for establishing the diagnosis of cancer. With a very small nodule, a negative biopsy may be in question because of the difficulty of being sure that the needle is indeed within the nodule. A few cases of implantation of tumor in the needle tract have been reported. This is rare.

Aspiration of bone marrow from the posterior iliac crest will show more evidence of malignant spread than either the bone scan or radiograms (Gursel & others, 1974). Nelson and his co-workers (1973) are less enthusiastic, finding relatively few positive bone marrow biopsies in those patients with known lymph node metastases.

I. Lymphangiography: This procedure is increasingly used to seek evidence of metastases to the pelvic nodes. Positive nodes preclude radical prostatectomy, though a few urologists feel that radical pelvic node dissection may cure a few of these patients. Radiotherapists employ this technic before institution of therapy in order to better stage the tumor.

Differential Diagnosis

Benign prostatic hyperplasia can usually be differ-

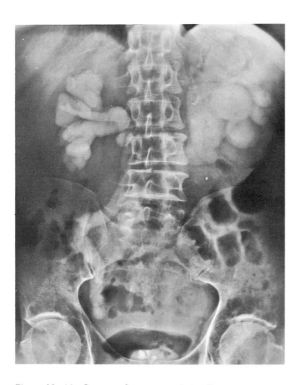

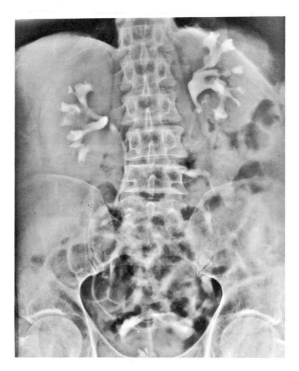

Figure 18—16. Cancer of prostate. *Left:* Excretory urogram at 75 minutes showing bilateral hydroureteronephrosis. *Right:* Fifteen-minute urogram after 3 months of diethylstilbestrol. Significant reduction of obstruction.

entiated by palpation of the prostate. Osteoblastic metastases in the pelvic bones as shown on x-ray or scan or an elevated serum acid phosphatase establishes the diagnosis of advanced cancer. At times only biopsy will clarify it.

Benign firm nodules may present difficulties in differential diagnosis. They may be caused by tuberculosis, chronic infection with fibrosis, granulomatous prostatitis, or calculi. The early cancerous nodule is usually not raised above the surface of the gland (Fig 4–2). The change in consistency from malignant to normal tissue is abrupt. Biopsy, however, is often necessary to make the diagnosis.

(1) Tuberculous nodules are often multiple. One or both seminal vesicles may be thickened. A nontender, thickened epididymis suggests tuberculosis. "Sterile" pyuria with the finding of tubercle bacilli establishes the diagnosis. Urograms may reveal the renal tuberculous lesion.

(2) The fibrous nodule associated with chronic prostatitis is usually raised above the surface of the gland. The induration gradually lessens as the finger approaches normal tissue. Pus is found in the prostatic secretion. Biopsy, however, may be necessary.

(3) Granulomatous prostatitis will cause development of a hard nodular prostate. A recent history of an acute prostatic infection can usually be elicited. Biopsy, however, may be needed for differentiation.

(4) Prostatic calculi often cause crepitation on palpation. An x-ray will usually reveal their presence just above or behind the symphysis. Occasionally a patient may have both calculi and cancer, however.

Paget's disease may present a mottled area of increased density of the pelvic bones on a radiogram which must be differentiated from metastatic prostatic cancer. Although Paget's disease may cause a slight increase in serum acid phosphatase, it is less than 10 King-Armstrong units. Higher levels mean prostatic cancer. X-rays of the skull and long bones will show the typical lesion of Paget's disease. Rectal examination should settle the diagnosis.

Mastocytosis, a benign disease, may resemble the osteoblastic prostatic lesion.

Prolonged intake of fluoride (in drinking water) has been reported to cause osteosclerosis that simulates the x-ray appearance of osseous metastases from carcinoma of the prostate.

Complications

Obstruction of the prostatic urethra may cause the formation of vesical diverticula or stones. Infection is common.

Renal damage may be due to functional obstruction of the ureterovesical junction secondary to trigonal hypertrophy, invasion of the intramural portion of the ureters by tumor, or compression of the ureters at the pelvic brim by iliac nodes containing metastatic tumor. Infection may further impair renal function.

Edema of the legs—even of the genitalia—may occur as a result of pressure of involved iliac nodes upon the great vessels or blockage of lymph channels.

Spontaneous fractures can develop at the site of bony metastases. Sudden spinal cord compression is not uncommon and may require immediate laminectomy.

Prevention

At present, only 5% of men, when first seen by the urologist, have lesions that are amenable to cure by radical surgery. In order that this percentage may be significantly increased, careful palpation of the prostate in all men over 50 years of age is mandatory. Any suspicious induration requires immediate exploration.

Treatment

A. Curative (Radical) Measures: If, on palpating an indurated nodule in the prostate of a well-preserved man less than age 70, the clinician is unable to say that the patient does not have an early malignancy (and unless there is evidence of metastases to bone by x-ray or scan, elevations of the serum acid phosphatase, or a positive bone marrow biopsy), radical prostatectomy should be considered. If a needle biopsy has not been done, tissue can be subjected to immediate frozen section. This may be accomplished either by the perineal or retropubic routes. The entire prostate, including its capsule, the seminal vesicles, and a portion of the bladder neck are removed. The retropubic approach makes possible discovery of lymph node metastases. Lymph node dissection is feasible. Prostatovesiculectomy will cure about 75% of these favorable stage B cases. Urinary control is usually normal after the operation, but impotence is to be expected. Some advise preliminary estrogen for 3–6 months before radical prostatectomy is performed, feeling that the overall control is thereby enhanced.

Gill & others (1974) advise preoperative radiotherapy, radical retropubic prostatectomy, and pelvic lymph node dissection for stage C lesions, hoping to convert them to stage B tumors. McCullough & Leadbetter (1972) practice radical prostatocystectomy and lymph node dissection—even pelvic exenteration—for stage C lesions.

B. Palliative Measures:

1. Radiation therapy—There is increasing (and justified) enthusiasm for radiation therapy in the management of prostatic carcinoma. Clinicians who believe that stage B lesions should be subjected to radical prostatectomy give irradiation to patients with stage C lesions in the hope of cure and to those with stage D tumors for the purpose of palliation. The usual dose is 6000–7000 rads as a curative dose and 4000–5000 rads for palliation. The regimen is extended over a period of 5–6 weeks. Some proctitis, diarrhea, and urinary frequency is experienced toward the end of therapy in most cases, but chronic disability is rare. Impotence occurs in 30%. Obstructive symptoms usually diminish; ureteral obstruction improves; and the prostate usually becomes softer. Ray & others (1973) have reported on 310 patients subjected to radiotherapy. In those with an isolated nodule (stage B), the 5-year survival rate was 72%; at 10 years, the rate was 48%. In more advanced lesions, 48% survived to 5 years and 30% to 10 years.

Rhamy & others (1972) treated 15 patients with stage B tumors (suitable for radical prostatectomy). Thirteen (87%) had residual tumor 4–38 months later as shown by needle biopsy. Radiotherapy, however, is certainly the treatment of choice for the more advanced lesions. For stage D tumors, antiandrogen therapy should also be used.

2. Antiandrogen therapy—About 85% of prostatic cancers are androgen-dependent. These will show definite regression in size after a few weeks of antiandrogen therapy. The consistency of the gland tends to approach normal, the degree of urinary obstruction lessens, and bone pain disappears or decreases. The patient gains weight and strength, and anemia tends to correct itself. X-ray films often show healing of the metastatic lesions in bone. The price the patient must pay for this palliation includes impotence with loss of sexual desire, tender gynecomastia, and, at times, edema of the ankles. The edema can be controlled by restricted salt intake. Painful gynecomastia can usually be prevented by directing x-ray therapy to the region of the areola before estrogen treatment is begun.

There is no doubt that this mode of therapy affords much comfort to patients who formerly suffered greatly. It is also true that the life of these patients is slightly prolonged.

Although there is little doubt that antiandrogen therapy has a palliative effect on surgically incurable prostatic carcinoma, it has been shown that the administration of large doses of estrogen significantly increases the incidence of death from thromboembolic phenomena. Therefore, estrogens should be withheld until the patient develops symptoms or signs of metastases; when this happens, estorgens can be expected to cause regression of metastases in most patients.

Antiandrogen therapy includes orchiectomy and medical neutralization of testicular (and adrenal) androgens. The latter may be accomplished in the following ways:

a. Estrogen medication—Diethylstilbestrol, 1 mg/day, has proved effective and does not seem to be associated with secondary thromboembolic disorders. Other estrogens given in comparable dosage are equally efficient. A few advocate diethylstilbestrol, 5–100 mg/day for 3 months, and then 25 mg/day thereafter. Such large doses are of questionable value.

Therapy with massive doses of diethylstilbestrol diphosphate has been suggested for those patients with extensive disease or in those who are no longer being controlled by the usual dose of estrogen. The drug is given intravenously, undiluted. The following dosage schedule has been recommended: 500 mg 3 times a day for 10 days, 500 mg 2 times a day for 10 days, and then a similar dose daily for the next 10 days followed by 500 mg every week. Possibly half of patients will experience significant improvement.

Smith & others (1973) note that cyproterone acetate also inhibits elaboration of testosterone and

believe that it is superior to estrogens. Barnes & Ninen (1972) believe that in the treatment of stage B tumors the results of antiandrogen therapy rival those obtained by radical surgery.

b. Orchiectomy—Orchiectomy is similar in action to the administration of estrogens. Bone pain is relieved more promptly when this procedure is used. The combination of diethylstilbestrol and orchiectomy adds little to therapy. Both suppress plasma testosterone.

c. Medical adrenalectomy—This can be accomplished by the administration of cortisone (or an equivalent drug), 50 mg/day in divided doses. Salt must be restricted (0.3 g/day) and potassium added to the diet (3 g/day). This should be tried when the effectiveness of estrogen therapy begins to wane.

d. Surgical adrenalectomy—This rather rigorous procedure offers so little more relief than is afforded by cortisone that it is seldom indicated.

e. Hypophysectomy—Hypophysectomy has few advocates (West & others, 1973), but [99]yttrium or cryosurgical hypophysectomy has been shown to afford relief from diffuse bone pain in 75% of such patients when all other methods of therapy have been exhausted.

3. Resection—If the degree of obstruction is severe or if antiandrogenic therapy fails to afford much relief, transurethral resection of the prostate will be necessary. Since cancer of the prostate invades the hyperplastic tissue, there is no longer any cleavage plane which will permit intracapsular enucleation, as is ordinarily practiced for benign hyperplasia (eg, suprapubic prostatectomy).

4. Cryosurgery—This technic has been used in the poor-risk patient instead of transurethral resection with some measure of successful relief of obstruction. Gursel & others (1972) have recorded relief of bone pain following prostatic cryosurgery. The implication is that the procedure enhances the immunologic response to the tumor. Flocks & others (1972), however, failed to notice such an effect.

5. Testosterone and radioisotope therapy—If the tumor becomes androgen-independent and metastases are widespread, some regression may be obtained on the following regimen. Discontinue estrogens and steroids. Give testosterone, 100 mg/day for 17 days. Beginning on the sixth day of this course administer 1.8 mCi of ^{32}P per day orally or IV for 7 days. The latter should be followed by therapy with iron, vitamin B complex, and liver extract to maintain an adequate hemogram. Dicalcium phosphate will contribute to reossification of healing bone. Estrogen therapy should then be resumed. Such a course of therapy can be repeated.

Tong & Finkelstein (1973) report impressive results by giving parathyroid hormone followed by [32]P. The parathyroid hormone leaches calcium from the bones. When it is suddenly stopped and ^{32}P is administered, the uptake of the latter is enhanced. Fractures healed, the clinical state improved, and both serum acid and alkaline phosphatases decreased. When the administration of parathyroid hormone is stopped, the patient should be given 3 g of calcium glucomate, 100 mg of vitamin C, and one multivitamin tablet containing B_{12} 3 times a day. The schedule recommended by these authors is as follows:

Parathyroid hormone, 100 units IM 3 times daily for 7 days.
^{32}P (sodium phosphate) orally:
3 mCi on the 9th day
2 mCi on the 10th and 11th days, then twice a week for 2 more weeks (total, 6 doses)
1 mCi twice a week beginning on the 28th day (total, 6 doses)

Pinck & Alexander (1973) report similar results.

6. Testosterone alone—When all else fails, the administration of testosterone alone can be tried. In most, it increases existing pain, but in a few cases relief may be afforded. The mechanism for this effect is not clear.

7. Injection of radioisotopes—The results of direct injection of radioactive isotopes (eg, gold) into the cancerous glands are equivocal, though Carlton & others (1972) recommend suprapubic placement of radioactive gold seeds (2500–4500 rads) followed by 4500 rads delivered by either linear accelerator or cobalt for stage B and small stage C lesions. Their results are encouraging. In the majority, their prostatic biopsies were negative at 1 year.

C. Follow-Up Care: Following radical prostatectomy, periodic rectal examination should be done to seek local recurrence. Serum acid phosphatase levels should be monitored. A rise in this value would imply the presence of metastatic tumor. Serial chest films should be obtained, as well as a plain film of the bones of the lumbar spine, pelvis, and femoral heads in search of metastatic deposits.

A similar regimen should be followed for those given palliative therapy. If indicated, a bone scan should be ordered. A rising serum creatinine suggests progressive obstruction.

Prognosis

Of the 10% of men with prostatic carcinoma whose illness is diagnosed early enough so that radical surgery would offer a reasonable hope of cure, at least half are over 70 years of age and may suffer from other infirmities of age. For this reason they are not good subjects for radical procedures and most of them will live more comfortably and just as long with palliative treatment and will die of other causes. The cure rate for radical prostatectomy for stage B lesions is 60–70%. For stage C lesions, following radiotherapy, the control rate is about 50% at 5 years. When the effect of irradiation wears off, the physician still has a number of treatment modalities to offer.

SARCOMA OF THE PROSTATE

Sarcoma of the prostate is rare. Two-thirds of them are embryonal rhabdomyosarcomas, seen in young boys, and leiomyosarcomas, which occur in older men. The remainder are lymphomas. Most sarcomas grow rapidly; all are highly malignant. They may extend into the base of the bladder and finally occlude the urethra. They may compress the rectum and cause obstipation. These tumors metastasize by way of the lymphatics to the pelvic and lumbar lymph nodes. Venous spread may occur, in which case the lungs, liver, and bone may become involved.

Clinical Findings

A. Symptoms: Symptoms are largely those of urinary obstruction. Rectal obstruction may cause increasing constipation and symptoms of bowel obstruction.

B. Signs: Since these tumors often grow to large size, they may be felt suprapubically. Rectal examination reveals a very large mass in the prostatic area. It may be firm, or may be soft enough to suggest abscess. Considerable residual urine is usually recovered upon catheterization.

C. X-Ray Findings: Cystograms or excretory urograms may show that the bladder has been lifted up by the tumor. A urethrogram will demonstrate the compression and elongation of the posterior urethra.

D. Instrumental Examination: Cystoscopy or panendoscopy will demonstrate the prostatic enlargement. Grapelike masses often fill the prostatic urethra and bladder neck in children.

Treatment & Prognosis

Sarcoma of the prostate is radioresistant, and attempts at treatment have so far been of little avail. Total prostatocystectomy has cured a very few. Postoperative radiotherapy has been advocated.

TUMORS OF THE SEMINAL VESICLES

About 30 cases of primary carcinoma of the seminal vesicles have been reported in the literature; sarcoma and benign lesions are even rarer. The tumors cause symptoms suggesting obstruction from an enlarged prostate. Bloody ejaculation may be noted. Rectal examination will reveal a mass above the prostate and involving one vesicle. Angiography reveals neovascularity. Radical extirpation of the lesion is indicated, but cure is rare.

TUMORS OF THE URETHRA

BENIGN TUMORS

Benign tumors of the urethra are not common in men or women. A few cases of congenital urethral polyps have been described. They are usually papillary and may be found anywhere between the bladder neck and the external orifice. The most distal tumors may be visible; the others may make their presence known by bloody spotting. If the tumor is large enough, symptoms of urinary obstruction may develop. If the tumor arises in the prostatic urethra, bleeding may be noted in the last portion of the urine. If obstructive, infection is apt to be a complication. The diagnosis is made by biopsy. Transurethral electrocoagulation cures these lesions.

MALIGNANT TUMORS

Malignant tumors of the urethra are not common; they occur more often in women than in men. Those arising from the most distal portion of the urethra are epidermoid carcinomas. Those originating more proximally are of the transitional cell type, though a few adenocarcinomas have been reported. Tumors involving the region of the external meatus metastasize to the superficial and deep subinguinal lymph nodes. The more proximal tumors spread to the vesical, sacral, hypogastric, and external iliac nodes (Figs 18−1 and 18−2). They may infiltrate the vulva or vagina.

If distal, either in men or women, these tumors may first present themselves as visible or palpable masses. Bloody discharge may be noted. Urinary obstruction may occur. The deeper tumors may be quite obstructive and are often complicated by infection. In men, they may be misdiagnosed and treated as urethral strictures. At times these tumors are complicated by periurethral abscesses which may lead to the formation of urinary fistulas.

The diagnosis is made by biopsy of the tumor, which is either palpated externally or seen directly by panendoscopy or on urethrograms (Fig 6−9).

Tumors of the distal urethra in women can often be cured by local excision, though Taggart & others (1972) as well as Chu (1973) recommend the insertion of radium needles or radiotherapy for the smaller tumors. Similar tumors in men require amputation of the penis. Radical inguinal node dissection (which includes the superficial and deep subinguinal and the superficial inguinal nodes) is indicated if the nodes are involved.

Cancer of the perineal urethra may require radical penectomy with the formation of a perineal urethral orifice. If the bulb is involved, prostatocystectomy must be performed as well and the urinary stream diverted. In the female, if the deep urethra or all of the urethra is involved, consideration should be given to urethrocystectomy with urinary diversion.

Radiotherapy or surgical excision of small distal lesions offers a 5-year control rate of about 50%. The prognosis is poor for proximal tumors.

On the whole, these tumors are very malignant, and few cures are obtained in those patients whose lesions involve the proximal urethra.

TUMORS OF THE SPERMATIC CORD

More than 300 cases of tumors of the spermatic cord have been reported. Most are benign and are composed of connective tissue elements. The malignant tumors (eg, rhabdomyosarcoma, fibrosarcoma) spread by both the hematogenous and lymphatic routes. The latter is the most common. They involve the iliac and preaortic lymph nodes as well as the liver and lungs.

These tumors present palpable masses which may be associated with local pain. A blow to the area may bring the lesion to the attention of the patient. They must be differentiated from hernias, hydrocele of the cord, and spermatocele.

Benign tumors require orchiectomy with division of the cord at the internal inguinal ring just in case the pathologist should find a malignant focus. Sarcomas require a similar procedure. If no hematogenous spread can be demonstrated, radical retroperitoneal lymphadenectomy should be done. The latter operation has afforded cures in some patients with positive nodes. As an alternative, some authorities advocate radiotherapy to these nodes, but this appears to be less efficacious. Sarcomas are highly malignant and prognosis must be guarded.

TUMORS OF THE TESTIS

With rare exception, all tumors of the testes are malignant. While most develop between the ages of 18−35 years, Smith (1973) has found over 600 instances of such tumors in childhood, the majority occurring during the first year of life. Most are embryonal carcinomas, benign teratomas, and teratocarcinomas. Tsuji & others (1973) report a high incidence of such new growths in Japanese children. Most of those seen after the age of 60 years are reticulum cell sarcomas, Sertoli cell tumors, or interstitial cell tumors; only 25% arise from germ cells. Testis tumors account for about 0.5% of all malignancies in men and

4% of all tumors affecting the genitourinary tract. About 30 instances of bilateral tumors have been reported. Metastasis occurs relatively early. Some elaborate chorionic gonadotropins, and the prognosis in this type is poor. Retroperitoneal and mediastinal tumors without evidence of testicular involvement are occasionally seen.

Testicular tumors are relatively rare in blacks.

Etiology

The cause of testicular tumors is not known. It may be significant, however, that they usually develop during the age of greatest sexual activity. Many authorities believe that the undescended testis, particularly in the pseudohermaphrodite, has a definite tendency to undergo carcinomatous change. Whether maldescent is the cause or whether some unknown factor causes both the lack of descent and tumor formation is not decided. Twenty-eight instances of bilateral tumors have been reported.

Pathogenesis & Pathology

A. Classification: Many classifications of tumor of the testis have been offered, most of them based upon morphology. Since about 30% of these tumors elaborate chorionic gonadotropin (Wilson & Woodhead, 1972), a morphologic-endocrine grouping is feasible.

1. Teratoma—Most authorities agree that all of the teratomatous tumors of the testis, mixed or pure, arise from a totipotent cell which can develop in many directions. These cells have been likened to a twin of the host—a twin which develops in the host's own testis. Mixed tumors (teratomas) contain both mesenchymal and epithelial tissues. Fewer than 5% are benign, and most of those occur in children, the rest are malignant. The malignant epithelial cells may overgrow the other elements and appear as the only cell in the tumor unless serial secretions are studied. However, one tumor frequently contains elements of 2 or even 3 of the common types.

a. Seminoma pattern (30%)—These tumors are made up of sheets of round epithelial cells with clear cytoplasm and large nuclei. Fibrous septa course through the tumor; these may be infiltrated with lymphocytes. Mitoses are common. Thirteen percent are chromatin-positive (female). The modal chromosome numbers are usually 50 or more. Twelve percent secrete chorionic gonadotropin.

b. Carcinoma pattern (40%)—This type tends to secrete chorionic gonadotropin and is often associated with hyperplasia of the interstitial cells. These tumors may therefore have arisen from primitive chorionic tissues. These embryonal epithelial cells may take on a papillary pattern. The cytoplasm is often granular. There is considerable variation in the size of the cells. Many mitoses are present. In some, syncytial cells are apparent; in others, the small Langhans' cells are seen. Typical choriocarcinoma may be observed (2% of all testis tumors). Almost all secrete gonadotropin. Embryonal carcinoma is the most common tumor in this group and is the type most often seen in children.

Twenty-five percent elaborate chorionic gonadotropins.

c. Teratoma pattern (25%)—These tumors contain numerous types of immature and mature mesenchymal and epithelial structures, including muscle, cartilage, nerve, and mucosa. One or more of these may predominate and present malignant change. These tumors probably represent malformed embryos. The pure teratoma does not elaborate chorionic gonadotropin, so hyperplasia of Leydig cells is not seen. This hormone, however, is secreted in 37% of patients whose tumors contain embryonal carcinoma or choriocarcinoma. Positive chromosome patterns are seen in 32% of this group. Many have 50 or more chromosomes.

2. Interstitial cell tumors—More than 170 cases have been reported (Selvaggi & others, 1973). About 75% are seen after the age of 30; 90% are benign. They secrete an increased amount of estrogens; 17-ketosteroids are normal or low. When the tumor develops before puberty, macrogenitosomia occurs. About 20% of adults develop gynecomastia and most are impotent and sterile. The malignant form metastasizes widely, but particularly to bone.

3. Sertoli cell tumors—These rare, usually benign tumors are feminizing. Gynecomastia is a cardinal finding.

4. Lymphoma and reticulum cell sarcoma—These tumor types are occasionally observed. Leukemic infiltration has been reported.

5. Adrenal rests are occasionally seen.

6. Metastatic testis tumors—Tumors metastatic to the testis include tumors of the lung, prostate, and gastrointestinal tract and malignant melanoma (skin).

B. Chorionic Gonadotropins: These substances may be found in the urine in abnormal amounts in about 30% of patients with testicular tumors. The prognosis in those with positive hormone titers is relatively poor. Usually such tumors have a carcinomatous pattern. If a positive hormone test is found in what seems to be a seminoma or teratoma, further sectioning will often reveal tumor of the carcinoma type. If the level of this hormone drops to normal after orchiectomy, the prognosis is improved. If, however, it rises again or if, after orchiectomy, it fails to drop, the presumption is that metastatic tumor is present. Clinically, these tumors must be considered choriocarcinomas even though typical cells cannot be found in the testis. At autopsy, many of these patients will be found to have the hemorrhagic metastases typical of choriocarcinoma.

C. Metastases: Except for choriocarcinoma, the major route for metastases is lymphatic. The lumbar and mediastinal nodes are most commonly involved. The left and occasionally the right supraclavicular nodes are at times affected. The lesion will spread to the superficial inguinal and subinguinal nodes only if the scrotum becomes invaded (and this is unusual) or if previous orchiectomy or hernioplasty has been performed. In 20% of cases with lymph node metastases, the abdominal (lumbar) lymph nodes on the side opposite the primary tumor will contain metastatic cancer.

It is for this reason that lymph node dissection should be bilateral.

Masses of lumbar lymph nodes may displace the ureters or kidneys. Ureteral occlusion occasionally is observed. Bowel may also be displaced.

Metastases are commonly found in the lungs and liver; other organs are involved less frequently. Probably 30–40% of the patients have metastases when they are first seen.

Staging of Testicular Tumors

The following is the Walter Reed General Hospital staging system (Buck & others, 1972):

Stage IA: Tumor confined to testis; no clinical or radiographic evidence of spread.

Stage IB: Tumor confined to testis; no clinical or radiographic evidence of spread but histologic evidence of metastasis to iliac or para-aortic nodes at time of retroperitoneal lymphadenectomy.

Stage II: Clinical or radiographic evidence of metastasis to nodes below the diaphragm; no demonstrable metastasis above the diaphragm or to viscera.

Stage III: Clinical or radiographic evidence of metastasis above the diaphragm or to viscera.

Clinical Findings

A painless lump in the testis must be regarded as tumor until proved otherwise. The common sites of metastases are the preaortic lymph nodes and the lungs. Gynecomastia suggests the presence of a functioning tumor and is a bad prognostic sign. About 10% of tumors produce this symptom. If carcinoma of the testis cannot be unequivocally ruled out, orchiectomy must be done immediately.

A. Symptoms: The most common presenting symptom is enlargement of the testis. It may be discovered quite by accident, or attention may be drawn to it because of mild discomfort caused by its weight. On rare occasion it can be quite painful if bleeding occurs into its own substance.

If the tumor is elaborating large amounts of chorionic gonadotropins, gynecomastia may be seen. This change is also seen with Sertoli and Leydig cell tumors, both of which cause secretion of estrogen.

Symptoms from metastases include a supraclavicular or abdominal mass (lymph nodes), abdominal pain from bowel or ureteral obstruction, cough from metastases to the lung, and nonspecific symptoms of loss of weight and anorexia.

In the rare instance of a Leydig cell tumor, a preadolescent boy may undergo precocious development of sexual organs and secondary sexual characteristics. The adult experiences no accentuation of sex characteristics; in fact, he is apt to become impotent. The boy with Sertoli cell tumor may develop a female escutcheon and gynecomastia.

B. Signs: The testis is usually definitely enlarged and diffusely involved. The tumor is ordinarily smooth and in general maintains the ovoid shape of the testis. It is firm and gives the sensation of abnormal weight. It does not transilluminate. Of the greatest importance is the fact that pressure on the organ fails to cause the typical sickening testicular discomfort. The epididymis can be distinguished from the testis in the early stages, but later it is lost in the mass. A very early tumor may present as a firm, nontender nodule embedded in the testis.

The spermatic cord is usually normal on palpation. It is rare for the scrotum to be involved except in the last stage of the disease unless previous orchiopexy, herniorrhaphy, or removal of the tumor through a scrotal incision has been done (Herr & others, 1973). Hydrocele develops secondary to tumor in about 10% of cases. In such instances in young men, if adequate palpation of the testis cannot be done, the hydrocele must be aspirated.

Metastases without an evident primary source occurring in a young cryptorchid should suggest the possibility of tumor of that testis. A hard mass in the left supraclavicular area in a young man should be regarded as testicular malignancy until proved otherwise, since tumor of the testis is the most common malignancy in that age group. Gynecomastia should suggest the presence of a functioning testicular neoplasm. Metastases should be sought along the aorta; masses of involved lymph nodes are often palpable.

In the later stages, evidence of weight loss and even cachexia may be seen.

C. Laboratory Findings: The patient may be anemic if metastases are widespread. Urinalysis is of no help in diagnosis. Renal function is usually normal even though unilateral ureteral occlusion develops. An estimate of the level of urinary chorionic gonadotropins should be done. Its presence means testicular tumor of the carcinoma type or choriocarcinoma, and is a grave prognostic sign. A negative test has no diagnostic significance.

The 17-ketosteroids are normal or low with Leydig cell tumor. Urinary estrogens may be increased with both Leydig cell and Sertoli cell neoplasms.

D. X-Ray Findings: A chest film may show evidence of metastases. Excretory urograms are indicated in all cases of testicular tumor; masses of carcinomatous lumbar nodes may displace the ureter or kidney (Fig 18–17) and may cause ureteral stenosis. Retrograde ureterograms (Fig 18–17) or venacavagrams (Fig 6–16) may more clearly delineate an extraureteral mass. Lymphangiography is an excellent method for demonstrating lymph node metastases (Fig 18–17), although a number of false-positives and a few false-negatives have been observed. A liver scan should be done.

E. Biopsy: Buck & others (1972) recommend that stage II patients have bilateral supraclavicular lymph node biopsy. In 13% of their ostensibly stage II patients, the biopsy was positive, thus moving them to the stage III group.

F. Total Body Scanning With Gallium-67 Citrate: Bailey & others (1973) have studied the usefulness of this technic in the diagnosis of metastases to lymph nodes. This substance is deposited in reticuloendothelial tissues, the nasopharynx, bone marrow, liver,

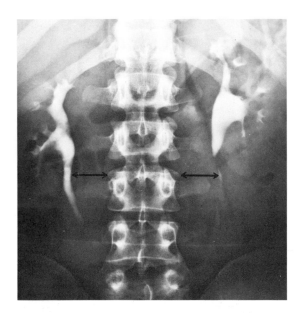

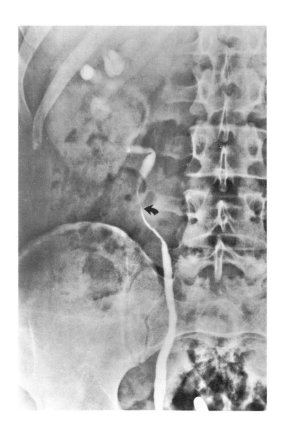

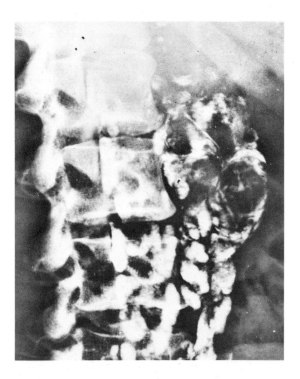

Figure 18—17. Carcinoma of the testis. **Above left:** Excretory urogram showing lateral displacement of both upper ureters by metastases to lumbar lymph nodes. **Above right:** Retrograde bulb ureterogram showing hydrone-phrosis and ureteral deviation at L4 secondary to metas-tases in right lumbar lymph nodes. (See Fig 7—16 for venacavagram on same patient.) **Left:** Lymphangiogram demonstrating enlarged lumbar lymph nodes involved by metastatic tumor.

spleen, and inflammatory tissue. They found that it was more accurate than lymphangiography or chest x-ray in revealing such spread.

G. Plasma or Urinary Carcinoembryonic Antigen (CEA): Javadpour (1973) found increased levels of this antigen in 80% of patients with teratocarcinoma.

Differential Diagnosis

A. Painless Scrotal Swellings: Hydrocele may be quite tense and even firm if the tunica vaginalis is thickened. It will transilluminate. Hydrocele, it must be remembered, develops secondary to some testicular malignancies. In case of doubt, aspirate the hydroceles of young men to afford adequate palpation of the testis.

A spermatocele is a free cystic mass lying above and behind the testis.

Tuberculosis of the epididymis may present itself as an enlargement, but palpation should reveal that the testis is separate from the mass. If the testis has become secondarily involved, differentiation may be more difficult. The diagnosis of tuberculosis will be enhanced by finding beading of the vas, induration of the prostate or seminal vesicles, and pus and tubercle bacilli in the urine.

Gumma is a very rare nontender testicular lesion which causes enlargement. A history of syphilis and a positive serologic test should suggest this diagnosis.

About 75 instances of epidermoid cyst of the testis have been reported. The correct diagnosis is made by the pathologist. Occasionally other tumors may metastasize to the testes. The primary sites are the prostate, lung, gastrointestinal tract, and skin (melanoma).

B. Painful Scrotal Swellings: It is rare for testicular tumors to be exquisitely painful, but moderate discomfort is present in 40% of patients. Nonspecific epididymitis, if acute, is exceedingly painful. If seen early it is obvious that only the epididymis is involved. After some hours, the entire testis becomes swollen. Pyuria and symptoms of lower tract infection are usually present. Chronic epididymitis should not be confusing, for the induration will involve the epididymis only.

Mumps orchitis is usually much more painful than tumor and is quite tender. Parotitis is almost always evident, and fever may be quite high.

Torsion of the spermatic cord is a disease of childhood, at which age tumor is unusual. Torsion is suggested if the epididymis can be felt anterior to the testis. Also, elevation of the testis onto the pubis increases the torsion and therefore the pain.

Complications

Complications arise from the metastases. Rarely a ureter may become completely occluded by extrinsic pressure from involved lymph nodes.

Following bilateral retroperitoneal lymphadenectomy, most patients will produce no ejaculate with orgasm. This is caused by damage to the lumbar sympathetic trunks that govern seminal emission.

Treatment

A. Orchiectomy: If after careful examination a testicular tumor cannot be ruled out, the testicle should be removed. Orchiectomy is performed through an inguinal incision. It must not be done through the scrotum. This permits high ligation of the cord at the internal ring. Furthermore, the blood supply of the testis should be divided before the tumor itself is handled thus decreasing the risk of vascular or lymphatic dissemination.

B. Bilateral Radical Retroperitoneal Lymph Node Resection: Radical resection of the retroperitoneal (iliac and lumbar) lymph nodes is indicated for almost all testicular tumors except the seminoma, which is highly radiosensitive. It appears to be of little value in cases of choriocarcinoma because of its penchant for metastasizing via the bloodstream, but, on theoretical grounds, it might be worth trying. The presence of massive metastases in these nodes is considered a contraindication to resection. Preoperative lymphangiography allows radiograms to be taken on the operating table to be sure that all nodes have been removed.

About 75% of patients undergoing node dissection will have ejaculatory impotence because of sympathetic nerve damage. Hinman (personal commuication) has found that giving 25 mg of ephedrine one-half hour before intercourse is apt to lead to ejaculation. If this fails, he recommends increasing the dose to 50 mg.

Lobectomy has been successfully employed in a few patients with isolated pulmonary metastases.

C. X-Ray Therapy: Radiation therapy is given in all cases of testicular neoplasm, whether metastases have been discovered or not. It is the treatment of choice for seminoma. For the other tumors, radiotherapy is given following lymphadenectomy. A few clinicians advise radiation both before and after node dissection (Earle & others, 1973). There seems to be increasing interest in routine therapy to the mediastinum and supraclavicular regions despite lack of evidence of local disease, though Ytredel & Bradfield (1972) found no benefit from this procedure for stage I seminoma.

Without concomitant lymph node dissection (seminoma), those patients subjected to radiotherapy only are usually fertile (Smithers & others, 1973).

D. Chemotherapy: It has been shown that the employment of 3 cancericidal drugs is effective in palliation of metastatic testicular tumor. These comprise an alkylating agent (eg, chlorambucil), an antimetabolite (eg, methotrexate), and the antitumor antibiotic dactinomycin. Given in combination as a first course, they are repeated at intervals. Mithramycin and adriamycin are also reported to be effective in the treatment of embryonal carcinoma, teratocarcinoma, and choriocarcinoma.

This method of treatment is apt to cause subsidence of lumbar lymph node involvement and pulmonary metastases. In most cases the urinary chorionic gonadotropin titer falls sharply to normal; this demonstrates the effect of chemotherapy upon trophoblastic tissue.

Toxic effects include nausea and vomiting, stoma-

now PVB
D.D. Platinum, Vinblastine, Bleo —

titis, diarrhea, leukopenia, thrombocytopenia, skin eruptions, and loss of hair. Serious toxic symptoms necessitate withholding the drug until the side effects have cleared.

Bloom & Hendry (1973) found that, in a few patients who had not benefited from chemotherapy, some response was noted after the administration of medroxyprogesterone acetate.

E. Follow-Up Care: Periodic abdominal palpation in search of masses of lymph nodes or liver enlargement or nodule formation is essential. Examination for supraclavicular lymph node enlargement is also necessary, as well as serial chest films. If the patient had an increased level of chorionic gonadotropin before treatment, the titer should be checked at intervals. An increasing titer may indicate the need for chemotherapy.

Prognosis

The presence of demonstrable metastases implies a guarded prognosis, except in seminomas.

The type of tumor is of great prognostic significance. Seminomas are the least malignant, particularly if they contain lymphoid stroma microscopically (Javadpour, 1973). Only 5% of patients are dead 5 years after operation. Teratomas are more often fatal; 35% are dead 5 years after operation. Fifty-five percent of those with tumors of the carcinoma pattern are dead in 5 years. Almost all patients with choriocarcinoma are dead within 2 years of diagnosis.

In the nonseminoma group, Staubitz & others (1974) obtained a 5-year survival rate of 85% for stage I and 70% for stage II tumors.

Hyperplasia of interstitial cells is a bad prognostic sign. The majority of these patients also have increased levels of urinary gonadotropins. The finding of chorionic gonadotropin in the urine is a serious sign. Most of these patients die within 2 years.

TUMORS OF THE EPIDIDYMIS

Tumors of the epididymis are quite rare, but most are benign (adenomatoid tumors). They may arise from epithelial or connective tissue structures. The malignant group spreads by lymphatics (same as testis) and veins and offers a poor prognosis. Tumors metastasizing to the epididymis are rare.

These tumors often present as painless enlargement, although mild discomfort may be felt. Hydrocele may be the only change present; this, of course, is also true of tumors of the testis. Aspiration of hydroceles is imperative if the testicle cannot be properly palpated.

These lesions must be differentiated from tuberculous or nonspecific epididymitis; this may prove impossible without surgical exploration.

Treatment consists of epididymectomy if one can be sure the lesion is benign (frozen section). Orchiectomy must be undertaken for cancer or sarcoma. X-ray therapy to regional lymph nodes is also indicated. The prognosis is poor for the malignant tumors.

TUMORS OF THE PENIS

Almost all of the tumors of the penis are of epithelial origin and almost always involve the prepuce or glans. They are similar in all respects to epitheliomas elsewhere on the body.

Etiology

There seems to be no doubt that the most common cause of cancer of the penis is chronic inflammation from infection of the foreskin and glans. In China, Africa, and Southeast Asia, 10–15% of all tumors are of the penis. On the other hand, the incidence is less than 5% where circumcision is the rule. Kuruvilla & others (1971) note that the incidence of penile cancer is higher in Hindus than in Muslims. The latter practice circumcision; the former do not.

Pathogenesis & Pathology

Certain precancerous lesions can be recognized. Leukoplakia may rarely involve the penis. It consists of a white scaly lesion which causes some thickening of the skin. Microscopically, hyperplasia of the squamous cell layer is evident. There is no invasion of the subcutaneous tissue. Considerable small round cell infiltration is seen.

Erythroplasia of Queyrat is strictly a lesion of the penis. Its surface is ordinarily red and indurated and may ulcerate. On microscopic examination, considerable overdevelopment of the rete pegs is noted, yet their basement membranes remain intact. Mitoses are present, but the cells are fairly uniform in size. Some increase in vascularity is noticeable. It may respond to fluorouracil applied locally.

Bowen's disease, or carcinoma in situ, may be found on any skin surface. A raised indurated red plaque may be noted; its center may be ulcerated. Microscopic study reveals anaplasia of epithelial elements with considerable hyperplasia of the squamous cell layers and mitotic activity. The basement membrane, however, remains intact.

Epidermoid carcinoma of the penis is rarely found in a man who has been circumcised during infancy. The growth arises on the glans or the inner surface of the foreskin. It may first appear as a raised, red, firm plaque or as an ulcer. As it grows it may be proliferative or ulcerative. It is usually painless, although severe secondary infection may cause discomfort. Because of the tumor and the edema from infection, retraction of the prepuce may be impossible.

The microscopic picture in epidermoid carcinoma is the same as that of epidermoid cancer anywhere on the skin or mucous surfaces. Hyperkeratosis is prominent. Hyperplasia of the rete is marked, and mitoses are frequent. Invasion of the connective tissue is obvious. Metastases occur through lymph channels which drain to the superficial and deep subinguinal and superficial inguinal nodes; the iliac nodes may also become involved. Enlarged lymph nodes are commonly found in these patients; some are inflammatory and others contain metastatic tumor cells. Widespread metastases by way of veins are not common.

Among the rare growths reported are leiomyosarcoma, melanoma, Kaposi's sarcoma, and vascular tumors.

Metastatic tumors to the penis include the following primary sites: bladder, prostate, rectum, lung, nasopharynx, and skin.

Staging of Tumors of the Penis

Stage I: Lesion limited to glans or foreskin.
Stage II: Tumor invading shaft or corpora cavernosa. No nodes involved.
Stage III: Tumor invading shaft. Lymph node involvement.
Stage IV: Inoperable lymph nodes and distant metastases.

Clinical Findings

Neoplasms of the penis are usually epithelial and malignant. They involve the foreskin or glans and may be papillary or infiltrating. Metastases to the subinguinal and inguinal lymph nodes are common and imply a poor prognosis.

A. Symptoms: The patient may notice an enlarging warty growth or a spreading ulcer on the glans or foreskin. These lesions are usually painless unless secondary infection is marked. Tumors of the shaft are rare.

If the foreskin cannot be retracted, the patient may complain of local pain from infection; a foul, often bloody discharge emanating from the preputial pouch; and a firm lump in the region of the glans.

Masses in the inguinal region may be noted. They can be quite painful and tender if inflammatory, although this finding does not rule out the presence of metastases. In the late stages the metastatic nodes may be quite large, may ulcerate, and can cause hemorrhage which may be difficult to control.

B. Signs: A papillary or ulcerating tumor may be seen. The latter type may be quite destructive. If tumor is suspected and the foreskin cannot be retracted, a dorsal slit of the prepuce should be done.

Enlarged lymph nodes may be found both above and below the inguinal ligament. These can be due to metastases, infection, or both. In the advanced stage, these masses may be quite large. They may ulcerate through the skin.

C. Laboratory Findings: Anemia may be evident in the later stages of the disease. Leukocytosis may be secondary to local infection. The urine bathing an un-

retractable foreskin will show pus, bacteria, and often red cells. Biopsy is necessary in all patients suspected of having tumors. This can usually be done under local anesthesia. A slit in the dorsal surface of the foreskin may be necessary to properly visualize the lesion.

D. X-Ray Findings: A lymphangiogram may show metastases to the iliac lymph nodes (Fig 6–15). They are indicated when positive nodes are present in the groin.

Differential Diagnosis

Syphilitic chancre may simulate a small ulcerating epithelioma. Dark-field examination should reveal *Treponema pallidum.* In case of doubt, biopsy is indicated.

Chancroid can at times cause some confusion in diagnosis. It is ordinarily a rapidly spreading ulcerative lesion which is quite painful. Complement fixation tests or the finding of *Haemophilus ducreyi* on smears from the lesion is diagnostic.

Condylomata acuminata are soft warty growths usually of venereal origin and probably caused by a virus. They are usually not invasive. If any doubt exists, biopsy should be done.

Complications

The common complications of tumors of the penis are infection of the tumor and inguinal adenitis, metastatic involvement to the ilioinguinal and iliac nodes, and, rarely, invasion of the urethra with urinary obstruction.

Prevention

The evidence seems to be quite clear that circumcision in infancy will almost certainly prevent carcinoma of the penis in later life.

Treatment

Before treatment is instituted, a biopsy must be obtained and a positive diagnosis of cancer established.

A. The Local Lesion: Small lesions without evidence of metastases, (stage I) can be destroyed by local excision or by x-ray or radium therapy. More extensive lesions (stage II) may require partial amputation, though evidence is mounting that irradiation offers a comparable cure rate (50%). Amputation should be done at a level 2 cm proximal to the tumor. Local recurrence after amputation is rare.

B. The Inguinal and Subinguinal Lymph Nodes: If the primary lesion is small and no adenopathy is demonstrable (stage I), radical resection of the inguinal areas is not indicated. These wounds are often slow to heal, and considerable lymphedema of the area develops.

If a few metastatic inguinal nodes are evident (stage III) as judged by examination or biopsy and if the lymphangiogram shows no involvement of the iliac nodes, bilateral radical inguinal and subinguinal node dissection must be done because of the cross-connection between the 2 sides.

In the presence of advanced metastases, either

local or general, excision of these nodes is valueless.

C. The Iliac Lymph Nodes: If lymphangiography or exploratory laparotomy reveals involvement of the iliac nodes, radical resection of these nodes should be considered (Skinner & others, 1972).

D. X-Ray Therapy: Gursel & others (1973) found that lymph node dissection contributed little to their cure rates. They advise irradiation of the inguinal and subinguinal nodes should they be involved (stage III) and similar therapy to the deep pelvic nodes should laparotomy or lymphangiography reveal their involvement (stage IV). Most authors, however, would only irradiate inoperable lymph nodes for palliation.

E. Chemotherapy: Bleomycin has been employed in the more advanced cases. It is quite toxic and occasionally causes pulmonary fibrosis (de Kernion & others, 1973).

Prognosis

When a small tumor is localized to the penis and there are no metastases (stage I), the 5-year control rate is 70–90%. If the tumor invades the penile shaft or corpora cavernosa (without lymph node involvement), the cure rate drops to about 70%. Should there be moderate lymph node spread, cure is obtained in only 30%. When there are distant metastases, the cure rate is zero.

TUMORS OF THE SCROTUM

Tumors of the scrotal skin are rare. Most of them arise from occupational exposure to various carcino-gens, including soot, tars, creosote, and petroleum products. While a few benign tumors of the skin or subcutaneous tissues occur, most are epitheliomas. Also encountered are reticulum cell sarcoma, melanoma, rhabdomyosarcoma, leiomyosarcoma, and liposarcoma. They metastasize by lymphatic channels to the superficial inguinal and subinguinal nodes.

The diagnosis should be considered in any lesion of the scrotal skin in a man who gives a history of prolonged exposure to carcinogens. Biopsy is necessary if any doubt exists. Treatment consists of wide excision of the primary tumor. If a few inguinal metastases are noted, bilateral inguinal node dissection is indicated.

In the absence of lymph node metastasis, the cure rate is 50%. When lymph node spread is found, only 25% survive.

RETROPERITONEAL EXTRARENAL TUMORS

Although these tumors and cysts are rare, they must be considered in the differential diagnosis of renal and suprarenal masses since they present as masses in the flank. Most of these noeplasms arise from mesothelial tissues of the retroperitoneum and are therefore of connective tissue origin. They may be comprised of a single type of cell (eg, lipoma, fibroma), but more commonly are mixed tumors (eg, chondrolipomyxoma). Many are malignant (eg, lipomyxorhabdomyosarcoma). Others, for the most part, arise from the mesonephros and its duct, and the gonads.

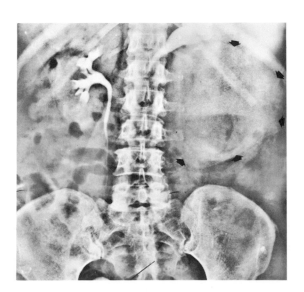 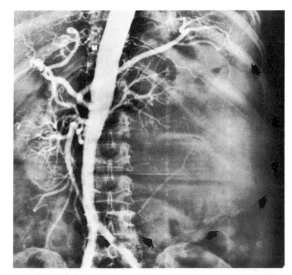

Figure 18–18. Retroperitoneal lipoma. *Left:* Excretory urogram showing large soft tissue mass in left upper quadrant displacing kidney superomedially. Right kidney is normal. *Right:* Renal angiogram, same patient, revealing large, relatively avascular mass in left abdomen. Left renal vasculature displaced medially and superiorly.

The cystic tumors are benign; the solid growths may be benign or malignant. Even if benign, however, they tend to grow to large size and to surround and displace adjacent organs.

The most common finding is the discovery of a mass in the flank. Gastrointestinal symptoms caused by displacement or invasion of intraperitoneal organs may also be noted. Edema of the legs may occur if the vena cava is occluded. A plain film of the abdomen may show a large soft tissue mass in the upper abdomen. The kidney may be displaced, yet its calyceal system is not distorted; this is a cardinal sign of retroperitoneal extrarenal tumor (Fig 18–18). Hydronephrosis may develop from ureteral compression. Gastrointestinal studies may reveal displacement of the stomach or colon. Renal tumors or cysts cause distortion of the pelvis and calyces. Extrarenal tumors ordinarily do not. Angiography shows a relatively avascular mass whose blood supply is largely derived from the lumbar arteries.

Adrenal tumors are rarely large enough to be palpable. The x-ray findings are the same in both, but most adrenal tumors are associated with symptoms and signs of hyperfunction. Angiography will differentiate the two.

An enlarged spleen may present as a mass in the left upper abdomen and at times can displace the kidney. Hematologic changes may accompany splenomegaly; findings elsewhere consistent with lymphoma may be helpful. Again, angiography will make the diagnosis.

The main complication is displacement, envelopment, or invasion of adjacent organs (eg, spleen, stomach, liver, ureter, kidney, vena cava, and aorta).

Surgical removal of the cyst or tumor is the only method of cure. The solid tumors are difficult to remove in toto because of their penchant for invading and surrounding vital structures. These tumors are radioresistant.

The prognosis after the excision of cysts is good. The recurrence rate after removal of the solid tumors is high even though the neoplasm is benign.

• • •

References

General

Proceedings of The American Cancer Society's National Conference on Urologic Cancer. Cancer 32:1017, 1973.

Benign Tumors of the Renal Parenchyma

Antoine JE, Kopperman M: Renal adenoma: Retrospect and prospect. Am J Roentgenol 119:727, 1973.

Becker JA & others: Angiomyolipoma (hamartoma) of the kidney: An angiographic review. Acta radiol diag 14:561, 1973.

Berdon WE, Wigger HJ, Baker DH: Fetal renal hamartoma: A benign tumor to be distinguished from Wilms' tumor. Am J Roentgenol 118:18, 1973.

Bernie JE: Renal angiomyolipoma in an adolescent: A case report. J Urol 109:492, 1973.

Bredin HC, Lauengood RW Jr, Barondess JA: Renal hamartoma: Arteriographic findings suggesting hypernephroma. Urology 2:574, 1973.

Charlot-Charles J, Jones GW: Renal angiomyolipoma associated with tuberous sclerosis: Review of literature. Urology 3:465, 1974.

Chonko AM & others: Renal involvement in tuberous sclerosis. Am J Med 56:124, 1974.

Clark RE, Palubinskas AJ: The angiographic spectrum of renal hamartoma. Am J Roentgenol 114:715, 1972.

Conn JW, Bookstein JJ, Cohen EL: Renin-secreting juxtaglomerular-cell adenoma: Preoperative clinical and angiographic diagnosis. Radiology 106:543, 1973.

Fois A, Pindinelli CA, Berardi R: Early signs of tuberous sclerosis in infancy and childhood. Helv paediat acta 28:313, 1973.

Hajdu SI, Koss LG: Endometriosis of the kidney. Am J Obst Gynec 106:314, 1970.

Hilton C, Keeling JW: Neonatal renal tumours. Brit J Urol 46:157, 1974.

Loening S, Richardson JR Jr: Papillary cystadenoma of kidney. Urology 1:593, 1973.

McCullough DL: Renal hamartoma: Current concepts of diagnosis and surgical treatment. Urology 4:235, 1974.

Murphy GP, Mostofi FK: Histologic assessment and clinical prognosis of renal adenoma. J Urol 103:31, 1970.

Neonatal kidney tumors. Brit MJ 4:627, 1973.

Peters HJ, Nuri M, Münzenmaier R: Hemangioendothelioma of the kidney: A case report and review of the literature. J Urol 112:723, 1974.

Peterson NE, Thompson HT: Renal hemangioma. J Urol 105:27, 1971.

Phillips G, Mukherjee TM: A juxtaglomerular cell tumour: Light and electron microscopic studies of a renin-secreting kidney tumour containing both juxtaglomerular cells and mast cells. Pathology 4:194, 1972.

Sareen CK & others: Tuberous sclerosis: Clinical, endocrine, and metabolic studies. Am J Dis Child 123:34, 1972.

Walker D, Richard GA: Fetal hamartoma of the kidney: Recurrence and death of a patient. J Urol 110:352, 1973.

Adenocarcinoma

Alberto P, Senn HJ: Hormonal therapy of renal carcinoma alone and in association with cytostatic drugs. Cancer 33:1226, 1974.

Almgård LE & others: Treatment of renal adenocarcinoma by embolic occlusion of the renal circulation. Brit J Urol 45:474, 1973.

Aron BS, Gross M: Renal adenocarcinoma in infancy and childhood: Evaluation of therapy and prognosis. J Urol 102:497, 1969.

Block NL, Jaksy J, Tessler AN: Carcinoma of urinary tract: Clinical significance of urinary phosphokinase activity in diagnosis. Urology 4:174, 1974.

Bloom HJG: Adjuvant therapy for adenocarcinoma of the kidney: Present position and prospects. Brit J Urol 45:237, 1973.

Bloom HJG: Medroxyprogesterone acetate (Provera) in the treatment of metastatic renal cancer. Brit J Cancer 25:250, 1971.

Brandstetter LH, Schwentker FN: Palliative treatment of renal tumor by infarction. Urology 2:196, 1973.

Cassady JR & others: Carcinoma of the kidney in children: Results of an interdisciplinary approach to management. Radiology 112:619, 1974.

Castellanos RD, Aron BS, Evans AT: Renal adenocarcinoma in children: Incidence, therapy and prognosis. J Urol 111:534, 1974.

Chisholm GD: The systemic effects of malignant renal tumors. Brit J Urol 43:687, 1971.

Chu TM & others: Plasma carcinoembryonic antigen in renal cell carcinoma patients. J Urol 111:742, 1974.

Dehner LP, Leestma JE, Price EB Jr: Renal cell carcinoma in children: A clinicopathologic study of 15 cases and review of the literature. J Pediat 76:358, 1970.

Dorr RP, Cerny JC, Hoskins PA: Inferior venacavagrams and renal venograms in the management of renal tumors. J Urol 110:280, 1973.

Doust VL, Doust BD, Redman HC: Evaluation of ultrasonic B-mode scanning in the diagnosis of renal masses. Am J Roentgenol 117:112, 1973.

Felson B, Moskowitz M: Renal pseudotumors: The regenerated nodule and other lumps, bumps, and dromedary humps. Am J Roentgenol 107:720, 1969.

Fenlon JW, Silber I, Koehler PR: Perirenal masses simulating renal tumors. J Urol 106:448, 1971.

Finney R: An evaluation of postoperative radiotherapy in hypernephroma treatment: A clinical trial. Cancer 32:1332, 1973.

Finney R: The value of radiotherapy in the treatment of hypernephroma: A clinical trial. Brit J Urol 45:258, 1973.

Franksson C & others: Renal carcinoma (hypernephroma) occurring in 5 siblings. J Urol 108:58, 1972.

Freed SZ, Gliedman ML: The removal of renal carcinoma thrombus extending into the right atrium. J Urology 113:163, 1975.

Friedenberg MJ, Spjut HJ: Xanthogranulomatous pyelonephritis. Am J Roentgenol 90:97, 1963.

Garfield DH, Kennedy BJ: Regression of metastatic renal cell carcinoma following nephrectomy. Cancer 30:190, 1972.

Ghose MK, Berman LB: Adenocarcinoma of the kidney: Report of a cured case in childhood. Cancer 30:197, 1972.

Gittes RF, McCullough DL: Bench surgery for tumor in solitary kidney. J Urol 113:12, 1975.

Golde DW & others: Gonadotropin-secreting renal carcinoma. Cancer 33:1048, 1974.

Gooding CA: Childhood renal pseudotumor. Radiology 98:79, 1971.

Gorder JL, Stargardter FL: Pancreatic pseudocysts simulating intrarenal masses. Am J Roentgenol 107:65, 1969.

Green WM & others: "Column of Bertin": Diagnosis by nephrotomography. Am J Roentgenol 116:714, 1972.

Gross M, Minkowitz S: Ureteral metastasis from renal adenocarcinoma. J Urol 106:23, 1971.

Guinan PD & others: Carcinoembryonic antigen test in renal cell carcinoma. Urology 5:185, 1975.

Javadpour N: Immunologic features of genitourinary cancer. Urology 2:103, 1973.

Kiely JM, Wagoner RD, Holley KE: Renal complications of lymphoma. Ann Int Med 71:1159, 1969.

Kikkawa K, Lasser EC: "Ring-like" or "rim-like" calcification in renal cell carcinoma. Am J Roentgenol 107:737, 1969.

King DL: Renal ultrasonography: An aid in the clinical evaluation of renal masses. Radiology 105:633, 1972.

Klugo RC, Farah RN, Cerny JC: Renal malignant hystiocytoma. J Urol 112:727, 1974.

Kölln CP & others: Bilateral partial nephrectomy for bilateral renal cell carcinoma: A case report. J Urol 105:45, 1971.

Kvartstein B, Lindemann R, Mathisen W: Renal carcinoma with increased erythropoietin production and secondary polycythemia. Scandinav J Urol Nephrol 7:178, 1973.

Leitner WA & others: Limitations of arteriography in renal mass lesions. Arch Int Med 130:868, 1972.

Marshall VF & others: Surgery for renal cell carcinoma in the vena cava. J Urol 103:414, 1970.

McAninch LN, Reid-Smith A: The radiologic differentiation of benign and malignant tumors of the kidney. J Urol 107:550, 1972.

McCullough DL, Talner LB: Inferior vena caval extension of renal carcinoma: A lost cause? Am J Roentgenol 121:819, 1974.

McFarland WL, Wallace S, Johnson DE: Renal carcinoma and polycystic disease. J Urol 107:530, 1972.

McLaughlin AP III & others: Avascular primary renal cell carcinoma: Varied pathologic and angiographic features. J Urol 111:587, 1974.

Merrin C & others: Chemotherapy of advanced renal cell carcinoma with vinblastine and CCNU. J Urol 113:21, 1975.

Middleton RG, Presto AJ III: Radical thoracoabdominal nephrectomy for renal cell carcinoma. J Urol 110:36, 1973.

Mount BM & others: Cytologic diagnosis of renal-cell carcinoma: Reassessment of fat-soluble staining. Urology 2:421, 1973.

Nygaard KK, Simon HB: Hypernephroma in children. Arch Surg 108:97, 1974.

Olsson CA, Moyer JD, Laferte RO: Pulmonary cancer metastatic to the kidney: A common renal neoplasm. J Urol 105:492, 1971.

Peterson LJ & others: Hormonal therapy in metastatic hypernephroma. Urology 4:669, 1974.

Pfister RR, Husberg B: Renal salvage through autotransplantation. Urology 4:703, 1974.

Pollack HM, Popky G: Spontaneous subcapsular hemorrhage: Its significance and roentgenographic diagnosis. J Urol 108:530, 1972.

Rafla S: Renal cell carcinoma: Natural history and results of treatment. Cancer 25:26, 1970.

Ram MD, Chisholm GD: Hypertension due to hypernephroma. Brit MJ 4:87, 1969.

Ravich L, Lerman PH, Drabkin JW: Metastatic disease to kidney from lung. Urology 5:239, 1975.

Richards RD, Mebust WK, Schimke RN: A prospective study on Von Hippel-Lindau disease. J Urol 110:27, 1973.

Riding GR: Renal adenocarcinoma: Regression of pulmonary metastases following irradiation of primary tumor. Cancer 27:936, 1971.

Sanford EJ & others: Preliminary evaluation of urinary polyamines in the diagnosis of genitourinary tract malignancy. J Urol 113:218, 1975.

Schoenfeld MR, Bernstein R: Hypernephroma, marked renal vein dilatation and the Bernoulli phenomenon. Am J Med 50:845, 1971.

Schwarz GR, Borden TA, Bergreen PW: Follow-up studies in renal adenocarcinoma: The use of abdominal aortography. J Urol 111:445, 1974.

Seltzer RA, Wenlund DE: Renal lymphoma: Arteriographic studies. Am J Roentgenol 101:692, 1967.

Skinner DG & others: Diagnosis and management of renal cell carcinoma. Cancer 28:1165, 1971.

Sondag TJ & others: Hypernephromas with massive arteriovenous fistulas. Am J Roentgenol 117:97, 1973.

Tveter KJ: Unusual manifestations of renal carcinoma: A review of the literature. Acta chir scandinav 139:401, 1973.

Van der Werf-Messing A, Van Gilse HA: Hormonal treatment of metastases of renal carcinoma. Brit J Cancer 25:423, 1971.

Vermillion CD, Skinner DG, Pfister RC: Bilateral renal cell carcinoma. J Urol 108:219, 1974.

von Micsky LI: Clinical sonography in urology. Urology 1:506, 1973.

Wagle DG: Vagaries of renal cell carcinoma. J Med (Basel) 3:178, 1972.

Warren MM, Utz DC, Kelalis PP: Concurrence of hypernephroma and hypercalcemia. Ann Surg 174:863, 1971.

Weigensberg IJ: The many faces of metastatic renal carcinoma. Radiology 98:353, 1971.

White AA, Palubinskas AJ: Renal Hodgkin's disease: Angiographic demonstration. Radiology 96:551, 1970.

Yates-Bell AJ, Cardell BS: Adenocarcinoma of the kidney in children. Brit J Urol 43:399, 1971.

Young JM, Morrow JW: Problems in interpretation of angiograms in renal mass lesions. J Urol 107:925, 1972.

Zusman RM & others: Antihypertensive function of a renal-cell carcinoma: Evidence for a prostaglandin-A-secreting tumor. New England J Med 290:843, 1974.

Embryoma

Aron BS: Wilms' tumor: A clinical study of eighty-one patients. Cancer 33:637, 1974.

Bannayan GA, Huvos AG D'Angio GJ: Effect of irradiation on the maturation of Wilms' tumor. Cancer 27:812, 1971.

Brown WT & others: Wilms' tumor in three successive generations. Surgery 72:756, 1972.

Burger R, Guthrie TH, Fernbach DJ: An approach to metastatic nephroblastoma. J Urol 109:104, 1973.

Canale VC, Muecke EC: Wilms' tumor. Urology 3:675, 1974.

Canale VC, Muecke EC: Wilms' tumor: A clinical review. CA:24:66, 1974.

Cassady JR & others: Considerations in the radiation therapy of Wilms' tumor. Cancer 32:598, 1973.

Clark RE & others: Arteriography of Wilms' tumor. Am J Roentgenol 113:476, 1971.

Cox D: Chromosome constitution of nephroblastomas. Cancer 19:1217, 1966.

Ehrlich RM, Goldman R, Kaufman JJ: Surgery of bilateral Wilms' tumors: The role of renal transplantation. J Urol 111:277, 1974.

Fay R, Brosman S, Williams DI: Bilateral nephroblastoma. J Urol 110:119, 1973.

Fleming ID, Johnson WW: Clinical and pathologic staging as a guide in the management of Wilms' tumor. Cancer 26:660, 1970.

Fraumeni JF, Glass AG: Wilms' tumor and congenital aniridia. JAMA 206:825, 1968.

Gammill S, Puyau F, Neizschman H: Phlebo-arterio-urography in the assessment of abdominal masses in children. Am J Roentgenol 120:389, 1974.

Ganguly A & others: Renin-secreting Wilms' tumor with severe hypertension: Report of a case and brief review of renin-secreting tumors. Ann Int Med 79:835, 1973.

Hidai H, Fukuoka H, Murayama T: Arteriography of Wilms' tumor. J Urol 110:347, 1973.

Jereb B: Metastases and recurrences in nephroblastoma. Acta radiol therap 12:289, 1973.

Kenny GM & others: Erythropoietin levels in Wilms' tumor patients. J Urol 104:758, 1970.

Loomis RC: Primary leiomyosarcoma of the kidney: Report of a case and review of the literature. J Urol 107:557, 1972.

Margolis LW & others: Wilms' tumor: An interdisciplinary treatment program with and without dactinomycin. Cancer 32:618, 1973.

Martin J, Rickham PP: Wilms's tumour: An improved prognosis report of 22 consecutive children seen from 1967–1971. Arch Dis Childhood 49:459, 1974.

Newman D, Vellios F: Adult carcinosarcoma (adult Wilms' tumor) of the kidney. Clin Path 42:45, 1964.

Perez CA & others: Treatment of Wilms' tumor and factors affecting prognosis. Cancer 32:609, 1973.

Rios JT: Renal liposarcoma with hypertension. Urology 1:246, 1973.

Sanders RC: B-scan ultrasound in the management of abdominal masses in children. JAMA 231:81, 1975.

Silber SJ, Chang CY: Primary lymphoma of kidney. J Urol 110:282, 1973.

Tremblay M: Ultrastructure of a Wilms' tumour and myogenesis J Pathol 105:269, 1971.

Vietti TJ & others: Vincristine sulfate and radiation therapy in metastatic Wilms' tumor. Cancer 25:12, 1970.

Wara WM & others: Treatment of Wilms's tumor. Radiology 112:695, 1974.

Wedemeyer PP & others: Resection of metastases in Wilms' tumor: A report of three cases cured of pulmonary and hepatic metastases. Pediatrics 41:446, 1968.

Wolff JA & others: Long-term evaluation of single versus multiple courses of actinomycin D therapy of Wilms's tumors New England J Med 290:84, 1974.

Sarcoma

Gupta OP, Dube MK: Rare primary renal sarcoma. Brit J Urol 43:546, 1971

Helmbrecht LJ, Cosgrove MD: Triple therapy for leiomyosarcoma of kidney. J Urol 112:581, 1974.

Jenkins JD, Anderson CK, Williams RE: Renal sarcoma. Brit J Urol 43:263, 1971.

Niceta P & others: Leiomyosarcoma of kidney: Review of the literature. Urology 3:270, 1974.

Tumors of the Renal Pelvis

Aufderheide AC, Streitz JM: Mucinous adenocarcinoma of the renal pelvis. Cancer 33:167, 1974.

Binder R & others: Aberrant papillae and other filling defects of the renal pelvis. Am J Roentgenol 114:746, 1972.

Brown RC & others: Lesions causing radiolucent defects in the renal pelvis. Am J Roentgenol 119:770, 1973.

Burünner S: Angiographic and conventional radiographic examination of renal pelvic carcinoma. Scandinav J Urol Nephrol (Suppl 15):97, 1972.

Cummings KB & others: Renal pelvic tumors. J Urol 113:158, 1975.

Johansson S & others: Uroepithelial tumors of the renal pelvis associated with abuse of phenacetin-containing analgesics. Cancer 33:743, 1974.

Latham HS, Kay S: Malignant tumors of the renal pelvis. Surg Gynec Obst 138:613, 1974.

Myrvold H, Fritjofsson Å, Magnusson P: Cholesteatoma of the renal pelvis. Scandinav J Urol Nephrol 8:69, 1974.

Newman LB & others: Small round cell sarcoma of the renal pelvis: A case report. J Urol 108:227, 1972.

Ochsner MG & others: Transitional-cell carcinoma of renal pelvis and ureter: Retrospective review of 40 patients. Urology 4:392, 1974.

Petković SD: Conservation of the kidney in operations for tumours of the renal pelvis and calyces: A report of 26 cases. Brit J Urol 44:1, 1972.

Poole-Wilson DS: Occupational tumours of the renal pelvis and ureter arising in dye-making industry. Proc Roy Soc Med 62:93, 1969.

Rabinowitz JG & others: Renal pelvic carcinoma: An angiographic reevaluation. Radiology 102:551, 1972.

Say CC, Hori JM: Transitional cell carcinoma of the renal pelvis: Experience from 1940 to 1972 and literature review. J Urol 112:438, 1974.

Sherwood T: Upper urinary tract tumours following on bladder carcinoma: Natural history of urothelial neoplastic disease. Brit J Radiol 44:137, 1971.

Summers JL, Keitzer A: Radiographic clue to the diagnosis of hemangioma of the kidney. J Urol 108:852, 1972.

Tolia BM, Hajdu SI, Whitmore WF Jr: Leiomyosarcoma of the renal pelvis. J Urol 109:974, 1973.

Wagle DC, Moore RH, Murphy GP: Primary carcinoma of the renal pelvis. Cancer 33:1642, 1974.

Wagle DC, Moore RH, Murphy GP: Squamous cell carcinoma of the renal pelvis. J Urol 111:453, 1974.

Williams CB, Mitchell JP: Carcinoma of the renal pelvis: A review of 43 cases. Brit J Urol 45:370, 1973.

Tumors of the Ureter

Alexander S & others: Metastatic ureteral tumors. J Urol 110:288, 1973.

Arger PH, Stolz JL: Ureteral tumors: The radiologic evaluation of a differential diagnosis "throw-in." Am J Roentgenol 116:812, 1972.

Cancelmo JJ Jr & others: Tumors of the ureter: Problems in diagnosis. Am J Roentgenol 117:132, 1973.

Cohen WM, Freed SZ, Hasson J: Metastatic cancer to the ureter: A review of the literature and case presentations. J Urol 112:188, 1974.

Colgan JR III, Skaist L, Morrow JW: Benign ureteral tumors in childhood: A case report and a plea for conservative management. J Urol 109:308, 1973.

DeWolf WC, Rogers R, Blackard C: Conservative management of ureteral tumors. Urology 4:44, 1974.

Graham JB: Delayed recognition of ureteral tumors. J Urol 110:191, 1973.

Hawtrey CE: Fifty-two cases of primary ureteral carcinoma: A clinical-pathologic study. J Urol 105:188, 1971.

Hussaini MA, Marden HE Jr, Woodruff MW: Multiple fibrous polyps of ureter. Urology 2:563, 1973.

Kim YH, Leiter E, Brendler H: Primary tumors of the ureter. J Urol 107:955, 1972.

Kretkowski RC, Derrick FC Jr: Primary ureteral tumors: Reconsideration of management. Urology 1:36, 1973.

Magri J, Atkinson EA: Primary amyloidosis of the ureter. Brit J Urol 42:37, 1970.

Malek RS: Primary tumours of the ureteric stump. Brit J Urol 45:391, 1973.

Petković SD: A plea for conservative operation for ureteral tumors. J Urol 107:220, 1972.

Stiehm WD, Becker JA, Weiss RM: Ureteral endometriosis. Radiology 102:563, 1972.

Stuppler SA, Kandzari SJ: Fibroepithelial polyps of the ureter: A benign ureteral tumor. Urology 5:553, 1975.

Takaha M, Nagata H, Sonoda T: Localized amyloid tumor of the ureter: Report of a case. J Urol 105:502, 1971.

Tveter KJ, Mathisen W, Enge I: Primary tumours of the ureter. Scandinav J Urol Nephrol 6:299, 1972.

Williams CB, Mitchell JP: Carcinoma of the ureter: A review of 54 cases. Brit J Urol 45:377, 1973.

Tumors of the Bladder

Al-Hadithi NA: The role of some tryptophan metabolites in certain diseases of the genito-urinary system. Brit J Urol 46:337, 1974.

Aquilina JN, Bugeja TJ: Primary malignant lymphoma of the bladder: Case report and review of literature. J Urol 112:64, 1974.

Barnes RW & others: Control of bladder tumors by endoscopic surgery. J Urol 97:864, 1967.

Beck AD, Gaudin HJ, Bonham DG: Carcinoma of the urachus. Brit J Urol 42:555, 1970.

Berg RA, Chan YS: Diagnosis of bladder cancer on intravenous pyelography. Urology 1:230, 1973.

Bessette PL, Abell MR, Herwig KR: A clinicopathologic study of squamous cell carcinoma of the bladder. J Urol 112:66, 1974.

Blackard CE & others: Results of a clinical trial of surgery and radiation in stages II and III carcinoma of the bladder. J Urol 108:875, 1972.

Bladder cancer and smoking. Brit MJ 1:763, 1972.

Boyland E: *The Biochemistry of Bladder Cancer.* Thomas, 1963.

Brannan W, Lucas TA, Mitchell WT Jr: Accuracy of cytologic examination of urinary sediment in the detection of urothelial tumors. J Urol 109:483, 1973.

Bruce PT: Colocystoplasty: Bladder replacement after total cystectomy. Australian New Zealand J Surg 43:270, 1973.

Carlson DH, Wilkinson RH: Neurofibromatosis of the bladder in children. Radiology 105:401, 1972.

Castellanos RD, Wakefield PB, Evans AT: Carcinoma of the bladder in children. J Urol 113:261, 1975.

Cattolica EV: Hydrostatic bladder distention for bladder tumor: A fatal outcome. Urology 5:115, 1975.

Cordonnier JJ: Simple cystectomy in the management of bladder carcinoma. Arch Surg 108:190, 1974.

Dann RH, Arger PH, Enterline HJ: Benign proliferation processes presenting as mass lesions in the urinary bladder. Am J Roentgenol 116:822, 1972.

DeWeerd JH, Colby MY Jr: Bladder carcinoma treated by irradiation and surgery: Interval report. J Urol 109:409, 1973.

Doctor VM, Phadke AG, Sirat MV: Pheochromocytoma of the urinary bladder. Brit J Urol 44:351, 1972.

Dretler SP, Bredin HC: Managing carcinoma of the bladder. Geriatrics 29:75, 1974.

Dretler SP, Ragsdale BD, Leadbetter WF: The value of pelvic lymphadenectomy in the surgical treatment of bladder cancer. J Urol 109:414, 1973.

Early K & others: Mitomycin C in the treatment of metastatic transitional cell carcinoma of urinary bladder. Cancer 31:1150, 1973.

Elliot GB, Moloney PJ, Anderson GH: "Denuding cystitis" and in situ urothelial carcinoma. Arch Path 96:91, 1973.

Ellis LR, Udall DA, Hodges CV: Further clinical experience with intestinal segments for urinary diversion. J Urol 105:354, 1971.

England HR & others: Evaluation of Helmstein's distention method for carcinoma of the bladder. Brit J Urol 45:593, 1973.

Exelby PR: Management of embryonal rhabdomyosarcoma in children. S Clin North America 54:849, 1974.

Fair WR: Formalin in the treatment of massive bladder hemorrhage: Techniques, results, and complications. Urology 3:573, 1974.

Falor WH: Chromosomes in noninvasive papillary carcinoma of the bladder. JAMA 216:791, 1971.

Feneley RCL & others: The treatment of advanced bladder cancer with sensitized pig lymphocytes. Brit J Surg 61:825, 1974.

Firlit CF: Intractable hemorrhagic cystitis secondary to extensive carcinomatosis: Management with formalin solution. J Urol 110:57, 1973.

Ghavimi F & others: Combination therapy of urogenital embryonal rhabdomyosarcoma in children. Cancer 32:1178, 1973.

Ghazali S: Embryonic rhabdomyosarcoma of the urogenital tract. Brit J Surg 60:124, 1973.

Ghoneim MA, Mansour MA, El Boulkany MN: Radical cystectomy for carcinoma of the bilharzial bladder. Brit J Urol 44:461, 1972.

Glashan RW, Brown PR: Initial experience with Helmstein's treatment by a hydrostatic pressure technique in carcinoma of the bladder. Brit J Surg 61:466, 1974.

Goldstein AG: Metastatic carcinoma to the bladder. J Urol 98:209, 1967.

Grosfeld JL, Smith JP, Clatworthy HW Jr: Pelvic rhabdomyosarcoma in infants and children. J Urol 107:673, 1972.

Guinan P & others: Urinary carcinoembryonic-like antigen levels in patients with bladder carcinoma. J Urol 111:350, 1974.

Halaka TR & others: Antibody induction of lymphocyte-mediated cytotoxicity against human transitional-cell carcinomas of the urinary tract. New England J Med 291:637, 1974.

Hald T, Mygind T: Control of life-threatening vesical hemorrhage by unilateral hypogastric artery muscle embolization. J Urol 112:60, 1974.

Hall RR, Schade ROK, Swinney J: Effects of hyperthermia on bladder cancer. Brit J Med 2:593, 1974.

Hall RR & others: Carcinoembryonic antigen and urothelial carcinoma. Brit J Urol 45:88, 1973.

Hall RR & others: Methotrexate treatment for advanced bladder cancer. Brit J Urol 46:431, 1974.

Hammonds JC, Williams JL, Fox M: The control of severe bleeding from the bladder by intravesical hyperbaric therapy. Brit J Urol 46:309, 1974.

Helmstein K: Treatment of bladder carcinoma by a hydrostatic technique: Report on 43 cases. Brit J Urol 44:434, 1972.

Hendricks ED & others: Radium in treatment of infiltrating carcinoma of urinary bladder. Urology 5:465, 1975.

Hewitt CB & others: Intercavitary radiation in the treatment of bladder tumors. J Urol 107:603, 1972.

Holtz F, Fox JE, Abell MR: Carcinosarcoma of the urinary bladder. Cancer 29:294, 1972.

Hoover R, Cole P: Temporal aspects of occupational bladder carcinogenesis. New England J Med 288:1040, 1973.

Jarman WD, Kenealy JC: Polypoid rhabdomyosarcoma of the bladder in children. J Urol 103:227, 1970.

Johnson DE, Hogan JM, Ayala AG: Primary adenocarcinoma of the urinary bladder. South MJ 65:527, 1972.

Kalish M, Silber SJ, Herwig KR: Papillary necroses: Result of intravesical instillation of formalin. Urology 2:315, 1973.

Kallet HA, Lapco L: Urine beta glucuronidase activity in urinary tract disease. J Urol 97:352, 1967.

Kenny GM & others: Current results from treatment of stages C and D bladder tumors at Roswell Park Memorial Institute. J Urol 107:56, 1972.

Kerr WK & others: The effect of cigarette smoking on bladder carcinogens in man. Canad MAJ 93:1, 1965.

Leestma JE, Price EB Jr: Paraganglioma of the urinary bladder. Cancer 28:1063, 1971.

Lindenauer SM, Cerny JC, Morley GW: Ureterosigmoid conduit urinary diversion. Surgery 75:705, 1974.

Matsumoto K & others: Accurate roentgenographic diagnosis of vesical tumors with double contrast cystography and arteriography. J Urol 107:46, 1972.

McGuire EJ, Lytton B, Mitchell MS: Treatment of metastatic transitional cell carcinoma with adriamycin: A case report. J Urol 110:384, 1973.

Melicow MM: Tumors of the bladder: A multifaceted problem. J Urol 112:467, 1974.

Miller SW, Pfister RC: Calcification in urothelial tumors of the bladder: Report of 5 cases and survey of the literature. Am J Roentgenol 121:827, 1974.

Million RR, Rutledge F, Fletcher GH: Stage IV carcinoma of the cervix with bladder invasion. Am J Obst Gynec 113:239, 1972.

Morales A: Haemangioma of the bladder. Postgrad MJ 48:117, 1972.

Mullin EM, Glenn JF, Paulson DF: Lesions of bone and bladder cancer. J Urol 113:45, 1975.

Nevin JE & others: Advanced carcinoma of bladder: Treatment using hypogastric artery infusion with 5-fluorouracil, either as a single agent or in combination with bleomycin or adriamycin and supravoltage radiation. J Urol 112:752, 1974.

Norehad EA & others: Endometriosis of the bladder: Case report. J Urol 96:901, 1966.

O'Boyle PJ, Cooper EH, Williams RE: Evaluation of immunological reactivity in bladder cancer. Brit J Urol 46:303, 1974.

O'Flynn JD, Mullaney J: Vesical leukoplakia progressing to carcinoma. Brit J Urol 46:31, 1974.

Ogata J, Migita N, Nakamura T: Treatment of carcinoma of the bladder by infusion of the anticancer agent (Mitomycin C) via the internal iliac artery. J Urol 110:667, 1973.

Orlin I: The role of cystography in thio-tepa toxicity. J Urol 108:257, 1972.

Oyasu R, Hopp ML: The etiology of cancer of the bladder. Surg Gynec Obst 138:97, 1974.

Poole-Wilson DS: Occupational tumours of the bladder. Proc Roy Soc Med 53:801, 1960.

Ray B & others: Bladder tumors in children. Urology 2:426, 1973.

Resnick MI, O'Conor VJ Jr: Segmental resection for carcinoma of the bladder: Review of 102 patients. J Urol 109:1007, 1973.

Reuter HJ: Endoscopic cryosurgery of prostate and bladder tumors. J Urol 107:389, 1972.

Richie JP, Skinner DG, Kaufman JJ: Radical cystectomy for carcinoma of the bladder: 16 years of experience. J Urol 113:186, 1975.

Riddle PR: The management of superficial bladder tumours with intravesical epodyl. Brit J Urol 45:84, 1973.

Rose DP: Aspects of tryptophan metabolism in health and disease: A review. J Clin Path 25:17, 1972.

Rose GA, Wallace DM: Observations on urinary chemiluminescence of normal smokers and non-smokers and of patients with bladder cancer. Brit J Urol 45:520, 1973.

Santino AM, Shumaker EJ, Garces J: Primary malignant lymphoma of the bladder. J Urol 103:310, 1970.

Schlegel JU & others: The role of ascorbic acid in the prevention of bladder tumor formation. J Urol 103:155, 1970.

Schmidt JD, Hawtrey CE, Buchbaum HJ: Transverse colon conduit: A preferred method of urinary diversion for radiation-treated pelvic malignancies. J Urol 113:308, 1975.

Scott R Jr & others: Preoperative irradiation in the surgical treatment of transitional cell cancer of the bladder: Preliminary report based on 12 years experience. J Urol 109:405, 1973.

Shah BC, Albert DJ: Intravesical instillation of formalin for the management of intractable hematuria. J Urol 110:519, 1973.

Siegel WH: Neoplasms in bladder diverticula. Urology 4:411, 1974.

Simpson W, Duncan AW, Clayton CB: A useful sign in the diagnosis of bladder tumours on intravenous urograms. Brit J Radiol 47:272, 1974.

Singh SM, Raghavaiah NV: Combined double contrast cystography and polycystography in the evaluation of bladder carcinoma. J Urol 110:70, 1973.

Smart JG: Renal and ureteric tumours in association with bladder tumours. Brit J Urol 36:380, 1964.

Sørensen BL & others: Ultraviolet light cystoscopy in patients with bladder cancer. Scandinav J Urol Nephrol 3:193, 1969.

Stams UK, Gursel EO, Veenema RJ: Prophylactic urethrectomy in male patients with bladder cancer. J Urol 111:177, 1974.

Strong GH, Kelsey D, Hoch W: Primary amyloid diseases of the bladder. J Urol 112:463, 1974.

Susan LP, Marsh RJ: Phenolization of bladder in treatment of massive intractable hematuria. Urology 5:119, 1975.

Tank ES & others: Treatment of urogenital tract rhabdomyosarcoma in infants and children. J Urol 107:324, 1972.

Tara HH, Mentus NL: Leiomyosarcoma of urinary bladder. Urology 2:460, 1973.

Thomas DG, Ward AM, Williams JL: A study of 52 cases of adenocarcinoma of the bladder. Brit J Urol 43:4, 1971.

Trott PA, Edwards L: Comparison of bladder washings and urine cytology in the diagnosis of bladder cancer. J Urol 110:665, 1973.

Troup CW, Thatcher G, Hodgson NB: Infiltrative lesion of the bladder presenting as gross hematuria in child with leukemia: Case report. J Urol 107:314, 1972.

Varkarakis MJ & others: Superficial bladder tumor: Aspects of clinical progression. Urology 4:414, 1974.

Veenema RJ, Romas NA, Fingerhut B: Chemotherapy for bladder cancer. Urology 3:135, 1974.

Walbom-Jørgensen S: Treatment of bladder carcinoma with 6 MeV linear accelerator. Scandinav J Urol Nephrol (Suppl 15):113, 1972.

Wendel RG, Hoegg UR, Zavon MR: Benzidine: A bladder carcinogen. J Urol 111:607, 1974.

Whitehead ED, Tessler AN: Carcinoma of the urachus. Brit J Urol 43:468, 1971.

Williams RE, Smith PH: Report on International Bladder Cancer Conference: Leeds 1971. Brit J Urol 45:310, 1973.

Yoshida O, Brown RR, Bryan GT: Relationship between tryptophan metabolism and heterotopic recurrences of human urinary bladder tumors. Cancer 25:773, 1970.

Benign Prostatic Hyperplasia

Blandy JP: Benign prostatic enlargement. Brit MJ 1:31, 1971.

Finestone AJ, Rosenthal RS: Silent prostatism. Geriatrics 26:89, 1971.

Hutch JA, Rambo ON Jr: A study of the anatomy of the prostate, prostatic urethra and the urinary sphincter system. J Urol 104:443, 1970.

Izumi AK, Edwards J Jr: Herpes zoster and neurogenic bladder dysfunction. JAMA 224:1748, 1973.

Lytton B, Kupfer DJ, Traurig AR: The vesicorenal reflex. Invest Urol 4:521, 1967.

Mad P & others: Human prostatic hyperplasia. Arch Path

79:270, 1965.

Marshall A & others: An assessment of cryosurgery in the treatment of prostatic obstruction. J Urol 109: 1026, 1973.

Melzer M: The urecholine test. J Urol 108:728, 1972.

Merrill DC, Markland C: Vesical dysfunction induced by the major tranquilizers. J Urol 107:769, 1972.

Michaels MM, Brown HE, Favino CJ: Leiomyoma of prostate. Urology 3:617, 1974.

Mostofi FK, Thomson RV: Benign hyperplasia of the prostate gland. In: *Urology,* 3rd ed. Cambell MF, Harrison JH (editors). Saunders, 1970.

Nicoll GA: Suprapubic prostatectomy: A comparative analysis of 525 consecutive cases. J Urol 111:213, 1974.

Richmond DE: Effects of alcohol on the kidney and blood electrolytes. New Zealand MJ 79:561, 1974.

Salvatierra O Jr, Rigdon WO, Malley JA: Modified retropubic prostatectomy: A new technique. J Urol 108:126, 1972.

Scott FB & others: Uroflowmetry before and after prostatectomy. South MJ 60:948, 1967.

Scott WW, Wade JC: Medical treatment of benign nodular prostatic hyperplasia with cyproterone acetate. J Urol 101:81, 1969.

Semple JE: Surgical capsule of the benign enlargement of the prostate: Its development and action. Brit MJ 1:1640, 1963.

Singh M, Tresidder GC, Blandy JP: The evaluation of transurethral resection for benign enlargement of the prostate. Brit J Urol 45:93, 1973.

Tanagho EA, Meyers FH: Trigonal hypertrophy: A cause of ureteral obstruction. J Urol 93:678, 1965.

Turner-Warwick R & others: A urodynamic view of prostatic obstruction and the results of prostatectomy. Brit J Urol 45:631, 1973.

Watanabe H & others: Diagnostic application of ultrasonotomography to the prostate. Invest Urol 8:548, 1971.

Wildbolz E: Elective prostatectomy. Proc Roy Soc Med 51:1029, 1958.

Witherington R, Shelor WC Jr: Suprapubic prostatectomy: Modified Hryntschak technique. Urology 4:550, 1974.

Zinman L, Flint LD, Libertino JA: Techniques of open prostatectomy. Geriatrics 29:107, 1974.

Carcinoma of the Prostate

Barnes RW, Ninan CA: Carcinoma of the prostate: Biopsy and conservative therapy. J Urol 108:897, 1972.

Barrett JJ, Smith PHS: Bone imaging with $^{99}Tc^m$ polyphosphate: A comparison with ^{18}F and skeletal radiography. Brit J Radiol 47:387, 1974.

Bärring NE, Holmér A, Rudé'BI: Interstitial irradiation of the pituitary gland with a ^{90}Sr-^{90}Y applicator having adjustable active length. Acta radiol ther 8:294, 1969.

Belt E, Schroeder FH: Total perineal prostatectomy for carcinoma of the prostate. J Urol 107:91, 1972.

Bhanalaph T, Varkarakis MJ, Murphy GP: Current status of bilateral adrenalectomy for advanced prostatic carcinoma. Ann Surg 179:17, 1974.

Bissada NK, Bell RA, Redman JF: Periureteral extension of prostatic carcinoma. Urology 5:514, 1975.

Blackard CE, Byar DP, Jordan WP Jr: Orchiectomy for advanced prostatic carcinoma. Urology 1:553, 1973.

Brown JS, Rubenfeld S: Irradiation in preventing gynecomastia induced by estrogens. Urology 3:51, 1974.

Butler MR, O'Flynn JD: Prostatic disease in the leukemic patient: With particular reference to leukemic infiltration of the prostate: A retrospective clinical study. Brit J Urol 45:179, 1973.

Byar DP, Mostofi FK: Carcinoma of the prostate: Prognostic evaluation of certain pathologic features in 208 radical prostatectomies. Cancer 30:5, 1972.

Byar DP & others: Survival of patients with incidentally found microscopic cancer of the prostate: Results of a clinical trial of conservative treatment. J Urol 108:908, 1972.

Carcinoma of the prostate. Brit MJ 2:566, 1973.

Carlton CE Jr & others: Irradiation treatment of carcinoma of the prostate: A preliminary report based on 8 years of experience. J Urol 108:924, 1972.

Catalona WJ: Effects of chemotherapy for prostatic carcinoma on T lymphocyte levels. J Urol 112:802, 1974.

Cerny JC & others: An evaluation of lymphangiography in staging carcinoma of the prostate. J Urol 113:367, 1975.

Chiu CL, Weber DL: Prostatic carcinoma in young adults. JAMA 230:724, 1974.

Cook S, Rodriguez-Antunez A: Pre-estrogen irradiation of the breast to prevent gynecomastia. Am J Roentgenol 117:662, 1973.

Cosgrove MD, Metzger CK: Lymphangiography in genitourinary cancer. J Urol 113:93, 1975.

Derrick FC Jr: Cancer of the prostate and other prostatic problems. Postgrad Med 54:123, 1973.

Desai SG, Woodruff LM: Carcinoma of the prostate: Local extension following perineal needle biopsy. Urology 3:87, 1974.

Edland RW: Testosterone potentiated radiophosphorus therapy of osseous metastases in prostatic cancer. Am J Roentgenol 120:678, 1974.

Fergusson JD, Hendry WF: Pituitary irradiation in advanced carcinoma of the prostate: Analysis of 100 cases. Brit J Urol 43:514, 1971.

Fletcher JW & others: Radioisotopic detection of osseous metastases: Evaluation of ^{99m}Tc polyphosphate and ^{99m}Tc pyrophosphate. Arch Int Med 135:553, 1975.

Gilbaugh JH Jr, Thompson GJ: Fluoride osteosclerosis simulating carcinoma of the prostate with widespread bony metastases: A case report. J Urol 96:944, 1966.

Gill WB & others: Radical retropubic prostatectomy and retroperitoneal lymphadenectomy following radiotherapy conversion of stage C to stage B carcinoma of the prostate. J Urol 111:656, 1974.

Green N & others: Radiation therapy of inoperable localized prostatic carcinoma: An assessment of tumor response and complications. J Urol 111:662, 1974.

Greene LF & others: Primary transitional cell carcinoma of the prostate. J Urol 110:235, 1973.

Gursel EO, Roberts MS, Veenema RJ: Cryotherapy in advanced prostatic cancer. Urology 1:392, 1973.

Gursel EO & others: Comparative evaluation of bone marrow acid phosphatase and bone scanning in staging of prostatic cancer. J Urol 111:53, 1974.

Hardy JG, Newble GM: The detection of bone lesions using $^{99}Tc^m$ labeled polyphosphate. Brit J Radiol 47:769, 1974.

Hendry WF, Williams JP: Transrectal prostatic biopsy. Brit MJ 4:595, 1971.

Hilaris BS & others: Radiation therapy and pelvic node dissection in the management of cancer of the prostate. Am J Roentgenol 121:832, 1974.

Hill DR, Crews QE Jr, Walsh PC: Prostate carcinoma: Radiation treatment of primary and regional lymphatics. Cancer 34:156, 1974.

Hudson HC, Howland RL Jr: Radical retropubic prostatectomy for cancer of the prostate. J Urol 108:944, 1972.

Jewett HJ, Eggleston JC, Yawn DH: Radical prostatectomy in the management of carcinoma of the prostate: Probable causes of some therapeutic failures. J Urol 107:1034, 1972.

Johnson DE, Chalbaud R, Ayala AG: Secondary tumors of the prostate. J Urol 112:507, 1974.

Jones LW: Cryosurgery for prostatic carcinoma. Urology 4:499, 1974.

Kilduff JT, Ansell JS: Mastocytosis: A benign mimic of malignant osteoblastic metastases. J Urol 110:104, 1973.

Kontturi MJ, Sotaniemi EO, Larmi TKI: Body fluid and electrolyte balance during estrogen therapy of prostatic cancer. J Urol 111:652, 1974.

Lentle BC, McGowan DG, Dierich H: Technetium-99m polyphosphate bone scanning in carcinoma. Brit J Urol 46:543, 1974.

Linsk JA & others: Transrectal cytologic aspiration in the diagnosis of prostatic carcinoma. J Urol 108:455, 1972.

Marks LS, Gallo DA: Ureteral obstruction in the patient with prostatic carcinoma. Brit J Urol 44:411, 1972.

Marshall S, Lyon RP, Scott MP Jr: Prostatic acid phosphatase levels. Urology 4:435, 1974.

McCullough DL, Leadbetter WF: Radical pelvic surgery for locally extensive carcinoma of the prostate. J Urol 108:939, 1972.

Merrin C & others: Carcinoma of prostate: Long-term survival after bilateral adrenalectomy. Urology 3: 223, 1974.

Mollenkamp JS, Cooper JF, Kagan AR: Clinical experience with supravoltage radiotherapy in carcinoma of the prostate: A preliminary report. J Urol 113:374, 1975.

Morales A, Connolly JG, Bruce AW: Androgen therapy in advanced carcinoma of the prostate. Canad MAJ 105:71, 1971.

Nelson CMK, Boatman DL, Flocks RH: Bone marrow examination in carcinoma of the prostate. J Urol 109:667, 1973.

Newmark SR, Dluhy RG, Bennett AH: Ectopic adrenocorticotropin syndrome with prostatic carcinoma. Urology 2:666, 1973.

Nussbaum M: Carcinoma of prostatic origin: Metastatic to cervical lymph nodes. New York J Med 73:2050, 1973.

O'Donoghue EPN & others: Cryosurgery for carcinoma of prostate. Urology 5:308, 1975.

Pinck BD, Alexander S: Parathormone-potentiated radiophosphorus therapy in prostatic cancer. Urology 1:201, 1973.

Pistenma DA, McDougall R, Kriss JP: Screening for bone metastases: Are only scans necessary? JAMA 231: 46, 1975.

Puigvert A, Elizalde C, Matz JA: Perineal implantation of carcinoma of the prostate following needle biopsy: A case report. J Urol 107:821, 1972.

Raskin P, McLain CJ, Medsger TA Jr: Hypocalcemia associated with metastatic bone disease. Arch Int Med 132:539, 1973.

Ray GR, Cassady JR, Bagshaw MA: Definitive radiation therapy of carcinoma of the prostate: A report on 15 years of experience. Radiology 106:407, 1973.

Rhamy RK, Buchanan RD, Spalding MJ: Intraductal carcinoma of the prostate gland. J Urol 109:457, 1973.

Rhamy RK, Wilson SK, Caldwell WL: Biopsy-proved tumor following definitive irradiation for resectable carcinoma of the prostate. J Urol 107:627, 1972.

Robinson MRG, Shearer RJ, Fergusson JD: Adrenal suppression in the treatment of carcinoma of the prostate. Brit J Urol 46:555, 1974.

Robinson MRG, Thomas BS: Effect of hormonal therapy on plasma testosterone levels in prostatic carcinoma. Brit MJ 4:391, 1971.

Rubin H, Lome LG, Presman D: Neurological manifestation of metastatic prostatic carcinoma. J Urol 111:799, 1974.

Sadoughi N & others: Cancer of the prostate: Relief of bone pain with levodopa. Urology 4:107, 1974.

Saglam S, Wilson CB, Seymour RJ: Indications for hypophysectomy in diabetic retinopathy and cancer of the breast and prostate. California Med 113:1, Feb 1970.

Schellhammer PF, Milsten R, Bunts RC: Prostatic carcinoma with cutaneous metastases. Brit J Urol 45: 169, 1973.

Sewell RA & others: Extended biopsy follow-up after full course radiation for resectable prostatic carcinoma. J Urol 113:371, 1975.

Sinha AA, Blackard CE: Ultrastructure of prostatic benign hyperplasia and carcinoma. Urology 2:114, 1973.

Shahmanesh M & others: Metabolic effects of oestrogen treatment in patients with carcinoma of the prostate: A comparison of stilboestrol and conjugated equine estrogens. Brit MJ 2:512, 1973.

Smith RB, Walsh PC, Goodwin WE: Cyproterone acetate in the treatment of advanced carcinoma of the prostate. J Urol 110:106, 1973.

Sy FA, Gursel EO, Veenema RJ: Positive random iliac bone biopsy in advanced prostatic cancer. Urology 2:125, 1973.

Tannenbaum M: Atypical epithelial hyperplasia or carcinoma of prostate gland: The surgical pathologist at an impasse? Urology 4:758, 1974.

Tong ECK, Finkelstein P: The treatment of prostatic bone metastases with parathormone and radioactive phosphorus. J Urol 109:71, 1973.

Varkarakis MJ & others: Lung metastases in prostatic carcinoma: Clinical significance. Urology 3:447, 1974.

Weber DA & others: Comparison of Tc^{99m} polyphosphate and F^{18} for bone imaging. Am J Roentgenol 121:184, 1974.

Weitzner S: Survival of patients with secondary carcinoma of prostate in the testes. Cancer 32:447, 1973.

Welvaart K & others: Stage D prostatic carcinoma: Survival rate in relapsed patients following new forms of palliation. Urology 4:283, 1974.

West CR, Murphy GP: Pituitary ablation and disseminated prostatic carcinoma. JAMA 225:253, 1973.

Whitmore WF Jr & others: Implantation of ^{125}I in prostatic cancer. S Clin North America 54:887, 1974.

Wynder EL, Mabuchi Y, Whitmore WF Jr: Epidemiology of cancer of the prostate. Cancer 28:344, 1971.

Zingg EJ, Hérither P, Gôthlin J: Lymphangiography in carcinoma of the prostate. Brit J Urol 46:549, 1974.

Sarcoma of the Prostate

Lemmon WT Jr, Holland JM, Ketcham AS: Rhabdomyosarcoma of the prostate. Surgery 59:736, 1966.

Siegel J: Sarcoma of the prostate: A report of four cases and a review of current therapy. J Urol 89:78, 1963.

Smith BH, Dehner LP: Sarcoma of the prostate gland. Am J Clin Pathol 58:43, 1972.

Tumors of the Seminal Vesicles

Damjanov I, Apić R: Cystadenoma of seminal vesicles. J Urol 111:808, 1974.

Goldstein AG, Wilson ES: Carcinoma of the seminal vesicle: With particular reference to the angiographic appearances. Brit J Urol 45:211, 1973.

Hajdu SI, Faruque AA: Adenocarcinoma of the seminal vesicle. J Urol 99:798, 1968.

Smith BA Jr, Webb EA, Price WE: Carcinoma of the seminal vesicle. J Urol 97:743, 1967.

Tumors of the Urethra

Blath RA, Boehm FH: Carcinoma of the female urethra. Surg Gynec Obst 136:574, 1973.

Chu AM: Female urethral carcinoma. Radiology 107:627, 1973.

De Wolf WC, Fraley EE: Congenital urethral polyp in the infant: Case report and review of the literature. J Urol 109:515, 1973.

Grabstald H: Tumors of the urethra in men and women. Cancer 32:1236, 1973.

Peterson DT & others: The peril of primary carcinoma of the urethra in women. J Urol 110:72, 1973.

Selikowitz SM, Olsson CA: Metastatic urethral obstruction. Radiology 107:906, 1973.

Taggart CG, Castro JR, Rutledge FN: Carcinoma of the female urethra. Am J Roentgenol 114:145, 1972.

Tumors of the Spermatic Cord

Arlen M, Grabstald H, Whitmore WF Jr: Malignant tumors of the spermatic cord. Cancer 23:525, 1969.

Banowsky LH, Shultz GN: Sarcoma of the spermatic cord and tunics: Review of the literature, case report and discussion of the role of retroperitoneal node dissection. J Urol 103:628, 1970.

Brosman SA, Cohen A, Fay R: Rhabdomyosarcoma of testis and spermatic cord in children. Urology 3:568, 1974.

Skeel DA, Drinker HR Jr, Witherington R: Rhabdomyosarcoma of the spermatic cord: Report of 3 cases with review of literature. J Urol 113:279, 1975.

Wacksman J, Case G, Glenn JF: Extragenital gonadal neoplasia and metastatic testicular tumor. Urology 5:221, 1975.

Williams G, Banerjee R: Paratesticular tumours. Brit J Urol 41:332, 1969.

Tumors of the Testis

Abell MR, Holtz F: Testicular and paratesticular neoplasms in patients 60 years of age and older. Cancer 21:852, 1968.

Asif S, Uehling OT: Microscopic tumor foci in testes. J Urol 99:776, 1968.

Atkin NB: High chromosome numbers of seminomata and malignant teratomata of the testis: A review of data on 103 tumors. Brit J Cancer 28:275, 1973.

Bailey TB & others: A new adjunct in testis tumor staging: Gallium-67 citrate. J Urol 110:307, 1973.

Bedsole DA, Shirley SW, Derrick WA Jr: Metastatic choriocarcinoma with 30 month survival. J Urol 112:783, 1974.

Bloom HJG, Hendry WF: Possible role of hormones in treatment of metastatic testicular teratomas: Tumor regression with medroxyprogesterone acetate. Brit MJ 3:563, 1973.

Boatman DL, Culp DA, Wilson VB: Testicular neoplasms in children. J Urol 109:315, 1973.

Bradfield JS, Hagen RO, Ytredel DO: Carcinoma of the testis: An analysis of 104 patients with germinal tumors of the testis other then seminoma. Cancer 31:633, 1973.

Buck AS & others: Supraclavicular node biopsy and malignant testicular tumors. J Urol 107:619, 1972.

Burke EF, Gilbert E, Uehling DT: Adrenal rest tumors of the testes. J Urol 109:649, 1973.

Cha EM: Ectopic seminoma (germinoma) in the retroperitoneum and mediastinum: With emphasis on the lymphangiogram. J Urol 110:47, 1973.

Collins DH, Pugh RCB: The pathology of testicular tumors. Brit J Urol 36 (Suppl):1, 1964.

Dahl DS: Torsion of intrabdominal seminoma of testis. Urology 4:590, 1974.

Earle JD, Bagshaw MA, Kaplan HS: Supervoltage radiation therapy of the testicular tumors. Am J Roentgenol 117:653, 1973.

Gagnon JH & others: Lymphography in germinal tumours of the testes. Brit J Urol 44:136, 1972.

Gehring GG, Rodriguez FR, Woodhead DM: Malignant degeneration of cryptorchid testes following orchiopexy. J Urol 112:354, 1974.

Giebink GS, Ruymann FB: Testicular tumors in children. Am J Dis Child 127:433, 1974.

Glover L, Frensilli FJ, Derrick FC Jr: Simultaneous adenomatoid tumors of epididymis and tunica vaginalis. Urology 2:192, 1973.

Gulley RM, Kowalski R, Neuhoff CF: Familial occurrence of testicular neoplasms: A case report. J Urol 112:620, 1974.

Haggar RA, MacMillan AB, Thompson DG: Leukemic infiltration of testes. Canad J Surg 12:197, 1969.

Henry SC, Walsh PC, Rotner MB: Choriocarcinoma of the testis. J Urol 112:105, 1974.

Herr HW, Silber I, Martin DC: Management of inguinal lymph nodes in patients with testicular tumors following orchiopexy, inguinal or scrotal operations. J Urol 110:223, 1973.

Hessl JM: Orchioblastoma or infantile embryonal carcinoma: Pediatric testis tumor. Urology 5:265, 1975.

Higby DJ & others: Diamminodichloroplatinum in the chemotherapy of testicular tumors. J Urol 112:100, 1974.

Jacobs EM: Combination chemotherapy of metastatic testicular germinal cell tumors and soft part sarcomas. Cancer 25:324, 1970.

Javadpour N: Immunologic features of genitourinary cancer. Urology 2:103, 1973.

Jonsson K, Ingemansson S, J Ling L: Lymphangiography

in patients with testicular tumor. Brit J Urol 45:548, 1973.

Kenny GM & others: Radiation therapy: Testicular tumors. J Urol 112:495, 1974.

Keough B & others: Urinary gonadotropins in management and prognosis of testicular tumor. Urology 5:496, 1975.

Koppikar DD, Sirat MV: A malignant Sertoli cell tumour of the testis. Brit J Urol 45:213, 1973.

Mahon FB Jr & others: Malignant interstitial cell testicular tumor. Cancer 31:1208, 1973.

Maier JG, Schamber DT: The role of lymphangiography in the diagnosis and treatment of malignant testicular tumor. Am J Roentgenol 114:482, 1972.

Marin-Padilla M: Histopathology of the embryonal carcinoma of the testis. Arch Path 85:614, 1968.

Markland C, Kedia K, Fraley EE: Inadequate orchiectomy for patients with testicular tumors. JAMA 224:1025, 1973.

Martini N & others: Primary mediastinal germ cell tumors. Cancer 33:763, 1974.

Meares EM Jr, Ho TL: Metastatic carcinomas involving the testis: A review. J Urol 109:653, 1973.

Monfardini S & others: Clinical use of adriamycin in advanced testicular cancer. J Urol 108:293, 1972.

Nefzger MD, Mostofi FK: Survival after surgery for germinal malignancies of the testis: 1. Rates of survival in tumor groups. 2. Effects of surgery and radiation therapy. (2 parts.) Cancer 30:1225, 1233, 1972.

Nicholson TC, Walsh PC, Rotner MB: Lymphadenectomy combined with preoperative and postoperative Cobalt 60 teletherapy in the management of embryonal carcinoma and teratocarcinoma of the testis. J Urol 112:109, 1974.

Price EB Jr: Epidermoid cysts of the testis: A clinical and pathologic analysis of 69 cases from the testicular tumor registry. J Urol 102:708, 1969.

Ray B, Hajdu SI, Whitmore WF Jr: Distribution of retroperitoneal lymph node metastases in testicular germinal tumors. Cancer 33:340, 1974.

Rubin P & others: Cancer of the urogenital tract: Testicular tumors. JAMA 213:89, 1970.

Sadoughi N & others: Bilateral germ-cell tumors of testis. Urology 2:452, 1973.

Selvaggi FP & others: Interstitial cell tumor of the testis in an adult: Two case reports. J Urol 109:436, 1973.

Sherman FP, Ciavarra VA, Cohen MJ: Testis tumors in negroes. Urology 2:318, 1973.

Sickles EA, Belliveau RE, Wiernik PH: Primary mediastinal choriocarcinoma in the male. Cancer 33:1196, 1974.

Skinner DG, Leadbetter WF, Wilkins EW Jr: The surgical management of testis tumors metastatic to the lung: A report of 10 cases with subsequent resection of from one to seven pulmonary metastases. J Urol 105:275, 1971.

Smith JP: Testicular tumors in infants and children. Urology 2:353, 1973.

Smithers DW: Chemotherapy for metastatic teratomas of the testis. Brit J Urol 44:217, 1972.

Smithers DW, Wallace DM, Austin DE: Fertility after unilateral orchidectomy and radiotherapy for patients with malignant tumours of the testis. Brit MJ 4:77, 1973.

Staubitz WJ & others: Surgical management of testis tumor. J Urol 111:205, 1974.

Tsuji I & others: Testicular tumors in children. J Urol 110:127, 1973.

Warikoo S, Gonick P: Testicular lymphoma. Urology 5:261, 1975.

Weiss JM, Hinman F: Factors affecting the success or failure of "sandwich therapy" for embryonal and teratocarcinoma of the testis. J Urol 112:779, 1974.

Wilson JM, Woodhead DM: Prognostic and therapeutic implications of urinary gonadotropin levels in the management of testicular neoplasia. J Urol 108:754, 1972.

Young PG & others: Embryonal adenocarcinoma in the prepubertal testis: A clinicopathologic study of 18 cases. Cancer 26:1065, 1970.

Ytredal DO, Bradfield JS: Seminoma of the testicle: Prophylactic mediastinal irradiation versus peri-aortic and pelvic irradiation alone. Cancer 30:628, 1972.

Tumors of the Epididymis

Broth G, Bullock WK, Morrow J: Epididymal tumors: 1. Report of 15 new cases including review of literature. 2. Histochemical study of the so-called adenomatoid tumor. J Urol 100:530, 1968.

Fisher ER, Klieger H: Epididymal carcinoma (malignant adenomatoid tumor, mesonephric, mesodermal carcinoma of epididymis). J Urol 95:568, 1966.

Spark RP: Leiomyoma of epididymis. Arch Path 93:18, 1972.

Viprakasit D, Tannenbaum M, Smith AM: Adenomatoid tumor of male genital tract. Urology 4:325, 1974.

Wachtel TL, Mehan DJ: Metastatic tumors of the epididymis. J Urol 103:624, 1970.

Williams G, Banerjee R: Paratesticular tumours. Brit J Urol 41:332, 1969.

Tumors of the Penis

Alexander LL & others: Radium management of tumors of penis. New York J Med 71:1946, 1971.

Almgård LE, Edsmyr F: Radiotherapy in treatment of patients with carcinoma of the penis. Scandinav J Urol Nephrol 7:1, 1973.

Bachrach P, Dahlen CP: Metastatic tumors to the penis. Urology 1:359, 1973.

DeKernion JB & others: Carcinoma of the penis. Cancer 32:1256, 1973.

Derrick FC Jr & others: Epidermoid carcinoma of the penis: Computer analysis of 87 cases. J Urol 110:303, 1973.

Fraley EE, Hutchens HC: Radical ilio-inguinal node dissection: The skin bridge technique. J Urol 108:279, 1972.

Groshong LE: A technique for radical groin dissection. Surg Gynec Obst 136:986, 1973.

Gursel EO & others: Penile cancer: Clinicopathologic study of 64 cases. Urology 1:569, 1973.

Hardner GJ & others: Carcinoma of the penis: Analysis of therapy in 100 consecutive cases. J Urol 108:428, 1972.

Hayes CW, Clark RM, Politano VA: Kaposi's sarcoma of the penis. J Urol 105:525, 1971.

Johnson DE, Ayala AG: Primary melanoma of penis. Urology 2:174, 1973.

Johnson DE, Fuerst DE, Ayala AG: Carcinoma of the penis: Experience with 153 cases. Urology 1:404, 1973.

Kelley CD & others: Radiation therapy of penile cancer. Urology 4:570, 1974.

Kossow JH, Hotchkiss RS, Morales PA: Carcinoma of penis treated surgically: Analysis of 100 cases. Urology 2:169, 1973.

Kuruvilla JT, Garlick FH, Mammen KE: Results of surgical treatment of carcinoma of the penis. Australian New Zealand J Surg 41:157, 1971.

Lewis RJ, Bendl BJ: Erythroplasia of Queyrat: Report of a patient successfully treated with topical 5-fluorouracil. Canad MAJ 104:148, 1971.

McAninch JW, Moore CA: Precancerous penile lesions in young men. J Urol 104:287, 1970.

Pratt RM, Ross RTA: Leiomyosarcoma of the penis. Brit J Surg 56:870, 1969.

Skinner DG, Leadbetter WF, Kelley SB: The surgical management of squamous cell carcinoma of the penis. J Urol 107:273, 1972.

Williams RD, Blackard CE: Chemotherapy for metastatic squamous-cell carcinoma of penis: Combination of vincristine and bleomycin. Urology 4:69, 1974.

Tumors of the Scrotum

El-Domeiri AA, Paglia MA: Carcinoma of the scrotum, radical excision and repair using ox fascia: Case report. J Urol 106:575, 1971.

Kickham CJE, Dufresne M: An assessment of carcinoma of the scrotum. J Urol 98:108, 1967.

Ray B, Huvos AG, Whitmore WF Jr: Unusual malignant tumors of the scrotum: Review of 5 cases. J Urol 108:760, 1972.

Tucci P, Haralambides G: Carcinoma of the scrotum: Review of literature and presentation of 2 cases. J Urol 89:585, 1963.

Retroperitoneal Extrarenal Tumors

Adlerman EJ & others: Primary retroperitoneal leiomyosarcoma. New York J Med 63:1709, 1963.

Armstrong JR, Cohn I Jr: Primary malignant retroperitoneal tumors. Am J Surg 100:937, 1965.

Braasch JW, Mon AB: Primary retroperitoneal tumors. S Clin North America 47:663, 1967.

Glenn F, Watson RC: Retroperitoneal liposarcoma. New York J Med 72:2789, 1972.

Kinne DW & others: Treatment of primary and recurrent retroperitoneal liposarcoma: Twenty-five-year experience at Memorial Hospital. Cancer 31:53, 1973.

Levin DC, Watson RC, Baltaxe HA: Arteriography of retroperitoneal masses. Radiology 108:543, 1973.

Lowman RM & others: The angiographic patterns of the primary retroperitoneal tumors. Radiology 104:259, 1972.

Polsky MS & others: Retrovesical liposarcoma. Urology 3:226, 1974.

Sadoughi N & others: Retroperitoneal xanthogranuloma. Urology 1:470, 1973.

Smith EH, Bartrum RJ Jr: Ultrasonic evaluation of pararenal masses. JAMA 231:51, 1975.

19 . . .
The Neurogenic Bladder

Normal vesical action depends upon an intact nerve supply. If either the sensory or motor nerves are interrupted, bladder function will be impaired. The type of abnormality is determined by the site and degree of the injury.

Spinal cord trauma secondary to vertebral fracture is the most common cause of neurogenic bladder dysfunction. Certain diseases (eg, tabes dorsalis, diabetes mellitus, multiple sclerosis) and cord tumors or herniated intervertebral disks also may cause abnormalities in micturition. Certain congenital anomalies (myelomeningocele, spina bifida, absence of the sacrum) are also associated with neurogenic vesical dysfunction. Cordotomy to relieve intractable pain may affect perception of the need for voiding; abdominoperineal resection of the rectum disturbs the innervation of the bladder and may be followed by at least temporary difficulty with urination. Herpes zoster may cause a transient neurologic deficit.

NORMAL VESICAL FUNCTION

ANATOMY

Detrusor Muscle

The bladder wall is composed of a mesh of muscle fibers running in every direction except when they approach the internal orifice, where they are rearranged to form 3 definite layers: internal longitudinal, middle circular, and external longitudinal. The outer layer extends down the whole length of the female urethra and to the distal end of the prostate but is circularly and spirally oriented; thus, it functions as the major involuntary sphincter. The middle circular detrusor muscle layer ends at the internal orifice of the bladder; it is best developed anteriorly. The internal component remains longitudinal and reaches the distal end of the urethra in the female and the end of the prostate in the male. These converging fibers cause a thickening that forms the so-called vesical neck, but anatomically there is no true sphincter at this point.

External Sphincters

There are 2 voluntary external sphincter mechanisms formed of striated muscle. The major one, which lies between the fascial layers of the urogenital diaphragm, is maximally condensed around the middle third of the female urethra (external to the external layer of urethral musculature), while in the male these fibers surround the distal portion of the prostate and the membranous urethra. The striated muscles of the pelvic floor (eg, levator ani) further contribute to sphincteric function.

Diaphragm & Abdominal Muscles

These play only secondary roles in micturition. Their contraction may further increase intravesical pressure in the female.

Nerve Supply

The sacral portion of the spinal cord, which contains the center controlling micturition (S2–4), is housed within the vertebral bodies T12 to L1. Fractures in the region of the twelfth thoracic and first lumbar vertebrae or below lead to flaccid neurogenic bladder because they destroy the voiding reflex center or the pelvic nerves (or both). Injuries above this level cause a spastic type of neurogenic bladder due to damage of the upper motor neurons.

A. **Motor Nerves:** (Fig 19–1.)

1. **To the detrusor**—These nerves are part of the parasympathetic nervous system. They arise from S2–4 and reach the bladder wall through the pelvic nerves. The trigonal portion of the bladder, because of its different embryologic origin, is innervated by motor fibers from the thoracolumbar outflow (T11 to L2) of the sympathetic nervous system. In dogs, intravenously administered epinephrine causes contraction of the trigone, the function of which is twofold. First, its tone pulls downward upon the ureterovesical junctions, thus combating possible reflux; second, its contracture helps open the bladder neck just before the detrusor is activated. Interruption of the sympathetic pathways may denervate the genital ducts and cause loss of the power of emission.

2. **To the external sphincter**—The motor nerve supply to the external sphincter and perineal muscles is somatic (voluntary) and reaches those structures through the pudendal nerves. They also arise from

S2–4. The motor fibers descend in the pyramidal tracts.

B. Sensory Nerves: Sensation from the urethra and bladder is returned to the central nervous system by fibers which travel with both the parasympathetic and somatic (S2–4) and the sympathetic motor nerves (T9 to L2). The parasympathetic nerves carry the sensory stretch perceptors. The sensory fibers ascend in the lateral spinothalamic tracts and fasciculus gracilis.

C. Voiding (Spinal) Reflex: The afferent and efferent fibers of the sacral portion of the cord (S2–4) form a simple spinal reflex arc which controls vesical function. Its activity is under the voluntary control of the cerebral cortex through the mediation of suprasegmental connections.

PHYSIOLOGY

Neurophysiology

Urinary control is largely centered in the simple reflex reaction between the bladder and the sacral cord. The normal bladder is able to distend gradually to normal capacity (400 ml) without appreciable increase in intravesical pressure. At this point, sensations of fullness are transmitted to the sacral cord where, if voluntary (cerebral) control is lacking (as in infants), discharges through the motor side of the reflex arc cause powerful, sustained detrusor contraction and spontaneous involuntary urination. As myelinization and training of the young child progress, cerebral inhibitory functions suppress the sacral reflex and the individual voids at his convenience.

Vesical Physiology

The normal act of urination is initiated by voluntary suppression of cerebral inhibition. Relaxation of the muscles of the pelvic floor and the striated external sphincter occur first. This operates to drop the vesical base, thereby further contributing to minimizing urethral resistance. Next, the trigone contracts, exerting increased pull on the ureterovesical junction and thus increasing ureteral occlusion. This prevents vesicoureteral reflux during the high intravesical pressure which develops with voiding. It also pulls the posterior portion of the bladder neck open, leading to its funneling. Only then do the muscle fibers (detrusor) of the bladder contract; intravesical pressure begins to rise. Because the vesical longitudinal muscles insert into the urethra, their contraction along with the trigone tends to pull the internal vesical sphincter open, further contributing to funneling of the vesical orifice. The increased hydrostatic pressure (30–40 cm of water) exerted by the detrusor is directed down the urethra. Reciprocally, the urethral counterpressure drops and voiding ensues. The detrusor maintains its contraction until complete emptying has occurred.

When the bladder is empty, the detrusor muscle relaxes and the bladder neck is allowed to close;

urethral and perineal muscle tone then returns to normal. Finally, the trigone resumes its normal tone. Should the person choose to interrupt the urinary stream, the external sphincter is contracted voluntarily. Detrusor muscle spasm then relaxes by reciprocal reflex action and the bladder neck closes.

CYSTOMETRIC STUDY

Cystometry has contributed much to our understanding of normal vesical function and is of value in diagnosing the types of nervous system lesions which cause neurogenic vesical dysfunction. A normal cystometrogram is shown in Fig 19–2. A cystometer is shown at left.

The normal bladder can usually perceive the first injection of fluid through a catheter. The desire to void is felt initially when 100–200 ml of fluid have been instilled. As fluid is introduced, intravesical pressure remains fairly constant at 8–10 cm of water. There are no sharp rises of pressure (uninhibited contractions) until 350–450 ml of fluid have been introduced, at which point a definite sensation of fullness (capacity) and distress is noted and the pressure increases sharply to 40–100 cm of water. This results in involuntary voiding around the catheter. If the catheter is withdrawn, the patient voids with a forceful, continuous stream. If bladder function is normal, there is no residual urine. Should the patient voluntarily strain to void, the resulting intravesical pressure recorded by the manometer will be a summation of true intravesical pressure and intra-abdominal pressure. The patient, therefore, should be cautioned against straining.

More sophisticated methods have been developed to study intravesical pressure and urethral resistance during the resting phase and while voiding, but these methods are not generally available for clinical use. Measurement of intravesical pressure and urethral resistance affords more information of a dynamic nature. Urinary continence requires that urethral pressure exceed intravesical pressure. In the normal person, during voiding, intravesical pressure rises to 30–40 cm of water, exceeding urethral resistance which drops reciprocally. If urethral resistance is high (eg, benign prostate hyperplasia, spasm of the striated periurethral muscles), voiding will require an abnormally high intravesical pressure. Should urethral resistance be low, even normal intravesical pressure or increased intra-abdominal pressure may be associated with incontinence.

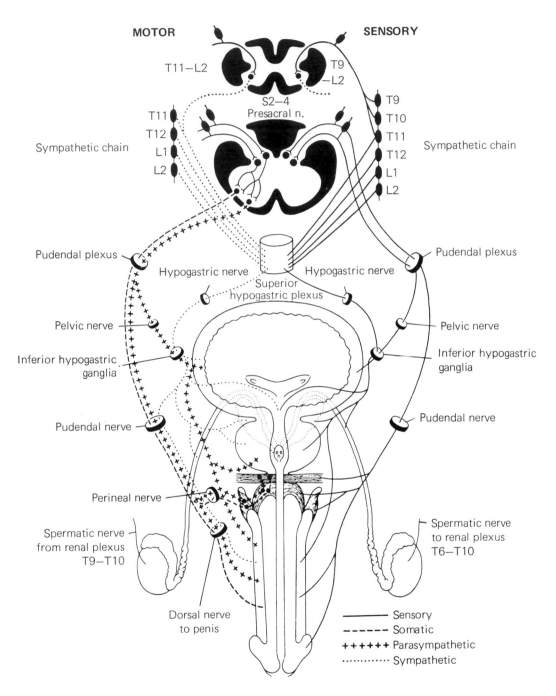

MOTOR

SENSORY

T11–L2

T9 –L2

S2–4
Presacral n.

T9
T10
T11
T12
L1
L2

T11
T12
L1
L2

Sympathetic chain

Sympathetic chain

Pudendal plexus

Pudendal plexus

Hypogastric nerve

Hypogastric nerve

Superior
hypogastric plexus

Pelvic nerve

Pelvic nerve

Inferior hypogastric
ganglia

Inferior hypogastric
ganglia

Pudendal nerve

Pudendal nerve

Perineal nerve

Spermatic nerve
from renal plexus
T9–T10

Spermatic nerve
to renal plexus
T6–T10

Dorsal nerve
to penis

———— Sensory
– – – – Somatic
+ + + + + Parasympathetic
·········· Sympathetic

Figure 19–1. Segmental and peripheral innervation of the urinary bladder, prostate, and external genitalia. (Reproduced, with permission, from Bors E: J Nerv Ment Dis 116:572, 1952.)

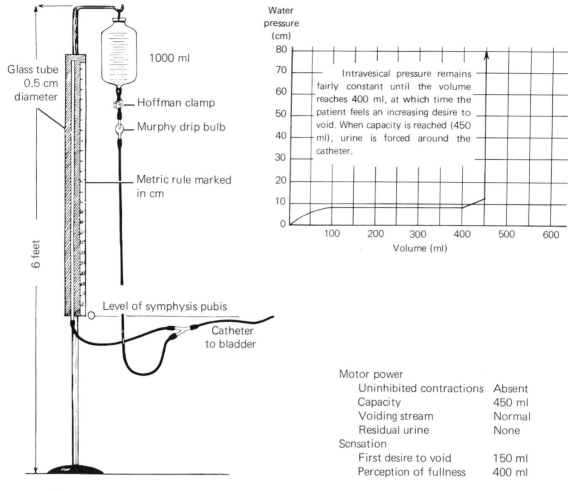

Figure 19–2. Cystometry. **Left:** A simple water manometer. **Right:** Normal cystometrogram. As fluid is slowly introduced into the bladder, the detrusor gradually relaxes to accept increasing amounts of fluid without change in intravesical pressure. At a volume of 400 ml, the patient felt an urge to void. Shortly thereafter, an involuntary contraction of the detrusor occurred which was reflected in a sharp increase in intravesical pressure.

ABNORMAL VESICAL FUNCTION

The following descriptions assume that the upper and lower motor neuron lesions are complete, but it must be realized that many incomplete lesions occur.

The bladder and the lower extremities respond similarly to injury or disease since their innervation arises from essentially the same segments of the spinal cord. Thus, an upper motor neuron (suprasegmental) lesion causes spasticity in both; lower motor neuron (segmental or infrasegmental) lesions cause flaccidity. Any lesion that damages the sacral cord on either side of the arc (sensory or motor) causes flaccidity.

There are, then, 2 main types of neurogenic bladder: spastic and flaccid. Each may be complete or incomplete. Mixed lesions are not uncommon.

SPASTIC (REFLEX OR AUTOMATIC) NEUROGENIC BLADDER
(Caused by Upper Motor Neuron Lesion)

This type of bladder disorder is caused by any lesion of the cord above the voiding reflex arc. Trauma is the most common cause, but the disorder may also be produced by tumor or multiple sclerosis. The lesion usually affects both the suprasegmental motor and sensory fibers (Fig 19–3). The sacral reflex arc remains intact, but the loss of conscious sensation and cerebral motor control lead to severe aberrations of function. This is potentially the most serious type of injury because the cord below the lesion is hyperirritable rather than "dead" and affects the bladder most adversely. For this reason, the incidence of renal damage is relatively high in this group. Injury to the pyramidal tracts deprives the bladder of cortical inhibition; uninhibited contractions then occur with filling, and vesical capac-

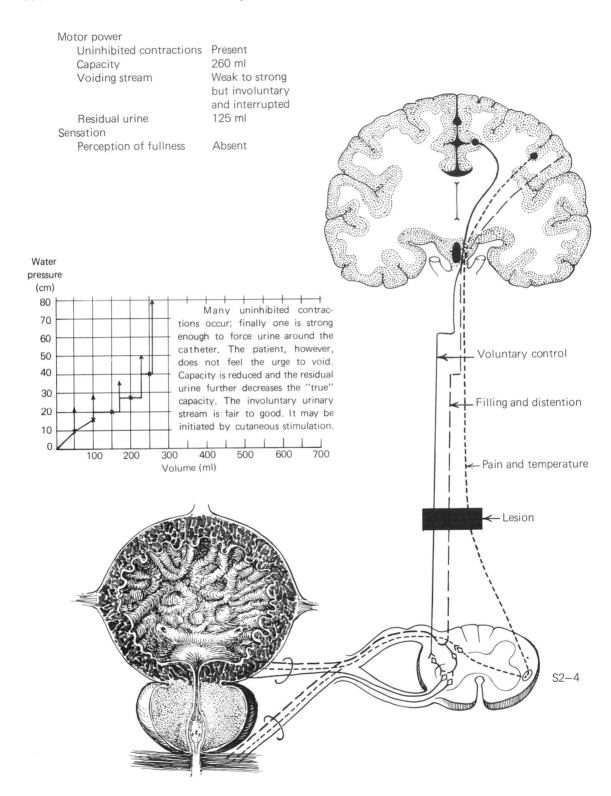

Motor power
    Uninhibited contractions   Present
    Capacity   260 ml
    Voiding stream   Weak to strong
                                but involuntary
                                and interrupted
    Residual urine   125 ml
Sensation
    Perception of fullness   Absent

Water
pressure
(cm)

Volume (ml)

Many uninhibited contractions occur; finally one is strong enough to force urine around the catheter. The patient, however, does not feel the urge to void. Capacity is reduced and the residual urine further decreases the "true" capacity. The involuntary urinary stream is fair to good. It may be initiated by cutaneous stimulation.

Voluntary control

Filling and distention

Pain and temperature

Lesion

S2–4

Figure 19–3. Complete spastic neurogenic bladder. Caused by a more or less complete transection of the spinal cord above S2. Cystometric study of a typical case shows function after recovery from spinal shock. (Modified after Nesbit, Lapides, & Baum: *Fundamentals of Urology*. Edwards, 1953.)

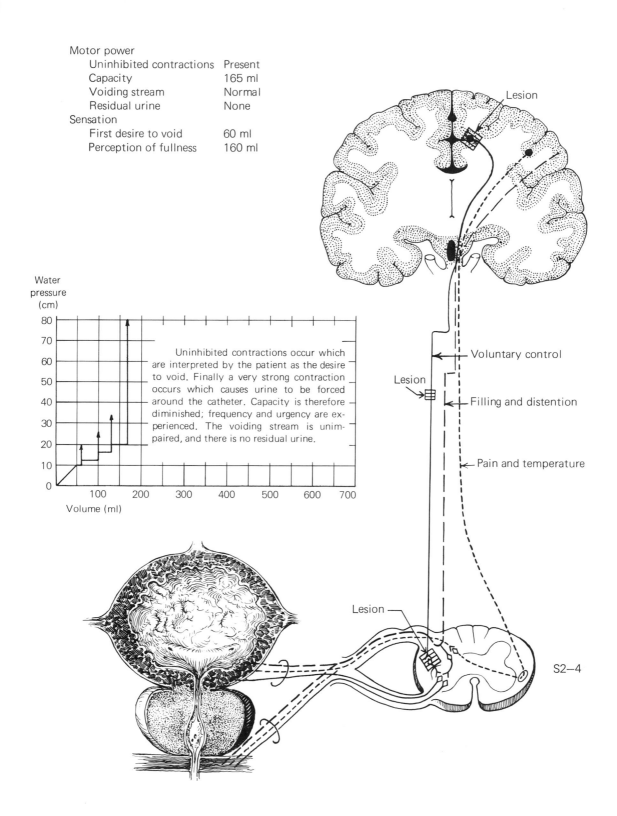

Motor power
    Uninhibited contractions   Present
    Capacity   165 ml
    Voiding stream   Normal
    Residual urine   None
Sensation
    First desire to void   60 ml
    Perception of fullness   160 ml

Water pressure (cm)

Uninhibited contractions occur which are interpreted by the patient as the desire to void. Finally a very strong contraction occurs which causes urine to be forced around the catheter. Capacity is therefore diminished; frequency and urgency are experienced. The voiding stream is unimpaired, and there is no residual urine.

Volume (ml)

Lesion

Voluntary control

Lesion

Filling and distention

Pain and temperature

Lesion

S2–4

Figure 19–4. Uninhibited neurogenic bladder. Caused by a lesion of the inhibitory centers of the cortex or pyramidal tracts. Cystometric study of a typical case. (Modified after Nesbit, Lapides, & Baum: *Fundamentals of Urology.* Edwards, 1953.)

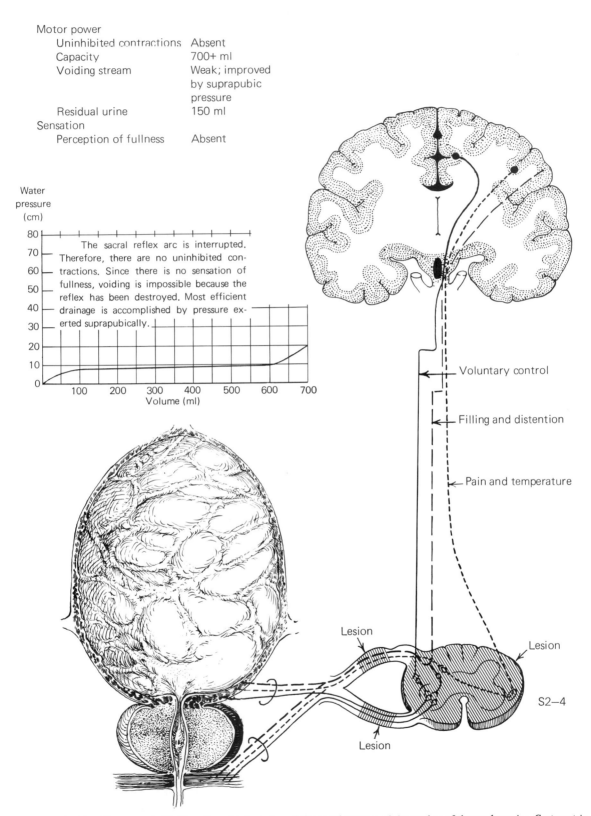

Motor power
Uninhibited contractions　Absent
Capacity　700+ ml
Voiding stream　Weak; improved by suprapubic pressure
Residual urine　150 ml
Sensation
Perception of fullness　Absent

Water pressure (cm)

The sacral reflex arc is interrupted. Therefore, there are no uninhibited contractions. Since there is no sensation of fullness, voiding is impossible because the reflex has been destroyed. Most efficient drainage is accomplished by pressure exerted suprapubically.

Volume (ml)

Voluntary control

Filling and distention

Pain and temperature

Lesion

Lesion

Lesion

S2–4

Figure 19–5. Flaccid neurogenic bladder. Caused by a lesion of the sacral portion of the cord or of the cauda equina. Cystometric study of a typical case shows function after recovery from spinal shock. (Modified after Nesbit, Lapides, & Baum: *Fundamentals of Urology*. Edwards, 1953.)

ity is diminished. Voiding is interrupted, involuntary, and incomplete. Hypertrophy of the detrusor develops, often leading to vesicoureteral reflux. Trigonal hypertrophy may cause functional obstruction of the ureterovesical junctions. Dilatation of the bladder neck occurs. The external sphincter and perineal muscles become spastic (upper motor neuron lesion) and obstructive. This causes increased resistance to the flow of urine and results in an impaired stream and residual urine. The sensory lesion deprives the patient of the perception of vesical fullness if the lesion is complete.

In summary, the spastic neurogenic bladder is typified by (1) reduced capacity, (2) involuntary detrusor contractions, (3) high intravesical voiding pressure, (4) marked hypertrophy of the bladder wall (trabeculation), and (5) spasm of the striated urinary sphincters. The diagram in Fig 19—3 illustrates these findings.

UNINHIBITED NEUROGENIC BLADDER
(Mild Spastic Neurogenic Bladder)

The uninhibited neurogenic bladder, a mild form of the spastic neurogenic bladder, may develop following a cerebrovascular accident or arteriosclerotic degeneration in the spinal cord. A prolapsed intervertebral disk may cause this reaction. It may also occur as the first sign of multiple sclerosis. It is associated with Parkinson's disease, and a similar reaction is seen with the spastic type of psychosomatic bladder reaction (see Chapter 34). The lesion is centered either in the inhibitory centers of the cortex or in the pyramidal tracts (upper neuron). Minor lesions due to myelomeningocele or spina bifida may occasionally affect the suprasegmental motor fibers, in which case the cortical inhibition to the vesical stretch reflex is lost and voiding may become precipitate and involuntary. Because all other mechanisms, including the sacral reflex arc, are normal, the sensation of fullness is retained, the stream is free, and there is no residual urine. Capacity is, however, diminished. The cystometrogram and the site of the lesion are diagrammed in Fig 19—4.

FLACCID (ATONIC, NONREFLEX, OR AUTONOMOUS) NEUROGENIC BLADDER
(Caused by Lower Motor Neuron Lesion)

The most common cause of flaccid neurogenic bladder is trauma, although tumors, herniated intervertebral disks, tabes dorsalis, poliomyelitis, and certain congenital defects, including meningomyelocele, can affect the same centers. Tranquilizers may cause vesical atonicity, as do parasympathetic blocking agents also. Vesical dysfunction arises when there is injury to the center of micturition in the cord (S2—4),

cauda equina, or sacral roots or nerves (Fig 19—5), thereby interrupting the sacral reflex arc. Loss of the perception of fullness permits overstretching of the detrusor and atony of the muscle, and this further contributes to weak and inefficient detrusor contraction. Thus, capacity is increased and the amount of residual urine is often large. Mild to moderate trabeculation (hypertrophy) of the bladder wall develops, accompanied by dilatation of the vesical outlet. External sphincter and perineal muscle tone is usually diminished, as is typical of striated muscle when a lower motor neuron lesion is present. Voluntary urination does not occur, but fairly efficient emptying can be accomplished by increased intra-abdominal and suprapubic (manual) pressure. The vesical (motor) paralysis which occurs occasionally in poliomyelitis usually clears quickly and spontaneously.

Myelomeningocele and spina bifida are associated with mild to severe vesical dysfunction, usually of the flaccid type, because the lesion affects the cauda equina and at times the sacral portion of the cord. Incontinence is the major symptom because of atony of the pelvic floor (external spincter). Occasionally, in conjunction with somatic (external sphincter) flaccidity, there may be visceral (bladder) spasticity as well; this is a difficult combination to treat.

In summary, flaccid neurogenic bladder is typified by (1) large capacity, (2) no involuntary detrusor contractions, (3) low intravesical pressure, and (4) mild (but at times even marked) trabeculation (hypertrophy) of the bladder wall and decreased tone of the external sphincter.

RECOVERY OF VESICAL FUNCTION AFTER SPINAL CORD INJURY

Initial Phase

A. Spinal Shock: Immediately following a severe injury to the spinal cord or cauda equina, no matter at what level, there is complete anesthesia and flaccid paralysis below the level of the lesion. The bladder, innervated as it is from the lowest part of the spinal cord, is similarly affected. Perception of fullness and detrusor contraction are absent. The bladder gradually fills until overflow incontinence occurs.

The cystometrogram (Fig 19—6) shows a very large bladder capacity, no involuntary detrusor contractions, and low intravesical pressure.

B. Recovery From Spinal Shock: Spinal shock may last for a period of a few weeks to 6 months or more. The early clues to the return of reflex activity (upper neuron lesion) include movement of a toe, spontaneous spasm in a leg, return of sensation in some area, and spontaneous voiding around the indwelling catheter.

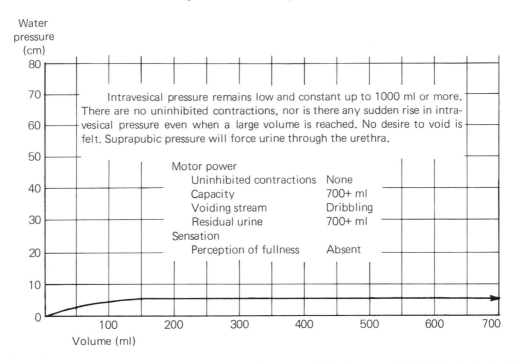

Figure 19–6. Stage of spinal shock. Cystometrogram showing flaccidity and lack of response of the bladder during the first few weeks or months after injury.

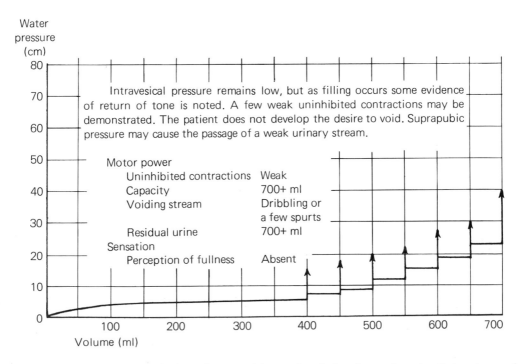

Figure 19–7. Stage of recovery of vesical function after severe injury to the spinal cord or cauda equina. Cystometrogram demonstrating the activity of the upper neuron bladder during the early stages of recovery from spinal shock.

Cystometric studies (Fig 19–7) may then demonstrate a large bladder capacity (but smaller than during the shock period), a few weak involuntary contractions of the detrusor, and the beginning of return of intravesical pressure (tone).

If the injury involves the cord above the sacral arc, anal sphincter tone and the bulbocavernosus reflex may return.

The "ice water test" should be tried periodically. Ninety ml of saline solution at 3 °C (38 °F) should be introduced forcefully into the bladder through a straight catheter. If the catheter is immediately ejected, the reaction is "positive." Should this not occur, the catheter should be removed quickly; if the fluid is ejected within 1 minute, this is also considered a "positive" test. "Negative" responses occur during the stage of spinal shock, but this reaction is one of the first to return with recovery if the sacral reflex arc is intact (upper neuron lesion). This test is therefore of value in differentiating an upper from a lower motor neuron lesion early in the recovery phase.

Final Phase

When spinal shock is over, the resulting condition of the bladder depends upon the level and extent of the lesion in the spinal cord.

A. Upper Motor Neuron (Suprasegmental) Lesion: Toward the end of the stage of spinal shock, more obvious evidence of reflex activity is observed: movement of an extremity; vigorous spasm of an extremity, often accompanied by voiding around the catheter; progressive return of sensation in one or more areas; and hyperactive peripheral reflex activity and muscle tone. On removal of the catheter, spontaneous though inefficient urination occurs.

Cystometry (Fig 19–3) will show the changes typical of a spastic neurogenic bladder: bladder capacity below normal (100–300 ml); forceful, involuntary detrusor contractions; and increased intravesical pressure.

B. Lower Motor Neuron (Segmental or Infrasegmental) Lesion: When spinal shock has cleared, the following may occur: progressive return of sensation in some areas, hypoactive peripheral reflexes, and flaccid muscle tone. It is difficult to know when the patient is coming out of shock, for this phase of recovery presents a similar picture. On removal of the catheter, spontaneous urination does not occur. As capacity is reached, overflow dribbling develops. The bladder can be partially emptied by manual pressure over the bladder.

The usual reactions seen with the flaccid neurogenic bladder are shown on cystometric study (Fig 19–5): bladder capacity above normal (600–1000 ml), absence of uninhibited detrusor contractions, and decreased intravesical pressure.

SPECIFIC TYPES OF NEUROGENIC BLADDERS

The diagnosis of neurogenic bladder depends upon a complete history and physical (including neurologic) examination and the application of such specialized urologic tests as cystoscopy, cystography, excretory urography, and cystometry, including determination of residual urine. These tests may have to be repeated several times as recovery progresses.

COMPLETE SPASTIC (REFLEX, AUTOMATIC) NEUROGENIC BLADDER

This type of cord bladder is the result of a partial or complete transection of the cord above the sacral level (above the lumbar spine) following recovery from spinal shock. The common causes are trauma, tumor, and multiple sclerosis. Cerebral control is lacking; the bladder functions in conjunction with its sacral reflex arc. The principal findings are diminished bladder capacity, increased intravesical pressure, spasm (obstruction) of the external urinary sphincters, and involuntary contractions of the vesical muscle.

Clinical Findings

A. Symptoms: The severity of symptoms depends on the site and extent of the lesion. Urinary symptoms include involuntary urination, often frequent and scanty, which may occur with involuntary spasm of the extremities. True sensation of fullness is lacking, although vague lower abdominal sensations due to stretching of the overlying peritoneum may be felt. The major nonurologic symptoms are spastic paralysis and objective sensory changes.

B. Signs: Complete neurologic examination will establish the site of the lesion. The anal sphincter tone is normal or increased; the bulbocavernosus reflex is intact or hyperactive (upper motor neuron lesion). Palpation and percussion usually do not reveal a distended bladder, since the bladder automatically discharges a portion of its contents when the urine volume reaches 150–300 ml. Stimulation of the skin of the abdomen, thigh, or genitals may initiate voiding. Such stimulation may also cause involuntary contraction of the extremities.

If the lesion is in the upper thoracic or cervical cord, distention of the bladder (plugged catheter, cystometry, cystoscopy) may excite hyperactive autonomic reflexes, which include severe hypertension, bradycardia, and pilomotor and sudomotor responses above the neurologic level. Headache may be severe; the hypertension may cause a cerebrovascular accident. Patients reacting in this manner should have an indwelling catheter open at all times. They are benefited by the administration of guanethidine (Ismelin), 10 mg

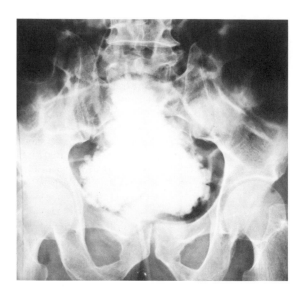
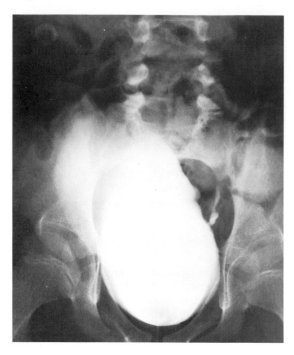

Figure 19–8. The spastic and flaccid neurogenic bladders as seen on cystography. *Left:* Spastic neurogenic bladder showing "Christmas tree" or "pine tree" effect. Heavy trabeculation, cellules, and small diverticula. ***Right:*** Flaccid neurogenic bladder showing oval-shaped bladder of large capacity in a boy 8 years old. The bladder, characteristically, is tipped to one side. Note severe spina bifida (myelomeningocele) and left ureteral reflux.

orally twice a day. Should instrumentation be necessary, spinal anesthesia or the administration of a ganglionic or postganglionic blocking agent will protect the patient from this reaction.

C. Laboratory Findings: Anemia may be found if infection of the urinary tract has been prolonged and poorly controlled. If secondary renal damage is severe and uremia has developed, anemia is to be expected. The urine is infected secondary to the indwelling catheter. Red cells may be found if calculi have developed. Renal function may be normal or impaired, depending on the efficacy of treatment and the absence of renal complications (hydronephrosis, pyelonephritis, calculosis).

D. X-Ray Findings: Excretory urograms and retrograde cystograms are essential since renal complications (eg, calculi, hydronephrosis) are common. Urinary stones may be seen. A trabeculated bladder of small capacity is typical of this type of neurogenic bladder. Ureteral reflux may be noted on the cystograms (Figs 11–5 and 19–8), which will almost certainly show a dilated bladder neck. If the cause of the neurogenic abnormality is undetermined, a plain film may reveal fracture or disease (eg, metastases) of the spine above the first lumbar vertebra.

E. Instrumental Examination: Cystoscopy and panendoscopy usually show moderate to severe trabeculation of the bladder wall, vesical diverticula, and changes compatible with infection. Stones may be visualized. The bladder is often hyperirritable to instrumentation.

The site of the lesion and the type of cystometrogram are diagrammed in Fig 19–3. As fluid is introduced into the bladder, strong, uninhibited contractions are noted until a contraction of such strength develops that involuntary urination occurs around the catheter. Capacity is diminished to 100–300 ml, and significant amounts of residual urine are found (50–150 ml). Although a true sense of fullness is lacking, various auras may be experienced (eg, sweating, vague low abdominal pain, intense spasm of the legs) when capacity is reached.

The "ice water test" is positive.

UNINHIBITED NEUROGENIC BLADDER
(Mild Spastic Neurogenic Bladder)

Incomplete lesions of the cortex or the pyramidal (motor) tracts may weaken or abolish cerebral restraint. The patient may have frequency and nocturia, and may suffer episodes of incontinence due to uncontrollable urgency. Brain tumors, multiple sclerosis, prolapsed lumbar disk, arteriosclerotic changes within the cord, and, at times, cerebrovascular accidents may be etiologic factors, but the cause is not always known. This type of reaction is often found in patients suffering from anxiety (see Chapter 34). The symptoms and clinical findings in adults are similar to those seen in normal infants.

Clinical Findings

A. Symptoms: Frequency, nocturia, and urgency are the principal symptoms and are similar to those of cystitis. If symptoms are due to organic neurologic disorders (eg, cerebrovascular accident, brain tumor), characteristic symptoms of these lesions may be found.

B. Signs: General and neurologic examinations are normal unless primary central nervous system disease is present, in which case hyperreflexia and abnormal peripheral reflexes may be elicited (eg, multiple sclerosis).

C. X-Ray Findings: Some patients with multiple sclerosis may develop vesicoureteral reflux or uretero-vesical obstruction. Urethrograms and cystograms are usually normal, but reflux may be seen.

D. Instrumental Examination: Cystoscopy and panendoscopy are normal, although some vesical irritability and diminished capacity may be demonstrated.

The sites of the possible lesions and the type of cystometrogram are diagrammed in Fig 19–4. As the bladder is filled, strong, uninhibited contractions are noted; long before "normal" capacity is reached, involuntary urination occurs around the catheter. Perception of sensation is normal, and there is no residual urine.

FLACCID (ATONIC, NONREFLEX, OR AUTONOMOUS) NEUROGENIC BLADDER

Injury to the sacral portion of the cord or to the motor or sensory roots of the cauda equina impairs the reflex arcs of the bladder. The common causes of this type of vesical reaction are trauma, tumors, tabes dorsalis, and congenital anomalies (eg, meningomyelocele). It may be seen following surgery in which the pelvic nerves are inadvertently injured (eg, abdominoperineal resection of the rectum). The bladder is also flaccid during the stage of spinal shock (Fig 19–6). This type of neurogenic bladder is characterized by large vesical capacity, low intravesical pressure, and the absence of involuntary detrusor contractions.

Clinical Findings

A. Symptoms: The patient complains of muscular paralysis and loss of peripheral sensation. The main urinary symptom is overflow incontinence. Suprapubic pressure may be required to initiate urination. Perception of fullness is absent.

B. Signs: Neurologic examination reveals evidence of a lower neuron lesion: absent or hypoactive peripheral reflexes, flaccid paralysis, absence of the bulbocavernosus reflex, and loss of anal sphincter tone. Sensation is diminished or absent. If perianal anesthesia alone is present, only one arm of the sacral reflex arc is damaged.

An overdistended bladder may be discovered on palpation or percussion. Pressure over the organ will cause passage of a stream of urine.

C. Laboratory Findings: Anemia may be noted, due either to chronic pyelonephritis or to uremia secondary to advanced renal damage (eg, infection, hydronephrosis, calculi). Pus cells and bacteria are found in the urine. Because of the amount of residual urine in the bladder, the PSP test must be performed with a catheter in place. Nitrogen retention may be associated with severe renal complications.

D. X-Ray Findings: A plain film of the abdomen may reveal a fracture of the lumbar spine or extensive spina bifida. Calcific shadows compatible with urinary stone may be visualized. Excretory urograms and retrograde cystograms should be performed routinely, since complications are common. These include vesical and renal calculi, renal scarring from pyelonephritis, and hydroureteronephrosis. However, the latter change is usually less marked than that seen with the spastic neurogenic bladder because the incidence of ureteral reflux and functional ureterovesical obstruction is lower. The bladder will appear large on the urogram.

E. Instrumental Examination: Cystoscopy and panendoscopy, when performed some weeks after the injury, reveal mild to moderate trabeculation (hypertrophy) of the detrusor. Vesical capacity is increased. Inflammatory changes may be present. The bladder neck is usually dilated. Stones may be visualized. The patient may experience little discomfort with instrumentation because of loss of local sensation.

Cystography will show a bladder of increased capacity (Fig 19–8). Reflux of the radiopaque fluid to the kidneys may be demonstrated.

Urethrography may reveal some laxness of the external urinary sphincter (lower neuron lesion). The bladder neck is usually wide open.

Cystometric examination and the site of the lesion are diagrammed in Fig 19–5. Vesical capacity is increased, the intravesical pressure is decreased, and there are no uninhibited contractions. Even after abdominal pressure is used to expel the bladder contents, as much as 250 ml of urine may be retained.

Lapides has described a simple test which is diagnostic of a lower motor neuron lesion. The intravesical pressure is noted after the instillation of 100 ml of water. Bethanechol chloride (Urecholine), 2.5 mg, is injected subcutaneously. A cystometric reading is made 10, 20, and 30 minutes later. If the rise is more than 15 cm of water, a lower motor neuron lesion is present.

DIFFERENTIAL DIAGNOSIS OF NEUROGENIC BLADDERS

The diagnosis of most cases of neurogenic bladder is obvious. Sacral nerve damage is evident, as judged by the bulbocavernosus reflex, anal sphincter tone, and perianal sensation. Too often the diagnosis of neurogenic bladder is made on very tenuous grounds.

Cystitis

Inflammations of the bladder, both nonspecific and tuberculous, also cause frequency of urination and urgency, even to the point of incontinence. Pyuria and bacteriuria are found, although it must be remembered that the neurogenic bladder is usually secondarily infected because of the presence of residual urine (or a retention catheter).

The cystometrogram of the inflamed bladder is similar to that obtained with uninhibited neurogenic bladder (Fig 19–4), but this reaction and the symptoms disappear after appropriate treatment. Should definitive antibiotic therapy not relieve symptoms, a primary neurologic lesion should be sought (eg, multiple sclerosis).

Chronic Urethritis

Symptoms of frequency, nocturia, and burning on urination may be due to chronic inflammation of the urethra. The urine is not infected. Panendoscopy will often reveal urethral stenosis and signs of urethral inflammation. Neurologic and cystometric studies are normal.

Vesical Irritation Due to Psychic Disturbance

The patient gives a long history of periodic bouts of urinary frequency, usually occurring only in the morning. Comparable nocturia is absent. The symptoms are precipitated by anxiety. The urine is normal.

Cystometric studies reveal a hyperirritable bladder of diminished capacity. The pressure curve is similar to that seen with the uninhibited neurogenic bladder (Fig 19–4). If the patient's anxiety can be allayed, the intravesical pressure and vesical capacity may return to normal.

Interstitial Cystitis

The patient with submucous fibrosis is almost always a woman over 40 years of age. She complains of great frequency, nocturia, urgency, and suprapubic pain when the bladder reaches its markedly limited capacity (60–100 ml). The urinalysis is usually normal, and there is no residual urine. Cystometry usually shows a hypertonic detrusor reaction with some uninhibited contractions. The voiding pressure is usually quite high, and voiding is involuntary. Cystoscopy shows typical scarring; the mucosa is apt to split and bleed with vesical distention.

Cystocele

Relaxation of the pelvic floor following childbirth may cause some frequency, nocturia, and stress incontinence. Since residual urine is often found, infection may be demonstrated on urinalysis.

Pelvic examination usually reveals relaxation of the anterior vaginal wall and descent of the urethra and bladder when the patient strains to urinate. Cystoscopy will reveal similar findings.

Infravesical Obstruction

Congenital urethral valves or strictures and benign or malignant enlargements of the prostate usually cause impairment of the urinary stream. Hypertrophy (trabeculation) of the detrusor occurs, and residual urine accumulates. During this compensatory stage, bladder neck obstruction may resemble the spastic neurogenic bladder.

If decompensation occurs, the vesical wall becomes attenuated and atonic and capacity may be markedly increased. Overflow incontinence may develop. The cystometrogram may simulate that of the flaccid neurogenic bladder (Fig 19–5).

If the difficulty is nonneurogenic, the anal sphincter tone is normal and the bulbocavernosus reflex is intact. Peripheral sensation, motor power, and reflexes are normal. Cystoscopy and panendoscopy will reveal the local lesion causing the obstruction. Even though appropriately treated, prolonged catheter drainage of the decompensated bladder may be necessary before the vesical tone returns to normal.

COMPLICATIONS OF NEUROGENIC BLADDER

The principal complications of neurogenic bladder are infection, hydronephrosis, and calculus formation. The primary factors which contribute to these complications are the presence of residual urine, ureteral reflux of urine, and confinement to bed. Sexual problems are common.

Infection

In neurovesical disease, the bladder loses the power to empty itself. Under these circumstances, infection is almost inevitable. With acute trauma to the spinal cord, the bladder is temporarily paralyzed and a retention catheter is therefore necessary. The introduction of an indwelling catheter always causes cystitis no matter what mechanical or medical measures are taken to prevent infection. The key to whether the kidneys will become involved is the ureterovesical junction. If the ureterovesical valves become incompetent, reflux of infected urine from the bladder reaches the kidneys. This may be caused by elevation of intravesical pressure from irrigations or expression of urine by the Credé maneuver, in which case these procedures must be discontinued.

If a large catheter is placed in the male bladder, periurethral abscess may ensue. This may rupture to the outside, producing a urinary fistula. If spontaneous drainage does not occur, urethral diverticulum may develop. Epididymitis secondary to prostatocystitis is not uncommon. The testis may become secondarily involved.

Hydronephrosis

The incidence of vesicoureteral reflux, particularly in the patient with a spastic neurogenic bladder, is significant. The etiologic factor appears to be the trabeculation which develops in association with this bladder condition. Secondary ureterohydronephrosis is the rule. Hypertrophy of the trigone is associated with vesical trabeculation. This causes an abnormal pull upon the ureterovesical junction which may lead to functional obstruction and therefore proximal dilatation.

Calculus

A number of factors may contribute to stone formation in the bladder or kidneys. Bed rest and inactivity cause demineralization of the skeleton and therefore hypercalciuria. Recumbency also contributes to urinary stasis.

If the infection is due to urea-splitting bacteria, the urine remains alkaline, in which medium calcium is less soluble.

In order to "build up" the injured patient, the physician may mistakenly encourage the drinking of milk (thereby increasing the calcium intake and urinary output) and prescribe vitamin preparations including vitamin D. The latter only increases the efficiency of the bowel to absorb calcium into the blood stream; increased urinary calcium excretion then occurs.

Renal Amyloidosis

Secondary amyloidosis of the kidneys is a common cause of death in patients with neurogenic bladder. Its incidence is highest in patients who have had decubitus ulcers or urethral infection.

Sexual Problems

Men who have suffered traumatic cord or cauda equina lesions experience varying degrees of sexual trouble. Those with upper motor lesions fare well; 95% will have psychic or reflex erections. In patients with complete lower neuron lesions, impotence occurs in 80%, but if the lesion is incomplete the incidence is 25%. The patient with an upper motor neuron defect has little chance of experiencing ejaculation or orgasm, although the patient with an incomplete lesion has a better prognosis.

TREATMENT OF NEUROGENIC BLADDER

The treatment of any form of neurogenic bladder is aimed at maintaining a relatively good functional capacity, combating infection, controlling incontinence, and preserving renal function. Functional capacity is measured by the difference between true capacity and the amount of urine retained after voiding. The desirable interval between voidings should be at least 2 and preferably 3 hours.

Urinary continence should not be sought at the expense of vesical capacity or renal function. Few paralytics are so confident of their control that they appear in public without some type of collecting apparatus (Fig 19—10).

Treatment of Stage of Spinal Shock

Following severe injury to the spinal cord, the bladder is temporarily paralyzed. During the next few months it undergoes gradual improvement. If the sacral cord or cauda equina is damaged, the end result is a flaccid bladder. If the injury is higher, the bladder becomes spastic in type.

During spinal shock, when the bladder is paralyzed, some type of vesical drainage must be instituted immediately and then maintained.

It has become increasingly clear that the presence of a permanent indwelling catheter always leads to persistent bacteriuria. Intermittent catheterization prevents this complication in a high percentage of cases, but it requires intensive nursing care. If this is not possible, an indwelling catheter must be used.

Either a No. 16F balloon (Foley) or a No. 8 or 10F Gibbon (polythene) catheter can be used. The latter, because of its small size, may decrease the incidence of urethral complications (eg, periurethral abscess, urethral diverticulum). The Foley catheter in the male should be taped to the abdomen so that sharp angulation does not occur at the penoscrotal junction. It should be changed every week. The Gibbon catheter usually need only be changed once a month.

Some advocate the use of cystostomy rather than a urethral catheter, thus circumventing the often serious urethral and genital tract complications. Should these develop in association with urethral catheter drainage, cystostomy should be seriously considered; it will allow removal of the offending urethral catheter.

Vesical hygiene contributes to the control of infection, lowers the incidence of vesical calculi, and possibly maintains optimum vesical capacity when a urethral catheter is used. A simple apparatus for closed irrigation and drainage is shown in Fig 19—9. Any sterile solution may be used. A 10% solution of hemiacridin (Renacidin) tends to prevent the precipitation of calcium salts in the lumen of the catheter. The capacity of the bladder should be determined by periodic cystometric observations and no more than this amount of fluid allowed to enter the bladder. It is then drained off. The bladder should be irrigated 3 times a day. If done faithfully, this is a much simpler procedure than tidal drainage and is probably just as efficient in maintaining vesical capacity. The Gibbon catheter is not irrigated.

Cystograms should be taken periodically. If they reveal ureteral reflux, forceful irrigation is contraindicated.

In order to control infection, a fluid intake of at least 3000 ml/day must be maintained (200 ml of fluid every hour when awake). This reduces stasis and decreases the concentration of calcium in the urine.

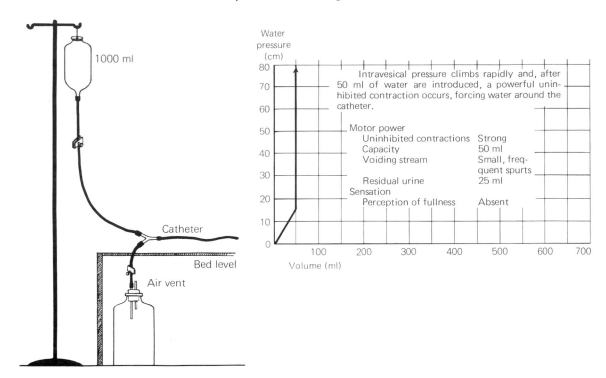

Figure 19–9. *Left:* Closed system for vesical irrigation and vesical drainage. *Right:* Cystometrogram typical of severely spastic bladder.

Renal and ureteral drainage are enhanced by raising the head of the bed, moving the patient frequently, and, above all, ambulating the patient in a wheel chair as early as possible. These measures lessen the incidence of acute pyelonephritis and renal and vesical calculosis. Sulfonamides or antibiotics should be vigorously administered if febrile reactions occur. Little is gained by prolonged prophylactic medication since sterilization of the urine is impossible when a catheter is in place.

Prevention of calculosis requires a low-calcium diet (eliminate dairy products) containing no vitamin D. As mentioned above, early ambulation in a wheel chair reduces the incidence of calculosis. If hypercalciuria is demonstrated by periodic Sulkowitch tests, other prophylactic measures should be considered (see Chapter 15).

TREATMENT OF SPECIFIC TYPES OF NEUROGENIC BLADDER

Once the specific type of neurogenic bladder is established (including the posttraumatic group after emergence from spinal shock), the following steps should be taken to attain optimum function.

Spastic Neurogenic Bladder

A. Patient With Large Bladder Capacity: To successfully train the spastic neurogenic bladder, the patient must be able to wait 2–3 hours between involuntary voidings. He should not leak during this period, and he must be able to initiate voiding by manual stimulation or squeezing of the abdomen, genitalia, or thighs. This can be done by the patient unless he is quadriplegic.

B. Patient With Markedly Diminished Functional Vesical Capacity: If the functional capacity is only 50–100 ml, involuntary voidings may occur as often as every 15–30 minutes; and satisfactory bladder training cannot be attained (see cystometrogram in Fig 19–9). The alternatives are:

1. Permanent retention catheter, cutaneous vesicostomy, cutaneous ureterostomy, ureteroileocutaneous anastomosis, or cystostomy, particularly if ureteral reflux can be demonstrated on cystograms.

2. Urinal or other collecting apparatus constantly in place.

3. If low functional capacity is due to the retention of a large volume of urine, transurethral resection of the bladder neck may be undertaken. If this fails to improve emptying power satisfactorily, transurethral destruction of the external sphincter may be necessary. It is quite efficacious in reducing the amount of residual urine. Since the patient will probably be incontinent, an external collecting device will be necessary.

4. If the true capacity is very low, and particularly if the patient suffers involuntary spasm of the extremities when he voids, his spastic bladder (and extremities) should be made flaccid.

If, despite catheter drainage, progressive ureterohydronephrosis develops, the conversion of an upper motor to a lower motor neuron lesion may cause regression of the upper tract changes. This can be accomplished by one of the following technics:

a. Subarachnoid injection of absolute alcohol—This should be preceded by spinal anesthesia. If voiding can be accomplished manually under spinal anesthesia, then the alcohol injection should be done. Alcohol injection acts by destroying the conus and the cauda equina.

b. Anterior and posterior rhizotomy from T12 to and including S5 also converts the lesion to a lower neuron type.

c. Sacral neurotomy of S2–4 has a similar effect upon the bladder but is not complete enough to eradicate annoying spasms of the extremities.

These procedures may have to be combined with resection of the bladder neck if stenosis of that structure is found.

5. Progressive upper tract deterioration may require urinary diversion.

C. Parasympatholytic Drugs: The quaternary ammonium amines methantheline bromide (Banthine), 50–100 mg 3–4 times daily orally, and propantheline bromide (Pro-Banthine), 15–30 mg 3–4 times daily orally, reduce vesical tone and thereby increase vesical capacity. Because of the prolonged nature of the disease, these agents have proved of little practical value except in patients with mildly spastic bladders (uninhibited neurogenic bladder).

Diokno & Lapides (1972) found that oxybutynin (Ditropan) has both analgesic and anticholinergic properties. The status of this drug is still investigational.

Flaccid Neurogenic Bladder

If the neurologic lesion is complete, volitional voiding cannot be accomplished without manual suprapubic pressure augmented, if possible, by abdominal and diaphragmatic contraction. If the lesion is incomplete, spontaneous voiding may occur but the size and force of the stream are impaired and residual urine remains in the bladder. Proper care of the flaccid bladder requires the following:

A. Bladder Training and Care: Voiding every 2 hours by the clock protects the bladder from overdistention, which the patient is unable to perceive, and preserves maximum tone. Intermittent catheterization has an excellent chance of rendering the urine sterile. Catheter drainage must be used for the patient who has ureteral reflux on cystography.

B. Surgery: Transurethral resection of the bladder neck is indicated for hypertrophy or spasm, which causes the retention of a large volume of residual urine. At times this operation may fail to reduce the amount of residual urine to a point where a proper interval

between voidings is afforded, in which case transurethral incision of the external sphincter may be considered (Gibbon, 1972). This will require the use of a collection device.

C. Parasympathomimetic Drugs: The stable derivatives of acetylcholine are at times of value in initiating and increasing the efficiency of the contraction of the detrusor. They may therefore be helpful in the symptomatic treatment of the milder types of flaccid neurogenic bladder. Their usefulness may be gauged during cystometric study. When the bladder has been filled to a volume of 400 ml, the minimal recommended dose should be given subcutaneously. If intravesical pressure rises appreciably within a few minutes, the drug can be expected to be helpful clinically.

Bethanechol chloride (Urecholine) is the drug of choice. It is given either orally, 10–50 mg every 4–6 hours (the latter dose is usually necessary), or subcutaneously, 5–10 mg every 4–6 hours. Methacholine chloride (Mecholyl) is given orally, 0.2–0.4 g every 4–6 hours, or subcutaneously, 10–20 mg every 4–6 hours.

D. Implanted Electrodes: An attempt is being made to implant electrodes into the bladder wall with an external stimulator mechanism in order to cause efficient detrusor action. Even more promising is the placement of electrodes into the sacral cord. Stimulation in this area is more efficient than that seen with vesical wall electrodes. When perfected, this technic may prove to be an important step in the treatment of the flaccid bladder.

Scott & others (1973) have designed an implantable prosthetic sphincter. Results so far are encouraging.

Neurogenic Bladder Associated With Spina Bifida

Following the repair of meningocele or myelomeningocele, the cauda equina and sacral cord are apt to be involved by scar tissue. These patients usually have neurogenic vesical dysfunction which may be of the atonic or spastic type but is often of the mixed type (spastic bladder—upper motor neuron lesion; atony of the pelvic floor—lower neuron lesion).

The goals of therapy are to control incontinence and to preserve renal function.

A. Conservative Treatment: Lyon, Scott, and Marshall (1975) find that clean intermittent catheterization will afford a sterile urine in most cases. The mother can be taught to do this for the child. Later, the patient can take over this function. It should be done 3 times a day. This will also control the incontinence in many of these patients.

1. Mild symptoms—If there is occasional dribbling or some residual urine associated with lack of desire to void, have the patient try to void every 2 hours when awake. Manual suprapubic pressure will enhance the efficiency of emptying. An external condom catheter (Fig 19–10) will protect the male who still suffers small losses. A similar complaint in a female will require an indwelling catheter.

2. More severe symptoms—If true urinary incontinence associated with residual urine and ureteral reflux is found, the following steps should be taken.

a. Mostly atonic bladder—If reflux is demonstrable, self-catheterization 3 times a day may protect the upper urinary tract from deterioration and the complication of pyelonephritis. Should this fail, an indwelling catheter is necessary.

b. Mostly spastic bladder—The problem with patients in this category is more serious because the bladder is hypertonic and has a small capacity but the external sphincter is atonic. Almost constant dribbling may result. In addition, a cystogram will reveal a heavily trabeculated bladder and, in many cases, reflux revealing advanced hydroureteronephrosis. Lyon recommends the placement of an indwelling catheter for many months. In most instances, the bladder assumes a normal smooth contour and the hydroureteronephrosis subsides. The patient is then able to resume intermittent self-catheterization. With time, many of these children develop a more balanced bladder and may continue to improve. Continence may finally be gained. Urinary diversion will not be necessary in most of these patients. Should vesicoureteral reflux persist, ureterovesicoplasty is highly successful once the bladder has smoothed out. Shochat & Perlmutter (1972) find that severe neonatal hydronephrosis may resolve after urethral dilatation.

B. Surgical Treatment: If significant residual urine is found and is associated with considerable dribbling, transurethral resection of the bladder neck or division of the external sphincter will reduce the residual urine and will cure some of these children. A few may notice increased incontinence, however.

If the bladder is of the spastic type with diminished capacity, sacral nerve block, internal pudendal neurectomy, or selective neurectomy (S3) may improve capacity and stop ureteral reflux.

Stanton & Edwards (1973) have had good success after implanting a stimulator in the bladder. Candidates must have good upper tracts and adequate bladder emptying; must be free of vesicoureteral reflux with good bladder capacity; and must have urethral incompetence.

If the refluxing patient suffers recurrent fever (pyelonephritis) despite the presence of an indwelling catheter, or if incontinence cannot be controlled, urinary diversion must be considered. The colonic conduit is the method of choice.

THE CONTROL OF URINARY INCONTINENCE

In the Hospital

Urinary incontinence is a distressing aspect of neurovesical dysfunction, particularly if the patient achieves a bladder which otherwise functions adequately. This difficulty is minimized in men under hospital conditions, for with close supervision and the ever-present urinal, the urine can usually be properly collected. Women have a greater problem because of the need for placement of the bedpan, and bedwetting may be frequent. Even an indwelling catheter does not guarantee dryness for the incontinent woman, since leakage around the catheter often occurs. No simple and satisfactory solution to this problem has yet been devised. Urinary diversion may be necessary.

After Discharge

When the time comes for discharge from the hospital almost all men, even though they have achieved "excellent" bladder control, must wear a "condom catheter" (Fig 19–10). This consists of a condom with a catheter at the distal end for drainage of any urine unexpectedly lost. The catheter drains into a leg urinal. The condom may be secured to the penis by elastoplast, cellulose tape, or cement.

A McGuire urinal (Fig 19–10) consists of a heavy condom incorporated into an athletic supporter. If there is considerable leakage of urine, the dependent end can be drained through a tube into a leg urinal.

Urethral compression by means of a Cunningham clamp is preferred by some patients. It may, however, lead to the development of a urethral diverticulum (Fig 19–11).

TREATMENT OF COMPLICATIONS

The most common and significant complications can be discovered by cystography, cystometry, cystoscopy, and excretory urography repeated at least once a year.

Hydronephrosis

Ureteral reflux, as shown by cystography, is an indication for an indwelling catheter. Over a period of months, the ureterovesical junction may again become competent. If, despite prolonged drainage, reflux persists, vesicoureteroplasty may be indicated, though it is difficult in the face of severe vesical trabeculation and trigonal hypertrophy. Progressive hydroureteronephrosis, found on urography, may require nephrostomy or urinary diversion as a lifesaving measure.

Pyelonephritis

Bouts of renal infection must be treated by antimicrobials. Intermittent self-catheterization may render the urine sterile. If the pyelonephritis is associated with ureteral reflux, constant vesical drainage must be instituted. Urinary diversion should be considered.

Epididymitis

In acute epididymitis secondary to prostatitis initiated by the urethral catheter, prophylactic vasoli-

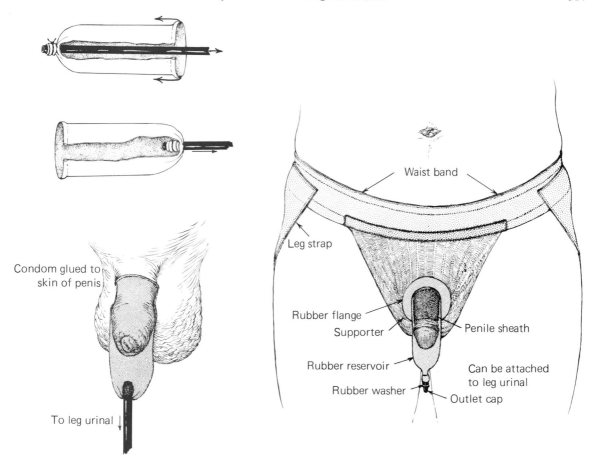

Figure 19–10. *Left:* Condom catheter. *Right:* McGuire urinal.

gation is indicated during a quiescent period. Should this not suffice, removal of the urethral catheter and placement of a suprapubic tube or intermittent catheterization will be necessary.

Calculi

A. Vesical: Vesical calculi, diagnosed by x-ray or cystoscopy, can usually be washed out through an instrument or crushed and removed transurethrally. If they are large, suprapubic removal will be required.

B. Ureteral: These can usually be diagnosed by excretory urograms; if no radiopaque fluid is excreted, cystoscopy and the passage of a ureteral catheter may be necessary. Most ureteral stones can be removed cystoscopically. Operative removal may at times be required.

C. Renal: The diagnosis of renal calculi is made by radiography. If the calculus is obstructive, it must be removed; if not, conservative treatment is the rule, for the recurrence rate is high because of the presence of urea-splitting organisms in the kidney.

If stones form despite the prophylactic steps listed on p 314, an even more rigorous regimen should be instituted (Chapter 15).

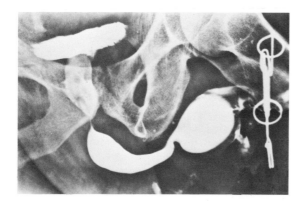

Figure 19–11. Urethral diverticulum. Atonic neurogenic bladder after transurethral resection. Diverticulum is a complication of prolonged use of a Cunningham clamp.

PROGNOSIS

The greatest threat to the patient with a neurogenic bladder is progressive renal damage (pyelonephritis, calculosis, and hydronephrosis). Some degree of hydronephrosis is found in 25% of these patients; a few will die because of it unless appropriate treatment is instituted.

The quadriplegic patient presents a serious problem. If his bladder is spastic, he cannot initiate voiding by self-stimulation; if his bladder has been made flaccid, he is unable to exert suprapubic pressure. An indwelling catheter may be the best solution. Most paraplegics can eventually achieve comfortable bladder function, although many must continue to wear some type of collecting apparatus.

•   •   •

References

Anderson RG: Results of social versus medical ileal conduit diversion in patients with myelodysplasia. J Urol 112:587, 1974.

Bors E, Comarr AE: *Neurological Urology: Physiology of Micturition, Its Neurological Disorders and Sequelae.* University Park Press, 1971.

Bradley WE, Timm GW, Scott FB: Cystometry. 2. Central nervous system organization of detrusor reflex. Urology 5:578, 1975.

Cass AS, Spence BR: Urinary incontinence in myelomeningocele. J Urol 110:136, 1973.

Chadduck WM, Loar CR, Denton IC: Vesical hypotonicity with diazepam. J Urol 109:1005, 1973.

Comarr AE: Intermittent catheterization for the traumatic cord bladder patient. J Urol 108:79, 1972.

Comarr AE: Sexual function among patients with spinal cord injury. Urol Internat 25:134, 1970.

Dalton JJ Jr, Hackler RH, Bunts RC: Amyloidosis in the paraplegic: Incidence and significance. J Urol 93:553, 1965.

Diokno AC, Koff SA, Bender LF: Periurethral striated muscle activity in neurogenic bladder dysfunction. J Urol 112:743, 1974.

Diokno AC, Lapides J: Oxybutynin: A new drug with analgesic and anticholinergic properties. J Urol 108:307, 1972.

Engel RME, Schirmer HKA: Pudendal neurectomy in neurogenic bladder. J Urol 112:57, 1974.

Ericsson NO & others: Micturition urethrocystography in children with myelomeningocele. Acta radiol diag 11:321, 1971.

Gibbon NOK: Division of the external sphincter. Brit J Urol 45:110, 1973.

Gottlieb RJ, Cuttner J: Vincristine-induced bladder atony. Cancer 28:674, 1971.

Greenberg M, Gordon HL, McCutchen JJ: Neurogenic bladder in Parkinson's disease. South MJ 65:446, 1972.

Grimes JH, Anderson EE, Currie DP: Surgical management of neurogenic bladder. Urology 2:500, 1973.

Grimes JH, Nashold BS, Anderson EE: Clinical application of electronic bladder stimulation in paraplegics. J Urol 113:338, 1975.

Hackler RH: Spinal cord injuries: Urologic care. Urology 2:13, 1973.

Halverstadt DB, Parry WL: Electronic stimulation of the human bladder: Nine years later. J Urol 113:341, 1975.

Herr HW, Engelman ER, Martin DC: External sphincterotomy in traumatic and non-traumatic neurogenic bladder dysfunction. J Urol 113:32, 1975.

Jones DL, Moore T: The types of neuropathic bladder dysfunction associated with prolapsed lumbar intervertebral discs. Brit J Urol 45:39, 1973.

Kahan M, Goldberg PD, Mandel EE: Neurogenic vesical dysfunction and diabetes mellitus. New York J Med 70:2448, 1970.

Kontturi M, Larmi TKI, Tuononen S: Bladder dysfunction and its manifestations following abdominoperineal extirpation of the rectum. Ann Surg 179:179, 1974.

Lapides J: Urecholine regimen for rehabilitating the atonic bladder. J Urol 91:658, 1964.

Lapides J & others: Clean, intermittent self-catheterization in the treatment of urinary tract disease. J Urol 107:458, 1972.

Linker DG, Tanagho EA: Complete external sphincterotomy: Correlation between endoscopic observation and the anatomic sphincter. J Urol 113:348, 1975.

Lyon RP, Scott MP, Marshall S: Intermittent catheterization rather than urinary diversion in children with meningomyelocele. J Urol 113:409, 1975.

Manfredi RA, Leal JF: Selective sacral rhizotomy for the spastic bladder syndrome in patients with spinal cord injuries. J Urol 100:17, 1968.

Masih BK, Brosman SA: Bladder dysfunction with herpes zoster. Urology 2:568, 1973.

Melzer M: The Urecholine test. J Urol 108:728, 1972.

Merrill DC: Clinical experience with the mentor bladder stimulator. 3. Patients with urinary vesical hypotonia. J Urol 113:335, 1975.

Merrill DC, Conway C, DeWolf W: Urinary incontinence: Treatment with electrical stimulation of the pelvic floor. Urology 5:67, 1975.

Merrill DC, Rotta J: A clinical evaluation of detrusor denervation supersensitivity using air cystometry. J Urol 111:27, 1974.

Miller H, Simpson CA, Yeates WK: Bladder dysfunction in multiple sclerosis. Brit MJ 1:1265, 1965.

Nanninga JB, Rosen J, O'Conor VJ: Experience with transurethral external sphincterotomy in patients with spinal cord injury. J Urol 112:72, 1974.

Pearman JW, England EJ: *The Urological Management of the Patient Following Spinal Cord Injury.* Thomas, 1972.

Perkash I: Intermittent catheterization: The urologist's point of view. J Urol 111:356, 1974.

Rabinovitch HH: Bladder evacuation in child with meningomyelocele. Urology 3:425, 1974.

Ray P, De Domenico I: Intestinal conduit urinary diversion in children. Brit J Urol 44:345, 1972.

Richmond W: The genito-urinary manifestations of herpes zoster. Brit J Urol 46:193, 1974.

Rossier AB, Ott R: Urinary manometry in spinal cord injury: A follow-up study. Value of cysto-sphincterometrography as an indicator for sphincterotomy. Brit J Urol 46:439, 1974.

Schoenfeld L, Carrion HM, Politano VA: Erectile impotence: Complication of external sphincterotomy. Urology 4:681, 1974.

Scott FB, Bradley WE, Timm GW: Treatment of urinary incontinence by implantable prosthetic sphincter. Urology 1:252, 1973.

Shea JD & others: Autonomic hyperreflexia in spinal cord injury. South MJ 66:869, 1973.

Shochat SJ, Perlmutter AD: Myelodysplasia with severe neonatal hydronephrosis: The value of urethral dilatation. J Urol 107:146, 1972.

Stanton SL, Edwards L: Treatment of paediatric urinary incontinence by stimulator implant. Brit J Urol 45:508, 1973.

Stark G: Pudendal neurectomy in management of neurogenic bladder in myelomeningocele. Arch Dis Childhood 44:698, 1969.

Symposium: The neurogenic bladder. Acta neurol scandinav, Supp 20, 1966.

Tanagho EA, Meyers FH, Smith DR: The trigone: Anatomical and physiological considerations. 1. In relation to the ureterovesical junction. J Urol 100:623, 1968.

Tanagho EA, Miller ER: Initiation of voiding. Brit J Urol 42:175, 1970.

Tarabulcy E: Neurogenic diseases of the bladder in the geriatric population. Geriatrics 29:123, 1974.

Thompson IM, Kirk RM, Dale M: Sacral agenesis. Pediatrics 54:236, 1974.

Williams JE: The renal tract in spina bifida cystica. Brit M Bull 28:250, 1972.

Zinke H & others: Neurovesical vesical dysfunction in diabetes mellitus: Another look at vesical neck resection. J Urol 111:488, 1974.

20 . . .
Disorders of the Adrenal Glands

Peter H. Forsham, MD

Diseases of the adrenal glands are accompanied by characteristic hormonal changes or, because of their size, give rise to pressure or pain and may be diagnosed by appropriate hormonal determinations and radiologic studies (Fig 20–1).

DISEASES OF THE ADRENAL CORTEX

CUSHING'S SYNDROME

Cushing's syndrome or Cushing's disease is caused by overproduction of cortisol (hydrocortisone). The majority of cases (85%) are due to bilateral adrenocortical hyperplasia stimulated by overproduction of pituitary adrenocorticotropic hormone (corticotropin, ACTH). A few cases are due to an undifferentiated ectopic ACTH-producing tumor that may be found (in decreasing order of incidence) in the lungs, the bronchial tree, the kidneys, the islets of the pancreas, or the thymus. Adrenal adenoma is the cause in 10% of cases and adenocarcinoma in 5%. In children, tumors are the most common cause.

Pathophysiology

Overproduction of cortisol or closely related glucocorticoids leads to a protein catabolic state. This causes liberation of amino acids from muscle tissue which are transformed into glucose and glycogen in the liver by glyconeogenesis. This results in weakened protein structures (muscle and elastic tissue), which causes a protuberant abdomen and poor wound healing, generalized muscle weakness, and marked osteoporosis; the latter is made worse by excessive urinary calcium loss and is irreversible in adults.

The protein catabolic state leads to a variety of secondary changes. Excess glucose is transformed

Peter H. Forsham is Professor of Medicine and Pediatrics and Director of the Metabolic Research Unit, University of California School of Medicine (San Francisco).

largely into fat and appears in characteristic sites such as the abdomen, supraclavicular fat pads, and cheeks. There is a diabetic tendency, with an elevated fasting plasma glucose in 20% of cases and a diabetic glucose tolerance curve in 80%, with insulinoplethora in the majority of cases.

Destruction of most of the lymphoid tissue leads to impairment of the immune mechanisms, which makes these patients susceptible to repeated infections. Inhibition of fibroplasia by excess cortisol further interferes with host defenses against infection. Hypertension is present in 99% of cases. Although aldosterone is not usually elevated, cortisol itself exerts a hypertensive effect when present in excessive amounts and favors the formation of angiotensinogen by the liver, resulting in production of angiotensin, the most potent hypertensive agent known.

The moderate rise in serum sodium with a marked fall in serum potassium is due to excess of cortisol and of the primary mineralocorticoid 11-deoxycorticosterone. The plasma bicarbonate is often elevated as a consequence of the low serum potassium.

An adrenal adenoma is stimulated to grow by the administration of ACTH in the same way as are hyperplastic adrenals. Adenocarcinoma of an adrenal gland, on the other hand, is independent of pituitary influence and does not respond to exogenous ACTH.

Pathology

The cells in adrenal hyperplasia resemble those of the zona fasciculata of the normal adrenal cortex. Frank adenocarcinoma reveals pleomorphism and invasion of its capsule or of the vascular system or both (Fig 20–2). Differentiation between adenoma and adenocarcinoma is sometimes difficult. The former is stimulated by the administration of exogenous ACTH, as reflected in an increased secretion of urinary or plasma hydroxycorticosteroids; this does not usually occur with adenocarcinoma. Local invasion may occur, and functional metastasis may occur to the liver, lungs, bone, or brain.

In the presence of adenoma or malignant tumor, atrophy of the cortices of both adrenals occurs because their main secretory product is cortisol, which inhibits the pituitary secretion of ACTH. Thus, although the tumor continues to grow, the contralateral adrenal undergoes atrophy.

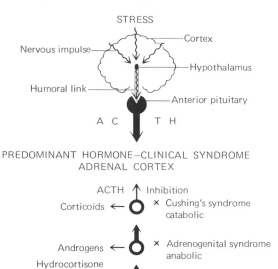

Figure 20—1. The hypothalamic pituitary-adrenocortical relationships in various adrenal syndromes.

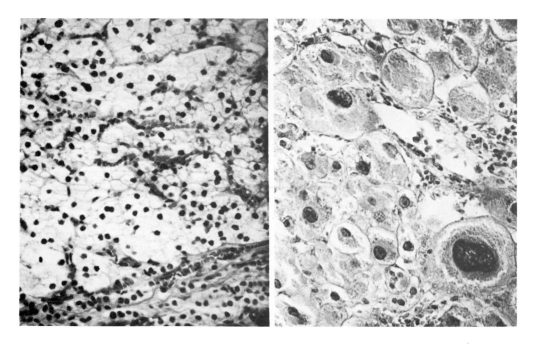

Figure 20—2. *Left:* Histologic appearance of a typical benign adenoma of the adrenal cortex made up of a large number of identical cells from the zona fasciculata removed from a 39-year-old female with Cushing's syndrome. *Right:* Section of an adenocarcinoma removed from a 36-year-old female with metastatic adenocarcinoma showing significant pleomorphism of the cells. Invasion of a large vein is not shown in this micrograph. Note that benign adenomas will occasionally have this appearance but without invasion of the bloodstream. (Reproduced, with permission, from Forsham PH: The adrenal cortex. In: *Textbook of Endocrinology,* 4th ed. Saunders, 1968.)

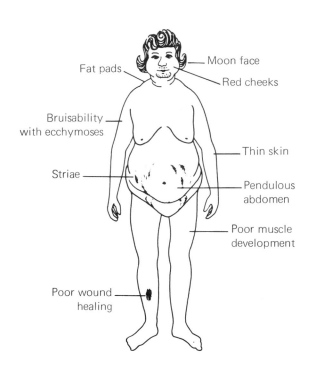

Figure 20—3. Drawing of a typical case of Cushing's syndrome showing the principal clinical features. (Reproduced, with permission, from Forsham PH: The adrenal cortex. In: *Textbook of Endocrinology*, 4th ed. Saunders, 1968.)

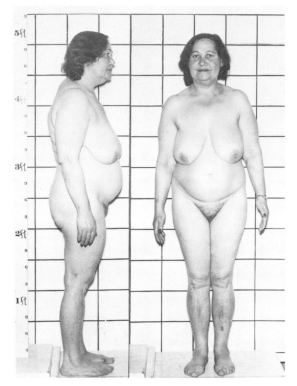

Figure 20—4. An actual case of Cushing's syndrome due to bilateral hyperplasia. Note the red moon face, receding hairline, buffalo hump over the seventh vertebra, protuberant abdomen, and inappropriately thin arms and legs. The combined adrenal weight was 20 g (as opposed to normal weight of 10 g).

Clinical Findings

A. Symptoms and Signs: (Figs 20—3 and 20—4.) The presence of at least 3 of the following strongly suggests Cushing's syndrome:

1. Obesity (with sparing of the extremities), moon face, and fat pads over the clavicles and the seventh cervical vertebra (buffalo hump). The abnormal distribution of fat is more characteristic than the actual body weight, which rarely exceeds 220 lb.

2. Striae (red and depressed) are seen over the abdomen and thighs. Festering ulcers of the skin may be present.

3. Weakness is marked, especially in the quadriceps femoris, making unaided rising from a chair impossible.

4. Hypertension is almost always present.

5. Osteoporosis is common, with back pain from compression fractures of the lumbar vertebrae as well as rib fractures.

6. In 80% of cases, a diabetic glucose tolerance curve is present, and in 20% there is an elevated plasma glucose.

7. The patient is irritable, has difficulty in sleeping, and may be psychotic.

8. To a variable extent there are features of the adrenogenital syndrome in cases of Cushing's syndrome—least marked in the case of adenoma, most severe with carcinoma, and to an intermediate degree with bilateral adrenocortical hyperplasia. They consist of recession of the hairline, hirsutism, small breasts, and generalized muscular overdevelopment with lowering of the voice. These relate to the excess of ketosteroids in general.

On the basis of the foregoing clinical findings alone, it is not possible to differentiate between bilateral adrenocortical hyperplasia, unilateral adenoma, and adenocarcinoma.

The most rapid onset is noted in cases due to an ectopic ACTH-producing tumor or adrenal adenocarcinoma. In the case of adenoma or adenocarcinoma, the tumor may be palpable.

B. Laboratory Findings: The white count is elevated to the range of 12—20 thousand/μl. Eosinophils are few in number or absent. Polycythemia is present in over half of cases, with the hemoglobin ranging from 14—16 g/100 ml. Anemia, however, is to be expected in association with ectopic ACTH-producing tumors.

Blood chemical analyses are apt to show increase in serum Na^+ and CO_2 and a decrease in serum K^+

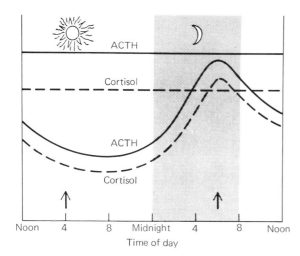

Figure 20–5. The circadian rhythm of ACTH and cortisol secretion which forms the basis of the dexamethasone suppression test for Cushing's syndrome.

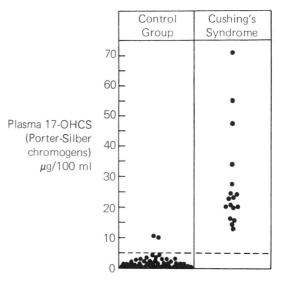

Figure 20–6. Results of the dexamethasone suppression test in obese individuals and patients with Cushing's syndrome. See text for procedure. 17-OHCS = 17-hydroxycorticosteroids. (Reproduced, with permission, from Pavlatos FC, Smilo RP, Forsham PH: A rapid screening test for Cushing's syndrome. JAMA 193:720, 1965.)

(metabolic alkalosis). A diabetic glucose tolerance curve is usually found.

1. Specific tests for Cushing's syndrome—

a. Suppression of ACTH by dexamethasone—In normal individuals, the ACTH level is twice as high at night as in the late afternoon (Fig 20–5). In patients with cortical hyperplasia, this diurnal variation does not occur. In those with cortical tumors producing hydrocortisone, there is suppression of ACTH. Thus, if dexamethasone is given at 11 p.m., ACTH is suppressed in normal persons but not in those with Cushing's syndrome. Dexamethasone is useful because it has 30 times the potency of hydrocortisone as an ACTH suppressant. It therefore can be used in such a small amount that it will have little effect upon the determination of circulating 17-hydroxycorticosteroids.

The procedure is to give 1–2 mg of dexamethasone by mouth at 11 p.m. with 0.2 g of pentobarbital to allay anxiety which might stimulate adrenocortical activity. Draw blood in the morning for measurement of plasma 11-hydroxycorticosteroids. If the level is below 5 μg/100 ml (normal is 5–20 μg/100 ml), Cushing's syndrome can be ruled out. If the value is above 10 μg/100 ml, Cushing's syndrome is present (Fig 20–6). A level in the range of 5–10 μg/100 ml is equivocal and the test should be repeated.

Women taking birth control pills will show elevated levels of plasma hydroxycorticosteroids because, as in pregnancy, the estrogen stimulates production of the cortisol-binding globulin. One must either discontinue medication for at least 3 weeks before giving the dexamethasone suppression test or obtain a baseline plasma 17-hydroxycorticosteroid level one morning shortly before the test. Normally, a greater than 50% suppression is observed.

b. Urinary 17-hydroxycorticosteroids and 17-ketosteroids—These constituents must be determined on a specimen collected for exactly 24 hours for comparison with normal levels (Table 20–1). In Cushing's syndrome, both 17-hydroxycorticosteroids and 17-ketosteroids are elevated if adrenal hyperplasia or adenocarcinoma is present; with adenoma, 17-ketosteroids remain normal or low. Since 17-hydroxycorticosteroids vary with body weight, a high level in an obese patient is significant only if the value (in mg) exceeds the body weight in pounds × 0.06.

c. Urinary cortisol level—Measure the urinary free cortisol level in a 24-hour specimen of urine. A value above 120 μg establishes the diagnosis of Cushing's syndrome.

2. Specific tests for differentiation of causes of Cushing's syndrome—

a. Plasma ACTH—If the diagnosis of Cushing's syndrome has been established, this test will differentiate between hyperplasia and tumor (Fig 20–7). Draw blood in the morning in a plastic syringe (glass absorbs ACTH). The blood must be stored in ice. The normal range is 40–100 pg/ml. A higher value indicates hyperplasia; a lower level means that tumor is present.

b. ACTH administration—Give ACTH (eg, Cortrosyn), 0.25–0.5 mg subcut. Collect blood at 1 and 2 hours for plasma hydroxycorticosteroid determinations. In the presence of an adenoma, there is usually a rise. With tumor, there is not.

c. 11-Deoxycortisol—A marked increase in the concentration of this substance in the urine suggests adenocarcinoma.

C. X-Ray Findings: Following catharsis, tomograms of the renal areas should be taken. The adrenals may be more clearly outlined if urographic medium

Hyperplasia   Adrenal tumor   Ectopic ACTH

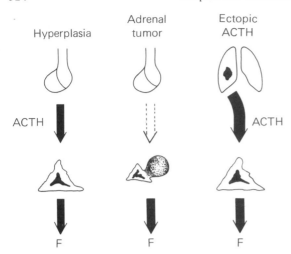

ACTH   ACTH

F   F   F

Figure 20–7. Schematic presentation of the pituitary-adrenal interrelationship in cases of hyperplasia, functional adrenocortical tumors, and ectopic ACTH syndrome. (Reproduced, with permission, from Forsham PH: The adrenal cortex. In: *Textbook of Endocrinology*, 4th ed. Saunders, 1968.)

Table 20–1. Normal "steroid" levels in plasma and urine.*

	Children	Adult Males	Adult Females
Plasma			
17-Hydroxycortico-steroids (μg/100 ml as cortisol)	5–20	5–20	5–20
Testosterone (ng/100 ml)	< 10	300–1200	30–120
Urine (mg/24 hours as cortisol or dehydroepiandrosterone†)			
17-Hydroxycortico-steroids (per kg body weight)	0.02–0.04	6–10	4–8
17-Ketogenic steroids‡	0.03–0.05	8–12	6–10
Cortisol (free)	1 μg/kg	20–120	20–120
17-Ketosteroids	Low, but rises to normal adult levels during puberty	8–20	5–15
Pregnanetriol		0.5–3	0.5–2.5

*There may be wide variations with different technics and as done by different laboratories.
†Except as noted in the case of cortisol in second column.
‡This artificially derived entity is used in many laboratories in lieu of 17-hydroxycorticosteroids.

has been given intravenously. Bilateral enlargement of the adrenals can usually be seen. When a tumor is present (Fig 20–8), it can be delineated by this method in almost 95% of cases. Atrophy of the contralateral adrenal is usually evident and diagnostic. Osteoporosis may be noted incidentally.

Adrenal venography or arteriography, while useful to show extremely small tumors, is usually not necessary since tumors causing Cushing's syndrome are in most cases large, varying in weight from 10–80 g. The size of the sella turcica should be determined by radiographic means. Enlargement of the sella may indicate the presence of a chromophobe adenoma.

Differential Diagnosis

An adrenal cyst may present as a suprarenal mass with displacement of the kidney on tomography. There is often some curvilinear calcification in its capsule. It is devoid of endocrinologic function.

A tumor or cyst of the upper pole of the kidney may give the appearance of a suprarenal mass, but excretory urograms will reveal the calyceal distortion of a space-occupying lesion while renal angiography will show its intrinsic nature.

Fluid in the cardiac end of the stomach may appear as a round opacity in the left suprarenal area on a plain x-ray film. It disappears on an upright film. Tomography will also settle the question.

Enlargement of the liver or spleen may displace the kidney downward, but physical examination and tomography should make the differentiation.

Complications

Hypertension may lead to cardiac failure or stroke. Diabetes may be a problem but is usually mild. Increased susceptibility to infections may be noted. Compression fractures of osteoporotic vertebrae and

rib fractures (often remarkably painless) may develop. Renal stone is not uncommon as a result of leaching of calcium from the bones. Gastric (stress) ulcer may become a problem. Psychosis is not uncommon. Chromophobe adenoma develops in up to 20% of treated patients.

Treatment

A. Bilateral Adrenocortical Hyperplasia: A significant reduction in total adrenocortical mass must be accomplished using the following methods: (1) Remove any anterior pituitary tumor (Cushing's disease) that is producing a fixed or increased amount of ACTH. The best treatment for an ACTH-producing pituitary tumor is transsphenoidal hypophysectomy. (2) Total bilateral adrenalectomy will produce Addison's disease, but this can be easily controlled by substitution therapy. (3) Irradiation of a known or suspected basophilic or chromophobe pituitary tumor requires 5000 rads delivered by linear accelerator or cobalt. The success rate with this treatment is 20–60%, though a 100% successful response is claimed when heavy particle irradiation (medical cyclotron) is delivered.

Total bilateral adrenalectomy is the preferred method of treatment for hyperplasia, but in 5% of cases ectopic adrenocortical tissue will lead to recrudescence of the disease. Following total adrenalectomy, growth of a chromophobe pituitary adenoma is observed in up to 20% of cases, leading to excessive ACTH secretion (Nelson's syndrome). This may be prevented or slowed by irradiation of the pituitary. For

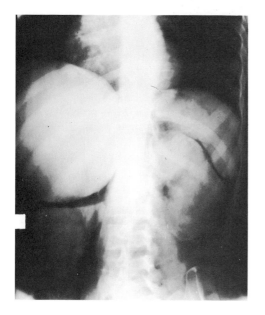

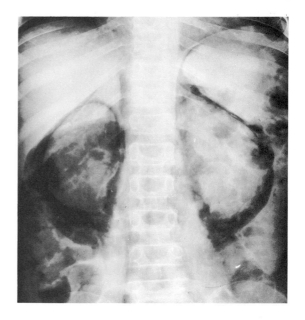

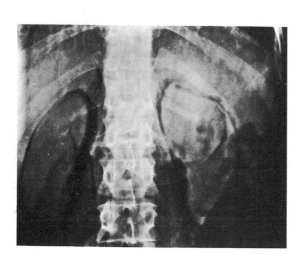

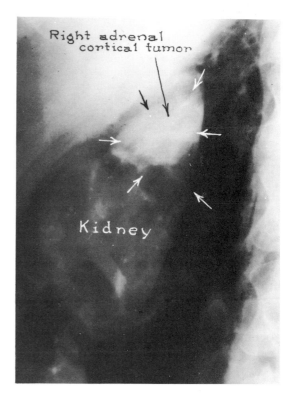

Figure 20—8. The adrenal gland and retroperitoneal insufflation. *Above left:* Pneumogram showing large androgenic tumor of right adrenal. Upper pole of kidney saucerized by pressure; kidney displaced downward. Spleen seen above left kidney. *Above right:* Pneumogram delineating small right adrenocortical tumor. *Below left:* Presacral oxygen showing large pheochromocytoma overlying upper half of left kidney. Upper renal pole has been displaced laterally. *Below right:* Pneumogram showing a large right adrenal tumor. (These illustrations show tumors delineated by retroperitoneal oxygen insufflation. This technic is rarely used today, but the x-rays show the reader what they look like.)

bilateral adrenalectomy, 2 surgical routes seem feasible: an anterior transverse transperitoneal (chevron) incision can be made just below the costal margin, or, with the patient in the prone position, both twelfth ribs are resected and the adrenals exposed. The latter route is associated with a lower morbidity rate.

1. Preoperative preparation—Inasmuch as removal of the source of excessive cortisol will inevitably lead to temporary or permanent adrenal insufficiency, it is of the utmost importance to administer cortisol preoperatively and to continue substitution therapy after surgery to control Addison's disease. In the postoperative period, the dose is tapered downward until the patient can be controlled by oral medication.

2. Postoperative status—After removal of the source of excess ACTH and while the patient is receiving a high dose of hydrocortisone in excess of the usual daily output of approximately 20 mg, the patient feels moderately well. It is when one approaches the upper limits of the physiologic dose of hydrocortisone that he may develop complaints of nausea, abdominal pain resembling that of pancreatitis (which in fact may occur), and extreme weakness. Thus, it is important to gradually reduce the steroid substitution over a period of several days.

3. Follow-up—Since one-third of administered cortisol is found in the urine, it follows that, while substitution therapy is being given, no decision can be made about the status of adrenocortical secretion. It is necessary to stop the usual cortisol replacement and give 1 mg of dexamethasone daily for 2 days while covering with additional sodium chloride in order to obtain a valid determination of 24-hour urinary 17-hydroxycorticosteroid levels.

Urinary 17-hydroxycorticosteroids or 17-ketogenic steroids should be measured at intervals of 3–6 months. The patient should cease taking cortisol temporarily and be given 1 mg of dexamethasone orally for only 2 days—one before and one after the urine collection—accompanied by a high sodium intake, in order to determine whether any reactivation of residual cortical tissue occurs. Plasma ACTH measurements, which are usually high when the patient is on standard replacement therapy, will show a significant further rise if a chromophobe adenoma develops.

A plain film of the sella turcica (anteroposterior and lateral) or, better still, tomograms of the fossa, when compared with preoperative films, will reveal an expanding tumor of the chromophobe variety. This study should be done every 6 months until the patient has remained asymptomatic for 1 year, especially if he shows increased melanin pigmentation due to excess ACTH and MSH secretion.

B. Adenoma and Adenocarcinoma: Preoperative preparation is the same as discussed above for treatment of bilateral hyperplasia because, with removal of one adrenal and the invariable atrophy of the contralateral gland, immediate hypoadrenalism is the rule.

1. Surgical technic—Depending on the size of the tumor and the patient's body habitus, the lesion can be approached through the flank with resection of the eleventh or twelfth rib. For large tumors, a transthoracic transdiaphragmatic incision affords ideal exposure of the mass.

2. Postoperative treatment and follow-up—Because of atrophy of the contralateral adrenal, postoperative substitution therapy must be designed to encourage return of function of the atrophic gland. Hydrocortisone is given orally in a dosage of 10 mg 3 times daily initially and reduced within 2 weeks to 10 mg daily given at 7 or 8 a.m. This may be necessary for 1 month to 2 years depending on the rate of recovery of the remaining adrenal.

Prognosis

Medical control after bilateral adrenalectomy is usually quite successful. Removal of an adenoma offers an excellent prognosis.

The outlook for the patient with adenocarcinoma is poor. In such cases, the use of the antineoplastic drug mitotane (o,p'DDD; Lysodren) in doses of up to 30 g orally daily reduces the symptoms and signs of Cushing's syndrome but does little to prolong survival.

ADRENAL ANDROGENIC SYNDROMES

These conditions are more common in females. Congenital bilateral adrenal hyperplasia and tumors, both benign and malignant, may be observed. They all represent an excessive or abnormal expression of

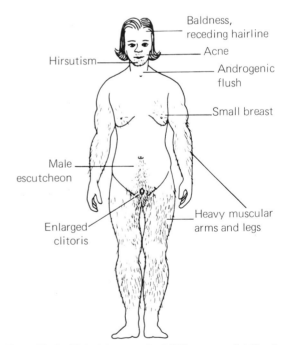

Figure 20–9. Clinical features of a full-blown case of virilism in a female with adrenogenital syndrome. (Reproduced, with permission, from Forsham PH: The adrenal cortex. In: *Textbook of Endocrinology,* 4th ed. Saunders, 1968.)

androgen excess. In contrast to Cushing's syndrome, which is protein catabolic, the androgenic syndromes are strongly anabolic. In untreated cases, there is a marked recession of the hairline, increased beard growth, and excessive growth of pubic and sexual hair in general in both sexes. In the male, there is enlargement of the penis, usually with atrophic testes; in the female (Fig 20–9), enlargement of the clitoris occurs, with atrophy of the breasts and amenorrhea. There is an increase in muscle mass and a definite decrease in fat content, leading to a powerful but trim figure. The voice becomes deeper, particularly in the female, and this feature is irreversible since it is due to enlargement of the larynx. The psyche of these patients is often deranged. In both sexes there is increased physical aggressiveness and libido.

1. CONGENITAL BILATERAL ANDROGENIC HYPERPLASIA

Pathophysiology

A congenital defect in certain adrenal enzymes results in the production of abnormal steroids (Fig 20–10), causing **pseudohermaphroditism** in females and **macrogenitosomia** in males. It is associated with excess androgen production in utero. While the Müllerian duct structures (eg, ovaries, uterus, and vagina) develop normally, the excess androgen exerts a masculinizing effect on the urogenital sinus and genital tubercle so that the vagina is connected to the urethra, which, in turn, opens at the base of an enlarged clitoris. The labia are often hypertrophied. Externally, then, the appearance is that of severe hypospadias with cryptorchism.

The adrenal cortex secretes mostly anabolic and androgenic steroids, leading to various degrees of cortisol deficiency depending on the nature of the enzyme block (Fig 20–10). This in turn increases the secretion of ACTH, which causes hyperplasia of both adrenal cortices. This may be accompanied by pigmentation due to an excess of ACTH associated with relative lack of cortisol. In extreme cases, adrenocortical insufficiency associated with hypertension due to excess 11-deoxycorticosterone may be observed.

In adult females, increased androgenicity manifested by hirsutism and amenorrhea may rarely develop after puberty, but this seldom leads to virilism in middle age. In such cases, one is dealing with a form of acquired mild enzyme abnormality of the adrenals known as **benign androgenic overactivity of the adrenal cortices.**

Clinical Findings

A. Symptoms and Signs: In the newborn female, the appearance of the external genitalia resembles severe hypospadias with cryptorchism. The male infant may appear quite normal at the outset. The earlier in intrauterine life the fetus has been exposed to excess

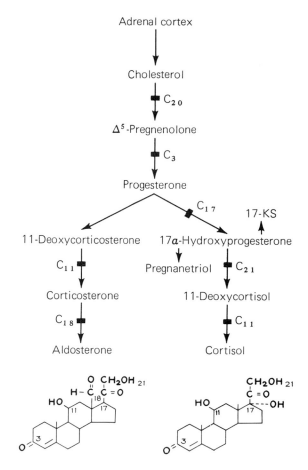

Figure 20–10. Deficiencies in hydroxylases and related enzymes in the adrenal cortex, giving rise to typical cases of adrenogenital syndrome.

androgen, the more marked the anomalies.

In untreated cases, hirsutism, excess muscle mass, and, eventually, amenorrhea are the rule. Breast development is poor. In males, growth of the phallus is excessive. The testes are often atrophic because of inhibition of gonadotropin secretion by the elevated androgens. On rare occasion, hyperplastic adrenocortical rests in the testes make them large and firm. In most instances, there is aspermia after puberty.

In both males and females with androgenic hyperplasia, growth rate is initially increased so that they are taller than their classmates. At about age 9–10 years, premature fusion of the epiphyses caused by excess androgen causes termination of growth so that these patients are short as adults. In both sexes, there is increased aggressiveness and libido which, particularly in some boys, present social and disciplinary problems.

B. Laboratory Findings: Urinary 17-ketosteroids are higher than normal for sex and age (Table 20–1). Urinary pregnanetriol is elevated early, and this is a more sensitive test than 17-ketosteroid levels since pregnanetriol is the precursor of the androgenic steroids. The most sensitive indicator of androgenic activ-

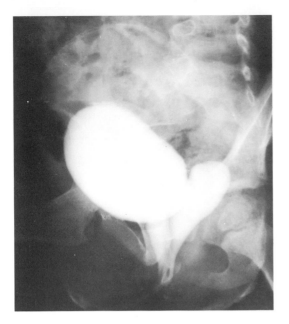

Figure 20–11. Urogenital sinus in congenital virilizing cortical hyperplasia. Oblique urethrogram showing connection of vagina with distal urethra. (Courtesy of F Hinman, Jr.)

corticoid dexamethasone, 0.5–1.5 mg orally at 11 p.m. every night, thereby suppressing the adrenal cortex at the time of its greatest activity, ie, from 2–8 a.m.

After puberty, it is feasible to surgically separate the vaginal opening from the urethra and cause it to open in the normal position on the perineum. If frequent clitoral erections occur, its resection or, preferably, recession should be considered. Judicious administration of estrogens or birth control pills will feminize the figure in pseudohermaphrodites and improve their psyche considerably.

Prognosis

Provided the condition is recognized early and ACTH suppression is begun even before surgical repair of the genital anomaly is started, the outlook for normal linear growth and development is excellent. Failure to do this early will inevitably result in stunted growth and a propensity to coronary artery disease, with early death due to myocardial infarction. In some female pseudohermaphrodites, menses may start after treatment, and conception and childbirth can occur when the anatomic abnormalities are minimal or have been surgically repaired.

ity is elevation of plasma 17-hydroxyprogesterone, and this test will prove particularly useful in children as it becomes more generally available in the future. The buccal smear is positive for Barr bodies in females. Chromosome studies are normal.

C. X-Ray Findings: X-rays will reveal acceleration of bone age. A lateral cystourethrogram may visualize the vagina as well as the urethra and bladder (Fig 20–11).

D. Instrumental Examination: Urethroscopy may permit visualization of the point at which the vagina opens into the posterior wall of the urethra. The vaginal tract can often be entered and the cervix seen.

Differential Diagnosis

A number of congenital anomalies that affect the development of the external genitalia resemble adrenal androgenic syndrome. These include (1) severe hypospadias with cryptorchism, (2) female pseudohermaphroditism of the nonadrenal type (caused by administration of androgens or progestational compounds during the pregnancy), (3) male pseudohermaphroditism, and (4) true hermaphroditism. These children show no hormonal abnormalities, however, and accelerated bone age and maturation do not occur.

Treatment

It is imperative to make the diagnosis early. Treatment of the underlying cause is medical. The basis of treatment is to suppress excessive ACTH secretion, thus minimizing excess androgenicity. This is accomplished by giving a single dose of the long-acting gluco-

2. ADRENOCORTICAL TUMORS

The differentiation between hyperplasia (a medical problem) and adrenocortical tumor (a surgical problem) is by means of the **dexamethasone suppression test.** The procedure is as follows: A 24-hour urine specimen is collected and 17-ketosteroids measured. The patient is then given dexamethasone, 2 g orally 4 times a day. On the second day, another 24-hour urine specimen is taken and the concentration of 17-ketosteroids is measured. If the second specimen contains less than half the 17-ketosteroids found in the first specimen, adrenal activity is suppressible and the condition is due to hyperplasia. Suppression does not occur in cases of adrenal overactivity due to tumor.

Localization of the tumor is best accomplished by excretory urography with tomograms (Fig 20–8). In these cases, there is no atrophy of the contralateral adrenal because there is no marked elevation of 17-hydroxycorticosteroids. Therefore, preoperative cortisol medication can be minimal, eg, 50 mg cortisol phosphate just before induction of anesthesia. The tumor can readily be removed through the flank. In contrast to patients with Cushing's syndrome, hemostasis is easy to obtain and wound healing is normal.

Adenocarcinoma is a highly malignant tumor that metastasizes to the liver, lungs, and brain. Successive determinations of urinary 17-ketosteroids will reveal the completeness of the resection and the presence or later development of metastases.

When metastases have occurred, hyperandrogenicity can be combated by giving up to 30 g of mitotane (o,p'DDD; Lysodren) orally daily. Unfortunately, this drug only temporarily halts tumor growth, and fluorouracil (5-FU; Efudex) is not successful either. X-ray treatment in large doses may postpone the inevitable death of these patients.

Prognosis

The removal of a benign adenoma is curative. Patients with adenocarcinoma rarely live more than 1 year after diagnosis—partly because diagnosis is delayed an average of 7 months after onset of symptoms.

THE HYPERTENSIVE, HYPOKALEMIC SYNDROME
(Primary Aldosteronism)

Excessive production of aldosterone, due either to aldosteronoma or to spontaneous bilateral hyperplasia of the zona glomerulosa of the adrenal cortex, leads to the combination of hypertension, hypokalemia, and, in some instances, diabetes insipidus. The low serum potassium may lead to muscular weakness with fully conscious collapse and postural hypotension due to baroreceptor paralysis, leading to syncope. A syndrome resembling diabetes insipidus may occur as a result of reversible damage to the renal collecting tubules. The alkalosis may produce tetany.

Pathophysiology

Excessive aldosterone, acting on most cell membranes in the body, produces typical changes in the distal renal tubule and the small bowel whereby there is urinary potassium loss and sodium reabsorption together with an increased renal hydrogen ion secretion. This results in potassium depletion, metabolic alkalosis, increased plasma sodium concentration, and hypervolemia. Potassium depletion affects baroreceptors, so that postural fall in blood pressure no longer results in reflex tachycardia. With low serum potassium, the concentrating ability of the kidney is lowered and the tubules no longer respond to the administration of vasopressin by increased reabsorption of water. Finally, potassium lack increases carbohydrate intolerance by impairment of insulin release secondary to potassium depletion in about 50% of cases.

Plasma renin and, secondarily, plasma angiotensin are depressed by excess aldosterone, presumably as a result of blood volume expansion (Fig 20–12). Early in the course of excess aldosterone production, there may be hypertension with a normal serum potassium. Later, potassium will be low as well, and this suggests the diagnosis.

Clinical Findings

A. Symptoms and Signs: Headaches are common, nocturia is invariably present, and rare episodes of paralysis occur with very low serum potassium levels. Numbness and tingling of the extremities are related to

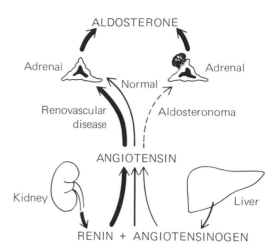

Figure 20–12. The angiotensin-aldosterone relationships in a case of aldosteronoma and hypertension due to renal vascular disease. (Reproduced, with permission, from Forsham PH: The adrenal cortex. In: *Textbook of Endocrinology,* 4th ed. Saunders, 1968.)

alkalosis that may lead to tetany. Hypertension is of varying degrees of severity. Orthostatic hypotension is common. Inappropriate control of vasomotor tone is usually demonstrable. Feel the patient's pulse while he is standing, have him crouch and straighten up, and take the pulse again. In a normal person, the pulse will be slower the second time; in the presence of hyperaldosteronism, it is not.

Ophthalmoscopic examination usually shows normal vessels inconsistent with the degree of hypertension. Unless acute heart failure is present, there is no edema. The Chvostek sign is often positive.

B. Laboratory Findings: Before the tests outlined below are done, one must ascertain that the patient is not taking oral contraceptives or other estrogen preparations since these may increase renin and angiotensin levels and therefore aldosterone levels, thus raising the blood pressure artificially. Withdrawal of these medications for 1 week is mandatory. Also, if the patient is taking a salt-restricted diet, aldosterone is normally elevated. Diuretics must be discontinued since they lower blood volume and induce secondary aldosteronism and hypokalemia.

Before serum electrolytes are measured, the patient is loaded with 6 g of salt for at least 2 days. This will furnish exchangeable sodium in the distal tubule and allow potassium to exchange with sodium, thus clearly revealing the electrolyte imbalance. Serum potassium must also be replenished because a very low level of this ion may decrease the secretory rate of aldosterone. If aldosterone excess is truly present, serum sodium will be slightly elevated and CO_2 increased, whereas serum potassium will be very low, eg, 3 mEq/liter or less.

Potassium wasting is considered to be established if the urinary potassium level is > 50 mEq/liter/24 hours but the serum potassium level is low (3 mEq/liter or less).

Definitive diagnosis rests on demonstration of an elevated urine or plasma aldosterone level or a positive desoxycorticosterone acetate test (Table 20–2). Before aldosterone is measured, the patient should be loaded with salt (6 g/day) to avoid a decrease in plasma volume, which by itself raises the aldosterone level. In the presence of hyperaldosteronism, urinary aldosterone is more than 10 μg/day after suppression with desoxycorticosterone acetate.

C. X-Ray Findings: Tomograms are of little value because aldosteronomas are too small to be seen. Visualization may, however, be accomplished by adrenal venography. The adrenal veins are catheterized and a contrast medium is injected. This examination will reveal a definite tumor blush on the affected side. Since these tumors are only 1–2 cm in diameter, this procedure is essential for their diagnosis (Fig 20–13).

Differential Diagnosis

Secondary hyperaldosteronism may accompany renovascular hypertension. An abdominal bruit will suggest this condition initially. This too is associated with hypokalemic alkalosis. Differentiation requires estimation of blood volume and serum sodium. In primary aldosteronism, both tend to be elevated. In the secondary form, both may be low.

Essential hypertension does not cause changes in the electrolyte pattern. Definitive tests for hyperaldosteronism are negative.

The diagnosis of pheochromocytoma (see below) is based on catecholamine measurements, which in patients suffering from paroxysmal hypertension are not elevated during normotensive intervals. Careful admin-

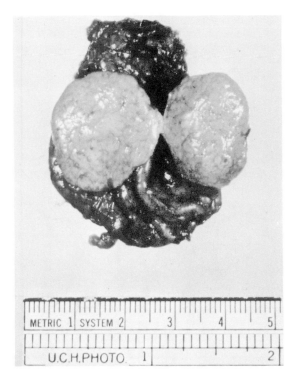

Figure 20–13. A typical canary yellow aldosteronoma associated with the syndrome of hypertension, hyperkalemia, and alkalosis. Note the relatively small size of this tumor compared to other types of adrenocortical neoplasms.

istration of glucagon, 1 mg IV, will cause a rise in both blood pressure and catecholamine levels. Aldosterone levels are normal.

Cushing's syndrome is associated with hypertension, but physical examination and appropriate hormonal assays will establish the diagnosis.

Treatment

A. Aldosteronoma: If localization of the tumor has been established, only that adrenal need be removed. A flank incision with resection of the eleventh or twelfth rib will afford good exposure. It is of interest that two-thirds of adenomas are in the left adrenal.

B. Bilateral Hyperplasia: Most authorities recommend total resection of both adrenals since the fall in blood pressure is usually only temporary and electrolyte imbalance may continue with subtotal resection. Total adrenalectomy relieves hypertension in 60–70% of patients, and addisonian replacement therapy is so satisfactory that total ablation is the treatment of choice.

C. Medical Treatment: If surgery must be postponed or the hypertension is mild in an older person, one may treat medically with spironolactone (Aldactone), 25–50 mg orally 4 times daily.

Prognosis

In rare cases, hypotension may persist for as long

Table 20–2. Desoxycorticosterone acetate test for primary aldosteronism.

Patient preparation
(1) Withdraw all hypotensive drugs for 1 week.
(2) Give 6+ g of salt for 3 days.
(3) Give 100 mEq (7 g) of potassium chloride for 3 days.

Test procedure
(1) Collect 24-hour urine sample for aldosterone determination.
(2) Give 5 mg of desoxycorticosterone acetate (eg, Percorten Acetate) IM daily for 3 days.
(3) On third day, repeat 24-hour urine test for aldosterone.

Results (aldosterone concentration in urine, μg/day)

	Normal	Primary Aldosteronism	Secondary Aldosteronism
Control day	9	18	25
Third day of suppression	3	17	9

as 2 years after removal of the adenoma. This can be controlled by increased sodium intake. Following removal of an adenomatous adrenal, the remission rate exceeds 85%, whereas the results with bilateral nodular hyperplasia are less favorable.

DISEASES OF THE ADRENAL MEDULLA

PHEOCHROMOCYTOMA

Pheochromocytoma, derived from the neural crest, is one of the surgically curable hypertensive syndromes. Pheochromocytoma accounts for fewer than 1% of cases of hypertension, but it is readily diagnosed if the possibility is kept in mind. It usually occurs spontaneously but may be a familial disease inherited as an autosomal dominant trait. There is no sex predilection. Rarely, pheochromocytoma occurs as part of a pluriglandular syndrome including medullary carcinoma of the thyroid, hyperparathyroidism (adenoma or hyperplasia), Cushing's syndrome with excess ACTH, and other exceedingly rare concurrences.

Neuroectodermal syndromes, including neurofibromatosis, are found in up to 5% of patients with pheochromocytoma. The tumor is bilateral or extra-adrenal in 10% of cases in adults and in an even greater percentage in children.

Clinical Findings

A. Symptoms and Signs: Hypertension is both systolic and diastolic. The appearance of the retinal vessels on ophthalmoscopic examination is commensurate with the severity of the hypertension and the duration of the disease state. Hypertension may be either sustained and indistinguishable from ordinary blood pressure elevation, or paroxysmal, coming on for variable lengths of time and then subsiding to normal levels. Such attacks are usually precipitated by trigger mechanisms of various sorts, eg, emotional upsets or straining at stool.

Headache is a frequent complaint and is commensurate in severity with the degree of hypertension. Increased sweating without appropriate causes such as exertion or environmental heat resembles the phenomenon seen during menopause and may be accompanied by flushing or blanching. Tachycardia with palpitations occurs mainly as a consequence of epinephrine excess. Postural hypotension is a frequent finding, partly as a result of diminished plasma volume and ganglionic blocking of normal pressor pathways by excess catecholamines.

Weight loss is common, partly because of the anorexia that results from elevated blood glucose and fatty acid levels—the former caused by increased glycogeno-

lysis and the latter by the increased lipolysis induced by elevated catecholamine levels.

Decreased gastrointestinal motility occurs, leading to nausea and vomiting, especially in children, and constipation. This effect is a direct pharmacologic consequence of excessive circulating catecholamines. Episodes of psychic instability verging on hysteria are frequent and are probably due to increased concentrations of catecholamines and other neurotransmitters in the brain, although circulating catecholamines penetrate the blood-brain barrier to only a limited extent.

In the 5% of patients that have associated neuroectodermal disease, café au lait spots are found with smooth outlines ("coast of California") rather than the ragged ones ("coast of Maine") that occur only with the unrelated fibrous dysplasia of bone. In neuroectodermal disease, telangiectasia and, rarely, cerebellar involvement coexist.

In a very few patients, the growth is palpable. Even if it is not palpable, pressure over the site of the tumor may cause an exacerbation of hypertension. Thus, in a tumor embedded in the bladder, blood pressure rise occurs with micturition.

B. Laboratory Findings: The hematocrit is usually elevated, and the white cell count is high, with few lymphocytes. Serum proteins are elevated. The fasting plasma glucose level is often elevated and accompanied by a diabetic glucose tolerance curve.

Urinary catecholamine levels must be measured. The patient must discontinue all medication except diuretics, digitalis, and barbiturates for at least 2 days. An exact 24-hour urine collection, in a bottle containing 15 ml of 6 N hydrochloric acid, is then obtained. The test must be performed within 48 hours. The normal limits are shown in Table 20–3.

In individual cases, epinephrine or norepinephrine (or both) may be elevated, but elevation of only epinephrine suggests that the tumor is in the adrenal medulla, in ectopic medullary tissue, or in the organ of Zuckerkandl, since the methylating enzyme necessary for transforming norepinephrine to epinephrine is present only in medullary tissue.

Urinary normetanephrine, metanephrine, and vanilmandelic acid (VMA) are breakdown products of

Table 20–3. Catecholamines in urine and plasma.*

Urine
Norepinephrine: 10–100 μg/24 hours
Epinephrine: Up to 20 μg/24 hours
Normetanephrine and metanephrine: < 1.5 mg/24 hours
Vanilmandelic acid (VMA): 2–9 mg/24 hours

Plasma
Norepinephrine: 0.1–0.2 μg/liter
Epinephrine: 0.03–0.05 μg/liter

*The values listed represent the means of the normal ranges, which vary for each laboratory.

epinephrine and norepinephrine. Whereas less than 5% of secreted catecholamines appear as such in the urine, over 50% appear as metabolites, and these are usually independent of any medication taken by the patient. Before collection of urine for measurement of VMA, the patient must have no vanilla ice cream, chocolate, coffee, tea, or citrus fruits for at least 48 hours. The range of normal values is shown in Table 20–3.

If estimations of both urinary catecholamines and VMA are performed, the diagnostic accuracy is 98%. In patients with paroxysmal hypertension, the urine must be collected during an attack. A spot urine specimen obtained during a brief paroxysm is suitable for determination of catecholamines and VMA, which may be compared to the amount of simultaneously determined creatinine. Since the average urinary excretion of creatinine per 24 hours is 1.4 g, a finding of 0.2 g of creatinine in the aliquot would mean that the amount of catecholamines and VMA should be multiplied by 7 to afford a rough estimate of the 24-hour excretion of these substances.

As a rule, a low ratio of VMA to catecholamines favors the presence of a large tumor; a high ratio favors the presence of a small one.

If pheochromocytoma as a cause of hypertension is suspected in a patient who may be in a period of remission (normotensive), excessive catecholamine secretion may be induced by the glucagon test. Give 1 mg of glucagon subcut. If pheochromocytoma is present, both blood pressure and catecholamine levels will rise markedly. A hormonal assay can then be done.

C. X-Ray Findings: Preoperative localization by x-ray may be attempted but is of limited importance since at least 10% of the tumors are multiple and require direct exploration. Since the tumors are often quite large (Fig 20–14), tomograms with or without excretory urograms often reveal the tumor (Fig 20–15 left).

A retrograde arteriogram (Fig 20–15 right) or venogram will reveal small or multiple tumors. Determination of plasma catecholamine concentrations at different levels during catheterization of the vena cava is quite helpful as a means of localizing ectopic tumors.

Differential Diagnosis

Thyrotoxicosis may be suggested because of the marked hypermetabolism, nervousness, and weight loss. However, normal thyroid indices, constipation rather than diarrhea, and a low rather than high blood lymphocyte count (as seen with pheochromocytoma) rule out a diagnosis of thyrotoxicosis.

Diabetes mellitus must always be suspected because of the elevated fasting plasma glucose. In the presence of pheochromocytoma, epinephrine directly inhibits insulin secretion from the beta cells while transforming liver glycogen to glucose by stimulating the process of glycogenolysis. Only persistence of hyperglycemia after removal of the pheochromocytoma demonstrates whether permanent diabetes mellitus is present.

Organic heart disease is often suggested by the

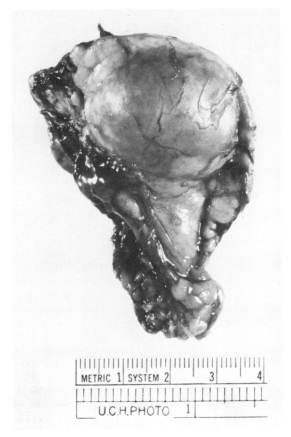

Figure 20–14. A typical large pheochromocytoma. Removal was followed by complete remission of hypertension.

clinical findings, including loud cardiac murmurs. Again, elimination of the hypertension must be established before a definitive diagnosis can be made inasmuch as many murmurs disappear following surgery.

Treatment

The sooner hypertension can be abolished, the better for the patient. Vascular accidents are common, and the longer the disease exists the more likely the hypertension is to become irreversible.

A. Preoperative Management: Oral administration of an alpha-adrenergic blocking agent such as phenoxybenzamine (Dibenzylene), 40–200 mg/day in 2 divided doses, will control the blood pressure. If this can be started at least 3 weeks before surgery, the dangerous hypovolemia that usually exists can be corrected. Hypovolemia has been noted in up to 80% of cases and may cause fatal postoperative vascular collapse. Blood and plasma volumes must be checked and normal volumes restored before surgery. For fine adjustment of blood pressure before and during induction of anesthesia, when the danger of development of hypertensive crisis is greatest, the alpha-adrenergic blocking agent phentolamine (Regitine), 5 mg in 200 ml of 5% dextrose in water, may be infused IV at a rate adjusted to maintain the blood pressure at a nearly normal level.

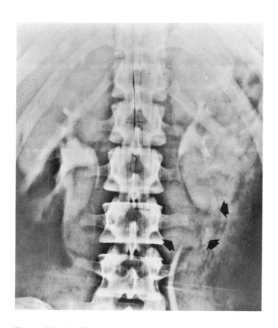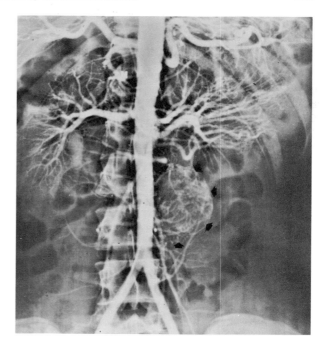

Figure 20—15. Extra-adrenal pheochromocytoma. *Left:* Excretory urogram showing normal kidneys but a soft tissue mass just below and medial to the left kidney. *Right:* Angiogram, same patient. Vascular mass below left renal arteries.

B. Anesthetic Management: Thiopental (Pentothal) sodium and nitrous oxide combined are used with curare or other muscle relaxants as necessary for muscle relaxation since they do not raise catecholamine secretion as some other agents do.

C. Operation: Since 15% of tumors (even more in children) may be multiple and ectopic, a transperitoneal approach is recommended. An anterior transverse (subcostal) incision affords the best exposure. When a tumor is found in one adrenal, early ligation of the adrenal vein is important if sudden blood pressure elevation from handling the tumor is to be avoided. Intravenous phentolamine during surgery will control such an eventuality. After removal of the tumor, there is always a fall in systemic blood pressure of variable severity and duration. This can be minimized by preoperative restoration of blood volume (as discussed above). Hypotension should be treated by infusion of norepinephrine or related pressor agents. If hypertension still persists, hydrocortisone phosphate, 100 mg IV, may reestablish the pressure or response. Only when both adrenals are removed is there an absolute need for cortisol replacement.

D. Immediate Postoperative Care: Two to 3 days following surgery, a 24-hour urinary VMA level should be obtained. If it is normal, similar tests every 6 months need be done only in patients with a family history of pheochromocytoma. If the VMA value is still elevated immediately after surgery, another site of pheochromocytoma exists. Malignancies (and, therefore, functional metastases) are very rare.

E. Medical Treatment: Drugs that limit the production of catecholamines such as alpha-methyl-

tyrosine, while often effective in decreasing catecholamine production, are not in general use because they do not prevent tumor growth and because numerous side-effects, including anxiety, sedation, diarrhea, lactation, and tremor, are reported. Antineoplastic drugs to inhibit the growth of metastases have been only moderately successful.

Prognosis

In general, the prognosis is good. With better understanding of the disease, surgical deaths are now rare. Blood pressure will fall to normal levels in about half of patients. In most of the remainder, blood pressure may remain elevated. In rare cases, the patient will become worse as a consequence of secondary vascular changes which have irreversibly activated various pressure systems. Although this persistent hypertension can be adequately controlled with medical therapy, it is much better to prevent this state of affairs by early diagnosis and operation.

OTHER TUMORS OF SYMPATHETIC ORIGIN

Because it is derived embryologically from the neural crest, the adrenal medulla is sometimes the site of tumors other than pheochromocytoma. Neuroblastoma (see Chapter 18) is the mother cell of either the chromaffin cell that gives rise to pheochromocytoma or the sympathetic ganglion cell that gives rise to ganglioneuroma. More primitive cell types in this line lead to ganglioneuroblastoma and neuroblastoma. The most common tumors of this type are neuroblastomas* and ganglioneuromas. Neuroblastomas are larger than ganglioneuromas and are found most frequently in children at any site along the neural crest, including the adrenal medulla, retroperitoneum, behind the pleura, in the brain, and in the sympathetic ganglia. They are quite malignant and prone to local invasion, and metastasize to local lymph nodes, liver, spleen, and brain.

Clinical Findings

A. Symptoms and Signs: Tumors of sympathetic origin are common in children but rare in adults. They present as a large, firm, fixed mass in the upper abdomen, and diarrhea is a common complaint. Hypertension is usually present. A familial incidence is characteristic of neuroblastoma.

B. Laboratory Findings: Anemia is usually present. Urinary VMA levels are elevated in a high percentage of cases. Bone marrow aspiration may reveal tumor cells.

C. X-Ray Findings: A plain film of the abdomen will reveal punctate calcification in the tumor in 50% of cases. Excretory urograms show that the otherwise normal kidney is markedly displaced. An inferior venacavogram may demonstrate occlusion of the vein by tumor, which is an indication for preoperative radiotherapy. A bone survey may reveal metastases to the skull or long bones.

*Neuroblastoma is discussed also in Chapter 18.

Differential Diagnosis

Wilms's tumor (nephroblastoma) is also a disease of childhood. Excretory urograms reveal distortion of the calyces, which is not the case with neuroblastoma. Urinary VMA levels are normal with Wilms's tumor but elevated in neuroblastoma. In the latter, excretory urograms may show diffuse punctate calcification of the tumor which displaces an otherwise normal kidney.

Hydronephrosis may also present as a mass in the flank. In infants and small children, it may transilluminate. Excretory urograms usually reveal the hydronephrotic nature of the mass. Sonography will settle the issue.

Treatment

Radical transperitoneal resection as early as possible followed by radiation therapy and the administration of antitumor agents is the treatment method of choice, but cures are rare. After operation and x-ray as well as medical treatment, there is a lessening of hypertension and diarrhea and the patient may become asymptomatic. The more localized the tumor and the younger the patient, the more hopeful the otherwise poor prognosis. In patients with increased levels of urinary catecholamines or VMA, such tests serve as an excellent way of following progress.

Prognosis

About 90% of patients die within a year. However, children less than 1 year old have a survival rate of 60%, and 80% survive if the tumor is localized.

•   •   •

References

Cushing's Syndrome & Adrenocortical Tumors

Bailey RE: Periodic hormonogenesis—a new phenomenon: Periodicity in function of a hormone-producing tumor in man. J Clin Endocrinol 32:317, 1971.

Baxter JD, Forsham PH: Tissue effects of glucocorticoids. Am J Med 53:573, 1972.

Bennett AH & others: Surgical treatment of adrenocortical hyperplasia: 20 years' experience. J Urol 109:321, 1973.

Besser GM, Landon J: Plasma levels of immunoreactive corticotrophin in patients with Cushing's syndrome. Brit MJ 4:552, 1968.

Birnholz JC: Ultrasound imaging of adrenal mass lesions. Radiology 109:163, 1973.

Bledsoe T: Surgery and the adrenal cortex. S Clin North America 54:449, 1974.

Christy NP: Cushing's syndrome: The natural disease. Pages 359–395 in: *The Human Adrenal Cortex.* Harper & Row, 1971.

Conn JW & others: Primary aldosteronism: Photoscanning of tumors after administration of [131]I-19-iodocholesterol. Arch Int Med 129:417, 1972.

Cushing H: The basophil adenomas of the pituitary body and their clinical manifestations (pituitary basophilism). Bull Johns Hopkins Hosp 50:137, 1932.

Eddy RL & others: Cushing's syndrome: A prospective study of diagnostic methods. Am J Med 55:621, 1973.

Flint LD: Surgical exposures for adrenal endocrinopathies. S Clin North America 53:445, 1973.

Gabrilove JL, Nicolis GL, Sohval AR: The testes in Cushing's syndrome. J Urol 112:95, 1974.

Glenn F & others: Total adrenalectomy for Cushing's disease. Ann Surg 175:948, 1972.

Graber AL & others: Natural history of pituitary-adrenal recovery following long-term suppression with corticosteroids. J Clin Endocrinol 15:11, 1965.

Herwig KR & others: Localization of adrenal tumors by photoscanning. J Urol 109:2, 1973.

Lee KR, Lin F, Sibala J: Adrenal adenoma and hyperplasia. Am J Roentgenol 119:796, 1973.

Liddle GW: The adrenal cortex. Pages 233–283 in: *Textbook of Endocrinology,* 5th ed. Williams RH (editor). Saunders, 1974.

Mattingly D: A simple fluorimetric method for the estimation of free 11-hydroxycorticoids in human plasma. J Clin Path 15:374, 1962.

Nelson DH & others: ACTH-producing pituitary tumors following adrenalectomy for Cushing's syndrome. Ann Int Med 52:560, 1960.

Netter FH: *The Ciba Collection of Medical Illustrations.* Vol IV: *Endocrine System and Selected Metabolic Diseases.* Section III: *The Suprarenal Glands (Adrenal Glands).* Ciba, 1965.

Norymberski JK: Determination of urinary corticosteroids. Nature 170:1074, 1952.

Porter CC, Silber RH: A quantitative color reaction for cortisone and related 17,21-dihydroxy-20-ketosteroids. J Biol Chem 185:201, 1950.

Schwartz DL, Gann DS, Haller JA Jr: Endocrine surgery in children. S Clin North America 54:363, 1974.

Wilson JM, Woodhead DM, Smith RB: Adrenal cysts: Diagnosis and management. Urology 4:248, 1974.

Adrenogenital Syndromes

Besser GM, Edwards CRW: Hirsuties and virilism. Clin Endocrinol Metab 1:491, 1972.

Biglieri EG, Herron MA, Brust N: 17-Hydroxylation deficiency in man. J Clin Invest 45:1946, 1966.

Bongiovanni AM & others: Disorders of adrenal steroid biogenesis. Recent Progr Hormone Res 23:375, 1967.

Bongiovanni AM, Root AW: The adrenogenital syndrome. (3 parts.) New England J Med 268:1283, 1342, 1391, 1963.

Hamilton HW: Congenital adrenal hyperplasia: Inborn errors of cortisol and aldosterone synthesis. Clin Endocrinol Metab 1:503, 1972.

Harrison JH, Mahoney E, Bennett AH: Tumors of the adrenal cortex. Cancer 32:1227, 1973.

Hoffman DL, Mattox VR: Treatment of adrenocortical carcinoma with o,p'DDD. M Clin North America 56:999, 1972.

Hutter AM Jr, Kayhoe DE: Adrenal cortical carcinoma. Am J Med 41:581, 1966.

Huvos AG & others: Adrenal cortical carcinoma: Clinicopathologic study of 34 cases. Cancer 25:354, 1970.

Liddle GW: The adrenal cortex. Pages 233–283 in: *Textbook of Endocrinology,* 5th ed. Williams RH (editor). Saunders, 1974.

Lipsett MB & others: Clinical and pathophysiologic aspects of adrenocortical carcinoma. Am J Med 35:374, 1963.

Mitty HA, Nicolis GL, Gabrilove JL: Adrenal renography: Clinical-roentgenographic correlation in 80 patients. Am J Roentgenol 119:564, 1973.

Shons AR, Gamble WG: Nonfunctioning carcinoma of the adrenal cortex. Surg Gynec Obst 138:705, 1974.

Hyperaldosteronism

Conn JW & others: Normokalemic primary aldosteronism. JAMA 195:21, 1966.

Horton R, Finck E: Diagnosis and localization in primary aldosteronism. Ann Int Med 76:885, 1972.

Liddle GW: The adrenal cortex. Pages 233–283 in: *Textbook of Endocrinology,* 5th ed. Williams RH (editor). Saunders, 1974.

Tarazi RC & others: Hemodynamic characteristics of primary aldosteronism. New England J Med 289:1330, 1973.

Weinberger MH, Donohue JP: Aldosterone updated. J Urol 110:1, 1973.

Pheochromocytomas & Related Tumors

Deoreo GA & others: Preoperative blood transfusion in the safe surgical management of pheochromocytoma: A review of 46 cases. J Urol 111:715, 1974.

Evans AE: Treatment of neuroblastoma. Cancer 30:1595, 1972.

Freier DT, Tank ES, Harrison TS: Pediatric and adult pheochromocytomas: A biochemical and clinical comparison. Arch Surg 107:252, 1973.

Funyu T & others: Familial pheochromocytoma: Case report and review of the literature. J Urol 110:151, 1973.

Gittes RF, Bendixen HH: Pheochromocytoma: Tumor localization and surgical management. California Med 118:1, June 1973.

Harrison J & others: Results of combination chemotherapy, surgery, and radiotherapy in children with neuroblastoma. Cancer 34:485, 1974.

Harrison TS, Freier DT: Pitfalls in the technique and interpretation of regional venous sampling for localizing pheochromocytoma. S Clin North America 54:338, 1974.

Himathongkam T & others: Pheochromocytoma: Medical emergency management. JAMA 230:1692, 1974.

James RE, Baker HL Jr, Scanlon PW: The roentgenologic aspects of metastatic pheochromocytoma. Am J Roentgenol 115:783, 1972.

Liebner EJ: Serial catecholamines in the radiation management of children with neuroblastoma. Cancer 32:623, 1973.

Mahoney EM & others: Adrenal and extra-adrenal pheochromocytomas: Localization by vena cava sampling and observations on renal juxtaglomerular apparatus. J Urol 108:4, 1972.

Melmon KL: Catecholamines and the adrenal medulla. Pages 283–322 in: *Textbook of Endocrinology,* 5th ed. Williams RH (editor). Saunders, 1974.

Remine WH & others: Current management of pheochromocytoma. Ann Surg 179:740, 1974.

Rogers LE, Lyon GM Jr, Porter FS: Spot test for vanillylmandelic acid and other guaiacols in urine of patients with neuroblastoma. Am J Clin Path 58:383, 1972.

Sturman MF & others: Radiocholesterol adrenal images for the localization of pheochromocytoma. Surg Gynec Obst 138:177, 1974.

Varkarakis MJ & others: Current status of prognostic criteria in neuroblastoma. J Urol 109:94, 1973.

Wilson LMK, Draper GJ: Neuroblastoma, its natural history and prognosis: A study of 487 cases. Brit MJ 3:301, 1974.

Zelch JV, Meany TF, Belhobek GH: Radiologic approach to the patient with suspected pheochromocytoma. Radiology 111:279, 1974.

21 . . .
Disorders of the Kidneys

CONGENITAL ANOMALIES OF THE KIDNEYS

Congenital anomalies occur more frequently in the kidney than in any other organ. Some cause no difficulty, but many (eg, hypoplasia, polycystic kidneys) cause impairment of renal function. It has been noted that the child with a gross deformity of an external ear associated with ipsilateral maldevelopment of the facial bones is apt to have a congenital abnormality of the kidney (eg, ectopy, hypoplasia) on the same side as the visible deformity. Lateral displacement of the nipples has been observed in association with bilateral renal hypoplasia.

In association with congenital scoliosis and kyphosis, a significant incidence of renal agenesis, ectopy, malrotation, and duplication has been observed. Unilateral agenesis, hypoplasia, and dysplasia are often seen in association with supralevator imperforate anus.

AGENESIS

One kidney may be absent. This is probably due to the fact that the ureteral bud (from the Wolffian duct) fails to develop or, if it does develop, does not reach the metanephros (adult kidney). Without a drainage system, the metanephric mass undergoes atrophy. The ureter is usually absent on the side of the unformed kidney, although a blind duct may be found. (See Chapter 2.)

Renal agenesis causes no symptoms; it is usually found by accident on urography. It is not an easy diagnosis to establish even though the ureteral ridge is absent and no orifice is visualized, for the kidney could be present but be drained by a ureter whose opening is ectopic (into the urethra, seminal vesicle, or vagina). A suggestive clue is the presence of low ears.

There appears to be an increased incidence of infection, hydronephrosis, and stones in the contralateral organ. Other congenital anomalies associated with this defect include cardiac, vertebral column, and anal anomalies as well as those of the long bones, hands, and genitalia.

HYPOPLASIA

Hypoplasia implies a small kidney. The total renal mass may be divided in an unequal manner, in which case one kidney is small and the other kidney correspondingly larger than normal. Some of these congenitally small kidneys prove, on pathologic examination, to be dysplastic.

Differentiation from acquired atrophy is difficult. Atrophic pyelonephritis usually reveals typical distortion of the calyces. Vesicoureteral reflux in the infant may cause a dwarfed kidney even in the absence of infection. Stenosis of the renal artery leads to shrinkage of the kidney.

Cha, Kandzari, & Khoury (1972) have noted that such kidneys have small renal arteries and branches and are associated with hypertension, which is relieved by nephrectomy. Selective renal venography is helpful in differentiating between a congenitally absent and a small, nonvisualized kidney.

SUPERNUMERARY KIDNEYS

The presence of a third kidney is very rare; the presence of 4 separate kidneys in one individual has only been reported once. This anomaly must not be confused with duplication (or triplication) of the pelvis in one kidney, which is not uncommon.

DYSPLASIA & MULTICYSTIC KIDNEY

Renal dysplasia presents protean manifestations. Multicystic kidney of the newborn is almost always unilateral, nonhereditary, and characterized by an irregularly lobulated mass of cysts; the ureter is usually absent or atretic. It may develop because of faulty union of the nephron and the collecting system. At most, only a few embryonic glomeruli and tubules are observed. The only finding is the discovery of an irregular mass in the flank. Nothing is shown on urography. Cystoscopy usually fails to reveal the ipsilateral ureteral orifice. In order to rule out tumor, surgical exploration is indicated.

Dysplasia of the renal parenchyma is also seen in association with ureteral obstruction or reflux which was probably present early in pregnancy. It is relatively common as a segmental renal lesion involving the upper pole of a duplicated kidney whose ureter is obstructed by a congenital ureterocele. It may also be found in urinary tracts severely obstructed by posterior urethral valves; in this instance, the lesion may be bilateral.

Microscopically, the renal parenchyma is "disorganized." Tubular and glomerular cysts may be noted; these elements are fetal in type. Islands of metaplastic cartilage are often seen. The common denominator seems to be fetal obstruction.

POLYCYSTIC KIDNEYS

Polycystic kidney disease is hereditary and almost always bilateral (95% of cases). The disease encountered in infancy is different from that seen in the adult. The former is an autosomal recessive disease and life expectancy is short, whereas those diagnosed in adulthood are autosomal dominant; symptoms ordinarily do not appear until after age 40. In association with both forms, cysts of the liver, spleen, and pancreas may be noted. The kidneys are larger than normal and are studded with cysts of various sizes.

Etiology & Pathogenesis

The evidence suggests that the cysts occur because of defects in the development of the collecting and uriniferous tubules and in the mechanism of their joining. Blind secretory tubules which are connected to functioning glomeruli become cystic. As these cysts enlarge, they compress adjacent parenchyma, destroy it by ischemia, and occlude normal tubules. The result is progressive functional impairment. It would appear that medullary sponge kidney is part of the spectrum but a milder form.

Pathology

Grossly, the kidneys are usually much enlarged. Their surfaces are studded with cysts of various sizes (Fig 21–1). On section, the cysts are found to be scattered throughout the parenchyma. The fluid in the cyst is usually amber-colored but may be hemorrhagic. Microscopically, the lining of the cysts consists of a single layer of cells. The renal parenchyma may show peritubular fibrosis and evidence of secondary infection. There appears to be a reduction in the number of glomeruli, some of which may be hyalinized. Renal arteriolar thickening is a prominent finding in the adult.

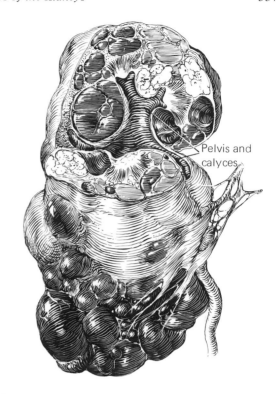

Figure 21–1. Polycystic kidney. Multiple cysts deep in the parenchyma and on the surface. Note distortion of the calyces by the cysts.

Clinical Findings

A. Symptoms: Pain over one or both kidneys may occur because of the drag on the vascular pedicles by the heavy kidneys or from hemorrhage into a cyst. Gross total hematuria is not uncommon and may be severe; the cause for this is not clear. Colic may be present if blood clots are passed. The patient may notice an abdominal mass.

Infection (chills, fever, renal pain) commonly complicates polycystic disease. Symptoms of vesical irritability may be the first complaint. When renal insufficiency ensues, headache, nausea and vomiting, weakness, and loss of weight occur.

B. Signs: One or both kidneys are usually palpable. They may feel nodular. If infected, they may be tender. Hypertension is found in 60–70% of these patients. Evidence of cardiac enlargement is then noted.

Fever may be present if pyelonephritis exists or if cysts have become infected. In the stage of uremia, anemia and loss of weight may be evident. Ophthalmoscopic examination may show changes typical of moderate or severe hypertension.

C. Laboratory Findings: Anemia may be noted, either caused by chronic loss of blood or, more commonly, by the hematopoietic depression which accompanies uremia. Proteinuria and microscopic (if not gross) hematuria are the rule. Pus cells and bacteria are commonly found.

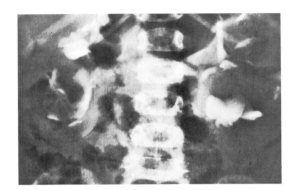

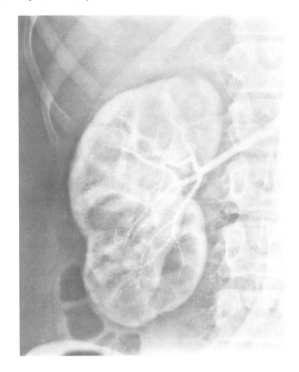

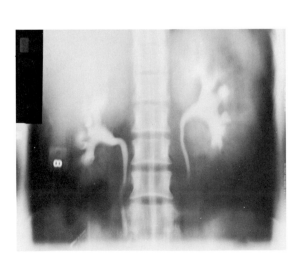

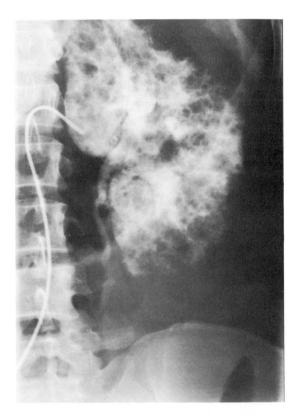

Figure 21–2. Polycystic kidneys. *Above left:* Excretory urogram in a child showing elongation, broadening, and bending of the calyces around cysts. Good renal function. *Above right:* Angiogram of right kidney showing "negative" shadows of cysts. *Below left:* Angionephrotomogram showing kidneys of essentially normal size. All infundibula on left and infundibulum of right upper calyx are widened, suggesting polycystic kidneys. *Below right:* Nephrogram phase of left selective angiogram showing multiple small negative shadows representing the cysts.

Progressive loss of concentrating power occurs. The PSP and clearance tests will show varying degrees of renal impairment. About a third of patients with polycystic kidney disease are uremic when first seen.

D. X-Ray Findings: Both renal shadows are usually enlarged on a plain film of the abdomen, even as much as 5 times normal size. Kidneys more than 16 cm in length are suspect.

Excretory infusion urograms with tomography are helpful if, as is true in most cases, the PSP excretion is better than 30% in 1 hour, in which event excretion of the medium may be sufficient to delineate the calceal system and thus establish the diagnosis. Tomography will reveal multiple lucencies representing cysts. On these or on retrograde urography the renal masses are usually enlarged, and the calyceal pattern is quite bizarre (spider deformity). The calyces are broadened and flattened, enlarged, and often curved, as they tend to hug the periphery of adjacent cysts (Fig 21-2). Often the changes are only slight or may even be absent on one side, leading to the erroneous diagnosis of tumor of the other kidney.

If cysts are infected, perinephritis may obscure the renal and even the psoas shadows.

Angiography will reveal bending of small vessels around the cysts and the "negative" shadows (nonvascular) of the cysts (Fig 21-2).

Photoscan (see Chapter 8) will reveal multiple "cold" avascular spots in large renal shadows.

E. Sonography: B-scan sonography appears to be superior to both excretory urography and isotope scanning in diagnosis of the polycystic disorders (Lufkin & others, 1974).

F. Instrumental Examination: Cystoscopy may show evidence of cystitis, in which case the urine will contain abnormal elements. Bleeding from a ureteral orifice may be noted.

After catheterization of the ureters, the collected pelvic urine may be found to contain pus and bacteria microscopically and by culture. The PSP test will usually reveal bilateral impairment of kidney function.

Differential Diagnosis

Bilateral hydronephrosis (on the basis of congenital or acquired ureteral obstruction) may present bilateral flank masses and signs of impairment of renal function, but urography will show changes quite different from those of the polycystic kidney.

Bilateral renal tumor is rare but may mimic polycystic kidney disease perfectly on urography. Differentiation of a unilateral tumor may be quite difficult if one of the polycystic kidneys shows little or no distortion on urography. However, tumors are usually localized to one portion of the kidney, whereas cysts are quite diffusely distributed. The total renal function should be normal with unilateral tumor but is usually depressed in the patient with polycystic kidney disease. Nephrotomograms or renal angiography may be needed at times, to differentiate between the 2 conditions (Fig 21-2). Photoscans or sonograms may also prove helpful in differentiation.

In **Lindau's disease** (angiomatous cerebellar cyst, angiomatosis of the retina, tumors or cysts of the pancreas), multiple bilateral cysts or adenocarcinomas of both kidneys may develop. Urograms or nephrotomograms may suggest polycystic kidney disease. The presence of other stigmas should make the diagnosis. Angiography, sonography, or scintophotography should be definitive.

Tuberous sclerosis (convulsive seizures, mental retardation, and adenoma sebaceum) is typified by hamartomatous tumors often involving the skin, brain, retinas, bones, liver, heart, and kidneys. (See Chapter 18.) The renal lesions are usually multiple and bilateral and microscopically are angiomyolipomas. If seen in the stage of uremia, the urograms are apt to suggest polycystic disease; the presence of other stigmas and angiography or scintillation imaging should make the differentiation.

Simple cyst (see below) is usually unilateral and single; total renal function should be normal. Urograms will show a single lesion (Fig 21-3), whereas polycystic kidney disease is bilateral and the filling defects are multiple.

Complications

Pyelonephritis, for reasons which are not clear, is a common complication of polycystic kidney disease. It may be asymptomatic; pus cells in the urine may be few or absent. Stained smears or quantitative cultures make the diagnosis.

Infection of cysts will be associated with pain and tenderness over the kidney and a febrile response. The differential diagnosis between infection of cysts and pyelonephritis may be difficult.

In rare instances gross hematuria may be so brisk and persistent as to endanger life.

Treatment

Except for unusual complications, the treatment is conservative and supportive.

A. General Measures: Place the patient on a low-protein diet (0.5-0.75 g/kg/day of protein) and force fluids to 3000 ml or more per day. Physical activity may be permitted within reason, but strenuous overexercise is contraindicated. When the patient is in the state of absolute renal insufficiency, treat as for uremia from any cause. Hemodialysis may be indicated.

B. Surgery: There is no evidence that excision or decompression of cysts improves renal function. Should a large cyst be found to be compressing the upper ureter, causing obstruction and further embarrassing renal function, it should be resected. When the degree of renal insufficiency becomes life-threatening, renal transplantation should be considered.

C. Treatment of Complications: Pyelonephritis must be rigorously treated to prevent further renal damage. Infection of cysts requires surgical drainage. If bleeding from one kidney is so severe as to threaten exsanguination, nephrectomy must be considered as a lifesaving measure.

Concomitant diseases (eg, tumor, obstructing stone) may require definitive surgical treatment.

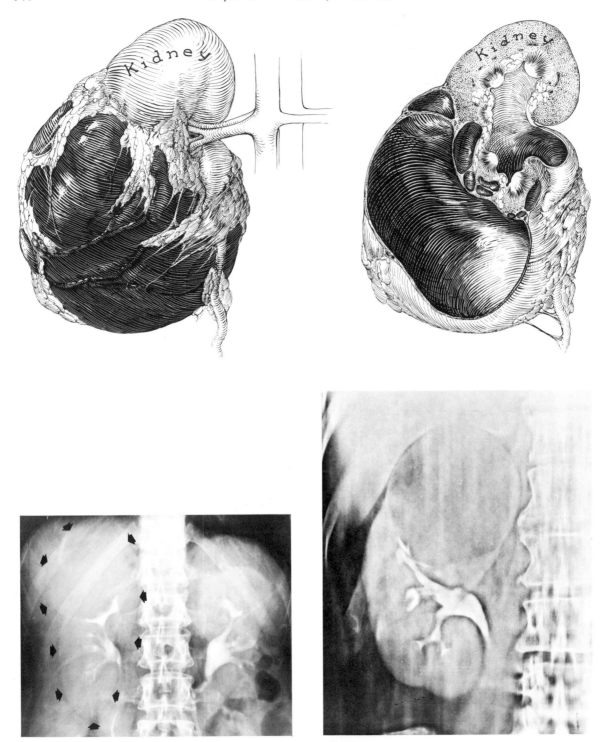

Figure 21–3. Simple cyst. *Above left:* Large cyst displacing lower pole laterally. *Above right:* Section of kidney showing one large and a few small cysts. *Below left:* Excretory urogram showing soft tissue mass in upper pole of right kidney. Elongation and distortion of upper calyces by cyst. *Below right:* Infusion nephrotomogram showing large cyst in upper renal pole distorting upper calyces and dislocating upper portion of kidney laterally.

Prognosis

If the disease is so severe as to present symptoms in infancy or childhood, the prognosis is very poor. The larger group, presenting clinical signs and symptoms after the age of 35–40 years, has a somewhat more favorable prognosis. Although there is wide variation, these patients usually do not live longer than 5 or 10 years after the diagnosis is made.

SIMPLE (SOLITARY) CYST

Simple cyst of the kidney is usually unilateral and single but may be multiple and multilocular and, more rarely, bilateral. It differs from polycystic kidneys both clinically and pathologically.

Etiology and Pathogenesis

Whether simple cyst is congenital or acquired is not clear. Its origin may be similar to that of polycystic kidneys, ie, the difference may be merely one of degree. On the other hand, simple cysts have been produced in animals by causing tubular obstruction and local ischemia, which suggests that the lesion can be acquired.

As a simple cyst grows it compresses and thereby destroys renal parenchyma, but rarely is a significant amount of renal tissue destroyed unless numerous cysts are present. A solitary cyst may be placed in such a position as to compress the ureter, causing progressive hydronephrosis. Infection may then complicate the picture.

Pathology

Simple cysts usually involve the lower pole of the kidney. They average about 10 cm in diameter when producing symptoms, but a few are large enough to fill the entire flank. They usually contain a clear amber fluid. Their walls are quite thin, and the cysts are "blue-domed" in appearance. Calcification of the sac is occasionally seen. About 5% contain hemorrhagic fluid, and possibly one-half of these have papillary cancers on their walls.

Simple cysts are usually superficial but may be deeply situated, in which case destruction of renal parenchyma is more extensive. When situated deep in the kidney, the cyst wall is adjacent to the epithelial lining of the pelvis or calyces, from which it may be separated only with great difficulty. Cysts do not communicate with the renal pelvis (Fig 21–3). Microscopic examination of the cyst wall shows heavy fibrosis and hyalinization; areas of calcification may be seen. The adjacent renal tissue is compressed and fibrosed.

Clinical Findings

A. Symptoms: Pain in the flank or back, usually intermittent and dull, is not uncommon. Should bleeding suddenly distend the cyst wall, pain may come on abruptly and be severe. Gastrointestinal symptoms are frequently noted and may suggest peptic ulcer or gallbladder disease. The patient may discover a mass in the abdomen, although cysts of this size are unusual. If the cyst becomes infected, the patient usually complains of pain in the flank, malaise, and fever.

B. Signs: Physical examination is usually normal, although occasionally a mass in the region of the kidney may be palpated or percussed. Tenderness in the flank may be noted if the cyst becomes infected.

C. Laboratory Findings: Urinalysis is usually normal. Microscopic hematuria is rare. Renal function tests are normal unless the cysts are multiple and bilateral (rare). Even in the face of extensive destruction of one kidney, compensatory hypertrophy of the other kidney will maintain normal total function.

D. X-Ray Findings: An expansion of a portion of the kidney shadow or a mass superimposed upon it can usually be seen on a plain film of the abdomen (Fig 6–2, top left). The axis of the kidney may be abnormal because of rotation due to the weight or position of the cyst. Streaks of calcium can sometimes be seen in the border of the mass.

Excretory urograms establish the presumptive diagnosis of cyst. On the film taken 1–2 minutes after infusion of the radiopaque fluid, the vascularized parenchyma becomes white while the space-occupying cyst does not because it is avascular. The urographic series will show changes compatible with a mass. One or more calyces or the pelvis will usually be indented or bent around the cyst and are often broadened and flattened, even obliterated (Figs 21–3 and 21–4). Oblique and lateral films may prove helpful. If a mass occupies the lower pole of the kidney, the upper part of the ureter may be displaced toward the spine. The kidney itself may be rotated. The psoas muscle may be seen through the radiolucent cyst fluid.

Should the routine urogram fail to significantly opacify the parenchyma, infusion nephrotomography should be done, thus increasing the contrast between vascular renal tissue and the cyst (Fig 21–3). Occasionally, a renal parenchymal tumor may be relatively avascular, thus being confused with cyst. In a few instances, carcinoma may grow on the cyst wall. Because of these phenomena, further steps in differential diagnosis should be performed.

Renal sonography is a noninvasive diagnostic technic which in a high percentage of cases differentiates between a cyst and a solid mass (see Chapter 7). If this study is also compatible with cyst, a needle can be introduced into the cyst under fluoroscopic or ultra-B-scanning control. The recovery of clear (urine-colored) fluid is compatible with cyst. This fluid, however, should be subjected to cytologic study to rule out intracystic tumor. The fat content of the fluid should be estimated, for its presence is compatible with tumor.

If the fluid is clear, a radiopaque fluid should be instilled and films taken in various positions to prove that the cyst wall is smooth or that there is an excrescence that might represent tumor. Injection of 3

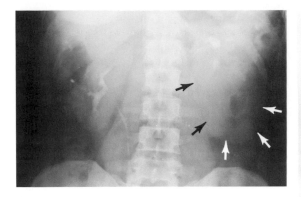

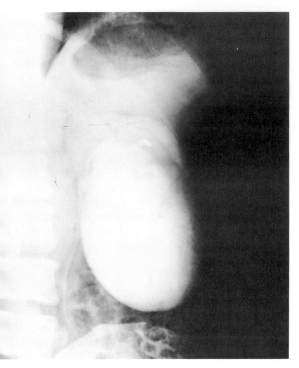

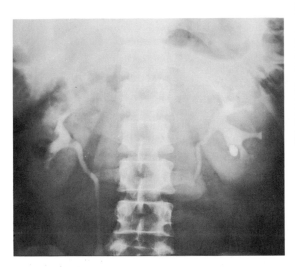

Figure 21—4. *Above left:* Excretory urogram showing large smooth mass in lower pole of left kidney with distortion of calyces. *Above right:* Cyst punctured and radiopaque fluid instilled. Cyst is smooth-walled. *Bottom:* Iophendylate then instilled. Excretory urogram 3 months later. Iophendylate occupies what is left of cyst. Urogram normal.

ml of iophendylate into the cavity before the cyst fluid is aspirated is said to decrease the chance of reaccumulation of fluid (Fig 21—24). If simple aspiration alone is utilized, some cysts will completely refill.

If the needle recovers blood from the mass or if the urographic and sonographic findings are equivocal for cyst, renal angiography should be done. If the mass is a cyst, it should be avascular and remain lucent. If it is a tumor, the mass will opacify and reveal neovascularity (Fig 18—3).

Renal cystography and renal angiography both involve a 5—10% risk of diagnostic error. In combination, they are definitive.

These studies have markedly decreased the need for surgical exploration. In case of doubt, however, exploration is recommended.

Isotope scanning. A rectilinear scan will clearly delineate the mass but does not differentiate cyst from tumor. The technetium scan, made with the camera, will reveal that the mass is, indeed, avascular (see Chapter 8).

Differential Diagnosis

Carcinoma of the kidney also occupies space but tends to lie more deeply in the organ and therefore causes more distortion of the calyces. Hematuria is common with tumor, rare with cyst. If a solid tumor overlies the psoas muscle, the edge of the muscle is obliterated on the plain film; it can be seen through a cyst, however. Evidence of metastases (ie, loss of weight and strength, palpable supraclavicular nodes, chest film showing metastatic nodules), erythrocytosis, hypercalcemia, and increased sedimentation rate suggest cancer. It must be remembered, however, that the walls of a simple cyst may undergo cancerous degeneration. If the renal vein is occluded by cancer, the excretory urogram may be visualized only faintly or not at all. Angiography (Fig 18—3) or nephrotomography (Fig 18—4) may reveal "pooling" of the medium in the highly vascularized tumor, whereas the density of a cyst is not affected. It is wise to assume that all space-occupying lesions of the kidneys are cancers. If metastases are not demonstrable, surgical exploration is indicated.

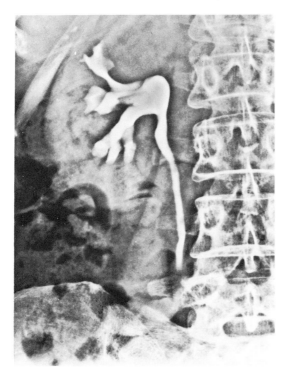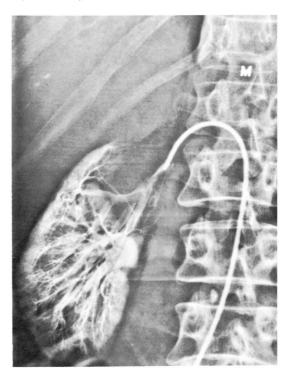

Figure 21–5. Diagnosis of simple renal cyst. *Left:* Excretory urogram showing lateral and inferior displacement and distortion of upper calyx, right kidney. Differential diagnosis: cyst versus tumor. *Right:* Same patient. Selective femoral angiogram showing a completely avascular mass typical of cyst.

Polycystic kidney disease is almost always bilateral, as shown by urography (Fig 21–2). Diffuse calyceal and pelvic distortion is the rule. Simple cyst is usually solitary and unilateral. Polycystic kidney disease is usually accompanied by impaired renal function and hypertension. Simple cyst is not.

Renal carbuncle is a rare disease. A history of skin infection a few weeks before the onset of fever and local pain may be obtained. Urograms may show changes similar to cyst or tumor, but the renal outline as well as the edge of the psoas muscle may be obscured because of perinephritis. The kidney may be fixed, as demonstrated by comparing the position of the kidney in the supine and upright positions. Angiography will demonstrate an avascular lesion (Fig 12–8). Surgery is indicated in either case.

Hydronephrosis may present the same symptoms and signs as simple cyst, but the urograms are quite different. Cyst causes calyceal distortion; with hydronephrosis, dilatation of the calyces and pelvis due to an obvious ureteral obstruction is present. Acute or subacute hydronephrosis usually produces more local pain because of increased intrapelvic pressure and is more apt to be complicated by infection.

Extrarenal tumor (eg, adrenal, mixed retroperitoneal sarcoma) may displace a kidney, but rarely does it invade it and distort its calyces.

If an echinococcus cyst of the kidney does not communicate with the pelvis it may be difficult to differentiate from solitary cyst, for no scoleces or hooklets will be present in the urine. The wall of a hydatid cyst often reveals calcification on x-ray examination (Fig 13–3). A skin sensitivity test (Casoni) for hydatid disease may prove helpful.

Complications (Rare)

Spontaneous infection in a simple cyst is rare, but when it occurs it is difficult to differentiate from carbuncle. Hemorrhage into the cyst sometimes occurs. If sudden, it causes severe pain. The bleeding may come from a complicating carcinoma arising on the wall of the cyst.

Hydronephrosis may develop if a cyst of the lower pole impinges upon the ureter. This in itself may cause pain from back pressure of urine in the pelvis. This obstruction may lead to renal infection.

Treatment

A. Specific Measures: Surgical exploration should be considered if the diagnosis is in doubt, for it is surprising how commonly cyst and renal tumor are confused. Furthermore, 3–5% of cysts have cancer on their walls, so all cysts must be assumed to be malignant until proved benign. Fortunately, they are not so dangerous as the parenchymal carcinoma.

It is rare for the kidney to be significantly damaged by a simple cyst. Therefore, only that portion

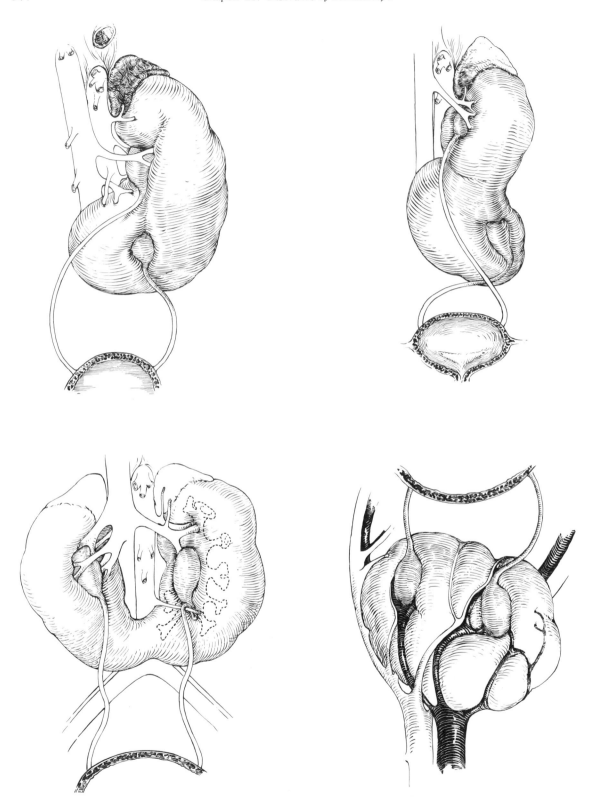

Figure 21–6. Renal fusion. *Above left:* Crossed renal ectopy with fusion. The renal mass lies in the left flank. The right ureter must cross over the midline. *Above right:* Example of "sigmoid" kidney. *Below left:* Horseshoe kidney. Pelves are anterior. Note aberrant artery obstructing left ureter; low position of renal mass. *Below right:* Pelvic "cake" kidney. Pelves are placed anteriorly. Note aberrant blood supply.

of the sac external to the kidney need be excised. If, however, the kidney is severely damaged (and if its mate is normal), nephrectomy may be indicated.

B. Treatment of Complications: If the cyst should become infected, intensive antibiotic therapy should be instituted. If this proves unsuccessful, surgical excision of the extrarenal portion of the cyst wall and drainage will prove curative.

If, on exploration, the cyst appears to contain blood (and the other kidney is normal), immediate nephrectomy should be strongly urged without preliminary incision into the cyst, for this finding makes the presence of neoplasm likely. Drainage of the contents of a cancerous cyst, either by incision or needle, invites growth of carcinoma in the wound.

If hydronephrosis is present, excision of the cyst will relieve the ureteral obstruction.

Pyelonephritis in the involved kidney should suggest urinary stasis secondary to impaired ureteral drainage. Removal of the cyst and consequent relief of urinary back pressure will make antimicrobial therapy more effective.

Prognosis

Without complications, the prognosis is excellent if the cyst is excised. If untreated, progressive damage to the kidney may occur.

RENAL FUSION

About one out of 1000 individuals has some type of renal fusion, the most common being the horseshoe kidney. The fused renal mass almost always contains 2 excretory systems and therefore 2 ureters. The renal tissue may be divided equally between the 2 flanks, or the entire mass may be on one side. Even in the latter case the 2 ureters open at their proper places in the bladder.

Etiology & Pathogenesis

It appears that this fusion of the 2 metanephroi occurs early in embryologic life when the kidneys lie low in the pelvis. For this reason, they seldom ascend to the high position which normal kidneys assume. They may even remain in the true pelvis. Under these circumstances such a kidney may derive its blood supply from many vessels in the area (eg, aorta, iliacs).

In association with both ectopia and fusion, 78% of the patients will have extraurologic anomalies and 65% will exhibit other genitourinary defects (Kelalis, Malek, & Segura, 1973).

Pathology (Fig 21–6)

Because the renal masses fuse early, normal rotation cannot occur; therefore, each pelvis lies on the anterior surface of its organ. Thus, the ureter must ride over the isthmus of a horseshoe kidney or traverse the anterior surface of the fused kidney. Some degree of

ureteral compression may arise from this or from obstruction by one or more aberrant blood vessels. The incidence of hydronephrosis and therefore infection is high. Vesicoureteral reflux has frequently been noted in association with fusion.

In horseshoe kidney the isthmus usually joins the lower poles of each kidney; each renal mass lies lower than normal. The axes of these masses are vertical, whereas the axes of normal kidneys are oblique to the spine since they lie along the edges of the psoas muscles.

On rare occasion the 2 nephric masses are fused into one mass ("cake kidney") containing 2 pelves and 2 ureters. The mass may lie in the midline to open into the bladder at the proper point (crossed renal ectopy with fusion).

Clinical Findings

A. Symptoms: Most patients with fused kidneys have no symptoms. Some, however, develop ureteral obstruction. Gastrointestinal symptoms (renodigestive reflex) mimicking peptic ulcer, cholelithiasis, or appendicitis may be noted. Infection is apt to occur if ureteral obstruction and hydronephrosis develop or if calculus develops.

B. Signs: Physical examination is usually negative unless the abnormally placed renal mass can be felt. With horseshoe kidney it may be possible to palpate a mass over the lower lumbar spine (the isthmus). In the case of crossed ectopy, a mass may be felt in the flank.

C. Laboratory Findings: Urinalysis is normal unless there is infection. Renal function is normal unless disease coexists in each of the fused renal masses.

D. X-Ray Findings: In the case of horseshoe kidney the axes of the 2 kidneys, if visible on a plain film, are parallel to the spine. At times the isthmus can be identified. The plain film may also reveal a large soft tissue mass in one flank yet not show a renal shadow on the other side ("cake kidney"). (Fig 21–7.)

Excretory urograms establish the diagnosis if the renal parenchyma has maintained good function. The increased density of the kidney tissue may make its position or configuration more distinct. Urograms will also visualize the pelves and ureters.

1. With horseshoe kidney, the renal pelves usually lie on the anterior surfaces of their respective kidney masses, whereas the normal kidney has its pelvis lying mesial to it. The most valuable clue to the diagnosis of horseshoe kidney is the presence of calyces in the region of the lower pole which point medially and overlie the psoas muscles or even reach the vertebrae (Figs 21–6 and 21–7).

2. Crossed renal ectopy with fusion shows 2 pelves and 2 ureters leading from it. One ureter must cross the midline in order to empty into the bladder at the proper point (Figs 21–6 and 21–7).

3. A cake or lump kidney may lie in the pelvis (fused pelvis kidney), but again its ureters and pelves will be shown (Figs 21–6 and 21–7).

Tomograms will clearly outline the renal mass but

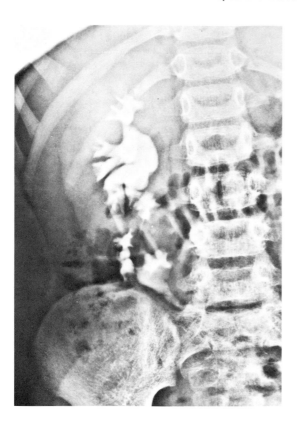
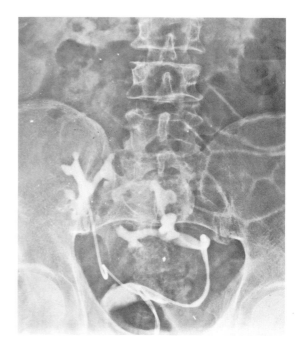
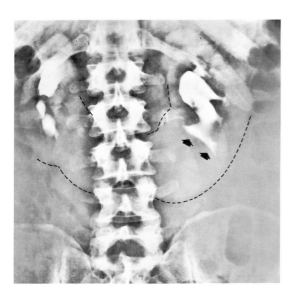
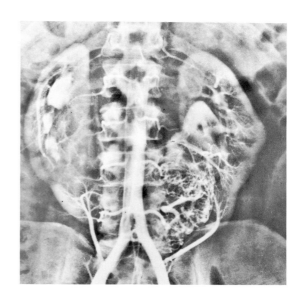

Figure 21–7. Renal fusion. *Above left:* Excretory urogram showing fused renal masses on the right side. Both kidneys are normal. Crossed renal ectopy. *Above right:* Retrograde urogram showing pelvic "cake" kidney. *Below left:* Excretory urogram showing horseshoe kidney with expansion of left side of isthmus and compression of lower left calyceal system. *Below right:* Angiogram on same patient. Hypervascular mass in left side of isthmus typical of adenocarcinoma.

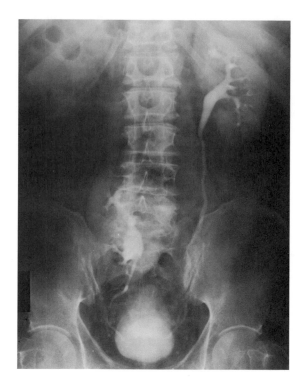

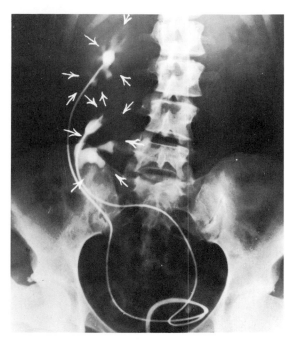

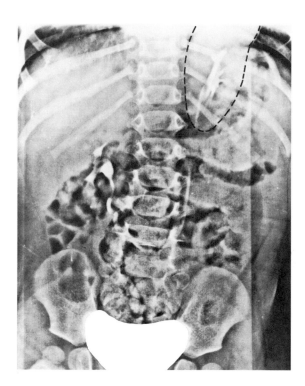

Figure 21–8. Renal ectopy. *Above left:* Excretory urogram showing congenital ectopy, right kidney. *Above right:* Retrograde urogram showing crossed renal ectopy. In this film the differentiation between fusion and nonfusion cannot be made. *Below:* Left kidney, ectopic in the chest.

are seldom necessary.

With pelvic fused kidney or one lying in the flank, the plain film taken with ureteral catheters in place will give the first hint of the diagnosis. Retrograde urograms will show the position of the pelves and demonstrate changes compatible with infection or obstruction (Fig 21–8). Renal scanning will delineate the renal mass and its contour (see Chapter 9).

Differential Diagnosis

Separate kidneys which fail to undergo the normal rotation may be confused with horseshoe kidney. They lie along the edges of the psoas muscles, whereas the poles of a horseshoe kidney lie parallel to the spine and their lower poles are placed on the psoas muscles. The calyces in the region of the isthmus of a horseshoe kidney point medially and lie close to the spine.

The diagnosis of cake or lump kidney may be missed on excretory urograms if one of its ureters is markedly obstructed so that a portion of the kidney and its pelvis and ureter fail to visualize. Catheterization of the ureters and retrograde urograms will demonstrate both excretory tracts in the renal mass.

Complications

Fused kidneys are prone to ureteral obstruction because of a high incidence of aberrant renal vessels and the necessity for one or both ureters to arch around or over the renal tissue. Hydronephrosis, stone, and infection therefore are common.

A large cake kidney occupying the concavity of the sacrum may cause dystocia.

Treatment

No treatment is necessary unless obstruction or infection is present. Drainage of a horseshoe kidney may be improved by dividing its isthmus. If one pole of a horseshoe is badly damaged, it may require surgical resection.

Prognosis

In most cases, the outlook is excellent. Should ureteral obstruction and infection occur, renal drainage must be improved by surgical means so that antimicrobial therapy will be effective.

ECTOPIC KIDNEY

Congenital ectopic kidney usually causes no symptoms unless complications such as ureteral obstruction or infection develop.

Simple Ectopy

Simple congenital ectopy is a low kidney on the proper side which failed to ascend normally. It may lie over the pelvic brim or in the pelvis. (Rarely, it may be found in the chest.) It takes its blood supply from adjacent vessels, and its ureter is short. It is prone to ureteral obstruction and infection, which may lead to pain or fever. At times such a kidney may be palpable, leading to an erroneous presumptive diagnosis (eg, cancer of the bowel, appendiceal abscess).

Excretory or retrograde urograms (Fig 21–8) will reveal the true position. Hydronephrosis, if present, will be evident. There is no redundancy of the ureter, as is the case with nephroptosis or acquired ectopy (eg, displacement by large suprarenal tumor).

Obstruction and infection may complicate simple ectopy and should be treated by appropriate means.

Crossed Ectopy Without Fusion

In crossed ectopy without fusion the kidney lies on the opposite side of the body but is not attached to its normally placed mate. Unless 2 distinct renal shadows can be seen, it may be difficult to differentiate this condition from crossed ectopy with fusion (Fig 21–6).

ABNORMAL ROTATION

Normally, when the kidney ascends to the lumbar region the pelvis lies on its anterior surface. Later, the pelvis comes to lie mesially. Such rotation may fail to occur, although this seldom leads to renal disease. Urography demonstrates the abnormal position.

MEDULLARY SPONGE KIDNEY
(Cystic Dilatation of the Renal Collecting Tubules)

Medullary sponge kidney is a congenital autosomal recessive defect characterized by widening of the distal collecting tubules. It is usually bilateral, affecting all of the papillae, but it may be unilateral. At times, only one papilla is involved. Cystic dilatation of the tubules is often present also. Infection and calculi are occasionally seen as a result of urinary stasis in the tubules. Potter believes that medullary sponge kidney is related to polycystic renal disease. Its occasional association with hemihypertrophy of the body has been noted.

The only symptoms are those arising from infection and stone formation. The diagnosis is made on the basis of excretory urograms (Fig 21–9). The pelvis and calyces are normal, but dilated (streaked) tubules are seen just lateral to them; many of the dilated tubules contain round masses of radiopaque material (the cystic dilatation). If stones are present, a plain film will reveal small round calculi in the pyramidal regions just beyond the calyces. Retrograde urograms often do not reveal the lesion unless the mouths of the collecting ducts are widely dilated.

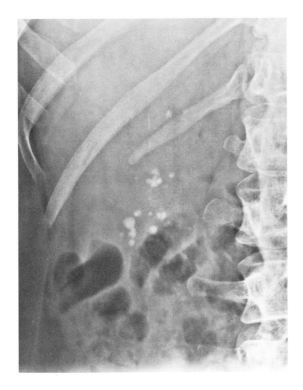
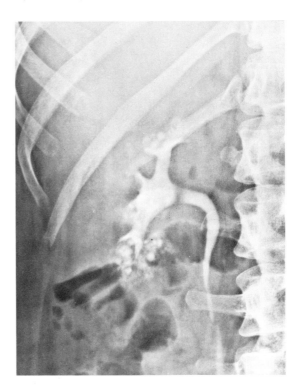

Figure 21—9. Medullary sponge kidneys. *Left:* Plain film of right kidney showing multiple small stones in its midportion. *Right:* Excretory urogram showing relationship of calculi to calyces. Typically, the calyces are large; the stones are located in the dilated collecting tubules.

The differential diagnosis includes tuberculosis, healed papillary necrosis, and nephrocalcinosis. Tuberculosis is usually unilateral, and urography shows ulceration of calyces; tubercle bacilli are found on bacteriologic study. Papillary necrosis may be complicated by calcification in the healed stage but may be distinguished by its typical calyceal deformity, the presence of infection, and, usually, impaired renal function (Fig 12—6). The tubular and parenchymal calcification seen in nephrocalcinosis is more diffuse than that seen with sponge kidney (Fig 15—12); the symptoms and signs of primary hyperparathyroidism or renal tubular acidosis may be found.

There is no treatment for medullary sponge kidney. Therapy is directed toward the complications (eg, pyelonephritis and renal calculi). Only a small percentage of people with sponge kidney develop complications. The overall prognosis is good. A few patients may pass small stones occasionally.

ABNORMALITIES OF RENAL VESSELS

As a rule, each kidney receives one renal artery from the aorta and has one vein passing to the vena cava. Aberrant veins and especially arteries are common. Three or 4 renal arteries may be depicted on angiography. An aberrant artery passing to the lower pole of the kidney may compress and thereby obstruct the ureter, causing hydronephrosis. On urography it is impossible to differentiate between an obstructing vessel and an intrinsic ureteral stenosis. The final diagnosis is made at the operating table.

ACQUIRED LESIONS OF THE KIDNEYS

RENOALIMENTARY FISTULA

Over 100 instances of renoalimentary fistula have been reported. They usually involve the stomach, duodenum, or adjacent colon, although fistula formation with the esophagus, small bowel, appendix, and rectum has been reported.

The underlying cause is usually a pyonephrotic kidney which becomes adherent to a portion of the alimentary tract and then ruptures spontaneously, thus creating a fistula (Fig 21—10). A few cases following trauma have been reported. The patient is therefore apt to suffer symptoms and signs of acute pyelonephri-

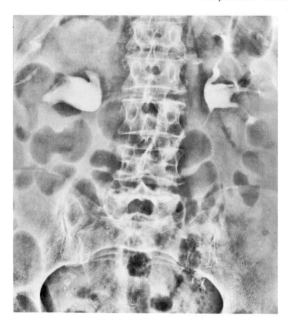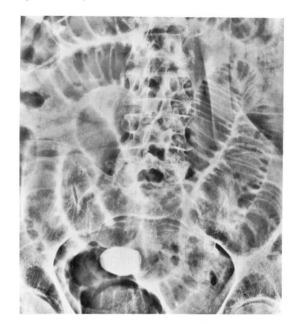

Figure 21–10. Nephroduodenal fistula and small bowel obstruction from renal staghorn calculus. *Left:* Excretory urogram showing nonfunction of right kidney; staghorn stone. *Right:* Patient presented with symptoms and signs of bowel obstruction 4 years later. Plain film showing dilated loops of small bowel down to a point just proximal to ileocecal valve. Obstruction due to stone which was extruded into duodenum. (Courtesy of CD King.)

tis. Urography may show radiopaque material escaping into the gastrointestinal tract. Gastrointestinal series may also reveal the connection with the kidney. The treatment is nephrectomy with closure of the opening into the gut.

ANEURYSM OF THE RENAL ARTERY

Aneurysm of the renal artery usually results from degenerative arterial disease which weakens the wall of the artery so that intravascular pressure may balloon it out. It is most commonly caused by arteriosclerosis or polyarteritis nodosa, but it may develop secondary to trauma or syphilis. Well over 300 cases have been reported. Congenital aneurysm has been recorded.

Aneurysmal dilatation has no deleterious effect upon the kidney unless the mass compresses the renal artery, in which case some renal ischemia and therefore atrophy is to be expected. A true aneurysm may rupture, thus producing a false aneurysm. This is especially likely to happen during pregnancy. The extravasated blood occupying the retroperitoneal space finally becomes encapsulated by a fibrous covering as organization occurs. An aneurysm may involve a small artery within the renal parenchyma. It may rupture into the renal pelvis or a calyx.

Most aneurysms cause no symptoms unless they rupture, in which case there may be severe flank pain and even shock. If an aneurysm ruptures into the renal

pelvis, marked hematuria occurs. The common cause of death is severe hemorrhage from rupture of the aneurysm. Hypertension is not usually present. A bruit should be sought over the costovertebral angle or over the renal artery anteriorly. If spontaneous or traumatic rupture has occurred, a mass may be palpated in the flank.

A plain film of the abdomen may show a ringlike calcification (Fig 21–11), either intra- or extrarenal. Urograms may be normal or reveal renal atrophy. Some impairment of renal function may be noted if compression or partial obstruction of the renal artery has developed. Aortography will delineate the aneurysm. The renal scan may show changes compatible with a renovascular lesion.

The differential diagnosis of rupture of an aneurysm and injury to the kidney is difficult unless a history or evidence of trauma is obtained. A hydronephrotic kidney may present a mass, but urography will clarify the issue.

Since the incidence of spontaneous rupture of noncalcified and large calcified aneurysms is significant, the presence of such a lesion is an indication for surgical intervention. The repair of extrarenal aneurysms may be considered, but complications (eg, thrombosis) are not uncommon. If an intrarenal aneurysm is situated in one pole, heminephrectomy may be feasible. If, however, it is in the center of the organ, nephrectomy will be required. Almgård & Fernström (1973) have reported therapeutic occlusion of an aneurysm by the intra-arterial injection of autologous muscle tissue. Those few patients found to have hyper-

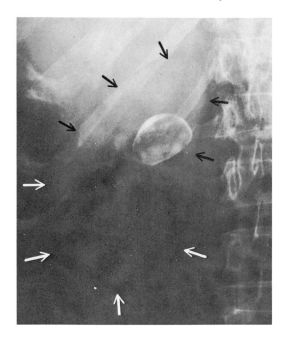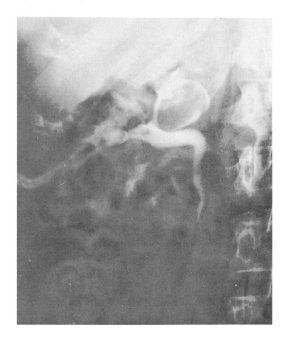

Figure 21–11. Intrarenal aneurysm of renal artery. *Left:* Plain film showing calcified structure over right renal shadow. *Right:* Excretory urogram which relates calcific mass to pelvis and upper calyx. (Courtesy of CD King.)

tension may become normotensive following definitive surgery.

RENAL INFARCTS

Renal infarcts are caused by arterial occlusion. The major causes are subacute bacterial endocarditis, atrial or ventricular thrombi, arteriosclerosis, polyarteritis nodosa, and trauma. A thrombotic process in the abdominal aorta may gradually extend upward to occlude the renal artery.

If smaller arteries or arterioles become obstructed, the tissue receiving blood from such a vessel will first become swollen and then undergo necrosis and fibrosis. Multiple infarcts are the rule. Should the main renal artery become occluded, the entire kidney will react in kind. The kidney may therefore become functionless and atrophic as it undergoes necrosis and fibrosis.

Partial renal infarction is usually a silent disease. Sudden and complete infarction may cause renal pain and at times gross or microscopic hematuria. Tenderness over the flank may then be elicited. The kidney is not significantly enlarged by arterial occlusion. Serum glutamic oxaloacetic transaminase will be elevated for 1 or 2 days after the incident.

Excretory urograms may fail to visualize a portion of the kidney with partial infarction; with complete infarction, none of the radiopaque fluid is excreted. In this instance, retrograde urography will reveal no obstruction—and in fact, ureteropyelograms will be normal—but no urine will drain from the ureteral catheter because the kidney has ceased to function. Even though complete loss of measurable function has occurred, renal circulation may be restored spontaneously in some instances.

Renal angiography makes the definitive diagnosis. A rectilinear scan may reveal no tubular function in a kidney of normal size. Lack of tracer activity may be noted in one pole if a segmental artery becomes occluded. A dynamic technetium scan will reveal no perfusion of the affected renal vasculature.

During the acute phase, infarction may mimic ureteral stone. With stone the excretory urogram may also show lack of renal function, but even so there is usually enough of the medium in the tubules so that a "nephrogram" is obtained (Fig 15–8). This will not occur with complete infarction. Evidence of a cardiac or vascular lesion is helpful in arriving at a proper diagnosis.

The complications are related to those arising from the primary cardiovascular disease. In a few cases, hypertension may develop a few days or weeks after the infarction. It may later subside.

If the diagnosis of thrombosis or embolism of the renal artery is made promptly, embolectomy should be considered. A few patients have undergone successful revascularization and autotransplantation. If this is not done, anticoagulants must be used as a means of preventing further thrombotic accidents; such treatment has a good chance of contributing to the return of some renal function. If permanent hypertension ensues in a patient with partial occlusion of the renal artery, renal endarterectomy or nephrectomy may cure the hypertension.

THROMBOSIS OF THE RENAL VEIN

Thrombosis of the renal vein is rare in the adult. It may develop secondary to various inflammatory lesions, including intrarenal or perirenal suppuration, or from ascending thrombosis of the vena cava associated with phlebothrombosis, or disseminated malignant disease. Thrombosis of the renal vein may occur as a complication of ileocolitis of infancy. The thrombosis may extend from the vena cava into the peripheral venules or may originate in the peripheral veins and propagate to the main renal vein. The severe passive congestion which develops causes the kidney to swell and to become engorged. Degeneration of the nephrons ensues. Pain in the flank is usually experienced, and symptoms and signs of sepsis are occasionally seen. Hematuria may be noted. A large tender mass is often felt in the flank. The blood count may reveal changes compatible with sepsis. Thrombocytopenia may be noted. The urine contains albumin, red cells, and frequently pus cells and bacteria. Urograms show poor or absent secretion of the radiopaque material in a large kidney. Stretching and thinning of the calyceal infundibula may be noted. Clots in the pelvis may cause filling defects. Later the kidney may undergo atrophy. Urograms may then show notching of the upper ureter by dilated collateral veins. The typical picture of nephrotic syndrome develops in many of these patients. Renal biopsy reveals findings compatible with membranous glomerulonephritis.

Renal angiography reveals stretching and bowing of small arterioles. In the nephrographic phase, the pyramids may become quite dense. Venacavography or, preferably, selective renal venography will demonstrate the thrombus in the renal vein (Fig 21–12) and, at times, in the vena cava. If washout from the vein affords poor filling, this may be enhanced by an injection of epinephrine into the renal artery.

The symptoms and signs may suggest acute renal infection or obstruction from a ureteral calculus. Acute pyelonephritis will cause the greatest difficulty in differential diagnosis, since the complaints and physical findings in the 2 diseases are similar. Excretory urography will prove helpful, for simple pyelonephritis will not appreciably depress renal function and there are no significant changes in the calyceal pattern. The presence of a stone in the ureter should be obvious; some degree of dilatation of the ureter and pelvis should then also be expected.

If the diagnosis of unilateral infected renal venous thrombosis can be established, immediate nephrectomy should be considered. Although this disease is a rare complication of thrombophlebitis of the iliac veins or vena cava, modern treatment of the latter by early vein ligation or the use of anticoagulants may be

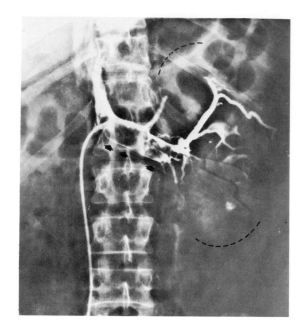

Figure 21–12. Thrombosis of renal vein. Selective left renal venogram showing almost complete occlusion of vein. Veins to lower pole failed to fill. Note large size of kidney.

expected to prevent propagation of the thrombosis. A few cases of successful thrombectomy have been reported. This appears to lead to some improvement in renal function. If nephrotic syndrome develops, appropriate treatment is indicated.

The prognosis is poor if bilateral renal vein thrombosis occurs. The outlook in the unilateral type is good if the primary cause can be controlled.

ARTERIOVENOUS FISTULA

Arteriovenous fistula may be congenital or acquired. A number of these fistulas have been reported following renal needle biopsy. A few have followed nephrectomy secondary to suture or ligature occlusion of the pedicle. These require surgical repair. A few have been recognized in association with adenocarcinoma of the kidney.

A thrill can often be palpated and a murmur heard both anteriorly and posteriorly. In cases with a wide communication, the systolic blood pressure is elevated and a widened pulse pressure is noted. Renal angiography establishes the diagnosis. Surgical repair is indicated, but nephrectomy is often necessary. A few have been occluded by the injection of autologous blood clot or fat into the appropriate branch of the renal artery. Those that develop secondary to renal biopsy tend to seal spontaneously.

ARTERIOVENOUS ANEURYSM

About 100 instances of this lesion have been reported (Fig 21–13). Most follow trauma. Hyper-

tension is to be expected and is associated with high-output cardiac failure. A bruit is usually present.

Nephrectomy is indicated.

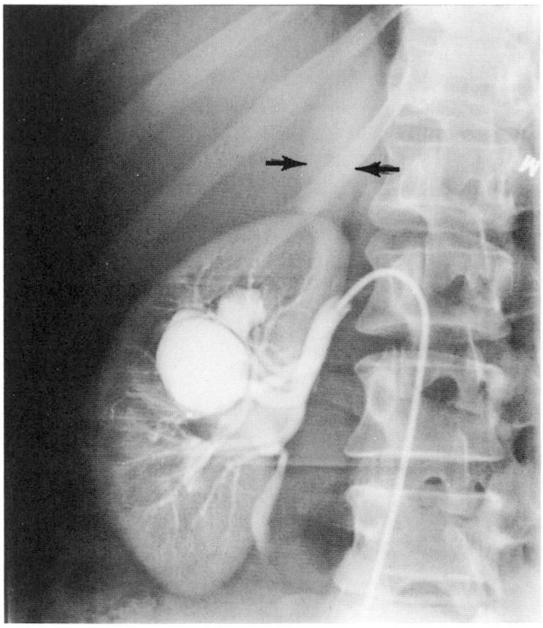

Figure 21–13. Arteriovenous aneurysm. Selective renal angiogram. Note aneurysm in center of kidney with prompt filling of the vena cava (shown by arrows).

RENAL CORTICAL NECROSIS

Acute necrosis of the renal cortex is, with few exceptions, a complication of severe hemorrhage, often occurring secondary to premature separation of the placenta in the third trimester of pregnancy. The entire cortex of each kidney commonly exhibits coagulation necrosis. The cause is thought to be spasm of the glomerular afferent arteries and disseminated intravascular coagulation. Microscopically, the glomeruli and proximal convoluted tubules are necrotic. The medulla is intact. After a few weeks, peripheral cortical calcification may be noted. It may be seen on laminagrams.

The onset is usually characterized by sudden severe abdominal pain secondary to severe uterine hemorrhage. Oliguria develops promptly and leads to progressive uremia. (For a discussion of the differential diagnosis and treatment of oliguria, see Chapter 23.)

Blood loss must be promptly replaced. Hyperkalemia may require dialysis. The use of ganglionic blocking agents, eg, trimethaphan (Arfonad), may relieve the cortical ischemia.

The prognosis depends upon the degree of renal damage. In many cases the renal lesion is irreversible. In most patients who recover, some degree of permanent renal damage is evident. Dialysis or renal transplantation may be necessary.

• • •

References

CONGENITAL ANOMALIES

General

Belman AB, King LR: Urinary tract abnormalities associated with imperforate anus. J Urol 108:823, 1972.

Fleisher DS: Lateral displacement of the nipples, a sign of bilateral renal hypoplasia. J Pediat 69:806, 1966.

Taylor WC: Deformity of ears and kidneys. Canad MAJ 93:107, 1965.

Vitko RJ, Cass AS, Winter RB: Anomalies of the genitourinary tract associated with congenital scoliosis and congenital kyphosis. J Urol 108:655, 1972.

Agenesis

Athanasoulis CA, Brown B, Baum S: Selective renal venography in differentiation between congenitally absent and small contracted kidney. Radiology 108:301, 1973.

Cain DR & others: Familial renal agenesis and total

dysplasia. Am J Dis Child 128:377, 1974.

Emanuel B & others: Congenital solitary kidney: A review of 74 cases. J Urol 111:394, 1974.

Kohn G, Borns PF: The association of bilateral and unilateral renal aplasia in the same family. J Pediat 83:95, 1973.

Mauer SM, Dobrin RS, Vernier RL: Unilateral and bilateral renal agenesis in monoamniotic twins. J Pediat 84:236, 1974.

Hypoplasia

Cha EM, Kandzari S, Khoury GH: Congenital renal hypoplasia: Angiographic study. Am J Roentgenol 114:710, 1972.

Kanasawa M & others: Dwarfed kidneys in children. Am J Dis Child 109:130, 1965.

Dysplasia & Multicystic Kidney

Bernstein J: The morphogenesis of renal parenchymal maldevelopment (renal dysplasia). P Clin North

America 18:395, 1971.

Johnson DE & others: Multilocular renal cystic disease in children. J Urol 109:101, 1973.

Kyaw MM: Roentgenologic triad of congenital multicystic kidney. Am J Roentgenol 119:710, 1973.

Miranda D, Schinella RA, Finegold MJ: Familial renal dysplasia: Microdissection studies in siblings with associated central nervous system and hepatic malformations. Arch Path 93:483, 1972.

Newman L & others: Unilateral total renal dysplasia in children. Am J Roentgenol 116:778, 1972.

Perrin EV & others: Renal duplication and dysplasia. Urology 4:660, 1974.

Risdon RA: Renal dysplasia. 1. A clinicopathological study of 76 cases. 2. A necropsy study of 41 cases. J Clin Path 24:57, 1971.

Stecker JF Jr, Rose JG, Gillenwater JY: Dysplastic kidneys associated with vesicoureteral reflux. J Urol 110:341, 1973.

Polycystic Kidneys

Bernstein J: Heritable cystic disorders of the kidney: The mythology of polycystic disease. P Clin North America 18:435, 1971.

Hatfield PM, Pfister RC: Adult polycystic disease of the kidneys (Potter type 3). JAMA 222:1527, 1972.

Igawa K-I, Miyagishi T: The use of scintillation and ultrasonic scanning to disclose polycystic kidneys and liver. J Urol 108:685, 1972.

Ivemark BI, Lagergren C, Lindvall N: Roentgenologic diagnosis of polycystic kidney and medullary sponge kidney. Acta radiol (diag) 10:225, 1970.

Kendall AR, Pollack HM, Karafin L: Congenital cystic disease of kidney: Classification and manifestations. Urology 4:635, 1974.

Lauritsen JG: Lindau's disease: A study of one family through six generations. Acta chir scandinav 139:482, 1973.

Lazarus JM & others: Hemodialysis and transplantation in adults with polycystic renal disease. JAMA 217:1821, 1971.

Lieberman E & others: Infantile polycystic disease of the kidneys and liver. Medicine 50:277, 1971.

Lufkin EG & others: Polycystic kidney disease: Earlier diagnosis using ultrasound. Urology 4:5, 1974.

Milam JH, Magee JH, Bunts RC: Evaluation of surgical decompression of polycystic kidneys by differential renal clearances. J Urol 90:144, 1963.

Osathanondh V, Potter EL: Pathogenesis of polycystic kidneys. Arch Path 77:459, 1964.

Salvatierra O Jr, Kountz SL, Belzer FO: Polycystic renal disease treated by renal transplantation. Surg Gynec Obst 137:431, 1973.

Sellers AL, Winfield A, Rosen V: Unilateral polycystic disease. J Urol 107:527, 1972.

Vuthibhagdee A, Singleton EB: Infantile polycystic disease of the kidney. Am J Dis Child 125:167, 1973.

Wallack HI, Kandel G, Presman DC: Polycystic kidneys: Indications for surgical intervention. Urology 3:552, 1974.

Wenzl JE, Lagos JC, Albers DD: Tuberous sclerosis presenting as polycystic kidneys and seizures in an infant. J Pediat 77:673, 1970.

Simple Cyst

Deliveliotis A, Zorzos S, Varkarkis M: Suppuration of soli-

tary cyst of the kidney. Brit J Urol 39:472, 1967.

Doust BD, Maklad NF: Control of renal cyst puncture by transverse ultrasonic B scanning. Radiol 109:679, 1973.

Evans AT, Coughlin JP: Urinary obstruction due to renal cysts. J Urol 103:277, 1970.

Firstater M, Farkas A: Simple renal cyst in a newborn. Brit J Urol 45:366, 1973.

Harp GE, Goldstein AMB, Morrow JW: Bleeding solitary renal cysts. Urology 3:649, 1974.

Jackman RJ, Stevens GM: Benign hemorrhagic renal cysts. Radiology 110:7, 1974.

Johanson K-E & others: Management of intrarenal peripelvic cysts. Urology 4:514, 1974.

Lalli AF: Argument for renal cyst aspiration. Urology 1:523, 1973.

Lang EK & others: Assessment of avascular renal mass lesions: The use of nephrotomography, arteriography, cyst puncture, double contrast study and histochemical and histopathologic examination. South MJ 65:1, 1972.

Leopold GR & others: Renal ultrasound: An updated approach to the diagnosis of renal cyst. Radiology 109:671, 1973.

McLaughlin AP III, Pfister RC: Spontaneous rupture of renal cysts into pyelocalyceal system. J Urol 113:2, 1975.

Pollack HM, Goldberg BB, Bogash M: Changing concepts in the diagnosis and management of renal cysts. J Urol 111:326, 1974.

Raskin MM, Roen SA, Serafini AN: Renal cyst puncture: Combined fluoroscopic and ultrasonic technique. Radiology 113:425, 1974.

Romeiser RS, Walls WJ, Valk WL: B-scan ultrasound in the evaluation of renal mass lesions. J Urol 112:8, 1974.

Stables DP, Jackson RS: Management of an infected simple renal cyst. Brit J Radiol 47:290, 1974.

Stahl EL Jr, Stutzman RE: Renal cystography with triple-contrast material. Urology 2:160, 1973.

Thornbury JR: Needle aspiration of avascular renal lesions: Correlation of contrast medium injection with cytologic and arteriographic diagnosis. Radiology 105:299, 1972.

Varma KR & others: Papillary carcinoma in wall of simple renal cyst. Urology 3:762, 1974.

Weitzner S: Clear cell carcinoma of the free wall of a simple renal cyst. J Urol 106:515, 1971.

Woesner ME, Lang DW, Selvaggi FP: Contralateral displacement of the kidney by solitary renal cyst. Am J Roentgenol 116:766, 1972.

Renal Fusion

Blackard CE, Mellinger GT: Cancer in a horseshoe kidney: Report of 2 cases. Arch Surg 97:616, 1968.

Boatman DL, Cornell SH, Kölln, C-P: The arterial supply of horseshoe kidneys. Am J Roentgenol 113:447, 1971.

Downs RA, Lane JW, Burns E: Solitary pelvic kidney: Its clinical implications. Urology 1:51, 1973.

Dworin JW: Crossed ectopia of a solitary kidney. J Urol 102:289, 1969.

Kelalis PP, Malek RS, Segura JW: Observations on renal ectopia and fusion in children. J Urol 110:588, 1973.

Kvarstein B, Mathisen W: Surgical treatment of horseshoe

kidney: A followup study. Scand J Urol Nephrol 8:10, 1974.

Segura JW, Kelalis PP, Burke EC: Horseshoe kidney in children. J Urol 108:333, 1972.

Ectopic Kidney

Arduino LJ: Crossed renal ectopia without fusion. J Urol 93:125, 1965.

Malkin RB, Dodson AI Jr, Koontz WW Jr: Adenocarcinoma in a sigmoid kidney. Urology 4:713, 1974.

Matteo IJ, Stanley RJ: The intrathoracic kidney, with a review of the literature. J Urol 107:538, 1972.

Vargas AD, Carlton FE, Scardino PL: Crossed renal ectopia. South MJ 67:1080, 1974.

Ward JN, Nathanson B, Draper JW: The pelvic kidney. J Urol 94:36, 1965.

Medullary Sponge Kidney

Eisenberg RL, Pfister RC: Medullary sponge kidney associated with congenital hemihypertrophy (asymmetry): A case report and survey of the literature. Am J Roentgenol 116:773, 1972.

Hayt DB & others: Direct magnification intravenous pyelography in re-evaluation of medullary sponge kidney. Am J Roentgenol 119:701, 1973.

Pòtter EL, Osathanondh V: Medullary sponge kidney: Two cases in young infants. J Pediat 62:901, 1963.

Spence HM, Singleton R: What is sponge kidney disease and where does it fit in the spectrum of cystic disorders? J Urol 107:176, 1972.

Swenson RS, Kempson RL, Friedland GW: Cystic disease of the renal medulla in the elderly. JAMA 228:1404, 1974.

ACQUIRED LESIONS

Renoalimentary Fistulas

Bissada NK, Cole AT, Fried FA: Reno-alimentary fistula: An unusual urological problem. J Urol 110:273, 1973.

Chowdhury SD, Higgins PM: An intrarenal foreign body. Brit J Urol 44:133, 1972.

Dunn M, Kirk D: Renogastric fistula: Case report and review of the literature. J Urol 109:785, 1973.

Newman JH, Jeans WD: Reno-colic fistula demonstrated by antegrade pyelography. Brit J Urol 44:692, 1972.

Schwartz DT & others: Pyeloduodenal fistula due to tuberculosis. J Urol 104:373, 1970.

Aneurysm of the Renal Artery

Almgård LE, Fernström I: Embolic occlusion of an intrarenal aneurism: A case report. Brit J Urol 45:485, 1973.

Carron J & others: Renal artery aneurysm: Polyaneurysmal lesion of kidney. Urology 5:1, 1975.

Cohen SG, Cashdan A, Berger R: Spontaneous rupture of a renal artery aneurism during pregnancy. Obst Gynec 39:897, 1972.

Cummings KB, Lecky JW, Kaufman JJ: Renal artery aneurisms and hypertension. J Urol 109:144, 1973.

DeBakey ME & others: Aneurism of the renal artery. Arch Surg 106:438, 1973.

McClure PH, Westcott JL: Periarteritis nodosa with perirenal hemorrhage: A case report with angiographic findings. J Urol 102:126, 1969.

Renal Infarcts

Fay R & others: Renal artery thrombosis: A successful revascularization by autotransplantation. J Urol 111:572, 1974.

Fergus JN, Jones NF, Thomas ML: Kidney function after arterial embolism. Brit MJ 4:587, 1969.

Grablowsky OM & others: Renal artery thrombosis following blunt trauma: Report of four cases. Surgery 67:895, 1970.

Lang EK, Mertz JHO, Nourse M: Renal arteriography in the assessment of renal infarction. J Urol 99:506, 1968.

Mounger EJ: Hypertension resulting from segmental renal artery infarction. Urology 1:189, 1973.

Moyer JD & others: Conservative management of renal artery embolus. J Urol 109:138, 1973.

Ranniger K, Abrams E, Borden TA: Pseudotumor resulting from a fresh renal infarct. Radiology 92:343, 1969.

Schramek A & others: Survival following late renal embolectomy in a patient with a single functioning kidney. J Urol 109:342, 1973.

Smith SP Jr & others: Occlusion of the artery to a solitary kidney: Restoration of renal function after prolonged anuria. JAMA 230:1306, 1974.

Tse RL, Leberman PR: Acute renal artery occlusion—etiology, diagnosis and treatment: Report of a case with subsequent revascularization. J Urol 108:32, 1972.

Thrombosis of the Renal Vein

Belman AB, King LR: The pathology and treatment of renal vein thrombosis in the newborn. J Urol 107:852, 1972.

Bernie JE & others: Left renal vein thrombosis treated conservatively. J Urol 107:517, 1972.

Duffy JL & others: Renal vein thrombosis and the nephrotic syndrome: Report of two cases with successful treatment in one. Am J Med 54:663, 1973.

Kees CJ, Harrell RS: Radiographic manifestations of renal vein thrombosis. J Urol 108:831, 1972.

Lewy PR, Jao W: Nephrotic syndrome in association with renal vein thrombosis in infancy. J Pediat 85:359, 1974.

Mauer SM & others: Bilateral renal vein thrombosis in infancy: Report of a survivor following surgical intervention. J Pediat 78:509, 1971.

McDonald P & others: Some radiologic observations on renal vein thrombosis. Am J Roentgenol 120:368, 1974.

Miller RA, Tremann JA, Ansell JS: The conservative management of renal vein thrombosis. J Urol 111:568, 1974.

Moore HL & others: Unilateral renal vein thrombosis and the nephrotic syndrome. Pediatrics 50:598, 1972.

Rosenmann E, Pollak VE, Pirani CL: Renal vein thrombosis in the adult: A clinical and pathologic study based on renal biopsies. Medicine 47:269, 1968.

Thompson IM, Schneider R, Lababidi Z: Thrombectomy for neonatal renal vein thrombosis. J Urol 113:396, 1975.

Weiner PL & others: Retrograde pyelography in renal vein thrombosis. Radiology 111:77, 1974.

Arteriovenous Fistula

Bookstein JJ, Goldstein HM: Successful management of postbiopsy arteriovenous fistula with selective arterial embolization. Radiology 109:535, 1973.

Chew QT, Madayag MA: Post-nephrectomy arteriovenous fistula. J Urol 109:546, 1973.

DeWeerd JH: Arteriovenous fistula in hypernephroma. J Urol 93:666, 1965.

Ekelund L, Lindholm T: Arteriovenous fistulae following percutaneous renal biopsy. Acta radiol (diag) 11:38, 1971.

Hart PL, Ingram DW, Peckham GB: Postnephrectomy arteriovenous fistula causing "stroke" and congestive heart failure. Canad MAJ 108:1400, 1973.

Javadpour N & others: Intrarenal arteriovenous fistula: Early surgical repair with preservation of renal parenchyma. Urology 1:457, 1973.

Kostiner AI, Burnett LL: Intrarenal arteriovenous fistula: Documented increase in size during an eight-year interval in one case and surgical treatment with renal salvage in another. Radiology 109:531, 1973.

Mark LK: Arteriovenous malformations of kidney. Urology 4:706, 1974.

Nelson BD, Brosman SA, Goodwin WE: Renal arteriovenous fistulas. J Urol 109:779, 1973.

O'Conor VJ Jr, Bergan JJ: Surgical repair in a solitary kidney of a large intrarenal arteriovenous fistula resulting from needle biopsy. J Urol 109:934, 1973.

Rizk GK, Atallah NK, Bridi GI: Renal arteriovenous fistula treated by catheter embolism. Brit J Radiol 46:222, 1973.

Tunner WS & others: Repair of an intrarenal arteriovenous fistula with preservation of the kidney. J Urol 103:286, 1970.

Tynes WV & others: Surgical treatment of renal arteriovenous fistulas: Report of 5 cases. J Urol 103:692, 1970.

Arteriovenous Aneurysm

Merritt BA, Middleton RG: Repair of a huge renal arteriovenous aneurysm with preservation of the kidney. J Urol 107:521, 1972.

Renal Cortical Necrosis

Bloom R, Swenson RS, Coplon NS: Acute renal cortical necrosis: Variable course and changing prognosis. California Med 119:1, Oct 1973.

Kleinknecht D & others: Diagnostic procedures and long-term prognosis in bilateral cortical necrosis. Kidney Internat 4:390, 1973.

Leonidas JC, Berdon WE, Gribetz D: Bilateral renal cortical necrosis in the newborn infant: Roentgenographic diagnosis. J Pediat 79:623, 1971.

Matlin RA, Gary NE: Acute cortical necrosis. Am J Med 56:110, 1974.

Ramachandran S, Perera MVF: Survival in renal cortical necrosis due to snake bite. Postgrad MJ 50:314, 1974.

22...
Diagnosis of
Medical Renal Diseases

Marcus A. Krupp, MD

The medical renal diseases are those that involve principally the parenchyma of the kidneys. Many of the symptoms and signs of urinary tract disease are common to both medical and surgical diseases of the kidneys and other urologic organs. Hematuria, proteinuria, pyuria, oliguria, polyuria, pain, renal insufficiency with azotemia, acidosis, anemia, electrolyte abnormalities, hypertension, headache, and ocular involvement may occur in a wide variety of disorders affecting any portion of the parenchyma of the kidney, its blood vessels, or the excretory tract.

Every effort must be made to rule out nonsurgical disease of the urinary tract before resorting to diagnostic or therapeutic procedures which may prove to be unnecessary or dangerous.

A complete medical history and physical examination, a thorough examination of the urine, and blood chemistry examinations as indicated are essential initial steps in the work-up of any patient.

History

A. Family History: The family history may reveal disease of genetic origin, eg, tubular metabolic anomalies, polycystic kidneys, unusual types of nephritis, or vascular or coagulation defects which may be essential clues to the diagnosis.

B. Past History: The past history should cover infections, injuries, and exposure to toxic agents, anticoagulants, or drugs that may produce toxic or sensitivity reactions, including blood dyscrasias. A history of diabetes, hypertensive disease, and collagen disease may be obtained. The inquiry must also elicit symptoms of uremia, debilitation, and the vascular complications of chronic renal disease.

Physical Examination

One must look for such physical signs as pallor, edema, hypertension, retinopathy, and the stigmas of congenital disease (eg, enlarged kidneys with polycystic disease).

Urinalysis

Examination of the urine (see Chapter 5) is the

Dr Krupp is Clinical Professor of Medicine, Stanford University School of Medicine, Stanford, California, and Director, Palo Alto Medical Research Foundation, Palo Alto, California.

most essential single part of the investigation.

A. Proteinuria: Proteinuria of any significant degree (2–4+) is suggestive of "medical" renal disease (parenchymal involvement). Proteinuria should be interpreted with consideration of the urine specific gravity, since a proteinuria of 1+ in a dilute urine may indicate a significantly great protein loss. Formed elements present in the urine usually establish the diagnosis. Only after careful examination of the patient and suitable urine specimens, as well as analysis of the chemical constituents of the blood, is urography or cystoscopy justified.

1. "Pathologic" proteinurias—Significant proteinuria is present in glomerulonephritis, subacute or chronic nephritis, nephrotic syndrome, collagen disease, diabetic nephropathy, myeloma of the kidney, and polycystic kidney disease.

2. "Nonpathologic" proteinurias—When investigating causes, one must be careful not to overlook mild cases of glomerulonephritis or other parenchymal disease.

a. "Physiologic" proteinuria—After vigorous exercise or protracted physical effort, protein, erythrocytes, casts, and tubule cells may appear transiently in the urine. Repeat examination of the urine after a period of rest usually resolves the problem.

b. Orthostatic proteinuria—Some persons have proteinuria when they are up and about but not while recumbent. In any patient with proteinuria, the degree of proteinuria is usually more pronounced when the patient is upright, and especially when he is active. Absence of proteinuria when the patient is supine during the period of urine formation confirms the diagnosis of orthostatic proteinuria.

B. Red Cell Casts: Although red cells in the urine indicate extravasation of blood anywhere along the urinary tract, the occurrence of red cells in casts proves the renal origin of the bleeding. The erythrocytes forming typical red cell casts are from the glomeruli or the upper portions of the nephron.

C. Fatty Casts and Oval Fat Bodies: Tubule cells showing fatty changes occur in degenerative diseases of the kidney (nephrosis, glomerulonephritis, collagen disease, amyloidosis, and damage due to such toxins as mercury).

D. Other Findings: The presence of abnormal urinary chemical constituents indicative of metabolic disorders involving the kidneys may be the only evidence of such disease. These include diabetes mellitus, renal glycosuria, aminoacidurias (including cystinuria), oxaluria, gout, hyperparathyroidism, hemoglobinuria, and myoglobinuria.

Renal Biopsy

Renal biopsy is a valuable diagnostic procedure which also serves as a guide to rational treatment. The technic has become well established, frequently providing sufficient tissue for light and electron microscopy and for immunofluorescent examination. Absolute contraindications include anatomic presence of only one kidney, severe malfunction of one kidney even though function is adequate in the other, bleeding diathesis, the presence of hemangioma, tumor, or large cysts, abscess or infection, hydronephrosis, and an uncooperative patient. Relative contraindications are the presence of serious hypertension, uremia, severe arteriosclerosis, and unusual difficulty in doing a biopsy due to obesity, anasarca, or inability of the patient to lie flat.

Clinical indications for renal biopsy, in addition to the necessity for establishing a diagnosis, include the need to determine prognosis, to follow progression of a lesion and response to treatment, to confirm the presence of a generalized disease (collagen disorder, amyloidosis, sarcoidosis), and to follow rejection response in a transplanted kidney.

GLOMERULONEPHRITIS

Information obtained from experimentally induced glomerular disease in animals and from correlations with evidence derived by modern methods of examination of tissue obtained by biopsy and at necropsy have provided a new concept of glomerulonephritis.

The clinical manifestations of renal disease are apt to consist only of varying degrees of hematuria, excretion of characteristic formed elements in the urine, proteinuria, and renal insufficiency and its complications. Alterations in glomerular architecture as observed in tissue examined by light microscopy are also apt to be minimal and difficult to interpret. For these reasons, attempts to correlate clinical syndromes with histologic features of renal tissue have failed to provide

Table 22—1. Common patterns of abnormal urine composition in disease.*

Disease	Specific Gravity	Protein†	Red Cells†	Casts†	Microscopic (Casts and Cells) and Other Findings
Normal	1.003–1.030	0 to trace (up to 0.05 g)	0 to occ	0 to occ	Hyaline casts (urine must be acid and fresh or preserved).
Diseases with high fevers	Increased	Trace or +	0	0 to few	Hyaline casts, tubule cells.
Congestive heart failure	High; varies with renal function	1–2+	0 to +	+	Hyaline and granular casts.
Eclampsia	Increased	3–4+	0 to +	3–4+	Hyaline casts.
Diabetic coma	High	+	0	0 to +	Hyaline casts, glucose, ketone bodies.
Acute glomerulo-nephritis‡	Increased	2–4+	1–4+	2–4+	Blood, cellular, granular, hyaline casts; renal tubule epithelium.
Degenerative phase glomerulonephritis	Normal or increased	4+	1–2+	4+	Granular, waxy, hyaline, fatty casts; fatty tubule cells.
Terminal phase glomerulonephritis	Low, fixed	1–2+	Trace to +	1–3+	Granular, hyaline, fatty, broad casts.
Lipoid nephrosis	Very high	4+	0 to trace	4+	Hyaline, granular, fatty, waxy casts; fatty tubule cells.
Collagen diseases	Normal or decreased	1–4+	1–4+	1–4+	Blood, cellular, granular, hyaline, waxy, fatty, broad casts, fatty tubule cells.
Pyelonephritis	Normal or decreased	0 to +	0 to +	0 to +	Leukocyte and hyaline cases, pus cells, bacteria.
Benign hypertension (late)	Normal or low	0 to +	0 to trace	0 to +	Hyaline and granular casts.
Malignant hypertension	Low, fixed	1–2+	Trace to +	1–2+	Hyaline and granular casts.

*Modified from Krupp & others: *Physician's Handbook,* 17th ed. Lange, 1973.
†Scale of 0–4+.
‡May be anuric, or have low, fixed specific gravity.

a satisfactory basis for precise diagnosis, treatment, and prognosis.

More recently, however, immunologic technics for demonstrating a variety of antigens, antibodies, and complement fractions have led to new concepts of the origins and pathogenesis of glomerular disease. Electron microscopy has complemented the immunologic methods.

Briefly, then, glomerular disease resulting from immunologic reactions may be divided into 2 groups:

(1) Immune complex disease, in which soluble antigen-antibody complexes in the circulation are trapped in the glomeruli. The antigens are not derived from glomerular components; they may be exogenous (bacterial, viral, chemical) or endogenous (circulating native DNA, thyroglobulin). Factors in the pathogenic potential of the antigen include its origin, quantity, and route of entry and the host's duration of exposure to it. The immune response to the antigen depends on the severity of inflammation or infection and the host's capacity to respond (immunocompetency).

In the presence of antigen excess, antigen-antibody complexes form in the circulation and are trapped in the glomeruli as they are filtered through capillaries rendered permeable by the action of vasoactive amines. The antigen-antibody complexes bind components of complement, particularly C3. Activated complement provides chemoactive factors which attract leukocytes whose lysosomal enzymes incite the injury to the glomerulus.

By immunofluorescent methods and by electron microscopy, these complexes appear as lumpy deposits between the epithelial cells and the glomerular basement. IgG, IgM, occasionally IgA, β1C, and C3 are demonstrable.

(2) Anti-GBM (glomerular basement membrane) disease, in which antibodies are generated against the glomerular basement membrane of the kidney and often against lung basement membrane, which appears to be antigenically similar to GBM. The autoantibodies may be stimulated by autologous GBM altered in some way or combined with an exogenous agent. The reaction of antibody with GBM is accompanied by activation of complement, the attraction of leukocytes, and the release of lysosomal enzymes. The presence of thrombi in glomerular capillaries is often accompanied by leakage of fibrinogen and precipitation of fibrin in Bowman's space with subsequent development of epithelial "crescents" in the space.

Immunofluorescent technics and electron microscopy show the anti-GBM complexes as linear deposits outlining the GBM. IgG and C3 are usually demonstrable.

The current classification of glomerulonephritis is based on the immunologic concepts described above. However, the discussions in the following pages will be organized according to traditional clinical categories.

I. Immunologic Mechanisms Likely
  A. Immune Complex Disease:
    Glomerulonephritis associated with infectious agents, including staphylococci, pneumococci, bacterial endocarditis, secondary syphilis, malaria, viruses of hepatitis (HB-Ag) and measles
    Lupus erythematosus
    Glomerulonephritis associated with other systemic (?autoimmune) disease such as polyarteritis nodosa, scleroderma, and idiopathic cryoglobulinemia
    Membranous glomerulonephritis, cause unknown
    Membranoproliferative glomerulonephritis, cause unknown
    Focal glomerulonephritis
    Rapidly progressive glomerulonephritis (some cases)
  B. Anti-GBM Disease:
    Goodpasture's syndrome
    Rapidly progressive glomerulonephritis (some cases)
II. Immunologic Mechanisms Not Clearly Demonstrated
    Lipoid nephrosis
    Focal glomerulonephritis (some cases)
    Chronic sclerosing glomerulonephritis
    Diabetic glomerulosclerosis
    Amyloidosis
    Hemolytic-uremic syndrome and thrombohemolytic thrombocytopenic purpura
    Wegener's granulomatosis
    Alport's syndrome
    Sickle cell disease

1. POSTSTREPTOCOCCAL GLOMERULONEPHRITIS

Essentials of Diagnosis

- History of preceding streptococcal infection.
- Malaise, headache, anorexia, low-grade fever.
- Mild generalized edema, mild hypertension, retinal hemorrhages.
- Gross hematuria; protein, red cell casts, granular and hyaline casts, white cells, and renal epithelial cells in urine.
- Elevated antistreptolysin O titer, variable nitrogen retention.

General Considerations

Glomerulonephritis is a disease affecting both kidneys. In most cases recovery from the acute stage is complete, but progressive involvement may destroy renal tissue and renal insufficiency results. Acute glomerulonephritis is most common in children 3−10 years of age, although 5% or more of initial attacks occur in adults over the age of 50. By far the most common cause is an antecedent infection of the pharynx and tonsils or of the skin with group A β-hemolytic streptococci, certain strains of which are nephritogenic. Nephritis occurs in 10–15% of children and young adults who have clinically evident infection with a nephritogenic strain. In children under age 6, pyoderma (impetigo) is the most common antecedent; in older children and young adults, pharyngitis is a common and skin infection a rare antecedent. Nephritogenic strains commonly encountered include, for the skin, M types 49 (Red Lake), 2, and provisional 55; for pharyngitis, types 12, 1, and 4. Rarely, nephritis may follow infections due to pneumococci, staphylococci, some bacilli and viruses, or *Plasmodium malariae* and exposure to some drugs. Rhus dermatitis and reactions to venom or chemical agents may be associated with renal disease clinically indistinguishable from glomerulonephritis.

The pathogenesis of the glomerular lesion has been further elucidated by the use of new immunologic technics (immunofluorescence) and electron microscopy. A likely sequel to infection by nephritogenic strains of β-hemolytic streptococci is injury to the mesangial cells in the intercapillary space. The glomerulus may then become more easily damaged by antigen-antibody complexes developing from the immune response to the streptococcal infection. β1C globulin of complement is deposited in association with IgG or alone in a granular pattern on the epithelial side of the basement membrane, and occasionally in subendothelial sites as well.

Gross examination of the involved kidney shows only punctate hemorrhages throughout the cortex. Microscopically, the primary alteration is in the glomeruli, which show proliferation and swelling of the mesangial and endothelial cells of the capillary tuft. The proliferation of capsular epithelium produces a thickened crescent about the tuft, and in the space between the capsule and the tuft there are collections of leukocytes, red cells, and exudate. Edema of the interstitial tissue and cloudy swelling of the tubule epithelium are common. As the disease progresses, the kidneys may enlarge. The typical histologic findings in glomerulitis are enlarging crescents which become hyalinized and converted into scar tissue and obstruct the circulation through the glomerulus. Degenerative changes occur in the tubules, with fatty degeneration and necrosis and ultimate scarring of the nephron. Arteriolar thickening and obliteration become prominent.

Clinical Findings

A. Symptoms and Signs: Often the disease is very mild, and there may be no reason to suspect renal involvement unless the urine is examined. In severe cases, about 2 weeks following the acute streptococcal infection, the patient develops headache, malaise, mild fever, puffiness around the eyes and face, flank pain, and oliguria. Hematuria is usually noted as "bloody" or, if the urine is acid, as "brown" or "coffee-colored." Respiratory difficulty with shortness of breath may occur as a result of salt and water retention and circulatory congestion. There may be moderate tachycardia and moderate to marked elevation of blood pressure.

Tenderness in the costovertebral angle is common.

B. Laboratory Findings: The diagnosis is confirmed by examination of the urine, which may be grossly bloody or coffee-colored (acid hematin) or may show only microscopic hematuria. In addition, the urine contains protein (1–3+) and casts. Hyaline and granular cases are commonly found in large numbers, but the classical sign of glomerulitis, the erythrocyte cast (blood cast), may be found only occasionally in the urinary sediment. The erythrocyte cast resembles a blood clot formed in the lumen of a renal tubule; it is usually of small caliber, intensely orange or red, and under high power with proper lighting may show the mosaic pattern of the packed red cells held together by the clot of fibrin and plasma protein.

With the impairment of renal function (decrease in GFR and blood flow) and with oliguria, plasma or serum urea nitrogen and creatinine become elevated, the levels varying with the severity of the renal lesion. The sedimentation rate is rapid. A mild normochromic anemia may result from fluid retention and dilution. Infection of the throat with nephritogenic streptococci is frequently followed by increasing antistreptolysin O (ASO) titers in the serum, whereas high titers are usually not demonstrable following skin infections. Production of antibody against streptococcal deoxyribonuclease B (anti-DNase B) is more regularly observed following both throat and skin infections. Serum complement levels are usually low.

Confirmation of diagnosis is made by examination of the urine, although the history and clinical findings in typical cases leave little doubt. The finding of erythrocytes in a cast is proof that erythrocytes were present in the renal tubules and did not arise from elsewhere in the genitourinary tract.

Differential Diagnosis

Although considered to be the hallmark of glomerulonephritis, erythrocyte casts also occur along with other abnormal elements in any disease in which glomerular inflammation and tubule damage are present, ie, polyarteritis nodosa, disseminated lupus erythematosus, dermatomyositis, sarcoidosis, subacute bacterial endocarditis, "focal" nephritis, Goodpasture's syndrome, Henoch's purpura, or poisoning with chemicals toxic to the kidney.

Treatment

There is no specific treatment. Eradication of infection, prevention of overhydration and hypertension, and prompt treatment of complications such as hypertensive encephalopathy and heart failure require careful observation and management.

Prognosis

The progression of glomerulonephritis to healing or advancing disease is depicted in Fig 22–1. Most patients with the acute disease recover completely within 1–2 years; 5–20% show progressive renal damage. If oliguria, heart failure, or hypertensive encephalopathy is severe, death may occur during the acute

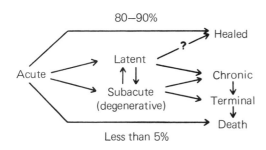

Figure 22–1. Prognosis in glomerulonephritis.

attack. Even with severe acute disease, however, recovery is the rule, particularly in children.

2. CHRONIC GLOMERULONEPHRITIS

Progressive destruction of the kidney may continue for many years in a clinically latent or subacute form. The subacute form is similar to the latent form (see below) except that symptoms occur, ie, malaise, mild fever, and sometimes flank pain and oliguria. Treatment is as for the acute attack. Exacerbations may appear from time to time, reflecting the stage of evolution of the disease.

3. LATENT GLOMERULONEPHRITIS

If acute glomerulonephritis does not heal within 1–2 years, the vascular and glomerular lesions continue to progress and tubular changes occur. In the presence of smoldering, active nephritis, the patient is usually asymptomatic and the evidence of disease consists only of the excretion of abnormal urinary elements.

The urinary excretion of protein, red cells, white cells, epithelial cells, and casts (including erythrocyte casts, granular casts, and hyaline and waxy casts) continues at levels above normal. As renal impairment progresses, signs of renal insufficiency appear (see below).

The differential diagnosis is the same as that given for acute glomerulonephritis. Recent studies of tissue obtained by renal biopsy in cases of recurrent or persistent hematuria indicate a high incidence of mesangial deposition of immune complexes made up of IgM or IgA (rarely IgG) and fractions of complement.

Prevention

Treat intercurrent infections promptly and vigorously as indicated. Avoid unnecessary vaccinations.

Prognosis

Worsening of the urinary findings may occur with infection, trauma, or fatigue. Exacerbations may resemble the acute attack and may be associated with intercurrent infection or trauma. Other exacerbations may be typical of the nephrotic syndrome (see below). Death in uremia is the usual outcome, but the course is variable and the patient may live a reasonably normal life for 20–30 years.

4. ANTI-GLOMERULAR BASEMENT MEMBRANE NEPHRITIS (Goodpasture's Syndrome)

The patient usually gives a history of recent hemoptysis and often of malaise, anorexia, and headache. The clinical syndrome is that of a severe acute glomerulonephritis accompanied by diffuse hemorrhagic inflammation of the lungs. The urine shows gross or microscopic hematuria, and laboratory findings of severely suppressed renal function are usually evident. Biopsy shows glomerular crescents, glomerular adhesions, and inflammatory infiltration interstitially. Electron microscopic examination shows an increase in basement membrane material and deposition of fibrin beneath the capillary endothelium. In some cases, circulating antibody against glomerular basement membrane can be identified. IgG and a1C complement can be demonstrated as linear deposits on the basement membranes of the glomeruli and the lung. Antiglomerular basement membrane antibody also reacts with lung basement membrane.

Only rare cases of survival have been documented. Adrenal corticosteroid therapy in combination with immunosuppressive therapy may be useful. Hemodialysis and nephrectomy with renal transplantation may offer the only hope for rescue. Transplantation should be delayed until circulating antiglomerular antibodies have disappeared.

Occasionally, acute renal disease with a similar clinical and immunologic pattern may occur without associated lung disease. Termed **idiopathic rapidly progressive glomerulonephritis**, it characteristically progresses to severe renal insufficiency in a few weeks.

NEPHROTIC SYNDROME

Essentials of Diagnosis

- Massive edema.
- Proteinuria > 3.5 g/day.
- Hypoalbuminemia < 3 g/100 ml.
- Hyperlipidemia: Cholesterol > 300 mg/100 ml.
- Lipiduria: Free fat, oval fat bodies, fatty casts.

General Considerations

Because treatment and prognosis vary with the cause of nephrotic syndrome (nephrosis), renal biopsy and appropriate examination of an adequate tissue specimen are important. Light microscopy, electron microscopy, and immunofluorescent identification of immune mechanisms provide critical information for identification of most of the causes of nephrosis.

Glomerular diseases associated with nephrosis include the following:

(1) Minimal glomerular lesions: Lipoid nephrosis accounts for about 20% of cases of nephrosis in adults. No abnormality is visible by examination of biopsy material with the light microscope. With the electron microscope, alterations of the glomerular basement membrane with swelling and vacuolization and loss of organization of foot processes of the epithelial cells (foot process disease) are evident. There is no evidence of immune disease by immunofluorescent studies. The response to treatment with adrenocortical steroids is satisfactory. Renal function remains good.

(2) Membranous glomerulonephritis: (About 25–27% of cases.) Examination of biopsy material with the light microscope shows thickening of the glomerular capillary walls and some swelling of mesangial cells but no cellular proliferation. With the electron microscope, irregular lumpy deposits appear between the basement membrane and the epithelial cells and new basement membrane material protrudes from the glomerular basement membrane as spikes or domes. Immunofluorescent studies show diffuse granular deposits of immunoglobulins (especially IgG) and complement (C3 component). As the membrane thickens, glomeruli become sclerosed and hyalinized.

This form of disease does not respond to any form of therapy. It usually progresses to renal failure in the course of a few to 10 years.

(3) Membranoproliferative (hypocomplement-emic) glomerulonephritis: (About 5% of cases.) Light microscopy shows thickening of glomerular capillaries accompanied by mesangial proliferation and obliteration of glomeruli. With the electron microscope, subendothelial deposits and growth of mesangium into capillary walls are demonstrable. Immunofluorescent studies show the presence of the C3 component of complement and, rarely, the presence of immunoglobulins. There is no known treatment.

(4) Proliferative glomerulonephritis: (About 5% of cases.) This is considered to be a stage in the course of poststreptococcal nephritis.

Clinical Findings

A. Symptoms and Signs: Edema may appear insidiously and increase slowly; often it appears suddenly and accumulates rapidly. As fluid collects in the serous cavities, the abdomen becomes protuberant and the patient may complain of anorexia and become short of breath. Symptoms other than those related to the mechanical effects of edema and serous sac fluid accumulation are not remarkable.

On physical examination, massive edema is apparent. Signs of hydrothorax and ascites are common. Pallor is often accentuated by the edema, and striae commonly appear in the stretched skin of the extremities. Hypertension, changes in the retina and retinal vessels, and cardiac and cerebral manifestations of hypertension may be demonstrated more often when collagen disease, diabetes mellitus, or renal insufficiency is present.

B. Laboratory Findings: The urine contains large amounts of protein, 4–10 g/24 hours or more. The sediment contains casts, including the characteristic fatty and waxy varieties; renal tubule cells, some of which contain fatty droplets (oval fat bodies); and variable numbers of erythrocytes. A mild normochromic anemia is common, but anemia may be more severe if renal damage is great. Nitrogen retention varies with the severity of impairment of renal function. The plasma is often lipemic, and the blood cholesterol is usually greatly elevated. Plasma protein is greatly reduced. The albumin fraction may fall to less than 2 g or even below 1 g/100 ml. Some reduction of gamma globulin occurs in pure nephrosis, whereas in systemic lupus erythematosus the protein of the gamma fraction may be greatly elevated. Serum complement is usually low in active disease. The serum electrolyte concentrations are often normal, although the serum sodium may be slightly low; total serum calcium may be low, in keeping with the degree of hypoalbuminemia and decrease in the protein-bound calcium moiety. During edema-forming periods, urinary sodium excretion is very low and urinary aldosterone excretion elevated. If renal insufficiency (see above) is present, the blood and urine findings are usually altered accordingly.

Renal biopsy is essential to confirm the diagnosis and to indicate prognosis.

Differential Diagnosis

The nephrotic syndrome (nephrosis) may be associated with a variety of renal diseases, including glomerulonephritis (membranous and proliferative), collagen diseases (disseminated lupus erythematosus, polyarteritis, etc), amyloid disease, thrombosis of the renal vein, diabetic nephropathy, myxedema, multiple myeloma, malaria, syphilis, reaction to toxins such as bee venom, Rhus antigen, drugs such as trimethadione, heavy metals, and constrictive pericarditis. In small children, nephrosis may occur without clear evidence of any cause.

Treatment

An adequate diet with restricted sodium intake (0.5–1 g/day) and prompt treatment of intercurrent infection are the basis of therapy. Other measures may be added as required.

The corticosteroids have been shown to be of value in treating nephrotic syndrome in children and in adults when the underlying disease is the minimal glomerular lesion (lipoid nephrosis), systemic lupus erythematosus, proliferative glomerulonephritis, or idiosyncrasy to toxin or venom. These drugs are less often effective in the treatment of membranous disease and membranoproliferative lesions of the glomerulus. They are of little or no value in amyloidosis or renal vein thrombosis and are contraindicated in diabetic nephropathy.

Diuretics may be given but are often ineffective. The most useful are the thiazide derivatives, eg, hydrochlorothiazide, 50–100 mg every 12 hours; other thiazides, chlorthalidone, and other diuretics may be employed in comparable effective dose levels. Spironolactone may be helpful when employed concurrently with thiazides. Salt-free albumin, dextran, and other oncotic agents are of little help, and their effects are transient.

Immunosuppressive drugs (alkylating agents, cyclophosphamide, mercaptopurine, azathioprine, etc) are under trial in the treatment of nephrotic syndrome. Combination therapy with corticosteroids is similar to that employed in reversing rejection of homotransplants in man. Encouraging early results have been reported in children and adults with proliferative or membranous lesions and with systemic lupus erythematosus. Those with minimal lesions refractory to corticosteroid therapy did no better when immunosuppressive agents were added. Improvement was noted in the glomerular changes and renal function in many patients responding well to treatment. It is not known what percentage of patients can be expected to benefit from these drugs.

Both the corticosteroids and the cytotoxic agents are commonly associated with serious side-effects. At present, this form of therapy should be employed only by those experienced in treating nephrotic syndrome in patients who have proved refractory to well-established treatment regimens.

For renal vein thrombosis, treatment is directed against progress of thrombus formation with heparin and long-term use of coumarin drugs.

Prognosis

The course and prognosis depend upon the basic disease responsible for nephrotic syndrome. In about 50% of cases of childhood nephrosis, the disease appears to run a rather benign course when properly treated and to leave insignificant sequelae. Of the others, most go inexorably into the terminal state with renal insufficiency. Adults with nephrosis fare less well, particularly when the fundamental disease is glomerulonephritis, systemic lupus erythematosus, amyloidosis, renal vein thrombosis, or diabetic nephropathy. In those with minimal lesions, remissions, either spontaneous or following corticosteroid therapy, are common. Treatment is more often unsuccessful or only ameliorative when other glomerular lesions are present. Hypertension and nitrogen retention are serious signs.

RENAL INVOLVEMENT IN COLLAGEN DISEASES

The collagen diseases often produce symptoms and signs of renal disease indistinguishable from acute or chronic glomerulonephritis, nephrosis, renal vein thrombosis, and renal infarction. Although it may not be accurate to classify all of these disorders as collagen diseases, acute disseminated lupus erythematosus, polyarteritis nodosa, scleroderma, dermatomyositis, Wegener's granulomatosis, and thrombotic thrombocytopenic purpura have been implicated in producing a syndrome resembling glomerulonephritis. In about one-third to one-half of cases, the urine sediment is diagnostic, containing red blood cells and red blood cell casts; renal tubule cells, including some filled with fat droplets; and waxy and granular broad casts. The presence of these formed elements is indicative of active glomerular and tubular disease with extensive focal destruction of nephrons. The symptoms and signs of the primary disease and a variety of new tests of autoimmune disease help to differentiate the form of collagen disease present. When collagen disease involves the kidneys, complete recovery from the disease is not likely to occur, although steroid and immunosuppressive drugs (alone or in combination) may be effective for long-term amelioration.

DISEASES OF THE RENAL TUBULES & INTERSTITIUM

1. INTERSTITIAL NEPHRITIS

Acute interstitial disease may be due to systemic infections such as syphilis and sensitivity to drugs, including antibiotics (penicillins, colistin, sulfonamides), phenindione, and diphenylhydantoin. Recovery may be complete.

Chronic interstitial nephritis is characterized by focal or diffuse interstitial fibrosis accompanied by infiltration with inflammatory cells ultimately associated with extensive atrophy of renal tubules. It represents a nonspecific reaction to a variety of causes: analgesic abuse, lead and cadmium toxicity, nephrocalcinosis, urate nephropathy, radiation nephritis, sarcoidosis, Balkan nephritis, and some instances of obstructive uropathy. There are a few cases in which antitubule basement membrane antibodies have been identified.

2. ANALGESIC NEPHROPATHY

Renal papillary necrosis has usually been associated with fulminating urinary tract infection in the presence of diabetes mellitus. Since 1953, however, increasing numbers of cases have been associated with long-term ingestion of phenacetin alone or in analgesic mixtures. The typical patient is a middle-aged woman with chronic and recurrent headaches or a patient with chronic arthritis who habitually consumes large amounts of analgesic mixtures containing phenacetin. The ensuing damage to the kidneys usually is detected late, after renal insufficiency has developed.

The kidney lesion is pathologically nonspecific, consisting of peritubular and perivascular inflammation with degenerative changes of the tubule cells (chronic interstitial nephritis). There are no glomerular changes. Renal papillary necrosis extending into the medulla may involve many papillae.

Hematuria is a common presenting complaint. Renal colic occurs when necrotic renal papillae slough away. Polyuria may be prominent. Signs of acidosis (hyperpnea), dehydration, and pallor of anemia are common. Infection is a frequent complication. The history of phenacetin ingestion may be concealed by the patient.

The urine usually is remarkable only for the presence of blood and small amounts of protein. Hemolytic anemia is usually evident. Elevated BUN and creatinine and the electrolyte changes characteristic of renal failure are typically present.

Urograms show typical cavities and ring shadows of areas of destruction of papillae.

Treatment consists of withholding analgesics containing phenacetin and aspirin. Renal failure and infection are treated as outlined elsewhere in this chapter.

3. URIC ACID NEPHROPATHY

Crystals of urate produce an interstitial inflammatory reaction. Urate may precipitate out in acid urine in the calyces distally in the ureters to form uric acid stones. Patients with myeloproliferative disease under treatment may develop hyperuricemia and are subject to occlusion of the upper urinary tract by uric acid crystals. Alkalinization of the urine and a liberal fluid intake will help prevent crystal formation. Allopurinol is a useful drug to prevent hyperuricemia and hyperuricosuria.

4. OBSTRUCTIVE UROPATHY

Interstitial nephritis due to obstruction may not be associated with infection. Tubular conservation of salt and water is impaired. Following relief of obstruction, diuresis may be massive and may require vigorous but judicious replacement of water and electrolyte.

5. MYELOMATOSIS

Features of myelomatosis which contribute to renal disease include proteinuria (including filtrable Bence Jones protein and κ and λ chains) with precipitation in the tubules leading to accumulation of abnormal proteins in the tubule cells, hypercalcemia, and occasionally increase in viscosity of the blood associated with macroglobulinemia. A Fanconi-like syndrome may develop.

Plugging of tubules, giant cell reaction around tubules, tubular atrophy, and, occasionally, the accumulation of amyloid are evident on examination of renal tissue.

Renal failure may occur acutely or may develop slowly. Hemodialysis may rescue the patient during efforts to control the myeloma with chemical agents.

HEREDITARY RENAL DISEASES

The importance of inheritance and the familial incidence of disease warrants inclusion of the classification of hereditary renal diseases suggested by Perkoff (see reference below). Although relatively uncommon in the population at large, hereditary renal disease must be recognized to permit early diagnosis and treatment in other family members and to prepare the way for genetic counseling.

1. HEREDITARY CHRONIC NEPHRITIS

Evidence of the disease usually appears in childhood, with episodes of hematuria often following an upper respiratory infection. Renal insufficiency commonly develops in males but only rarely in females. Survival beyond age 40 is rare.

In many families, deafness and abnormalities of the eyes accompany the renal disease. Another form of the disease is accompanied by polyneuropathy. Infection of the urinary tract is a common complication.

The anatomic features in some cases resemble proliferative glomerulonephritis; in others, there is thickening of the glomerular basement membrane or podocyte proliferation and thickening of Bowman's capsule. In a few cases there are fat-filled cells (foam cells) in the interstitial tissue or in the glomeruli.

Laboratory findings are commensurate with existing renal function.

Treatment is symptomatic.

2. CYSTIC DISEASES OF THE KIDNEY

Congenital structural anomalies of the kidney must always be considered in any patient with hypertension, pyelonephritis, or renal insufficiency. The manifestations of structural renal abnormalities are related to the superimposed disease, but management and prognosis are modified by the structural anomaly.

Polycystic Kidneys

Polycystic kidney disease is familial and often involves not only the kidney but the liver and pancreas as well.

The formation of cysts in the cortex of the kidney is thought to result from failure of union of the collecting tubules and convoluted tubules of some nephrons. New cysts do not form, but those present enlarge and, by exerting pressure, cause destruction of adjacent tissue. Cysts may be found in the liver and pancreas. The incidence of cerebral vessel aneurysms is higher than normal.

Cases of polycystic disease are discovered during the investigation of hypertension, by diagnostic study in patients presenting with pyelonephritis or hematuria, or by investigating the families of patients with polycystic disease. At times, flank pain due to hemorrhage into a cyst will call attention to a kidney disorder. Otherwise the symptoms and signs are those commonly seen in hypertension or renal insufficiency. On physical examination the enlarged, irregular kidneys are easily palpable.

The urine may contain leukocytes and red cells. With bleeding into the cysts there may also be bleeding into the urinary tract. The blood chemical findings reflect the degree of renal insufficiency. X-ray examination shows the enlarged kidneys, and urography demonstrates the classical elongated calyces and renal pelves stretched over the surface of the cysts.

No specific therapy is available, and surgical interference is contraindicated unless ureteral obstruction is produced by an adjacent cyst. Hypertension, infection, and uremia are treated in the conventional manner.

Because persons with polycystic kidneys may live in reasonable comfort with slowly advancing uremia, it is difficult to determine when renal transplantation is in order. Hemodialysis can extend the life of the patient, but recurrent bleeding and continuous pain indicate the need for a transplant.

Although the disease may become symptomatic in childhood or early in early adult life, it usually is discovered in the fourth or fifth decades. Unless fatal complications of hypertension or urinary tract infection are present, uremia develops very slowly and patients live longer than with other causes of renal insufficiency.

Cystic Disease of the Renal Medulla

Two syndromes have been recognized with increasing frequency as their diagnostic features have become better known.

Medullary cystic disease is a familial disease which may become symptomatic during adolescence. Anemia is usually the initial manifestation, but azotemia, acidosis, and hyperphosphatemia soon become evident. Hypertension may develop. The urine is not remark-able, although there is often an inability to produce a concentrated urine. Many small cysts are scattered through the renal medulla. Renal transplantation is indicated by the usual criteria for the operation.

Sponge kidney is asymptomatic and is discovered by the characteristic appearance of the urogram. Enlargement of the papillae and calyces and small cavities within the pyramids are demonstrated by the contrast media in the excretory urogram. Many small calculi often occupy the cysts, and infection may be troublesome. Life expectancy is not affected, and only symptomatic therapy for ureteral impaction of a stone or for infection is required.

3. ANOMALIES OF THE PROXIMAL TUBULE

Defects of Amino Acid Reabsorption

A. Congenital Cystinuria: Increased excretion of cystine results in the formation of cystine calculi in the urinary tract. Ornithine, arginine, and lysine are also excreted in abnormally large quantities. There is also a defect in absorption of these amino acids in the jejunum. Nonopaque stones should be examined chemically to provide a specific diagnosis.

Maintain a high urine volume by giving a large fluid intake. Maintain the urine pH above 7.0 by giving sodium bicarbonate and sodium citrate plus acetazolamide at bedtime to ensure an alkaline night urine. In refractory cases, a low-methionine (cystine precursor) diet may be necessary. Penicillamine has proved useful in some cases.

B. Aminoaciduria: Many amino acids may be poorly absorbed, resulting in unusual losses. Failure to thrive and the presence of other tubular deficits suggest the diagnosis.

There is no treatment.

C. Hepatolenticular Degeneration: In this congenital familial disease, aminoaciduria is associated with cirrhosis of the liver and neurologic manifestations. Hepatomegaly, evidence of impaired liver function, spasticity, athetosis, emotional disturbances, and Kayser-Fleischer rings around the cornea constitute a unique syndrome. There is a decrease in synthesis of ceruloplasmin with a deficit of plasma ceruloplasmin and an increase in free copper which may be etiologically specific.

Give penicillamine to chelate and remove excess copper. Edathamil (EDTA) may also be used to remove copper.

Multiple Defects of Tubular Function (De Toni-Fanconi-Debre syndrome)

Aminoaciduria, phosphaturia, glycosuria, and a variable degree of renal tubular acidosis characterize this syndrome. Osteomalacia is a prominent clinical feature; other clinical and laboratory manifestations are associated with specific tubular defects described separately above.

The proximal segment of the renal tubule is replaced by a thin tubular structure constituting the "swan neck" deformity. The proximal segment also is shortened to less than half the normal length.

Treatment consists of replacing cation deficits (especially potassium), correcting acidosis with bicarbonate or citrate, replacing phosphate loss with isotonic neutral phosphate (mono- and disodium salts) solution, and a liberal calcium intake. Vitamin D is usually useful, but the dose used must be controlled by monitoring serum calcium and phosphate.

Defects of Phosphorus & Calcium Absorption

A. Vitamin D-Resistant Rickets: Excessive loss of phosphorus and calcium results in rickets or osteomalacia which respond poorly to vitamin D therapy. Treatment consists of giving large doses of vitamin D and calcium supplementation of the diet.

B. Pseudohypoparathyroidism: As a result of excessive reabsorption of phosphorus, hyperphosphatemia and hypocalcemia occur. Symptoms include muscle cramps, fatigue, weakness, tetany, and mental retardation. The signs are those of hypocalcemia; in addition, the patients are short, round-faced, and characteristically have short fourth and fifth metacarpal and metatarsal bones. The serum phosphorus is high, serum calcium low, and serum alkaline phosphatase normal. There is no response to parathyroid hormone.

Vitamin D therapy and calcium supplementation may prevent tetany.

Defects of Glucose Absorption (Renal Glycosuria)

This results from an abnormally low ability to reabsorb glucose, so that glycosuria is present when blood glucose levels are normal. Ketosis is not present. The glucose tolerance response is usually normal. In some instances, renal glycosuria may precede the onset of true diabetes mellitus.

There is no treatment for renal glycosuria.

Defects of Glucose & Phosphate Absorption (Glycosuric Rickets)

The symptoms and signs are those of rickets or osteomalacia, with weakness, pain, or discomfort of the legs and spine, and tetany. The bones become deformed, with bowing of the weight-bearing long bones, kyphoscoliosis, and, in children, signs of rickets. X-ray shows markedly decreased density of the bone, with pseudofracture lines and other deformities. Nephrocalcinosis may occur with excessive phosphaturia, and renal insufficiency may follow. Urinary calcium and phosphorus are increased and glycosuria is present. Serum glucose is normal, serum calcium is normal or low, serum phosphorus is low, and serum alkaline phosphatase is elevated.

Treatment consists of giving large doses of vitamin D and calcium supplementation of the diet.

Defects of Bicarbonate Reabsorption

A form of renal tubular acidosis in which proximal tubular wasting of bicarbonate is the characteristic defect may be associated with multiple dysfunctions of the proximal tubule, often genetically transmitted. Excretion of excessive amounts of bicarbonate occurs even in the presence of low plasma bicarbonate.

For a complete discussion, see Morris RC Jr: New England J Med 281:1405, 1969.

4. ANOMALIES OF THE DISTAL TUBULE

Defects of Hydrogen Ion Secretion & Bicarbonate Reabsorption (Classical Renal Tubular Acidosis)

Failure to secrete hydrogen ion and to form ammonium ion results in loss of "fixed base": sodium, potassium, and calcium. There is also a high rate of excretion of phosphate. Vomiting, poor growth, and symptoms and signs of chronic metabolic acidosis are accompanied by weakness due to potassium deficit and the bone discomfort due to osteomalacia. Nephrocalcinosis, with calcification in the medullary portions of the kidney, occurs in about half of cases. The urine is alkaline and contains larger than normal quantities of sodium, potassium, calcium, and phosphate. The blood chemical findings are those of metabolic acidosis (low HCO_3^- or CO_2) with hyperchloremia, low serum calcium and phosphorus, low serum potassium, and, occasionally, low serum sodium.

Treatment consists of replacing deficits and increasing the intake of sodium potassium, calcium, and phosphorus. Sodium and potassium should be given as bicarbonate or citrate. Additional vitamin D may be required.

Excess Potassium Secretion (Potassium "Wastage" Syndrome)

Excessive renal secretion or loss of potassium may occur in 4 situations: (1) chronic renal insufficiency with diminished H^+ secretion; (2) renal tubular acidosis and the De Toni-Fanconi syndrome, with cation loss resulting from diminished H^+ and NH_4^+ secretion; (3) hyperaldosteronism and hyperadrenocorticism; and (4) tubular secretion of potassium, the cause of which is as yet unknown. Hypokalemia indicates that the deficit is severe. Muscle weakness, metabolic alkalosis, and polyuria with dilute urine are signs attributable to hypokalemia.

Treatment consists of correcting the primary disease and giving supplementary potassium.

Defects of Water Absorption (Renal Diabetes Insipidus)

Nephrogenic diabetes insipidus occurs more frequently in males. Unresponsiveness to antidiuretic hormone is the key to differentiation from pituitary diabetes insipidus.

In addition to congenital refractoriness to antidiuretic hormone, obstructive uropathy, lithium, methoxyflurane, and demeclocycline may also render the tubule refractory.

Symptoms are related to an inability to reabsorb water with resultant polyuria and polydipsia. The urine volume approaches 12 liters/day, and osmolality and specific gravity are low. Mental retardation, atonic bladder, and hydronephrosis occur frequently.

Treatment consists primarily of an adequate water intake. Chlorothiazide may ameliorate the diabetes; the mechanism of action is unknown, but the drug may act by increasing isosmotic reabsorption in the proximal segment of the tubule.

5. UNSPECIFIED RENAL TUBULAR ABNORMALITIES

In **idiopathic hypercalciuria**, decreased reabsorption of calcium predisposes to the formation of renal calculi. Serum calcium and phosphorus are normal. Urine calcium excretion is high; urine phosphorus excretion is low.

See treatment of urinary stones containing calcium.

● ● ●

References

General

Black DAK (editor): *Renal Disease,* 3rd ed. Oxford Univ Press, 1972.

De Wardener HE: *The Kidney: An Outline of Normal and Abnormal Structure and Function.* Little, Brown, 1961.

Earley LE & others: Nephrotic syndrome. California Med 115:23, Nov 1971. (Editorial by Relman AS: The nephrotic syndrome. California Med 115:58, Dec 1971.)

Krupp MA: Genitourinary tract. Chap 15 in: *Current Medical Diagnosis & Treatment 1975.* Krupp MA, Chatton MJ (editors). Lange, 1975.

Lindheimer MD & others: The kidney in pregnancy. New England J Med 283:1095, 1970.

Papper S: *Clinical Nephrology.* Little, Brown, 1971.

Pitts RF: *Physiology of the Kidney and Body Fluids,* 2nd ed. Year Book, 1968.

Smith HW: *The Kidney: Structure and Function in Health and Disease.* Oxford Univ Press, 1952.

Strauss MB, Welt G (editors): *Diseases of the Kidney,* 2nd ed. Little, Brown, 1971.

Symposium on diseases of the kidney. M Clin North America 55:1, 1971.

Symposium on glomerulonephritis. Bull New York Acad Med 46:747, 1970.

Urinalysis

Brody LH & others: Urinalysis and the urinary sediment. M Clin North America 55:243, 1971.

Lippman RW: *Urine and the Urinary Sediment; a Practical Manual and Atlas,* 2nd ed. Thomas, 1957.

Glomerulonephritis

Baldwin DS & others: The long-term course of post-streptococcal glomerulonephritis. Ann Int Med 80:342, 1974.

Carpenter CB: Immunologic aspects of renal disease. Ann Rev Med 21:1, 1970.

Dixon FJ: The pathogenesis of glomerulonephritis. Am J Med 44:493, 1968.

Fish AJ & others: Epidemic acute glomerulonephritis associated with type 49 streptococcal pyoderma. II. Correlative study of light, immunofluorescent and electron microscopic findings. Am J Med ·48:28, 1970.

Gutman RA & others: The immune complex glomerulonephritis of subacute bacterial endocarditis. Medicine 51:1, 1972.

Kaplan EL & others: Epidemic acute glomerulonephritis associated with type 49 streptococcal pyoderma. I. Clinical and laboratory findings. Am J Med 48:9, 1970.

Lewis EJ: Rapidly progressive glomerulonephritis. The Kidney 6:1, Jan 1973.

Lewis EJ & others: An immunopathologic study of rapidly progressive glomerulonephritis in the adult. Human Path 2:185, 1971.

Mahieu P & others: Detection of humoral and cell mediated immunity to kidney basement membrane in human renal disease. Am J Med 53:185, 1972.

Merrill JP: Glomerulonephritis. (3 parts.) New England J Med 290:257, 313, 374, 1974.

Morel-Maroger L, Leathem A, Richet G: Glomerular abnormalities in nonsystemic diseases. Am J Med 53:170, 1972.

Wannamaker LW: Streptococcal infections of the throat and skin. New England J Med 282:78, 1970.

Wilson CB: Immunological mechanisms of glomerulonephritis. California Med 116:47, Jan 1972.

Nephrotic Syndrome

Hayslett JP & others: Clinicopathological correlation in the nephrotic syndrome due to primary renal disease. Medicine 52:93, 1973.

Hopper J Jr & others: Lipoid nephrosis in 31 adult patients: Renal biopsy study by light, electron and fluorescence microscopy with experience in treatment. Medicine 49:321, 1970.

Medical Research Council Working Party: Controlled trial of azathioprine and prednisone in chronic renal disease. Brit MJ 2:239,.1971.

Rosen S: Membranous glomerulonephritis: Current status. Human Path 2:209, 1972.

Skinner MD, Schwartz RS: Immunosuppressive therapy. (2 parts.) New England J Med 287:221, 281, 1972.

Steinberg AD & others: Cytotoxic drugs in treatment of nonmalignant diseases. Ann Int Med 76:619, 1972.

White RHR, Cameron JS, Trounce JR: Immunosuppressive therapy in steroid-resistant proliferative glomerulonephritis accompanied by the nephrotic syndrome. Brit MJ 2:853, 1966.

Cystic Disease

Gardner KD Jr: Evolution of clinical signs in adult-onset cystic disease of the renal medulla. Ann Int Med 74:47, 1971.

Hatfield PM, Pfister RC: Adult polycystic disease of the kidneys (Potter type 3). JAMA 222:1527, 1972.

Medical Staff Conference: Renal cystic disease. California Med 119:36, Nov 1973.

Osathanondh V, Potter EL: Pathogenesis of polycystic kidneys. Arch Path 77:459, 1964.

Wahlqvist L: Cystic disorders of kidney: Review of pathogenesis and classification. J Urol 97:1, 1967.

Tubule Disorders

Courey WR, Pfister RC: The radiographic findings in renal tubular acidosis. Radiology 105:497, 1972.

Frimpter GW: Aminoacidurias due to inherited disorders of metabolism. (2 parts.) New England J Med 289:835, 895, 1974.

Lee DBN & others: The adult Fanconi syndrome. Medicine 51:107, 1972.

Perkoff GT: Hereditary renal diseases. (2 parts.) New England J Med 277:79, 129, 1967.

Stanbury JB, Wyngaarden JB, Fredrickson DS (editors): *The Metabolic Basis of Inherited Disease,* 3rd ed. McGraw-Hill, 1972.

23...
Oliguria

Richards P. Lyon, MD

When the urine output is so low that the end products of metabolism cannot be effectively excreted, the patient is said to be in a state of oliguria. It is not possible to define oliguria in terms of so many milliliters of urine excreted. A patient who can concentrate urine to a specific gravity of 1.040 does not become oliguric until his daily urine volume falls below 500 ml; the patient who can concentrate only to a specific gravity of 1.006 is oliguric when his daily urine volume falls below 1000 ml.

The causes of oliguria may be classified as follows: (1) organic renal lesions, eg, acute tubular necrosis (lower nephron syndrome), acute glomerulonephritis, and terminal chronic renal disease;* (2) severe fluid and electrolyte imbalance, eg, dilution or hypotonicity, hypertonic dehydration; and (3) urinary tract obstruction. This classification has clinical value since the diagnostic approach and the treatment of each are specific. For example, although groups (1) and (2) have in common a small urine volume and rising nitrogen levels, restriction of potassium and fluid is essential in the acute organic group whereas the administration of potassium and fluid may be lifesaving in the physiologic imbalance group.

ACUTE TUBULAR NECROSIS
(Lower Nephron Nephrosis; Acute Reversible Renal Failure)

The most common causes of acute tubular necrosis are shock, exposure to nephrotoxic chemicals (eg, carbon tetrachloride), intravascular hemolysis (eg, due to transfusion reactions or following transurethral resection), severe crushing injuries with myohemoglobinuria, and prolonged and severe fluid and electrolyte imbalances.† Most lesions are due to a combination of causes. Damage to the renal tubules is more prone to

*Only acute tubular necrosis will be discussed here.
†An increasing number of cases of hemolytic-uremic syndrome are being reported in the literature.

Dr. Lyon is Clinical Professor of Urology, University of California School of Medicine, San Francisco, California.

occur among elderly persons.

Acute tubular necrosis was at one time commonly termed "lower nephron nephrosis" because Lucké and others first observed the lesion in the distal tubule only. Subsequent studies have demonstrated that the proximal tubule and the glomerulus are often involved. The essential lesion is cellular necrosis which does not begin to heal for 6–10 days or longer. Repair is ultimately complete upon gross clinical examination, but more sensitive tests of renal function indicate that some residual damage is always present. In rare instances the basement membrane of the tubules sloughs away, in which case cellular replacement cannot take place and the lesion is irreversible. Anuria is a common finding in these cases and implies a much less favorable prognosis.

Clinical Findings

A. Symptoms and Signs: The clinical picture is not distinctive. The patient with carbon tetrachloride poisoning may have no complaint other than progressive edema, whereas a patient who has undergone abdominal surgery or one with severe hemorrhage resulting from a ruptured aortic aneurysm will present with all of the signs that follow surgical procedures in the abdomen. When acute tubular necrosis is suspected, the physician should survey renal function by means of the usual tests and observe body water changes (reflected by changes in body weight). A daily urine output of less than 400 ml in spite of adequate intake is the presenting complaint. Acute tubular necrosis must always be suspected following clinical shock.

In the presence of shock or following transurethral resection (but in the absence of cardiac failure), an early postoperative increase in body weight suggests oliguria due to acute tubular necrosis.

B. Laboratory Findings: The diagnosis may be established by simple laboratory tests.

1. Specific gravity of urine—The urine specific gravity is near 1.010 within 48 hours of the onset of shock or poisoning. This test may mislead the physician during the first 48 hours because the urine specific gravity may be as high as 1.026 during this interval. It is not known whether elevation of specific gravity in the first 48 hours is due to transudative material in the urine or whether it reflects the specific gravity of the urine already present in the bladder before renal shutdown occurred.

2. PSP excretion—0 to trace per hour, regardless of urine volume.

3. Urine chloride concentration*—Fixed between 30–40 mEq/liter in the classical case where the urine contains no blood. A urine chloride measurement between 40–100 mEq/liter is compatible with a partial tubular lesion. These concentrations tend to remain fixed throughout the oliguric period. A urine chloride of less than 20 mEq/liter or more than 100 mEq/liter rules out acute tubular necrosis. Urine sodium tends to remain fixed between 30–60 mEq/liter. Urine potassium tends to be 25 mEq/liter.

4. Serum electrolytes—Sodium and chloride concentrations may be low, normal, or high, depending on salt and water intake. Serum potassium concentration is rarely elevated during the first 72 hours except in the patient with severe crush injuries. Serum CO_2 will reflect the degree of acidosis, although this may not be significant in terms of need for correction.

5. Tests of retention—Serum creatinine and urea nitrogen tend to rise together at a 1:10 ratio. In rare instances, the serum creatinine may rise precipitously (possibly as a response to end products of muscle trauma) out of proportion to urea nitrogen. If the cause of the oliguria is obstruction, urea nitrogen tends to rise faster than serum creatinine. If oliguria results from intra- or extraperitoneal urinary extravasation, the rise in urea nitrogen is precipitous while serum creatinine stays close to normal.

6. Urine:plasma creatinine ratio < 10:1.

7. Urine urea concentration—A value of 1.1 g/100 ml or more in a random urine specimen seems to guarantee that acute tubular necrosis has not occurred.

8. Renograms—The radioisotope renogram can be diagnostic in differentiating the oliguria of obstruction from that of acute tubular necrosis. The tubular phase of concentration of radioactive material remains elevated, as is shown by comparing curve D with curve B in Fig 8–12.

9. Mannitol—The mannitol diuresis test has been suggested as a means of differentiating the oliguria of acute tubular necrosis from that caused by physiologic imbalance. If the above criteria in differential diagnosis of oliguria are followed, the mannitol test could be useful only when urine specific gravity is 1.010, PSP excretion is 0 to trace, and urine chloride is fixed in the range of 40–100 mEq/liter. If, after correction of the fluid-ion imbalance, diuresis does not occur, the mannitol test might be used to satisfy the physician's concern that the diagnosis was still being missed. If a diuresis is achieved in this manner, the fluid-ion imbalance posing the problem would still have to be discovered.

10. Other diuretics—If the mannitol diuresis test is inconclusive, 2 other powerful diuretic agents may

*Urine chloride is measured with Scribner's Bedside Chloride Set, which permits accurate determination of the chloride concentration in any body fluid (eg, serum, urine, gastrointestinal fluid) in less than 60 seconds. (See p 48.)

be tried—ethacrynic acid (Edecrin), 150–200 mg, or furosemide (Lasix), 160 mg, as single doses given IV.

Treatment

A. During the Phase of Oliguria:

1. Fluid intake and body weight—Attention to total body water is of primary importance. The patient who is taking no food by mouth produces 300–500 ml/day of water in the process of metabolism. This is termed water of oxidation or metabolic water. This water contains no electrolytes and is therefore analogous to an infusion or a drink of salt-free water. To prevent overhydration (and therefore dilution), this amount of water must be excreted by the body each day. Therefore, to maintain a normal water-electrolyte relationship, the patient must be allowed to lose 1 lb/day. A chart should be made and a declining "weight line" should be plotted beginning on the day of onset of oliguria. Parenteral water should be ordered only if body weight falls below this weight line. Because invisible cutaneous and respiratory losses are 800 ml/day, about 300 ml/day of parenteral water will maintain this balance. If too much water has been given before the diagnosis is made, water must be completely withheld until the desired weight is reached no matter how many days that requires.

Overhydration to the point of pulmonary edema ("drowning") rarely occurs during the first several days of oliguria if the patient is carefully watched. However, cardiac failure not uncommonly occurs between the eighth and twelfth days unless a regimen of relative dehydration is rigidly enforced. The danger of slight overhydration during this interval is greater than the danger of slight dehydration.

2. Extracellular electrolytes—Serum sodium, chloride, CO_2, and pH should be determined every 48 hours if possible, and serum potassium must be determined every 24 hours. A base line ECG should be taken immediately and should be repeated every 2 or 3 days or whenever serum potassium elevations occur (Fig 23–1). (*Note:* Dangerous hyperkalemia is most to be feared in the young patient with crush injury. It is rare in the elderly patient if close attention is given to body weight and water restriction.) Salt or sodium should be added to parenteral solutions only if the serum sodium falls below 126 mEq/liter. Sodium in the form of sodium lactate or sodium bicarbonate is indicated primarily where clinical acidosis is noted. Serum nitrogen or creatinine levels may be determined, but they have no practical value in treatment.

3. Osmotic diuresis—The usefulness of mannitol in therapy is open to question. If obstruction of the tubule by such a material as acid hematin is considered a possibility, osmotic diuresis by mannitol (or 50% dextrose) should be effective through its osmotic diuretic action.

4. Nutrition—100 g of dextrose daily (supplying 400 Cal) is accepted as the amount necessary to minimize protein catabolism. The concentration of dextrose in the parenteral solution must be adjusted so as not to require an excessive water intake. (*Note:* An

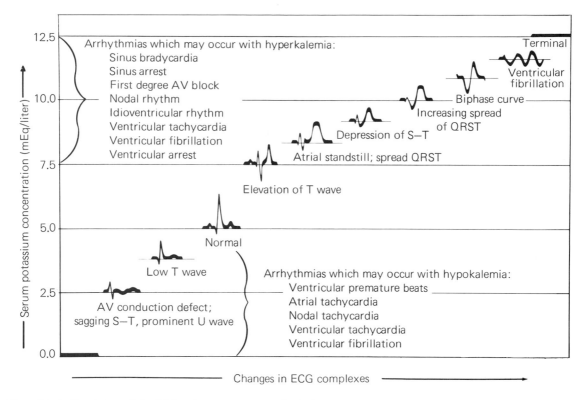

Figure 23–1. Correlation of the ECG with serum potassium levels (provided there is no parallel change in sodium and calcium). (Reproduced, with permission, from Krupp MA, Chatton MJ [editors]: *Current Medical Diagnosis & Treatment 1974.* Lange, 1974.)

increased rate of serum potassium elevation as a consequence of insufficient caloric intake has not been observed.)

B. Phase of Recovery: If close attention is paid to body weight and the patient loses 1 lb/day, intensive diuresis is rare. During the recovery phase, urine volume rapidly increases to 1500 ml/day at a specific gravity of 1.010, and removal of metabolic wastes again increases. At this point, urine chloride concentration will shift either up or down, depending upon serum chloride excess or lack. Tubular reabsorption of salt is still impaired at this time, and 2 g (35 mEq) of sodium chloride over normal intake should be allowed for every liter of urine to compensate the loss. The increasing urine volume will remove potassium (15 mEq or more per liter of urine) from the extracellular space rapidly, and hypokalemia may suddenly occur if oral or parenteral potassium is not supplied. In the usual case, oral intake is adequate and potassium supplements are sufficient. The body weight line will level out as the kidneys regain control of water and electrolyte balance and as oral intake supplies body needs. Attempts to force fluids at this time increase the danger of cardiac failure just when the patient is recovering. If urine volume falls off in the phase of diuresis, cardiac failure should be suspected rather than a reactivation of the renal tubular lesion.

Complications

Rapidly advancing acidosis is a rare complication which leads to fatiguing hyperventilation, movement of potassium from the cells with consequent hyperpotassemia, and other serious physiologic disturbances which are not fully understood. The most readily available emergency aid is parenteral sodium—preferably administered as $NaHCO_3$—which minimizes acidosis and thus favors the movement of potassium back into the cell. Insulin with 50% dextrose may be helpful if given aggressively by venous cannula. However, the rapidity with which peritoneal dialysis can be instituted makes it the most decisive treatment. Moderate serum potassium elevations may be controlled and further elevations prevented by oral administration of exchange resins, used in combination with sorbitol to promote evacuation.

In the rare instance where serious edema with overhydration has occurred, peritoneal dialysis with 7.5% dextrose solution may be lifesaving.

Prevention With Mannitol

The osmotic diuresis produced by mannitol is apparently effective in preventing acute tubular necrosis, particularly where poisons such as hemoglobin and myohemoglobin are presented to the kidney for filtration and excretion. Presumably, the osmotic property of mannitol prevents the usual absorption of H_2O from the filtrate and enables the drug to literally wash out the tubule. In this way, stasis of toxic materials is prevented.

Mannitol is most effective when used at the time of insult (as in intravascular hemolysis during cardiac bypass and as shock is controlled after injury or during surgery). An initial dose of 25 g of mannitol as a 20–50% solution may be followed by a 5% solution allowing a maximum 24-hour intake of 100 g of mannitol. Because salt tends to be lost at the rate of 4–6 g/liter of urine during mannitol diuresis, the drug should be administered in 0.45% saline. Where diuresis is in excess of the intake of the 5% mannitol solution, 0.45% saline is required by itself to compensate for the urine increment. If diuresis does not occur with the primary dose, mannitol should be promptly discontinued.

PHYSIOLOGIC IMBALANCES CAUSING OLIGURIA

Three-fourths of cases of oliguria are due to physiologic imbalances involving the body fluids, electrolytes, and blood volume rather than acute tubular necrosis or ureteral obstruction. In contrast to the organic lesion, functional renal failure requires prompt therapy with solutions that are usually withheld from a patient with acute tubular necrosis. The most common imbalances are (1) hypotonic dehydration or overhydration (dilutional syndrome), (2) acute normotonic dehydration, (3) hypertonic dehydration, and (4) circulatory failure.

Pathologic Physiology

Reasonably good kidney function is essential if fluid and electrolyte balance is to be maintained by the patient himself. The kidney excretes or retains various substances, including salt, potassium, water, and the end products of metabolism, thus maintaining a normal body water and electrolyte balance (or normotonicity) by means of the selective excretion of electrolytes with respect to water.

The second most important function of the kidney is the maintenance of normal body pH; the kidney accomplishes this by selectively excreting acid and base.

Unimpaired renal blood flow is necessary if these activities are to be carried out in the normal way. Any fluid or electrolyte imbalance affects all tissue cells; when the renal tubular cell is so affected, its ability to compensate losses (eg, from the gastrointestinal tract) becomes limited. Thus, decreased tubular function, when superimposed upon an existing water and electrolyte imbalance, compounds the clinical problem. The return of adequate renal function is necessary if normal fluid and electrolyte balance is to be maintained by the patient himself. The correction of tonic-ity (serum sodium concentration) is most important in returning renal tubular function to normal.

Diagnosis & Treatment

There are no characteristic clinical patterns for any particular fluid or electrolyte imbalance. Varying degrees of lethargy, weakness, ileus, and many other nonspecific symptoms are common to all. The physician must rely on a careful history of the route and volume of loss, must observe weight changes closely, and must use appropriate tests and measurements in order to establish a diagnosis and prescribe treatment.

A. **Dilutional Syndrome (Hypotonic Overhydration or Dehydration):** This is the most common fluid and electrolyte imbalance of iatrogenic origin and often leads to severe oliguria. It is due to the overzealous use of salt-free solutions in the immediate postoperative period, when the action of ADH leads to water retention. It is even more apt to develop if during the preoperative period the patient did not eat, lost electrolytes by vomiting, and was able to retain only water and thus came to surgery already in a mildly hypotonic state. The diagnosis is established by serum sodium and chloride levels 10 mEq/liter or more below normal, a PSP excretion of 5% or more per hour, and a history suggestive of salt deficit. Despite the low serum sodium and chloride levels, urine salt concentrations may be as high as 100 mEq/liter, which indicates that more salt is being lost by the kidney.

In the presence of overhydration, treatment requires at the least aggressive water restriction. Where a rapid recovery is important, as with the elderly patient immobilized in bed by the fluid-ion problem, 3–5% salt solution given slowly IV over a period of 24–48 hours will result in early diuresis. In the presence of dehydration (as measured by body weight), normal saline solution (0.9%) is indicated. The number of mEq of NaCl to make such a correction is determined by assuming that body water is 50% of body weight and that the administered salt will diffuse into this volume. Thus, the desired rise in serum sodium concentration, multiplied by the number of liters of estimated body water, provides the correction requirement.

B. **Simple Dehydration:** A diagnosis of simple dehydration can be made if weight loss is out of proportion to the severity of the illness (greater than 0.5–1 lb/day), the serum sodium and chloride concentrations are reasonably normal, and the urine specific gravity is 1.022 or higher. A normal serum creatinine or nitrogen level in the presence of oliguria is rare, but establishes the fact that kidney function is normal. If dehydration is severe and prolonged, the concentrating power of the kidney may have begun to fail; a specific gravity in the range of 1.010 suggests renal tubular damage. PSP excretion of 5% or more in 1 hour rules out acute tubular necrosis. The presence of anemia and a long history of chills and fever, nausea, weight loss, or pyuria suggest chronic renal failure. A urine chloride of less than 5 or more than 150 mEq/liter speaks against a chronic renal lesion.

Treatment consists of administering hypotonic

solutions such as 0.45% sodium chloride, with added potassium as urine volume increases. When rehydration is complete, the patient's weight will return to normal less starvation losses (0.5 lb/day).

C. Diminished Renal Blood Flow: Preclinical shock, cardiac failure, and a relative hypotension in a normally hypertensive patient are the most common disorders in this group. Shock, preclinical shock, and heart failure present no diagnostic difficulties. Oliguria may occur in the patient whose established systolic blood pressure is 200 mm Hg who, because of the administration of antipressor agents or serious primary disease, sustains a drop in systolic blood pressure to the usual normal range of 120 mm Hg.

Treatment is directed toward restoration of blood pressure, chiefly by blood volume replacement and on occasion with vasoconstrictors. Attempts to promote diuresis by the addition of fluids and salt are to be condemned except in cases where salt and water deficits are present. Digitalization of the patient with cardiac failure will lead to improved renal blood flow and diuresis.

BILATERAL URETERAL OBSTRUCTION*

The causes of bilateral ureteral stenosis are (1) occlusion by masses of metastatic (or lymphomatous) iliac or lumbar lymph nodes (eg, cancer of the cervix or prostate); (2) retroperitoneal fasciitis; (3) bilateral ureteral calculi (or ureteral calculus blocking an only kidney); and (4) trauma to or ligation of the ureters in conjunction with gynecologic surgery or abdominoperineal resection of the rectum. Ligation of only one ureter will not cause oliguria if the other kidney is normal.

Complete anuria (not oliguria) is rare with acute

---

*See also Injuries to the Ureter, Chapter 16; Acquired Diseases of the Ureter, Chapter 25; and the appropriate references in those chapters.

tubular necrosis and fluid and electrolyte aberrations and in association with diminished renal blood flow. Immediate anuria following surgery in the lower abdomen means bilateral ureteral injury until proved otherwise.

Clinical Findings

A. Symptoms and Signs: If obstruction is due to surgical injury, the patient suffers undue and prolonged ileus. If renal pain is present, renal tenderness may be elicited. If excess fluids have been given, edema may be noted. Signs of ileus are evident (eg, a quiet, distended abdomen, vomiting). A few days after surgical ureteral injury, urine may begin to leak through the wound or the vagina.

B. Laboratory Findings: The hematocrit may be low, particularly if edema is present. The urine specific gravity is often of no value, though it tends to be below 1.010 regardless of the state of hydration. If any urine is being secreted, some PSP will be recovered. The urine chloride concentration will depend upon water and salt relationships. Blood nitrogen may be elevated out of proportion to creatinine. The excretory urogram with "delayed" films taken up to 24 hours will often demonstrate adequate renal function and an increasing density of the kidney (nephrogram effect) typical of obstruction.

C. Instrumental Examination: Cystoscopy should be done and ureteral catheterization attempted. If the catheters are arrested in the lower ureters, radiopaque fluid can be introduced and x-rays taken. In this way the diagnosis of bilateral injury can be established.

Differential Diagnosis

If the patient has just undergone pelvic surgery and if there is no evidence of diminished renal blood flow (eg, cardiac failure, hemorrhage) or fluid-ion imbalance, bilateral ureteral obstruction should be suspected. A radioisotope renogram should clearly differentiate between acute renal failure and bilateral ureteral ligation (Fig 8–12).

Complications, Treatment, & Prognosis

For injuries to the ureter, see Chapter 16.

● ● ●

References

Acute Tubular Necrosis

Ajik M: Prevention of acute renal failure. Am J Surg 108:384, 1964.

Briggs JD & others: Renal function after acute tubular necrosis. Brit MJ 2:513, 1967.

Figueroa JE: Acute renal failure: Its unusual causes and manifestations. M Clin North America 51:995, 1967.

Flanagan WJ, Henderson LW, Merrill JP: The clinical application and technique of peritoneal dialysis. GP 28:98, Nov 1963.

Freeman RB & others: Renal tubular necrosis due to

nephrotoxicity of organic mercurial diuretics. Ann Int Med 57:34, 1962.

Gianantonio CA & others: The hemolytic-uremic syndrome. J Pediat 72:757, 1968.

Hall JW & others: Immediate and long-term prognosis in acute renal failure. Ann Int Med 73:515, 1970.

Hammond D & others: Hemolytic-uremic syndrome. Am J Dis Child 114:440, 1967.

Handa SP, Lazor MZ: Acute tubular necrosis: A review of 44 necropsied cases. Am J Med Sc 251:29, 1966.

Hedger RW: The conservative management of acute

oliguric renal function. M Clin North America 55:121, 1971.

Huffer JC, Lyon RP: The conservative management of acute renal failure by a controlled dehydration regimen. J Urol 85:459, 1961.

Lewers DJ & others: Long-term follow-up of renal function and histology after acute tubular necrosis. Ann Int Med 73:523, 1970.

Lunding M, Steiness L, Thaysen JH: Acute renal failure due to tubular necrosis. Acta med scandinav 176:103, 1964.

Lyon RP: Measurement of urine chloride as a test of renal function. J Urol 85:884, 1961.

Lyon RP: Nonobstructive oliguria: Differential diagnosis. California Med 99:83, 1963.

Maher JF, O'Connell JMB, Schreiner GE: Traumatic acute renal failure. Postgrad Med 39:70, 1966.

Merrill JP: Acute renal failure. JAMA 211:289, 1970.

Mueller CB: The mechanism of acute renal failure after injury and transfusion reaction and its prevention by solute diuresis. S Clin North America 45:499, 1965.

Myler RK, Lee JC, Hopper J Jr: Renal tubular necrosis caused by mushroom poisoning. Arch Int Med 114:196, 1964.

Nielsen VK, Larsen J: Acute renal failure due to carbon tetrachloride poisoning. Acta med scandinav 178:363, 1965.

Powers SR Jr & others: Prevention of postoperative acute renal failure with mannitol in 100 cases. Surgery 55:15, 1964.

Reidenberg MM & others: Acute renal failure due to nephrotoxins. Am J Med Sc 247:25, 1964.

Stahl WM: Effect of mannitol on the kidneys. New England J Med 272:381, 1965.

Stremple JF, Ellison EH, Carey LC: Osmolar diuresis: Success and/or failure. A collective review. Surgery 60:924, 1966.

Trinkle JK, Kiser WS: Acute renal failure: Diagnosis of etiology by radioisotope renography. J Urol 91:199, 1964.

Vertel RM, Knochel JP: Nonoliguric acute renal failure. JAMA 200:598, 1967.

Weeks RS: The crush syndrome. Surg Gynec Obst 127:369, 1968.

Wennberg JE & others: Renal toxicity of oral cholecystographic media. JAMA 186:461, 1963.

Physiologic Imbalances Causing Oliguria

Bell H, Hayes WL, Vosburgh J: Hyperkalemic paralysis due to adrenal insufficiency. Arch Int Med 115:418, 1965.

Berlyne GM & others: Treatment of hyperkalemia with a calcium-resin. Lancet 1:169, 1966.

Berman LB: The hypokalemic syndromes. GP 29:105, June 1964.

Bruck E, Abul G, Aceto T Jr: Pathogenesis and pathophysiology of hypertonic dehydration with diarrhea. Am J Dis Child 115:122, 1968.

Bruck E, Abul G, Aceto T Jr: Therapy of infants with hypertonic dehydration due to diarrhea. Am J Dis Child 115:281, 1968.

Burns RO & others: Peritoneal dialysis. New England J Med 267:1060, 1962.

Carpenter CCJ & others: Clinical evaluation of fluid requirements in Asiatic cholera. Lancet 1:726, 1965.

Cohn HE, Capelli JP: The diagnosis and management of oliguria in the postoperative period. S Clin North America 47:1187, 1967.

Davis BB Jr, Knox FG: Current concepts of the regulation of urinary sodium excretion: A review. Am J Med Sc 259:373, 1970.

Doolin RD & others: Evaluation of intermittent peritoneal lavage. Am J Med 26:831, 1959.

Flinn RB, Merrill JP, Welzant WR: Treatment of the oliguric patient with a new sodium-exchange resin and sorbitol. New England J Med 264:111, 1961.

Forland M, Pullman TN: Aspects of cardiac disease. M Clin North America 50:255, 1966.

Forland M, Pullman TN: Electrolyte complications of drug therapy. M Clin North America 47:113, 1963.

Gerst PH, Porter MR, Fishman RA: Symptomatic magnesium deficiency in surgical patients. Ann Surg 159:402, 1964.

Kassirer JP & others: The critical role of chloride in the correction of hypokalemic alkalosis in man. Am J Med 38:172, 1965.

Kleeman CR, Fichman MP: The clinical physiology of water metabolism. New England J Med 277:1300, 1967.

Klein DE, Wright HK, Persky L: Electrolyte and osmolality changes attending electroresection. Arch Surg 90:871, 1965.

Leaf A: The clinical and physiologic significance of the serum sodium concentration. (2 parts.) New England J Med 267:25, 77, 1962.

Leaf A, Santos RF: Physiologic mechanisms in potassium deficiency. New England J Med 264:335, 1961.

Levinsky NG: Management of emergencies. 6. Hyperkalemia. New England J Med 274:1076, 1966.

Lyon RP: Measurement of urine chloride as a test of renal function. J Urol 85:884, 1961.

Moore FD: Regulation of the serum sodium concentration: Origin and treatment of tonicity disorders in surgery. Am J Surg 103:302, 1962.

Moyer CA, Margraf HW, Monafo WW Jr: Burn shock and extravascular sodium deficiency: Treatment with Ringer's solution with lactate. Arch Surg 90:799, 1965.

Pullen H, Doig A, Lambie AT: Intensive intravenous potassium replacement therapy. Lancet 2:809, 1967.

Schwartz WB, Relman AS: Effects of electrolyte disorders on renal structure and function. (2 parts.) New England J Med 276:383, 452, 1967.

Symposium on fluid and electrolyte problems. P Clin North America 11:789, 1964.

Teree TM & others: Stool losses and acidosis in diarrheal disease of infancy. Pediatrics 36:704, 1965.

Winters RW: Studies of acid-base disturbances. Pediatrics 39:700, 1967.

Winters RW: Terminology of acid-base disorders. Ann Int Med 63:873, 1965.

Ziegler EE, Fomon SJ: Fluid intake, renal solute load, and water balance in infancy. J Pediat 78:561, 1971.

Zimmerman B: Pituitary and adrenal function in relation to surgery. S Clin North America 45:299, 1965.

24...
Chronic Renal Failure, Dialysis, & Renal Transplantation

William J.C. Amend, Jr., MD, Oscar Salvatierra, Jr., MD, & Folkert O. Belzer, MD

CHRONIC RENAL FAILURE & DIALYSIS

In renal failure, the clearance of endogenous solutes from the kidney is reduced and the concentrations of these solutes in the body become elevated. The most common solutes measured as indicators of renal failure are BUN and serum creatinine. However, marked elevation of BUN can occur from nonrenal causes such as prerenal azotemia, gastrointestinal hemorrhage, or high protein intake. If the serum creatinine has remained constant or risen to a new steady state, creatinine clearance can be measured as an indicator of glomerular filtration rate (GFR).

Renal failure may be classified as acute or chronic depending on the rapidity of onset and the subsequent course of azotemia. An analysis based on the acute or chronic development of renal failure is important in understanding physiologic adaptations, disease mechanisms, and ultimate therapy.

For a discussion of acute renal failure, see Chapter 23.

The general incidence of chronic renal failure in the USA, defined as "people who can benefit from hemodialysis or renal transplantation," is 50 per million population per year. The medical acceptance criteria are strict. All age groups are affected. The severity and the rapidity of development of uremia are hard to predict.

Historical Introduction

Various causes of progressive renal dysfunction lead eventually to end stage or terminal renal failure. Bright in the 1800s described several cases which presented with edema, hematuria, proteinuria, and eventual death. Early chemical analyses of patients'

The section on chronic renal failure and dialysis is contributed by William JC Amend, Jr, MD, Clinical Assistant Professor of Medicine, University of California School of Medicine, San Francisco. The section on renal transplantation is contributed by Oscar Salvatierra, Jr, MD, Associate Professor of Surgery and Urology and Director, Kidney Transplant Service, University of California School of Medicine, San Francisco; and Folkert O. Belzer, MD, Professor and Chairman, Department of Surgery, University of Wisconsin School of Medicine, Madison.

sera drew attention to retained nonprotein nitrogen (NPN) compounds and made the association between this and the clinical findings of uremia. Although the pathologic state of uremia was well described in the intervening years, it remained for technics of chronic dialysis and renal transplantation to solve the therapeutic problems.

Etiology

A variety of disorders are associated with end stage renal disease. Either a primary renal process (eg, glomerulonephritis, pyelonephritis, congenital hypoplasia) or a secondary one (eg, when the kidney is affected by a systemic process such as diabetes mellitus or lupus erythematosus) may be at fault. Minor physiologic alterations secondary to dehydration, infection, or hypertension often "tip the scale" and put a borderline patient into uncompensated, clinical uremia.

Clinical Findings

A. Symptoms and Signs: Symptoms such as pruritus, generalized malaise, lassitude, forgetfulness, loss of libido, nausea, and altered behavior patterns are subtle complaints in this chronic disorder. There is often a strong family history of renal disease. Growth failure is a primary complaint in preadolescent patients. Symptoms of a multisystem disorder (eg, arthritis in lupus erythematosus) may be present coincidentally. The blood pressure is usually elevated, especially when the patient is overhydrated or suffering from primary arteriolar nephropathy. The blood pressure may be normal or low, however, in the presence of a marked salt-losing nephritis (eg, medullary cystic disease). The pulse and respiratory rates are rapid as manifestations of anemia and metabolic acidosis. Clinical findings of uremic fetor, pericarditis, neurologic findings of asterixis, reduced mentation, and peripheral neuropathy are often present. Terry's nails—pallor of the proximal nail beds—can sometimes distinguish chronic from acute renal failure. Palpable kidneys suggest polycystic disease. Ophthalmoscopic examination may show diabetic retinopathy.

B. Laboratory Findings:

1. Urine composition—Urine volumes vary depending on the disease and—though to a lesser extent after end stage renal disease—become quite low on daily fluid intakes. Urine volumes are usually low as a consequence of reduced GFR but may exceed 1 liter/day in hydrated patients with polycystic disease. There is usually a fixed daily saline loss during the early phases, but with a GFR less than 5% of normal this loss will decrease and sodium retention will develop. If the patient has had proteinuria in the nephrotic range preceding the uremic stage, this degree of proteinuria will be absent as a result of reduced GFR.

2. Blood studies—Anemia is the rule, but the hematocrit may be normal in polycystic disease. Platelet dysfunction or thrombasthenia is characterized by abnormal bleeding times. Platelet counts and prothrombin content are normal.

Elevated serum creatinine, BUN, and NPN are the hallmarks of this disorder. Metabolic acidosis and hyperkalemia are present. Progressive reduction of body buffer stores and an inability to excrete titratable acids leads to progressive acidosis characterized by reduced serum bicarbonate and compensatory respiratory hyperventilation. Acidosis per se and reduced clearance of daily potassium loads produces elevated serum potassium. Serum phosphate is elevated and serum calcium is reduced secondary to multiple factors. Uremic patients have a reduced appetite and consequent reduced calcium ingestion. There is diminished activity of vitamin D from a reduction in conversion of vitamin D_2 to active vitamin D_3 in the kidney. Phosphate retention (from reduced phosphate clearance) is noted. These alterations may lead to uremic osteodystrophy with elements of both osteomalacia and secondary hyperparathyroidism. Creatinine clearance and urea clearance are markedly reduced.

C. X-Ray Findings: Infusion nephrotomograms are required if the serum creatinine is 3 mg/100 ml or more and will usually reveal small kidneys, congenital hypoplasia, polycystic disease, or some other structural disorder. Bone x-rays may show retarded growth, osteomalacia (renal rickets), or secondary hyperparathyroidism. Soft tissue calcification may be present.

D. Other Examinations: Renal biopsies may not reveal much except scarring and glomerulosclerosis. There may be pronounced vascular changes consisting of thickening of the media, fragmentation of elastic fibers, and intimal proliferation, which may be secondary to uremic hypertension or may be due to arteriolar nephrosclerosis.

Treatment

Conservative management should be offered until it becomes impossible for the patient to continue to enjoy life. This management would include dietary protein and potassium restriction as well as close sodium balance in the diet so that the patient does not retain sodium nor become sodium depleted. Transfusions are usually not helpful, but vitamin and iron supplementation might be offered. Prevention of possible uremic osteodystrophy requires close attention to calcium and phosphorus balance through phosphate-retaining antacids and administration of calcium or vitamin D supplementation. Extreme care must be paid to this management, however, since metastatic calcification can result from a Ca X P product of greater than 65 (mg/100 ml).

A. Chronic Peritoneal Dialysis: Peritoneal dialysis has been used primarily when hemodialysis facilities or a suitable access to the patient's vascular system is unavailable. Problems of reduced molecular clearances and infection make this method of chronic dialysis less desirable than hemodialysis, but improved soft catheters (Tenckhoff) have allowed for chronic use.

B. Chronic Hemodialysis: Chronic hemodialysis using semipermeable dialysis membranes is now widely used. Access to the vascular system is by means of Scribner shunts, arteriovenous fistulas, and grafts. The actual dialyzers may be of a parallel plate, coil, or hollow fiber type. Clearance of body solutes and excessive body fluids can be easily accomplished by using dialysate fluids of known chemical composition.

Treatment is intermittent—usually 5–8 hours 3 times weekly. It may be given in a kidney center, a satellite unit, or in the home. Very ill patients or those who for any reason cannot be trained in the use of the equipment with an assistant require treatment in a dialysis center. Home dialysis is optimal because it provides greater schedule flexibility and improved (psychologic) surroundings, but only 30–50% of a dialysis population meet the medical and training requirements for this type of hemodialysis therapy.

More widespread use of dialytic technics has permitted a more normal degree of patient mobility. Treatments on vacations, business, and other trips can be provided after pretrip arrangements are made.

Common problems of hemodialysis include infection, bone symptoms, technical accidents, persistent anemia, and psychologic disorders. Despite these difficulties, many patients lead productive lives while receiving treatment. Yearly costs range from an average of $6 thousand for home patients to $12–15 thousand for center-dialyzed patients, but much of this is now absorbed under HR-1 (Medicare) legislation. Long-term survival is possible on hemodialysis. The mortality rates are about 8–10% per year once maintenance therapy has been instituted.

C. Renal Transplantation:* After immunosuppression technics and genetic matching were developed, renal homotransplantation became an acceptable alternative to maintenance hemodialysis. The great advantage of transplantation is reestablishment of nearly normal constant body physiology and chemistry without intermittent dialysis. Diet can be more normal. The disadvantages include bone marrow suppression, susceptibility to infection, cushingoid body habitus, and the psychologic uncertainty of the homograft's future. Most of the disadvantages of transplantation are related to the medicines (azathioprine and corticosteroids) which are given to counteract the rejection. Later problems with transplantation include the formation of recurrent disease in the transplanted kidney. Genitourinary infection appears to be of minor importance if structural urologic complications (eg,

---

*For a more detailed review, see the next section.

leak) do not occur. Nephrology centers, with close cooperation between medical and surgical staff, attempt to use these treatment alternatives of dialysis and transplantation in an integrated fashion.

RENAL TRANSPLANTATION

Renal transplantation is an effective therapeutic modality for patients with end stage renal disease. Over 700 renal homotransplants have been performed at San Francisco Medical Center (UCSF), and many of the conclusions in this chapter are based on that experience. Although the immunologic problems of rejection remain unchanged, technical complications and patient mortality rates have been significantly reduced by detailed attention to organ procurement, preservation, surgical technics, and elimination of prolonged corticosteroid therapy in high doses. Prospective use of the mixed lymphocyte culture (MLC) in selecting living related donors has also improved graft survival.

Selection & Preparation of Recipients

The principal indication for renal transplantation is end stage renal failure. According to the Eleventh Report of the Human Renal Transplant Registry, the following are the most common diseases treated by renal transplantation: chronic glomerulonephritis (57%); chronic pyelonephritis (14%); polycystic renal disease (5%); and malignant nephrosclerosis (4%). Other diseases, including hereditary causes, account for 20% of cases.

A. Exclusions: Patients with active fungal or tuberculous infections, as well as those whose end stage renal failure is due to oxalosis, are not accepted for transplantation. Patients with systemic diseases such as juvenile diabetes mellitus and lupus erythematosus, however, are acceptable.

B. Preliminary Nephrectomy: Approximately 85% of all patients now receive transplants with their own kidneys left in situ. The only indications for preliminary nephrectomy are as follows:

1. Severe hypertension uncontrolled by dialysis.

2. Anatomic abnormalities of the urinary tract with or without infection, eg, hydronephrosis or ureteral reflux. In patients with refluxing ureters or ureteral abnormalities, nephroureterectomy should be performed with removal of the ureter to the ureterovesical junction.

3. Rapidly progressive glomerulonephritis, because of possible recurrent disease in the transplanted kidney. In patients with rapidly progressive glomerulonephritis, bilateral nephrectomy is performed and transplantation is delayed for 6 months.

4. Preliminary nephrectomy is used selectively in patients with polycystic renal disease. If the patient has a history of renal infection or significant hema-

turia, preparation by nephrectomy is an absolute prerequisite to transplantation. If the history is negative, transplantation without nephrectomy is preferred and has proved to be safe. The size of the polycystic kidneys is not an indication for preliminary nephrectomy in UCSF experience.

C. Splenectomy: Most transplant centers have abandoned splenectomy before transplantation since no clear evidence exists that it modifies the immunologic reaction.

Donor Selection

The kidney to be transplanted can be obtained from either a living related donor or a cadaver donor.

A. Living Related Donor: The only living related donors currently accepted are siblings or parents, and only after histocompatibility testing has shown a high probability of graft survival. Histocompatibility is determined as follows: (1) Determination of human leukocyte antigens (HL-A) establishes the inheritance pattern in a family group. (2) Mixed lymphocyte culture (MLC) measures the stimulation between donor and recipient lymphocytes incubated in the test tube by their uptake of tritiated thymidine. The best donor-recipient combinations are siblings who share all 4 possible HL-A antigens (HL-A identical) and who are nonstimulating on the mixed lymphocyte culture. The prognosis for long-term graft survival in this case is over 95%.

B. Cadaver Donor: If a suitable living related donor is not available, patients with end stage renal disease then must depend upon cadaver organs for transplantation.

1. Unacceptable cadaver donors—Cadaver kidneys are unacceptable in the following circumstances:

a. Newborns and those over the age of 55. Early thrombosis is the fate of most newborn kidneys, and data from the Renal Transplant Registry show that kidneys from donors over the age of 55 do not give results comparable to kidneys from young donors. Kidneys from children 10 months of age and older have provided excellent graft material, as renal hypertrophy occurs rapidly after transplantation.

b. Generalized or intra-abdominal sepsis.

c. Preexisting disease which imposes a risk of renal involvement, such as hypertension, diabetes, and lupus erythematosus.

d. Malignancy, except for brain tumors, because of the risk of transplanting tumor cells in the renal graft.

2. Donor-recipient matching—No correlation between the HL-A match and cadaver graft survival could be found in a recent evaluation at UCSF. We have also shown that sensitive cross-matching is especially important for recipients with preformed cytotoxic antibodies. Cross-matching implies incubation of recipient serum with donor lymphocytes. At UCSF, there has been no evidence of impaired graft survival in recipients with high levels of preformed cytotoxic antibodies. This indicates that every suitable cadaver kidney should be transplanted, no matter how poor the HL-A matching, even in sensitized patients. Although no correlation between HL-A typing and graft survival could be shown in our cadaver series, we did find an excellent correlation between the results of the MLC and subsequent graft survival. However, the 5-day incubation period required for the MLC still prevents prospective utilization of this test with cadaver kidneys.

Organ Preservation

Preservation of the cadaver kidney prior to transplantation can be accomplished in 2 basic ways: by simple hypothermic storage or by pulsatile perfusion.

A. Hypothermic Storage: In simple hypothermic storage, the kidneys are removed from the cadaver donor and then are rapidly cooled, usually by a combination of a flush-out solution and external cooling to reduce the renal core temperature. The kidneys are stored in a simple plastic container immersed in another container packed with crushed ice. The 2 disadvantages of this method are that the period of preservation is limited to about 24 hours, especially if warm ischemia has occurred at the time of organ retrieval, and that it provides no clues to the viability of the kidney.

B. Pulsatile Perfusion: The basic components of continuous pulsatile perfusion as used at UCSF are as follows: pulsatile flow, hypothermia, membrane oxygenation, and a perfusate containing albumin as well as lipids. The 2 major advantages of continuous pulsatile perfusion are that no kidneys need be discarded because of the time limitations of the storage method and that a sudden influx of several cadaver organs to a single transplant center can be satisfactorily transplanted by a small team. The average storage time at UCSF in over 450 cadaver transplants has been 31 hours, and some kidneys have been transplanted after storage periods of up to 3 days. Continuous perfusion also allows viability testing to be performed after donor nephrectomy and prior to transplantation. Viability testing is essential if donors are accepted who have been in prolonged shock or have abnormal renal function prior to death. The 3 criteria for organ viability are fully reliable if perfusion preservation is started immediately after donor nephrectomy. These criteria are a warm ischemia time of less than 1 hour, adequate perfusion characteristics, and a donor serum creatinine that is less than twice normal at the time of nephrectomy. These criteria are insufficient if the kidney has also been subjected to a period of simple cold storage prior to perfusion preservation.

When perfusion preservation was started immediately after donor nephrectomy, the postoperative dialysis rate following transplantation has been less than 20%.

The Human Renal Transplant Registry has shown that the choice between perfusion or cold storage has no influence on long-term survival of cadaver grafts.

Donor Nephrectomy

Strict adherence to technical detail during donor nephrectomy is of the utmost importance.

A. Technic of Donor Nephrectomy: Donor nephrectomy in both cadaver and living related donors should be performed so that the blood supply to the ureter from the renal vessels is preserved. Although the blood supply of the ureter in situ has multiple origins, the transplanted ureter receives its blood supply only from renal vessel branches that course in hilar and upper periureteral fat. Thus, no dissection should be performed in the area of the renal pelvis or the hilus of the kidney. As the ureteral blood supply courses in the adventitia, the ureter must also be meticulously removed with adequate surrounding tissue. For maximum assurance of preservation of the ureteral blood supply, a large mass of hilar and periureteral fatty tissue is removed en bloc with the kidney and ureter.

B. Management of Multiple Vessels: If multiple vessels are found in a cadaver kidney, the kidney is removed en bloc with the aorta, so that it can be perfused through the aorta. Subsequently, the kidney can be transplanted with a Carrel patch of aorta containing the multiple vessels. If the vessels are in close proximity to each other, a single Carrel patch will suffice, but if the vessels are some distance apart 2 Carrel patches are preferable. Since all living related donors have preoperative arteriograms, the presence of multiple arteries is determined prior to transplantation. Most donors have at least a single artery to one of their kidneys. Occasionally, a donor kidney with double arteries must be used, but without a Carrel patch because of the increased risk to the donor.

C. Treatment of Living Related Donor: Anesthesia is not started in the donor until rapid intravenous hydration has failed to result in excellent diuresis. If anesthesia is induced prior to diuresis, the ADH effect will make it difficult to obtain diuresis after induction of anesthesia. In donor nephrectomy, it is also important to avoid traction on the pedicle and to feel the kidney constantly during manipulation. It is stimulation of the nervous mechanism during dissection that produces vasospasm and causes the kidney to become soft, with no urine output. If the kidney becomes soft, dissection should be discontinued until the kidney has again become firm. Mannitol, 25 g IV, is given in 4 divided doses during dissection of the renal pedicle. It is imperative that the kidney be firm and that urine be spurting from the ureter prior to division of the renal vessels. By using this approach to donor nephrectomy, dialysis has not been necessary in any of our living related donor transplants the past 3 years, and all kidneys have functioned immediately after transplantation.

D. Treatment of the Cadaver Donor: The potential cadaver donor is often in shock and is receiving vasopressors, so that rapid infusion of normal saline is initially necessary to readjust the contracted blood volume. Subsequently, an alpha-adrenergic blocking agent such as phenoxybenzamine (Dibenzyline) or phentolamine (Regitine) is given to prevent agonal renal vasospasm. These agents are especially important when kidneys are removed after cardiac arrest. Once renal vasospasm is established, it will persist during preservation, resulting in inadequate tissue perfusion and organ damage.

Technic of Renal Transplantation

The surgical technic of renal transplantation involves vascular anastomoses and establishment of urinary tract continuity. Specific considerations may be outlined as follows:

In adults, the kidney is placed through an oblique lower abdominal incision and the iliac and hypogastric arteries are mobilized. The iliac veins are similarly mobilized so that an end-to-side renal vein-to-iliac vein anastomosis can be performed. An end-to-end renal artery-to-hypogastric artery anastomosis is usually accomplished unless the hypogastric artery is unsuitable because of arteriosclerotic changes, in which case the renal artery is transplanted end-to-side to the common iliac artery. (See Fig 24–1.)

When multiple arteries are present in cadaver donors, the kidneys are transplanted with anastomosis of a Carrel patch of aorta to the common iliac artery.

In small children, a midline abdominal incision is used and the cecum and ascending colon are mobilized, exposing the aorta and vena cava. An end-to-side anastomosis of the renal vessels to the vena cava and aorta is then easily accomplished, following which the kidney is placed retroperitoneally by resuturing the previously mobilized right colon.

When small pediatric kidneys are used, donor

nephrectomy is carried out en bloc with the aorta and vena cava. The kidneys are then stored by hypothermic pulsatile perfusion through the aorta. Subsequently, pediatric kidneys are transplanted as single units, with each donor providing kidneys for 2 recipients. Arterial anastomosis is performed by using a Carrel patch of donor aorta and, whenever possible, a Carrel patch of the vena cava for the venous anastomosis. If a Carrel patch of vena cava is not used, interrupted sutures for the venous anastomosis are used instead. Arterial and venous anastomoses are usually carried out on the iliac vessels, and the aorta and vena cava are utilized only in very small children.

Establishment of urinary tract continuity can be performed by pyeloureterostomy, ureteroureterostomy, or ureteroneocystostomy. Ureteroneocystostomy by a modified Politano-Leadbetter technic is used at UCSF. The primary ureteral leak rate with this method has been only 0.5%.

Immediate Posttransplant Care

Postoperative management does not differ essentially from that of other surgical patients except that emphasis is placed upon the following areas:

Foley catheter drainage is maintained for 1 week. This method has essentially eliminated urinary leakage from the bladder. If bacteriuria develops, it is detected by appropriate urinary cultures and specifically treated.

Intravenous fluids are given immediately after the operation and are maintained at a rate to equal urinary output but not to exceed 200 ml/hour so that urinary output is not "chased" with intravenous fluids. The urinary output in the immediate posttransplant patient may be considerable, primarily on the basis of preoperative overhydration of the recipient despite optimum dialysis.

Renal scintiphotography is useful in the immediate posttransplant period as a base line for future comparative studies and to evaluate the success of vascular and ureteral anastomoses. Good tracer uptake in the entire renal cortex indicates adequate perfusion, while normal drainage of urine confirms patency of the ureteral anastomosis. Renal scintiphotography with excretion of 131 I-orthoiodohippurate is the principal method used to evaluate the graft and to complement clinical impressions and chemical determinations.

As far as the transplanted kidney is concerned, the differential diagnosis of renal failure can be extremely difficult in 2 situations: (1) sudden decrease in urinary output shortly after transplantation, and (2) the diagnosis of rejection superimposed upon acute tubular necrosis. In our experience with almost 2000 scintiphotographic studies in renal transplant patients, serial 131 I-orthoiodohippurate scintiphotographic studies have proved to be of great value in the evaluation of the structure, function, and viability of the transplanted kidney. The study causes no discomfort or harm to the patient. Furthermore, good renal visualization is possible in patients with uremia.

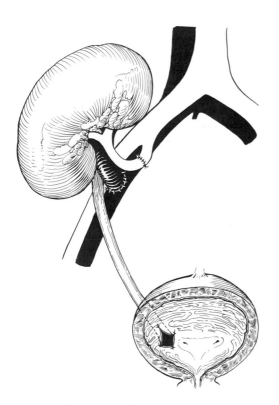

Figure 24–1. Renal transplantation.

Rejection

Rejection is generally classified as hyperacute, acute, or chronic.

Hyperacute rejection is mediated by humoral antibodies. It occurs in patients who have preexisting circulating cytotoxic antibodies which react with the donor kidney. The classical picture of hyperacute rejection is that, after release of the vascular clamps following vascular anastomoses, the kidney appears normal but very rapidly turns into a bluish-black, nonviable organ. The only treatment is immediate nephrectomy. Subliminal sensitization can also occur in which irreversible renal failure and graft nonviability take several days to become completely established.

Acute rejection is a cellular type of rejection process in which the allograft is usually at risk during the first several months following transplantation. This type of rejection process is usually characterized by fever, oliguria, weight gain, tenderness and enlargement of the graft, hypertension, and chemical evidence of renal functional impairment. This type of rejection process can be treated by increasing the corticosteroid dosage, and in most cases the process is reversible.

Chronic rejection is a late cause of renal deterioration on a humoral basis. Chronic rejection is most often diagnosed by evidence of slowly decreasing renal function in association with proteinuria and hypertension. This type of rejection process is resistant to standard methods of corticosteroid rejection treatment, and graft loss will eventually occur, though at times not for several years after inception of impaired renal function.

Immunosuppressive Therapy

The principal immunosuppressive drugs are prednisone in combination with either azathioprine (Imuran)—an antimetabolite—or cyclophosphamide (Cytoxan)—an alkylating agent. The latter is used instead of azathioprine only in patients with past or present hepatic dysfunction, and also when allopurinol (Zyloprim) is used concurrently. In general, the basic prednisone dosage at the time of transplantation is 120 mg daily in adults, with appropriate lower dosages in children. Dosage is then rapidly reduced to mainte-

nance levels. During an acute rejection episode, prednisone is increased to 2–3 mg/kg daily, followed by a rapidly progressive decrease to maintenance dosages.

Since 1972, emphasis at our transplant center has been on patient survival rather than graft survival. This has been accomplished by abolishing prolonged high-dose immunosuppressive therapy for graft rejection. Although graft rejection is now treated less vigorously, our results show that graft survival has not been jeopardized by emphasizing patient survival.

Complications

A. Urologic: The total urologic complication rate, including bladder urinary leaks, ureteral obstruction, and ureteral urinary leaks, is less than 4% in this center.

B. Vascular: Late renal artery stenosis has occurred in 12 of our patients, an incidence of less than 2%. Stenosis has been of 2 types: (1) that limited to the suture line and secondary to reaction to the suture material, and (2) generalized stenosis of the main renal artery to its bifurcation due to extensive periadventitial cicatricial formation, probably a part of the generalized reaction to the homograft. All 12 cases of renal artery stenosis were successfully corrected surgically.

C. Infection: The primary wound infection rate is 1%. Topical use of antibiotics, strict adherence to careful surgical technic, and omission of wound drainage are mainly responsible for this low incidence.

D. Complications Secondary to Immunosuppressive Therapy: These complications, such as infection and sepsis, can be kept to a minimum by emphasizing low-dose immunosuppressive therapy.

Results

A. Patient Survival: After a policy of low-dose immunosuppressive therapy was adopted in 1972, the patient mortality rate at 1 year has been reduced to 8%.

B. Graft Survival: Survival of primary cadaver grafts at 1, 2, and 3 years is 60%, 55%, and 50%, respectively. Survival of grafts from living related donors with a low-reacting MLC and followed from 6 months to 3 years is 89%.

•   •   •

References

Chronic Renal Failure & Dialysis

Anderson CF & others: Nutritional therapy for adults with renal disease. JAMA 223:68, 1973.

Bell PRF, Calman KC: *Surgical Aspects of Haemodialysis.* Churchill-Livingstone, 1974.

Bricker NS: Adaptations in chronic uremia: Pathophysiologic "trade-offs." Hosp Practice 9:119, July 1974.

Hampers CL, Schupak E: *Long-Term Hemodialysis,* 2nd ed. Grune & Stratton, 1973.

Merrill JP, Hampers CL: Uremia. (2 parts.) New England J Med 282:953, 1014, 1970.

Renal Transplantation

Belzer FO & others: Is HL-A typing of clinical significance in cadaver renal transplantation? Lancet 1:774, 1974.

Cochrum K, Salvatierra O, Belzer FO: The correlation between MLC stimulation and graft survival in living related and cadaver kidney transplants. Ann Surg 180:617, 1974.

Hamburger J & others: *Renal Transplantation.* Williams & Wilkins, 1972.

Najarian JS, Simmons RL: *Transplantation.* Lea & Febiger, 1972.

Salvatierra O, Kountz SL, Belzer FO: Prevention of ureteral fistula after renal transplantation. J Urol 112:445, 1974.

Salvatierra O, Kountz SL, Belzer FO: Polycystic renal disease treated by renal transplantation. Surg Gynec Obst 137:431, 1973.

Salvatierra O & others: The advantages of 131 I-orthoiodohippurate scintiphotography in the management of patients after renal transplantation. Ann Surg 180:336, 1974.

Starzl TE: *Experience in Renal Transplantation.* Saunders, 1964.

25 ...
Disorders of the Ureters

CONGENITAL ANOMALIES OF THE URETER

Congenital ureteral anomalies are common. Since most of them cause urinary obstruction or stasis, hydronephrosis with secondary renal infection is a common sequel.

INCOMPLETE URETER

The ureter may be entirely absent or may extend from the bladder only part way to the renal area. Either the ureteral bud fails to develop from the urogenital segment during embryologic development, or it is arrested in its development before it reaches the kidney. It is demonstrated by retrograde urography. Absence of the kidney or multicystic renal disease is to be expected.

DUPLICATION OF THE URETER

Complete or incomplete duplication of the ureter is one of the most common congenital ureteral anomalies. The family pattern of inheritance suggests an autosomal dominant gene of incomplete penetrance. The incomplete (Y) type (Fig 25—1) is more common than 2 complete ureters on one side (Figs 25—1, 25—3). The condition may be bilateral. Duplication presupposes 2 renal pelves in the renal mass. Most cases occur in females. An instance of 5 ureters on one side has been reported.

These abnormalities usually cause no difficulty; in the Y type, however, obstruction at the point where the 2 ureters join may be observed. One segment may become dilated because of retrograde flow (reflux) from one ureter into the other.

In complete duplication, the ureter from the upper pole opens at a point closest to the bladder neck. It follows that the ureter to the major lower pole has a relatively short intravesical ureteral segment. Thus, vesicoureteral reflux to the lower portion of the kidney may be seen (Fig 11—4). Most ureteroceles in children involve the ureter which drains the upper portion of the duplicated kidney. The ureter to the upper renal pole may open ectopically into the vulva, urethra, or seminal vesicle (Fig 25—3). Such ureters are always obstructed to some degree (Figs 25—1, 25—6).

Duplication of the ureter is clinically significant only when obstruction or reflux is present, in which case dilatation and tortuosity of the ureter and hydronephrosis are found (Fig 25—1).

The symptoms and signs are those of persistent or recurrent infection. Urologic investigation (urograms) will reveal the congenital abnormality. If complete hydronephrotic atrophy of one renal pole has occurred, excretory urograms may show only one normal pelvis and ureter (Fig 25—4). The clue to duplication will be the observation that the visualized pelvis and calyces fail to drain a relatively large area of the renal shadow. The visualized ureter may be displaced laterally by its dilated obstructed mate.

If the anomaly causes obstruction or reflux, surgical repair should be attempted if at all practicable. It may be necessary to resect the hydronephrotic pole of the kidney with its ureter. Nephrectomy may be indicated if renal damage is severe. Surgical repair offers a good prognosis.

URETEROCELE

A ureterocele is a ballooning of the submucosal ureter into the bladder, secondary probably to congenital stenosis of the epithelial lining at the vesical end of the ureter; thus the urine cannot easily escape into the bladder. The pressure produced by ureteral peristalsis pushes the periureteral vesical mucosa into the bladder, causing a cystic protrusion. This urine-filled cyst is covered by vesical mucosa on the outside and lined by ureteral mucosa internally (Fig 25—2). Its complications, basically caused by the obstruction, are hydroureter, hydronephrosis, and upper tract infection. Stones may develop in the cyst. If large enough, ureterocele may cause bladder neck obstruction

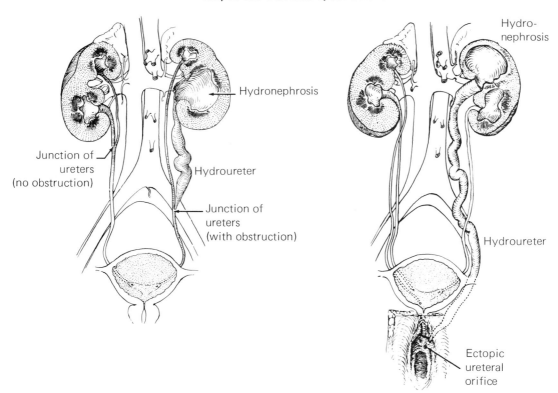

Figure 25–1. Duplication of ureters. *Left:* Incomplete Y type with hydroureteronephrosis on left. *Right:* Complete duplication with obstruction to one ureter with ectopic orifice on left. The ureter with the ectopic opening always drains the upper pole of the kidney.

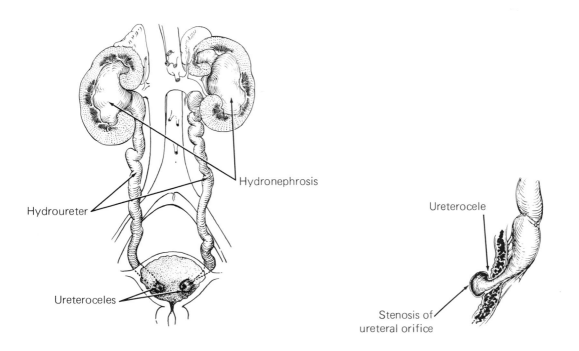

Figure 25–2. Ureterocele. *Left:* Obstructing ureteroceles (adult type) with hydroureteronephrosis. *Right:* Sagittal section through ureterocele and ureter to show pathologic changes. Resection of this ureterocele will be followed by vesicoureteral reflux.

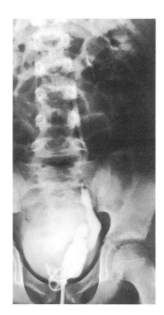
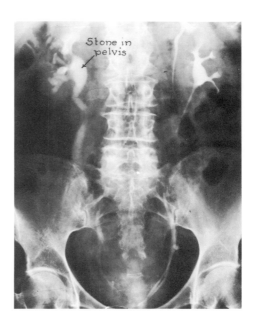

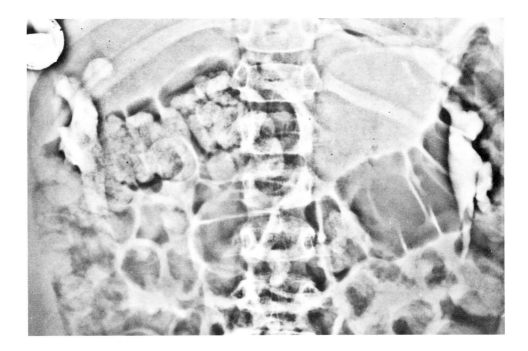

Figure 25—3. Duplication of ureters. *Above left:* Ureteral catheters passed through opening in region of verumontanum. Injection of radiopaque fluid reveals duplicated ureter to upper renal pole joining seminal vesicle (ectopic ureteral ostium). Second ureter not shown. *Above right:* Excretory urogram showing complete duplication of left ureters and renal pelves, which are otherwise normal. Staghorn calculus in right kidney; dilatation of upper ureter suggests possibility of presence of stone in lower portion of right ureter. *Below:* Excretory urogram showing marked displacement of visualized renal masses by giant functionless hydronephroses of upper renal segments. Ureters to upper poles opened into prostatic urethra.

(ectopic ureterocele) and may even prolapse through the female urethra.

Ureterocele is most commonly encountered in little girls and usually involves the ureter which drains the upper pole of a duplicated kidney (Figs 11—4 and 25—4). The obstructed portion is often dysplastic. Ureteroceles in adults tend to be bilateral, and are smaller and less obstructive than those seen in children.

The history and physical signs are compatible with ureteral obstruction or urinary tract infection. A history of an obstructed urinary stream, even incontinence, may be elicited if the ureterocele impinges on the bladder neck. Pyuria and bacteriuria may be present. Total renal function is normal unless both kidneys are affected. Excretory urograms may show cystic dilatation of the lower end of the ureter (Fig 25—4, left) or a round space-occupying lesion in a cystogram. Some changes from back pressure above this point are to be expected (eg, hydroureter, hydronephrosis, changes due to infection). A cystogram may reveal reflux into the lower renal pole.

Catheterization of the pinpoint ureteral opening may be impossible, but it is helpful in establishing the presence of infection in the kidney. If poor renal function has precluded adequate secretion of opaque material given intravenously, retrograde urography should be attempted.

The small, mildly obstructive ureterocele can usually be destroyed transurethrally. In children it may be necessary to open the bladder suprapubically so that the cyst can be resected. This may be followed, however, by vesicoureteral reflux because the obstruction has caused wide dilatation of the ureteral hiatus, thus shortening the intravesical ureter (Fig 11—4). At times, the obstructing ureterocele may so dilate the intramural ureter that reflux up the noninvolved ureter may occur. Excision of the cystic structure combined with simultaneous vesicoureteroplasty should, therefore, probably be done. Removal of this obstruction will usually cause the pathologic changes of the ureter and kidney to regress. Secondary infection can then more readily be controlled or cured. If the affected portion of a duplicated kidney is destroyed, heminephrectomy and complete ureterectomy are indicated.

POSTCAVAL URETER

The rare postcaval or retrocaval ureter is one which (from above downward) passes medially and behind the vena cava, turns forward along the great vein's left wall, and then passes laterally on the anterior surface of the vena cava and resumes its normal course to the bladder. It actually "hooks" around the cava. This anomalous position is due to an abnormal

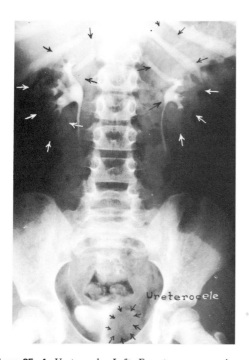 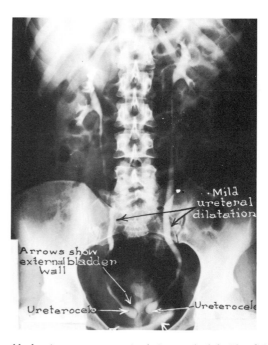

Figure 25—4. Ureterocele. *Left:* Excretory urogram in a girl 8 years old, showing a space-occupying lesion on the left side of the bladder caused by ureterocele. Absence of calyceal system in the upper portion of the left kidney implies duplication of the ureters and pelves and nonfunction (advanced hydronephrosis) of the upper pole; its dilated ureter drains into the obstructing ureterocele and displaces the visualized ureter laterally just below the kidney. *Right:* Excretory urogram in an adult female, showing "cobra head" deformity of the distal ends of both ureters; bilateral ureteroceles causing minimal obstruction; pressure on bladder from uterus. No treatment is indicated.

development of the vena cava.

The significance of postcaval ureter lies in the ureteral obstruction which is usually caused by the cava. This leads to hydronephrosis and, at times, infection. A catheter passed up such a ureter will take a course, in its midportion, overlying the spine. Excretory urograms will show deviation of the mid ureter over the spine. A retrograde ureterogram will show this defect graphically. A simultaneous venacavogram will relate the vena cava to the ureter (Fig 25–5).

Division of the ureter where it courses around the cava, with end-to-end anastomosis in the normal position, relieves the obstruction. It has also been recommended that the vena cava be divided, the ureter replaced in its normal position, and the vena cava then repaired. Nephrectomy may be necessary if secondary renal damage is advanced.

RETROILIAC URETER

A few cases of retroiliac ureter have been reported. They, too, are obstructed. On urography the ureter is deviated and compressed at the pelvic brim. The hydronephrosis is treated by division of the ureter with reanastomosis anterior to the vessels.

ECTOPIC URETERAL ORIFICE

In rare instances the ureter opens at a point other than the lateral horn of the interureteric ridge. If it drains distal to the external sphincter (this is seen only in the female), a constant dripping (incontinence) of urine is noted. Ectopy results from an abnormality of embryologic development (see Chapter 2). The Wolffian duct arises from the cloaca and acts as the drainage tube for the pronephros (primitive kidney) and the mesonephros. From this duct, at a point near the cloaca (which divides to form the rectum and lower urinary tract), the ureteral bud develops, then extends to and joins the metanephros. This junction forms the permanent kidney. As development progresses, the ureteral opening in the Wolffian duct gradually moves caudally until the Wolffian and ureteral ducts have separate openings in the urethrovesical area. Normally in the male the Wolffian ducts form the vasa deferentia and seminal vesicles. Their cranial ends drain the spermatogenic tubules of the testes. In the female, the superior portion atrophies and the caudal portion becomes Gartner's duct.

If abnormalities of development occur, the ureter may enter the urinary tract at a position below the normal point. In the male, its orifice may be found in the posterior urethra; in the female, just outside the bladder neck.

Should the ureteral orifice not disengage itself from the proximal end of the Wolffian duct, it is

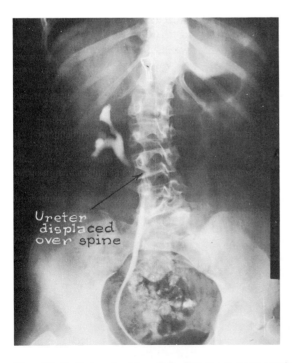

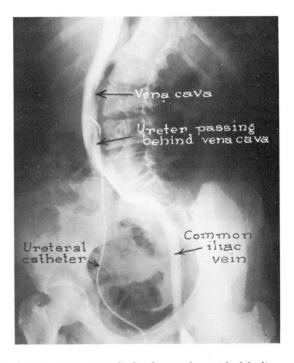

Figure 25–5. Postcaval ureter. *Left:* Retrograde ureteropyelogram showing upper ureter displaced onto the vertebral bodies, suggesting postcaval ureter. Note the congenital deformity of the spine. *Right:* Femoral venacavogram (right oblique view) showing ureter in retrocaval position.

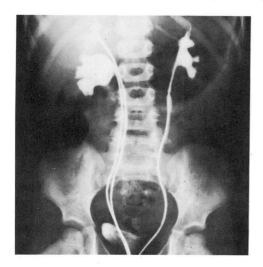 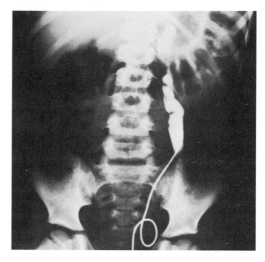

Figure 25—6. Ectopic ureter. (Girl, age 6, complained of partial urinary incontinence.) *Left:* Cystoscopy revealed 2 ureteral orifices on right, one on left; these were catheterized and urograms made. *Right:* Same patient. Ectopic ureteral orifice near urethral meatus catheterized. Retrograde urogram demonstrates second left hydronephrotic renal pelvis. Resection of upper pole and ureter cured incontinence.

obvious that in the male the ureter will drain into the seminal tract (eg, seminal vesicle, vas deferens). In the female it will drain into the remnants of Gartner's duct. In this instance urine will empty into the vagina, cervix, uterus, or the vaginal vestibule. The latter is the most common site (Figs 25–1, 25–6). Most ectopic orifices are seen in the female.

Most ureters with ectopic openings are one of a pair to a single kidney, and the ectopic ureter almost always drains the rudimentary upper renal pole. Since ureters which open in abnormal positions are usually obstructed at their terminations, hydroureter and hydronephrosis develop. Secondary infection is common. Those ureters opening in the proximal urethra usually reveal vesicoureteral reflux on cystography.

In the male, since all ectopic orifices are proximal to the external sphincter, no incontinence ensues. In the female, vaginal or vestibular ureters are devoid of sphincteric control, and a constant drainage of urine occurs in spite of normal voiding.

Symptoms therefore depend upon the site of the opening. If proximal to the external sphincter, there may be flank pain, fever, and vesical irritability. If the opening is distal to the external sphincter, "incontinence" is the complaint. Symptoms of renal infection and pain may also be experienced. In the female, careful inspection of the vestibule or anterior vaginal wall may reveal an orifice from which urine or purulent material may drain. Renal tenderness or enlargement may be present. Epididymitis is a common complication when the ureter drains into the seminal vesicle.

The urine may be infected. Excretory urograms will usually show duplication of the renal pelves with hydronephrosis of the upper pole whose ureter may be markedly dilated and tortuous. Distally it may be traced beyond the trigonal area. If renal destruction is

severe, no opaque medium may be excreted. Absence of calyces in the upper portion of the renal shadow and lateral displacement of the upper portion of the visualized ureter will suggest the diagnosis.

Cystoscopy may reveal the orifice in the urethra. If catheterization can be performed (it may be possible if a vaginal or vestibular orifice is identified), urine can be obtained for study and urograms made (Fig 25–6).

It may be feasible to resect the lowermost portion of the ureter and to implant the distal end of the ureter into the bladder. However, resection of the superior renal pole and its ureter is usually indicated because of the degree of parenchymal damage.

STRICTURE OF THE URETER
(See also Chapter 10.)

Evidence of obstruction at the ureteropelvic or ureterovesical junction has heretofore been interpreted as stricture. It is now clear that most cases of the latter type really represent changes secondary to ureterovesical reflux (Fig 25–7). Some ureteropelvic obstructions also develop as a complication of reflux. Most resolve when ureterovesicoplasty has been done. A few may require surgical correction. A similar picture develops secondary to hypertrophy of the trigone which arises in association with distal obstruction, eg, posterior urethral valves. Creevy has observed what he calls achalasia of the lower ureteral segment which produces a functional obstruction. Tanagho & others (1970) find that this obstruction is caused by congenital hypertrophy of the circular smooth musculature of the juxtavesical ureter. A few cases of ureteral-obstructing

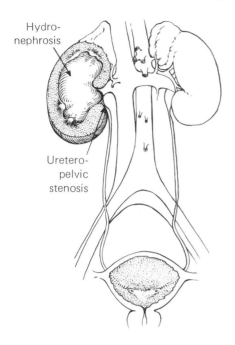

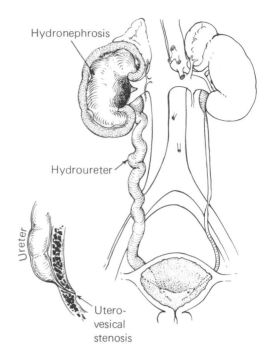

Figure 25–7. Congenital ureteral obstruction. *Left:* Right ureteropelvic stenosis with hydronephrosis. *Right:* Ureterovesical obstruction with hydroureteronephrosis. The common causes are (1) reflux, (2) hypertrophy of the ureterotrigonal complex secondary to distal obstruction, and (3) hypertrophy of the circular musculature of the juxtavesical ureter (Tanagho).

valves and aberrant vessels have been recorded.

Symptoms are often absent, for many of these strictures are so mild that sudden renal capsular distention does not take place even though the kidney is completely destroyed by hydronephrotic atrophy. Some patients, however, may have costovertebral angle pain from the obstruction; others may have only reflex gastrointestinal complaints; and some have both. Ureteral stricture on the right side not uncommonly simulates appendicitis. Symptoms of infection may be elicited. It should be remembered, however, that chronic pyelonephritis may cause no symptoms.

Physical examination may reveal nothing unless the hydronephrotic kidney is large and tense and can be felt or percussed. Tenderness may be present with complicating pyelonephritis. Urinalysis may provide evidence of urinary infection. Renal function will be normal unless there is bilateral renal disease.

A plain film of the abdomen may reveal an enlarged renal shadow. Excretory urograms will demonstrate dilatation of the excretory tract above the site of constant narrowing (Fig 25–8); one must not be confused by "pseudostrictures," which represent normal systolic ureteral contraction. Advanced renal damage may cause lack of excretion of the radiopaque medium. A voiding cystourethrogram may reveal ureterovesical reflux.

Retrograde passage of a ureteral catheter may be arrested by a severe stricture. It may, however, pass through the site of obstruction, only to be stopped by the acute ureteral angulations proximal to the stric-

ture. On the other hand, an area of functional obstruction may accept a large catheter easily although stasis persists. Retrograde ureteropyelograms will furnish a graphic picture of the obstruction and the changes secondary to it.

Little significance should be attached to the ease of passage of various sizes of catheters in the diagnosis of stricture. Unjustified diagnoses of stricture have also been made by passing a catheter with a fusiform bulge at its tip up the ureter. On withdrawal, a "hang" or sudden resistance to withdrawal is sometimes mistaken for evidence of stricture. It should be pointed out that it is the nature of the ureter to go into spasm even on being touched lightly during surgery. The diagnosis of true stricture is made on urographic study, preferably by the "nontraumatic" intravenous type. The point of narrowing should show in every film, and dilatation above this point should be demonstrated.

Repair of the stricture is usually indicated if the kidney retains some degree of function. Severe renal damage is treated by nephrectomy. Should the changes be secondary to vesicoureteral reflux or hypertrophy of the juxtavesical ureter, repair of this junction may be indicated.

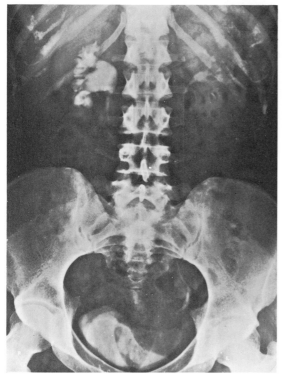 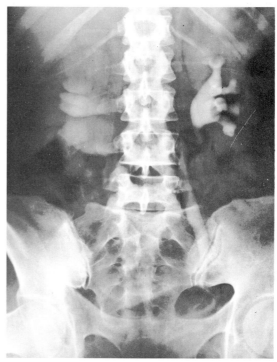

Figure 25—8. Ureteral obstruction. *Left:* Right ureteropelvic stenosis with mild hydronephrosis due to aberrant blood vessel. Pressure defect of left side of bladder from uterus. *Right:* Excretory urogram taken 2 weeks after Wertheim operation showing bilateral ureteral obstruction and advanced hydronephrosis on right.

ACQUIRED DISEASES OF THE URETER

ACQUIRED URETERAL STRICTURE

Most ureteral strictures are congenital, but some are acquired. The most common causes of acquired stenosis are the following:

(1) Injury to the ureters during extensive pelvic surgery or from intensive radiotherapy (Fig 25—8).

(2) Renal or ureteral injury secondary to external trauma with perirenal and periureteral hematoma which leaves periureteral scar tissue following absorption.

(3) Compression of the ureters by lymph nodes involved by cancer (metastases, lymphomas) (Fig 18—15).

(4) Contracture due to infection, and ischemia caused by prolonged impaction of a ureteral stone.

(5) Ureteral stenosis due to uterine prolapse.

(6) Tuberculous or bilharzial infection (pyeloureteritis) may cause fibrosis of the ureter, which may lead in turn to contracture (Fig 13—2).

(7) Retroperitoneal fibrosis.

(8) Aneurysm of the aorta or following aortofemoral bypass grafts.

(9) Ureteropelvic or ureterovesical obstruction secondary to vesicoureteral reflux (see Chapter 11).

(10) Occlusion of the ureterovesical junction by cancer of the bladder or prostate (Fig 18—14).

(11) Obstruction of the ureterovesical junction caused by hypertrophy of the trigone secondary to benign prostatic hyperplasia or posterior urethral valves.

(12) Compression of the lower ureters secondary to severe constipation in women and children.

(13) Endometriosis involving the ureter.

(14) Compression of the ureter by the right ovarian vein (rare).

(15) Retroperitoneal scarring with ureteral obstruction secondary to granulomatous bowel (Crohn's) disease.

The effects upon the kidney and the clinical findings, complications, and treatment of acquired ureteral stricture are the same as those described under congenital stricture and urinary obstruction and stasis.

RETROPERITONEAL FASCIITIS
(Chronic Retroperitoneal Fibroplasia, Retroperitoneal Fibrosis)

One or both ureters may be compressed by a chronic inflammatory process which involves the retroperitoneal tissues over the lower lumbar vertebrae. Patients treated for migraine with methysergide (Sansert), an ergot derivative, may also develop retroperitoneal fibrosis. Sclerosing Hodgkin's disease and other malignancies have occasionally been found to cause this reaction. Phils & others (1973) have observed the development of retroperitoneal fasciitis in 3 siblings with sickle cell trait. Recently, lysergic acid diethylamide (LSD; an ergot alkaloid) has been reported as a cause of retroperitoneal fibrosis (Stecker & others, 1974).

The symptoms, which are nonspecific, include renal pain, low back pain, and the syndrome of uremia. The only pathognomonic sign is the presence of a palpable firm mass over the sacral promontory.

Infection of the urinary tract is not usually present. Renal function tests are normal unless both ureters are obstructed; anemia may be found during the stage of uremia.

The diagnosis can be made if excretory urograms reveal medial deviation of the ureters involved in the fibrous plaque in the lumbar area (Fig 25–9). Secondary to obstruction, there is dilatation of the ureters and renal pelves proximal to that point. When uremia has supervened, retrograde urograms may be needed to delineate the excretory tracts.

If radiographic changes are moderate and the patient is not uremic, corticosteroid therapy should be instituted; rather dramatic response in a matter of a few weeks has been reported. Begin with 30–60 mg of prednisone per day. If serial urograms show lessening hydronephrosis, the dosage can be gradually decreased to a maintenance dose of 5–15 mg/day. If the degree of obstruction is severe, the ureters should be freed

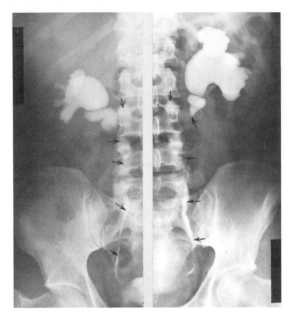

Figure 25–9. Retroperitoneal fasciitis. Right and left kidneys of same patient as shown by excretory urography. Note medial deviation of the upper portions of the ureters (see arrows) with marked obstruction. (Courtesy of JA Hutch.)

from the fibrous plaque, which should be subjected to multiple biopsies, and either transplanted intraperitoneally or displaced lateral to the psoas muscles so that they do not again become involved. Since there is a tendency for the disease to progress, prophylactic corticosteroid therapy should be instituted.

If the patient has been on methysergide, withdrawal of the drug is often followed by spontaneous regression of the obstruction.

Unless the cause is malignancy, the prognosis is fair to good. Autotransplantation has been accomplished in a few patients after failure of uterolysis.

● ● ●

References

Duplication of the Ureter

Amar AD: Lateral ureteral displacement: Sign of nonvisualized duplication. J Urol 105:638, 1971.

Amar AD, Chabra K: Reflux in duplicated ureters: Treatment in children. J Pediat Surg 5:419, 1970.

Atwell JD & others: Familial incidence of bifid and double ureters. Arch Dis Child 49:390, 1974.

Belman AB, Filmer RB, King LR: Surgical management of duplication of the collecting system. J Urol 112: 316, 1974.

Diaz-Ball FL & others: Pyeloureterostomy and ureteroureterostomy: Alternative procedures to partial nephrectomy for duplication of the ureter with only one pathological segment. J Urol 102:621, 1969.

Klauber GT, Reid EC: Inverted Y reduplication of the ureter. J Urol 107:362, 1972.

Perkins PJ, Kroovand RL, Evans AT: Ureteral triplication. Radiology 108:533, 1973.

Peterson C Jr, Silbiger ML: Five ureters: A case report. J Urol 100:160, 1968.

Whitaker J, Danks DM: A study of the inheritance of duplication of the kidneys and ureters. J Urol 95:176, 1966.

Ureterocele

Friedland GW, Cunningham J: The elusive ectopic ureteroceles. Am J Roentgenol 116:792, 1972.

Johnston JH, Johnson LM: Experiences with ectopic ureteroceles. Brit J Urol 41:61, 1969.

Malek RS & others: Simple and ectopic ureterocele in infancy and childhood. Surg Gynec Obst 134:611, 1972.

Nash AG, Knight M: Ureterocele calculi. Brit J Urol 45:404, 1973.

Newman LB McAlister WH, Kissane J: Segmented renal dysplasia associated with ectopic ureteroceles in children. Urology 3:23, 1974.

Shaw RE: Ureterocele. Brit J Surg 60:337, 1973.

Stephens FD: Caecoureterocele and concepts on the embryology and aetiology of ureteroceles. Australian New Zealand J Surg 40:239, 1971.

Tanagho EA: Anatomy and management of ureteroceles. J Urol 107:729, 1972.

Weiss RM, Spackman TJ: Everting ectopic ureterocele. J Urol 11:538, 1974.

Williams DI, Fay R, Lillie JG: The functional radiology of ectopic ureterocele. Brit J Urol 44:417, 1972.

Wines RD, O'Flynn JD: Transurethral treatment of ureteroceles: A report of 45 cases mostly treated by transurethral resection. Brit J Urol 44:207, 1972.

Postcaval Ureter

Brito RR & others: Retrocaval ureter. Brit J Urol 45:144, 1973.

Retroiliac Ureter

Hanna MK: Bilateral retroiliac-artery ureters. Brit J Urol 44:339, 1972.

Hock E, Purkayastha A, Jay BD: Retroiliac ureter: A case report. J Urol 107:37, 1972.

Ectopic Ureteral Orifice

Brannan W, Henry HH Jr: Ureteral ectopia: Report of 39 cases. J Urol 109:192, 1973.

Gordon HL, Kessler R: Ectopic ureter entering the seminal vesicle associated with renal dysplasia. J Urol 108:389, 1972.

Malek RS & others: Observations on ureteral ectopy in children. J Urol 107:308, 1972.

Mogg RA: The single ectopic ureter. Brit J Urol 46:3, 1974.

Williams DI, Lightwood RG: Bilateral single ectopic ureters. Brit J Urol 44:267, 1972.

Stricture of the Ureter

Albertson KW, Tainter LB: Valves of the ureter. Radiology 103:91, 1972.

Allen TD: Congenital ureteral strictures. J Urol 104:196, 1970.

Javadpour N, Solomon T, Bush IM: Obstruction of the lower ureter by aberrant vessels in children. J Urol 108:340, 1972.

Tanagho EA, Smith DR, Guthrie TH: Pathophysiology of functional ureteral obstruction. J Urol 104:73, 1970.

Acquired Ureteral Stricture

Alkema HD, Ratliff RK: Successful treatment of postradiation ureteral stricture by simple linear incision. J Urol 97:251, 1967.

Bagby RJ & others: Genitourinary complications of granulomatous bowel disease. Am J Roentgenol 117:297, 1973.

Berlin M: Ovarian vein thrombosis. Am J Obst Gynec 118:880, 1974.

Bissada NK, Redman JF: Ureteral complications in diverticulitis of the colon. J Urol 112:454, 1974.

Block GE, Enker WE, Kirsner JB: Significance and treatment of occult obstructive uropathy complicating Crohn's disease. Ann Surg 178:322, 1973.

Bosch A, Frias Z, de Valda GC: Prognostic significance of ureteral obstruction in carcinoma of the cervix uteri. Acta radiol ther 12:47, 1973.

Cussen LJ: The morphology of congenital dilatation of the ureter: Intrinsic ureteral lesions. Australia New Zealand J Surg 41:185, 1971.

Dick AL & others: Postmenopausal endometriosis with ureteral obstruction. Brit J Urol 45:153, 1973.

Fernandes M & others: Reconstruction of lower ureter and urethra, and closure of vesicovaginal fistula and other bladder defects: Various uses of bladder flap. Urology 1:444, 1973.

Heal MR: Primary obstructive megaloureter in adults. Brit J Urol 45:490, 1973.

Kaplan JH, Kudish HG: Endometrial obstruction of ureter. Urology 3:327, 1974.

Lang EK & others: Complications in the urinary tract related to treatment of carcinoma of the cervix. South MJ 66:228, 1973.

Mallouh C, Pellman CM: Scrotal herniation of the ureter. J Urol 106:38, 1971.

McLaughlin AP & others: The pathophysiology of primary megaloureter. J Urol 109:805, 1973.

Melnick GS, Bramwit DN: Bilateral ovarian vein syndrome. Am J Roentgenol 113:509, 1971.

Peck DR, Bhatt GM, Lowman RM: Traction displacement of the ureter: A sign of aortic aneurism. J Urol 109:983, 1973.

Petrone AF, Dudzinski PJ, Maniatis W: Ureteral obstruction secondary to aortic femoral bypass. Ann Surg 179:192, 1974.

Reddy AN, Evans AT: Endometriosis of the ureters. J Urol 111:474, 1974.

Rudin LJ, Megalli MR, Lattimer JK: Obstructive uropathy associated with uterine prolapse. Urology 4:73, 1974.

Schapira HE, Mitty HA: Right ovarian vein septic thrombophlebitis causing ureteral obstruction. J Urol 112:451, 1974.

Retroperitoneal Fasciitis

Arger PH, Stolz JL, Miller WT: Retroperitoneal fibrosis: An analysis of the clinical spectrum and roentgenographic signs. Am J Roentgenol 119:812, 1973.

Cerny JC, Scott T: Non-idiopathic retroperitoneal fibrosis. J Urol 105:49, 1971.

Jacobson JB, Redman HC: Ultrasound findings in a case of retroperitoneal fibrosis. Radiology 113:423, 1974.

Linke CA, May AG: Autotransplantation in retroperitoneal fibrosis. J Urol 107:196, 1972.

Mitchinson MJ, Withycombe JFR, Jones RA: The response of idiopathic retroperitoneal fibrosis to corticosteroids. Brit J Urol 43:444, 1971.

Morandi LP, Grob PJ: Retroperitoneal fibrosis: Response to corticosteroid therapy. Arch Int Med 128:295, 1971.

Nitz GL & others: Retroperitoneal malignancy masquer-

ading as benign retroperitoneal fibrosis. J Urol
103:46, 1970.

Phils JA & others: Retroperitoneal fibrosis in three siblings with sickle cell trait. Canad MAJ 108:1025,
1973.

Ross JC, Goldsmith HJ: The combined surgical and
medical treatment of retroperitoneal fibrosis. Brit J
Surg 58:422, 1971.

Stecker JF Jr & others: Retroperitoneal fibrosis and ergot
derivatives. J Urol 112:30, 1974.

Thomas MH, Chisholm GD: Retroperitoneal fibrosis
associated with malignant disease. Brit J Cancer
28:453, 1973.

Wright FW, Sanders RC: Is retroperitoneal fibrosis a self-
limiting disease? Brit J Surg 44:511, 1971.

26...
Disorders of the Bladder, Prostate, & Seminal Vesicles

CONGENITAL ANOMALIES OF THE BLADDER*

EXSTROPHY

Exstrophy of the bladder is a complete ventral defect of the urogenital sinus and the overlying skeletal system (see Chapter 2). Other congenital anomalies are frequently associated with it. The lower central abdomen is occupied by the inner surface of the posterior wall of the bladder, whose mucosal edges are fused with the skin. Urine spurts onto the abdominal wall from the ureteral orifices.

The rami of the pubic bones are widely separated. The pelvic ring thus lacks rigidity, the femurs are rotated externally, and the child "waddles like a duck." Since the rectus muscles insert on the rami, they are widely separated from each other inferiorly. A hernia, made up of the exstrophic bladder and surrounding skin, is therefore present. Epispadias almost always accompanies it.

Renal infection is common, and hydronephrosis caused by ureterovesical obstruction is often found on urography. These films also reveal the separation of the pubic bones.

Many attempts have been made to free the bladder from surrounding skin, close it primarily, and repair sphincteric mechanisms hoping for a continent bladder with protection of the upper urinary tract from progressive damage (Williams & Keeton, 1973). This goal has been achieved in a few girls but in boys only rarely. The exstrophic bladder for the most part reveals fibrosis, derangement of the muscularis mucosae, and chronic infection. Squamous metaplasia is often seen (Rudin, Tannenbaum, & Lattimer, 1972). These pathologic changes tend to defeat efforts to form a bladder of proper capacity and function. After surgical closure, detrusor contraction is subnormal and the incidence of vesicoureteral reflux is high, leading to pyelonephritis and hydronephrosis (Nisonson & Lattimer, 1972). About 60 cases of adenocarcinoma devel-

oping in such patients have been reported. Some form of urinary diversion is therefore the procedure of choice. An ileal loop conduit (Bricker operation) is usually done, but ureterosigmoidostomy has its proponents. Boyce (1972) performs vesicorectal anastomosis after closure of the bladder; proximal sigmoid colostomy is necessary. After other forms of urinary diversion, the bladder is resected and later the epispadiac defect must be closed. Sexual function is good, but the male will be infertile.

PERSISTENT URACHUS

Embryologically, the allantois connects the urogenital sinus with the umbilicus. Normally the allantois is obliterated and is represented by a fibrous cord (urachus) extending from the dome of the bladder to the navel (see Chapter 2).

Incomplete obliteration sometimes occurs. If obliteration is complete except at the superior end, a draining umbilical sinus may be noted. If it becomes infected, the drainage will be purulent. If the inferior end remains open it will communicate with the bladder, but this does not usually produce symptoms. Rarely, the entire tract remains patent, in which case urine drains constantly from the umbilicus. This is apt to become obvious within a few days of birth. If only the ends of the urachus seal off, a cyst of that body may form and may become quite large, presenting a low midline mass (Fig 26−1). If the cyst should become infected, signs of general and local sepsis will develop.

Adenocarcinoma may occur in a urachal cyst, particularly at its vesical extremity, and will tend to invade the tissues beneath the anterior abdominal wall. It may be seen cystoscopically. Stones may develop in a cyst of the urachus. These can be identified on a plain x-ray film.

Treatment consists of excision of the urachus, which lies on the peritoneal surface. If adenocarcinoma is present, radical resection is required.

Unless other serious congenital anomalies are present, the prognosis is good. The complication of adenocarcinoma offers a poor prognosis.

*Congenital vesicorectal fistulas are discussed with urethrorectal fistulas.

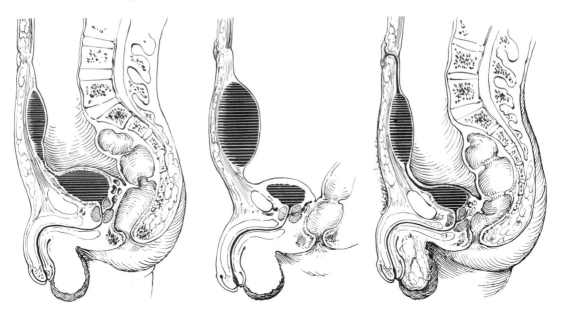

Figure 26–1. Types of persistent urachus. *Left:* Communicating urachus continuous with the bladder. This is a "pseudodiverticulum" and usually causes no symptoms. *Center:* Urachal cyst; usually causes no symptoms or signs unless it becomes larger or infected. *Right:* Patent urachus. There is constant drainage of urine from the umbilicus.

CONTRACTURE OF THE BLADDER NECK

There is considerable debate about the incidence of congenital narrowing of the bladder neck. Some feel that its presence is a common cause of vesicoureteral reflux, vesical diverticula, a bladder of large capacity, and the syndrome of irritable bladder associated with enuresis. A few observers consider this contracture a rare phenomenon and believe that the diagnosis is purely presumptive. The diagnosis is based upon endoscopic observation, which is an unreliable method. Voiding cystourethrography has been used to depict such narrowing, but interpretation of the films varies from urologist to urologist and radiologist to radiologist.

Nunn (1965) studied the intravesical and urethral pressures during voiding in · cases with the signs mentioned above. He found no evidence of bladder neck obstruction. The 2 recorded pressures were essentially equal. It appears that the bladder neck would have to be extremely stenotic to truly obstruct urine flow. It is becoming increasingly clear that, in the little girl, the obstructive lesion is spasm of the periurethral striated muscle which develops secondary to distal urethral stenosis (see Chapter 28).

Empirical treatment is often employed, consisting of suprapubic bladder neck revision or transurethral resection. Making the bladder neck incompetent in the male child may later cause retrograde ejaculation and, therefore, infertility. Revision of the bladder neck in the female may cause urinary incontinence. This diagnosis must therefore be made with caution.

ACQUIRED DISEASES OF THE BLADDER

INTERSTITIAL CYSTITIS
(Hunner's Ulcer, Submucous Fibrosis)

Interstitial cystitis is primarily a disease of middle-aged women. It is characterized by fibrosis of the vesical wall, with consequent loss of bladder capacity. Frequency is the principal symptom.

Pathogenesis & Pathology

Infection does not appear to be the cause of fibrosis of the bladder wall, for the urine is usually normal. It has been postulated that the fibrosis is due to obstruction of the vesical lymphatics secondary to pelvic surgery or infection, but many of these patients fail to give such a history. It may be secondary to thrombophlebitis complicating acute infections of the bladder or pelvic organs, or may be the result of prolonged intrinsic arteriolar spasm secondary to psychogenic impulses.

Recently, however, evidence has been adduced which suggests that interstitial cystitis is an autoimmune collagen disease. Oravisto & others (1970) studied 54 women afflicted with this disease. Antinuclear antibodies were found in 85%. A significant number had allergy of the reagin type or hypersensitivity to drugs. Jacobo & others (1974) and Gordon & others (1973) have confirmed these findings. An allergic cause would account for the favorable responses to corticosteroids.

The primary change is fibrosis in the deeper layers of the bladder. The capacity of the organ is decreased, sometimes markedly. The mucosa is thinned, especially where mobility is greatest as the bladder fills and empties (ie, over the dome), and small ulcers or cracks in the mucous membrane may be seen in this area. In the most severe cases, the normal mechanism of the ureterovesical junctions is destroyed, leading to vesicoureteral reflux. Hydroureteronephrosis and pyelonephritis may then ensue.

Microscopically, the mucosa may be thinned or even denuded. The capillaries of the tunica propria are often engorged, and signs of inflammation are apparent. The muscle is replaced by varying amounts of fibrous tissue, which is often quite avascular. The lymphatics may be engorged. Increased mast cells and lymphocytic infiltration are seen (Jacobo & others, 1974).

Clinical Findings

Interstitial cystitis should be considered when a middle-aged woman with clear urine complains of severe frequency and nocturia and suprapubic pain on vesical distention.

A. Symptoms: There is a long history of slowly progressive frequency and nocturia, both of which may be severe. The history does not suggest infection (burning on urination, cloudy urine). Suprapubic pain is usually marked when the bladder is full. Pain may also be experienced in the urethra or perineum. It is relieved on voiding. Gross hematuria is occasionally noted, usually when urination has had to be postponed (ie, following vesical overdistention). The patient is tense and anxious. Whether this is secondary to the prolonged and severe symptoms or is the primary cause of the vesical changes is not clear (see Chapter 34). A history of allergy may be obtained.

B. Signs: Physical examination is usually normal. Some tenderness in the suprapubic area may be noted. There may be some tenderness in the region of the bladder when palpated through the vagina.

C. Laboratory Findings: If the patient has had no previous treatment (eg, instrumentation), the urine is almost always free of infection. Microscopic hematuria may be noted. Renal function (as measured by the PSP test) is normal except in the occasional patient in whom vesical fibrosis has led to vesicoureteral reflux or obstruction.

D. X-Ray Findings: Excretory urograms are usually normal unless reflux has occurred, in which case hydronephrosis is found. The accompanying cystogram will reveal a bladder of small capacity; reflux into a dilated upper tract may be noted.

E. Instrumental Examination: Cystoscopy is usually diagnostic. As the bladder fills, increasing suprapubic pain is experienced. The vesical capacity may be as low as 60 ml. In a patient not previously treated (by fulguration or hydraulic overdistention), the bladder lining may look fairly normal. But if distention is continued in spite of increasing pain, punctate hemorrhagic areas may appear over the most distensible portion of the wall. With further distention, an arcuate split in the mucosa will occur and bleeding from it may be profuse.

Differential Diagnosis

Tuberculosis of the bladder may cause true ulceration but is most apt to involve the region of the ureteral orifice which drains the tuberculous kidney. Typical tubercles may be identified, pyuria is present, and tubercle bacilli can usually be found. Furthermore, urograms will often show the typical lesion of renal tuberculosis.

Nonspecific vesical infection seldom causes ulceration. Pus and bacteria will be found in the urine. Antimicrobial treatment will be effective.

Utz & Zinke (1974) have observed that 20% of their male patients who had been diagnosed as having interstitial cystitis actually had carcinoma. They stress the need for cytologic study and transurethral biopsy.

Complications

Gradual ureteral stenosis or reflux and its sequelae (eg, hydronephrosis) may develop.

Treatment

A. Specific Measures: There appears to be no definitive treatment for interstitial cystitis. The therapy usually employed frequently affords partial relief but may be completely ineffective.

Hydraulic overdistention, with or without anesthesia, in some cases gradually improves the bladder capacity. Vesical lavage with increasing strengths of silver nitrate (1:5000–1:100) may have the same effect. Superficial (transcystoscopic) electrocoagulation of the split mucosa is commonly practiced and may afford temporary relief of pain. Greenberg & others (1974) believe that transurethral resection of the lesion affords better results than fulguration.

Corticotropin causes an increase in vesical capacity in many patients and affords complete or partial relief from pain. The effective dose is in the range of 25 mg IM 4 times daily for 1 month.

Cortisone acetate, 100 mg, or prednisone (Meticorten), 10–20 mg/day, in divided doses orally for 21 days, followed by decreasing amounts for an additional 21 days, has also been found effective (Badenoch, 1971). Transcystoscopic injection of the lesions with prednisone has its proponents.

Antihistamines (eg, pyribenzamine, 50 mg 4 times a day) may also afford some relief. Heparin sodium (long-acting), 20,000 units/day IV, also blocks the action of histamine, and its use in the treatment of Hunner's ulcer is encouraging.

Bilateral section of the third sacral nerve may increase bladder capacity significantly and relieve the pain associated with vesical distention.

If corticosteroids fail to afford any relief, subtotal cystectomy and enlargement of the bladder by adding a patch of colon (colocystoplasty) should be considered.

B. General Measures: General or vesical sedatives

may be prescribed but seldom afford relief. If urinary infection is found (usually following instrumentation), it should be treated by appropriate antibiotics. If senile urethritis is discovered, diethylstilbestrol vaginal suppositories may prove helpful.

C. **Treatment of Complications**: If progressive hydronephrosis develops secondary to ureteral stenosis, little will be gained by ureteral dilatations. Diversion of the urinary stream (eg, ureteroileocutaneous anastomosis) may therefore be necessary.

Prognosis

Only a minority of patients are apparently cured or have their symptoms controlled by the treatment outlined above. Most are not relieved, and remain bladder invalids.

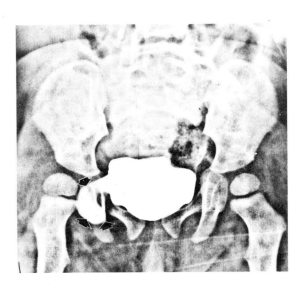

EXTERNAL VESICAL HERNIATION

The bladder of a young girl may protrude through a patulous urethra and present itself externally. Treatment requires gentle pressure upon the mass, with the patient in the Trendelenburg position. After reduction, a small urethral catheter should be left in the bladder for a few days. If herniation recurs, the bladder and urethra should be sutured to the linea alba.

INTERNAL VESICAL HERNIATION

One side of the bladder may become involved in an inguinal hernia (in men) or a femoral hernia (in women) (Fig 26–2). Such a mass may recede on urination. It is most often found as a previously unsuspected complication during the surgical correction of a hernia.

URINARY STRESS INCONTINENCE

Stress incontinence, the loss of urine with physical strain (eg, coughing, sneezing), is a common complaint of older women. Although it usually occurs as an aftermath of childbirth, it has been observed in girls and nulliparous women also.

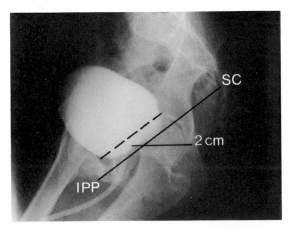

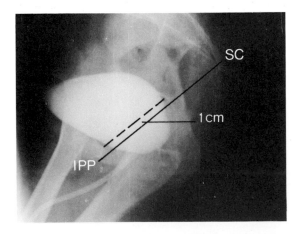

Figure 26–2. Internal vesical hernia; lateral cystograms in stress incontinence. *Above left:* Female, 6 months old. Cystogram of excretory urogram showing tongue of bladder in right femoral hernia (see arrows). In the 2 films shown below, the dashed line shows the normal position of the base of the normal bladder. Line SCIPP is a reference line drawn from the sacrococcygeal (SC) joint to the inferior point of the pubic bone (IPP). *Below left:* Resting cystogram in stress incontinence. The bladder base lies 2 cm below the normal position. *Right:* Cystogram taken with straining in a patient with stress incontinence. The base of the bladder descends about 4 cm, revealing poor support of the urethrovesical junction.

Normal urethral resistance is about 100 cm of water; this is the sum of the smooth muscle urethral sphincter (50 cm of water) and the striated midurethral sphincter (50 cm of water). Normally, with strain or cough, intraperitoneal pressure rises sharply but the resistance in the mid urethra rises also, thus maintaining the relatively high urethra-to-detrusor pressure ratio. In patients with stress incontinence, the basic lesion is loss of normal midurethral resistance caused by a severe sagging of the vesical base and urethra caused by poor support of these structures. The sphincter muscles are usually normal, but with the descent of the urethra and bladder they cannot work efficiently. Normally, the length of the urethra is 4 cm. Urethral pressure studies show that the proximal half of the urethra reveals little closure pressure. Thus, the functional length of their urethras is about 2 cm (Tanagho & Miller, 1973). In addition, the area of the posterior urethra and bladder neck has fallen out of the true pelvis so that the strain which suddenly increases intravesical pressure is associated with decreased resistance in the proximal and mid urethra thereby leading to incontinence.

Clinical Findings

The patient complains of loss of urine only with straining in the upright position. They remain dry while in bed. Some degree of urethrocele is usually noted. Of some diagnostic value is the demonstration that support to the bladder neck will cause the patient to be continent with cough or strain. This test must be performed with the patient standing. The region of the bladder neck is lifted well up under the symphysis pubis with 2 fingers or 2 clamps. (If clamps are used, infiltration with a local anesthetic is required.) False position tests, however, are sometimes elicited.

An important test in establishing the diagnosis of true stress incontinence is the lateral cystogram taken both with and without straining. A beaded chain or catheter should be placed in the bladder to dilineate the urethrovesical junction (Fig 26–2). In the normal female, the base of the bladder lies about 2 cm above a line drawn from the inferior margin of the pubis to the sacrococcygeal joint (the SCIPP line). With straining, the vesical base should descend no more than 1.5 cm. With true stress incontinence, the static lateral cystogram may reveal some sagging of the bladder, and this is markedly accentuated on the film taken when the patient strains to void (Noll & Hutch, 1969; Susset & others, 1974).

Differential Diagnosis

Careful history taking will usually differentiate between stress and urgency incontinence. The latter implies the presence of a local inflammatory disease. The following diseases must be differentiated from the lesion causing stress incontinence if good surgical results are to be obtained: ectopic ureteral orifice, neurogenic bladder, senile urethritis, urethral diverticulum, and local lesions of the urethra and bladder (eg, cystitis, urethritis). The history, physical examination, urinalysis, and PSP test as well as cystoscopy, excretory urography, lateral cystography, and cystometry should make the differentiation. None of these diseases exhibit the changes on cystourethrography described above.

Treatment

If hypoestrogenism of the vagina and urethra is discovered, give estrogens locally or by mouth. If this measure fails, either a vaginal repair with particular attention to support of the bladder neck or a urethrovesical suspension (Marshall-Marchetti) operation will usually be successful. In the type showing more severe derangement of urethrovesical relationships, urethrovesical suspension is the procedure of choice. It may be combined with vaginal repair if local conditions warrant. For the few failures, a sling of rectus fascia should be brought under the bladder neck in order to afford maximum support.

Prognosis

If the proper diagnosis has been made, the cure rate approaches 85%. Unfortunately, after a year or so, stress incontinence recurs in a few cases. Reoperation may therefore be necessary.

URINARY INCONTINENCE

Partial or complete urinary incontinence may develop after prostatectomy, particularly the transurethral type. Intrinsic damage to the smooth muscle urethral sphincter is implied. Though it is common to incriminate damage to or resection of the external voluntary sphincter, this is very rare. Such a patient can stop the voiding stream by contracture of the latter sphincter, but prolonged control is impossible because of fatigue of striated muscle. Only the smooth muscle with its constant tone can afford continence. Numerous operations for cure of total incontinence have been devised. Berry & Dahlen (1971) have employed a plastic device which is placed in the perineum so that it compresses the urethra. The success rate is less than 30%, and pain—even secondary infection—from the prosthesis is a problem. Hinman and co-workers (1970) have placed a segment of rib in the perineum in such manner that it compresses the perineal urethra. About 33% receive some benefit.

Kaufman (see references on p 402) has devised a number of procedures that apply pressure to the perineal urethra just distal to the prostate. These include apposition or transposition of the ischiocavernosus muscles and implantation of a plastic prosthesis. These procedures do not attempt to reconstruct the damaged sphincteric mechanism; they work by offering optimal obstruction to afford continence. Kaufman claims success in up to 70% of his cases.

Tanagho (1972) has designed a procedure based upon sound anatomic principles that has enjoyed significant success in restoring urinary continency. A strip of the heavy layer of the middle circular layer of the detrusor muscle, anteriorly, is formed into a tube, thus affording sphincteric action. This is anastomosed to the bladder neck or prostatic urethra. Preliminary results are encouraging.

FOREIGN BODIES INTRODUCED INTO THE BLADDER & URETHRA

Numerous objects have been found in the urethra and bladder of both men and women. Some of them find their way into the urethra in the course of inquisitive self-exploration. Others are introduced (in the male) as contraceptive devices in the hope that plugging the urethra will block the drainage of the ejaculate.

The presence of a foreign body causes cystitis. Hematuria is not uncommon. Embarrassment may cause the victim to delay medical consultation. A plain x-ray of the bladder area will disclose metal objects. Nonopaque objects sometimes become coated with calcium. Cystoscopy will visualize them all.

Cystoscopic or suprapubic removal of the foreign body is indicated. If not removed, the foreign body will lead to infection of the bladder. If the infecting organisms are urea-splitting, the alkaline urine (causing increased insolubility of calcium salts) contributes to rapid formation of stone upon the foreign object.

VESICAL MANIFESTATIONS OF ALLERGY

So many mucous membranes are affected by allergens that the possibility of allergic manifestations involving the bladder must be considered. Hypersensitivity is occasionally suggested in cases of recurrent symptoms of acute "cystitis" in the absence of urinary infection or other demonstrable abnormality. During the attack, general erythema of the vesical mucosa may be seen and some edema of the ureteral orifices noted.

A careful history may reveal that these attacks follow the ingestion of a certain food not ordinarily eaten (eg, fresh lobster). Sensitivity to spermicidal creams is occasionally observed. If vesical allergy is suspected, it may be aborted by the subcutaneous injection of 0.5–1 ml of 1:1000 epinephrine. Control may also be afforded by the use of one of the antihistamines. Skin testing has not generally proved helpful.

DIVERTICULUM

Most vesical diverticula are acquired and are secondary to either obstruction distal to the vesical neck or the upper motor neuron type of neurogenic bladder. Increased intravesical pressure causes vesical mucosa to insinuate itself between hypertrophied muscle bundles so that a mucosal extravesical sac develops. Often, this sac lies just superior to the ureter and causes vesicoureteral reflux (Hutch sacculi; see Chapter 11). The diverticulum is devoid of muscle and therefore has no expulsive power; residual urine is the rule, and infection is perpetuated. Reece & others (1974) suggest the use of a fiberoptic bronchoscope passed through a panendoscope sheath to inspect the wall of the diverticulum because carcinoma occasionally develops on its wall. At the time of open prostatectomy, resection of the diverticulum should be considered.

VESICAL FISTULAS

Vesical fistulas are common. The bladder may communicate with the skin, intestinal tract, or gynecologic organs. The primary disease is usually not urologic. The causes are as follows: (1) Primary intestinal disease—diverticulitis, 50–60%; cancer of the colon, 20–25%; and Crohn's disease, 10%. (2) Primary gynecologic disease—pressure necrosis during difficult labor; advanced cancer of the cervix. (3) Treatment for gynecologic disease following hysterectomy, low cesarian section, or radiotherapy for tumor. (4) Trauma.

Malignant tumors of the small or large bowel, uterus, or cervix may invade and perforate the bladder. Inflammations of adjacent organs may also erode through the vesical wall. Severe injuries involving the bladder may lead to perivesical abscess formation, and these abscesses may rupture through the skin of the perineum or abdomen. The bladder may be inadvertently injured during gynecologic or intestinal surgery; cystotomy for stone or prostatectomy may lead to a persistent cutaneous fistula.

Clinical Findings

A. Vesicointestinal Fistula: Symptoms arising from a vesicointestinal fistula include vesical irritability, the passage of feces and gas through the urethra, and usually a change in bowel habits (eg, obstipation, abdominal distention, diarrhea) caused by the primary intestinal disease. Signs of bowel obstruction may be elicited; abdominal tenderness may be found if the cause is inflammatory. The urine is always infected.

A barium enema, upper gastrointestinal series, or sigmoidoscopic examination may demonstrate the communication. Following a barium enema, centrifuged urine should be placed on an x-ray cassette and an exposure made. The presence of radiopaque barium will establish the diagnosis of vesicocolonic fistula.

Cystograms may reveal gas in the bladder or reflux of the opaque material into the bowel (Fig 26–3). Cystoscopic examination will show a severe localized inflammatory reaction from which bowel contents may exude. Catheterization of the fistulous tract may be feasible; the instillation of radiopaque fluid will often establish the diagnosis.

B. Vesicovaginal Fistula: This relatively common fistula is secondary to obstetric, surgical, or radiation injury or to invasive cancer of the cervix. The constant leakage of urine is most distressing to the patient. Pelvic examination usually reveals the fistulous opening, which can also be visualized with the cystoscope. It may be possible to pass a ureteral catheter through the fistula into the vagina. Vaginography often successfully shows ureterovaginal, vesicovaginal, and rectovaginal fistulas. A 30-ml Foley catheter is inserted into the vagina and the balloon is distended. A radiopaque solution is then instilled and appropriate x-rays are taken. Biopsy of the edges of the fistula may show carcinoma.

C. Vesicoadnexal Fistula: This rare fistula can be diagnosed by vaginal examination and by seeing the fistulous opening through the cystoscope.

Differential Diagnosis

It is necessary to differentiate ureterovaginal from vesicovaginal fistula. Instill methylene blue solution into the bladder and insert 3 cotton pledgets into the vagina; then have the patient ambulate. If the proximal cotton ball is wet but colorless, the lesion is ureterovaginal. If the deep cotton pledget contains blue fluid, the diagnosis is vesicovaginal fistula. If only the distal cotton is blue, the patient probably has urinary incontinence.

Treatment

A. Vesicointestinal Fistula: Treatment consists of proximal colostomy (if the lesion is in the rectosigmoid). When the inflammatory reaction has subsided, resection of the involved bowel may be done with closure of the opening in the bladder. Later the colostomy can be closed. Some authors recommend that the entire procedure be performed in one stage, thus avoiding the need for preliminary colostomy. Small bowel or appendiceal vesical fistulas require bowel or appendiceal resection and closure of the vesical defect.

B. Vesicovaginal Fistula: Those fistulas secondary to surgical or obstetric injury respond readily to surgical repair. Fistulas which develop following radiation therapy for cancer of the cervix are much more difficult to close because of the avascularity of the tissues. Surgical closure of fistulas which arise from direct invasion of the bladder by cervical carcinoma is impossible; diversion of the urinary stream above the level of the bladder (eg, ureterosigmoidostomy) is therefore necessary.

C. Vesicoadnexal Fistula: These fistulas are cured by removal of the involved gynecologic organs with closure of the opening in the bladder.

Prognosis

The surgical repair of fistulas caused by benign disease or operative trauma is highly successful. Postirradiation necrosis offers a more guarded prognosis. Fistulas secondary to invading cancers present difficult problems.

PERIVESICAL LIPOMATOSIS

About 50 cases of perivesical lipomatosis have been reported. The cause is not known. The disorder seems to affect principally black males in the 20–40 year age group. There are no pathognomonic symptoms. There may be some dysuria or mild urinary obstructive symptoms. Examination may demonstrate a distended or enlarged bladder. Excretory urograms and cystography may show dilatation of both upper tracts and an upward displacement and lateral compression of the bladder. In the perivesical area, x-ray reveals areas of radiolucency compatible with fatty tissue. A barium x-ray may show extrinsic pressure on the rectosigmoid. Angiography shows no evidence of neoplastic vessels.

On surgical exploration, lipomatous tissue surrounding the bladder at the lower ureteral zones is found. Wide excision of this tissue is indicated, but the results in terms of relief of ureteral obstruction have been equivocal for there are no cleavage planes.

RADIATION CYSTITIS

Many women receiving radiation treatment for carcinoma of the cervix develop some degree of vesical irritability. These symptoms may develop months after cessation of treatment. The urine may or may not be sterile. Vesical capacity is usually appreciably reduced. Cystoscopy will reveal a pale mucous membrane with multiple areas of telangiectatic blood vessels. Vesical ulceration may be noted, and vesicovaginal fistulas may develop. If symptoms are severe and prolonged, diversion of the urine from the bladder may be necessary.

NONINFECTIOUS HEMORRHAGIC CYSTITIS

Some patients, following radiotherapy for carcinoma of the cervix or bladder, are prone to intermittent, often serious vesical hemorrhage. The same is true of those given the chemotherapeutic agent cyclophosphamide.

In the case of the latter, the drug must be stopped. To control bleeding, cystoscopic fulguration

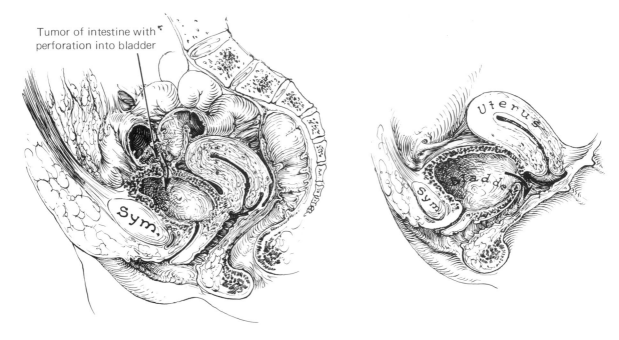

Tumor of intestine with
perforation into bladder

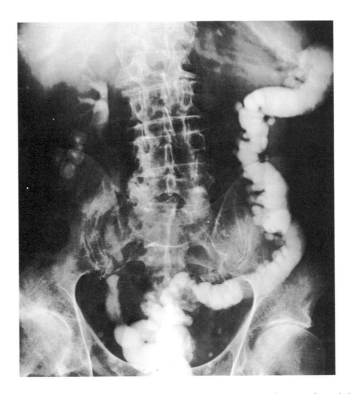

Figure 26–3. Vesical fistulas. ***Above left:*** Primary carcinoma of the sigmoid with perforation through bladder wall. ***Above right:*** Injury to base of bladder following delivery by forceps. ***Below:*** Cystogram showing radiopaque fluid entering sigmoid containing multiple diverticula; right urethral reflux, gallbladder calculi.

can be tried though it usually fails. The instillation of 3.9% formalin (prepared by diluting the standard 39% solution 10 times) is more efficacious. Clamp the catheter for 30 minutes and then lavage the bladder with 10% alcohol. A second or third instillation may be necessary on subsequent days. Holstein & others (1973) recommend the transurethral placement of a large balloon in the bladder. The balloon is filled to a pressure level equal to the systolic blood pressure and left in place for 6 hours. McGuire & others (1974) consider this the procedure of choice.

EMPYEMA OF THE BLADDER

If supravesical diversion of the urine is performed without cystectomy, severe infection of the bladder may develop because of lack of washout. In the male, cystostomy or cutaneous vesicostomy may be necessary. In the female, the formation of a vesicovaginal fistula will permit drainage. Occasionally, cystectomy may be necessary.

CONGENITAL ANOMALIES OF THE PROSTATE & SEMINAL VESICLES

Congenital anomalies of the prostate are rare. Cysts of the prostate and the seminal vesicles have been reported. Enlargements of the prostatic utricle are often found in association with penoscrotal or perineal hypospadias. They are usually small, lying in the midline posterior to the prostate and emptying through the verumontanum. These cysts represent embryologic remnants of the distal end of the Müllerian ducts (see Chapter 2). Rarely they become large enough to be easily palpable rectally or even abdominally. Through local pressure, they may cause symptoms of obstruction of the bladder neck.

BLOODY EJACULATION

The most common cause of bloody ejaculation is hypertrophy of the mucosa of the seminal vesicles. It usually responds to the administration of diethylstilbestrol, 5 mg/day for 1 week. Rare causes include prostatic ductal carcinoma and tumors of the seminal vesicles. It has also been postulated that there may be an anomalous venous communication with the seminal vesicles.

●   ●   ●

References

Exstrophy

Allen TD, Spence HM, Salyer KE: Reconstruction of the external genitalia in exstrophy of the bladder: Preliminary communication. J Urol 111:830, 1974.

Bennett AH: Exstrophy of bladder treated by ureterosigmoidostomies. Urology 2:165, 1973.

Boyce WH: A new concept concerning treatment of exstrophy of the bladder: 20 years later. J Urol 107:476, 1972.

Hanna MK, Williams DI: Genital function in males with vesical exstrophy and epispadias. Brit J Urol 44:169, 1972.

Kandzari SJ & others: Exstrophy of urinary bladder complicated by adenocarcinoma. Urology 3:496, 1974.

Megalli M, Lattimer JK: Review of the management of 140 cases of exstrophy of the bladder. J Urol 109:246, 1973.

Rudin L, Tannenbaum M, Lattimer JK: Histologic analysis of the exstrophied bladder after anatomical closure. J Urol 108:802, 1972.

Stanton SL: Gynecologic complications of epispadias and bladder exstrophy. Am J Obst Gynec 119:749, 1974.

Weed JC, McKee DM: Vulvoplasty in cases of exstrophy of the bladder. Obst Gynec 43:512, 1974.

Williams DI, Keeton JE: Further progress with reconstruction of the exstrophied bladder. Brit J Surg 60:203, 1973.

Persistent Urachus

Blichert-Toft M, Koch F, Nielsen OV: Anatomic variants of the urachus related to clinical appearance and surgical treatment of urachal lesions. Surg Gynec Obst 137:51, 1973.

Blichert-Toft M, Nielsen OV: Diseases of the urachus simulating intra-abdominal disorders. Am J Surg 122:123, 1971.

Constantian HM, Amaral EL: Urachal cyst: Case report. J Urol 106:429, 1971.

Nadjmi B & others: Carcinoma of the urachus: Report of two cases and review of the literature. J Urol 100:738, 1968.

Ney C, Friedenberg RM: Radiographic findings in anomalies of the urachus. J Urol 99:288, 1968.

Contracture of the Bladder Neck

Grieve J: Bladder neck stenosis in children: Is it important? Brit J Urol 39:13, 1967.

Kaplan GW, King LR: An evaluation of Y-V vesicourethroplasty in children. Surg Gynec Obst 130:1059, 1970.

Leadbetter GW Jr: Urinary tract infection and obstruction in children. Clin Pediat 5:377, 1966.

Moir JC: Vesicovaginal fistulae caused by wedge-resection of the bladder neck. Brit J Surg 53:102, 1966.

Nunn IN: Bladder neck obstruction in children. J Urol 93:693, 1965.

Ochsner MG, Burns E, Henry HH Jr: Incidence of retrograde ejaculation following bladder neck revision in the child. J Urol 104:596, 1970.

Shopfner CE: Roentgenologic evaluation of bladder neck obstruction. Am J Roentgenol 100:162, 1967.

Smith DR: Critique on the concept of vesical neck obstruction in children. JAMA 207:1686, 1969.

Interstitial Cystitis

Badenoch AW: Chronic interstitial cystitis. Brit J Urol 43:718, 1971.

Geist RW, Antolak SJ Jr: Interstitial cystitis in children. J Urol 104:922, 1970.

Gordon HL & others: Immunologic aspects of interstitial cystitis. J Urol 109:228, 1973.

Greenberg E & others: Transurethral resection of Hunner's ulcer. J Urol 111:764, 1974.

Jacobo EJ, Stamler FW, Culp DA: Interstitial cystitis followed by total cystectomy. Urology 3:481, 1974.

Jokinen EJ, Oravisto KJ, Alfthan OS: The effect of cystectomy on antitissue antibodies in interstitial cystitis. Clin Exper Immunol 15:457, 1973.

Oravisto KJ, Alfthan OS, Jokinen EJ: Interstitial cystitis: Clinical and immunological findings. Scandinav J Urol Nephrol 4:37, 1970.

Utz DC, Zinke H: The masquerade of bladder cancer as interstitial cystitis. J Urol 111:160, 1974.

Wallace HI, Lome LG, Presman D: Management of interstitial cystitis with ileocystoplasty. Urology 5:51, 1975.

Worth PHL, Turner-Warwick R: The treatment of interstitial cystitis by cystolysis with observations on cystoplasty. Brit J Urol 45:65, 1973.

Internal Vesical Herniation

Liebeskind AL, Elkin M, Goldman SH: Herniation of the bladder. Radiology 106:257, 1973.

Redman JF & others: The treatment of massive scrotal herniation of the bladder. J Urol 110:59, 1973.

Urinary Stress Incontinence

Ala-Ketola L: Roentgen diagnosis of female stress urinary incontinence: Roentgenological and clinical study. Acta obst gynec scandinav, Suppl 23, 1973.

Arnold EP & others: Urodynamics of female incontinence: Factors influencing the results of surgery. Am J Obst Gynec 117:805, 1973.

Bates CP & others: Synchronous cine/pressure/flow/cystourethrography with special reference to stress and urge incontinence. Brit J Urol 42:714, 1970.

Beck RP & others: Recurrent urinary stress incontinence

treated by the fascia lata sling procedure. Am J Obst Gynec 120:613, 1974.

Grout D, O'Conor VJ Jr: Long-term results of suprapubic vesicourethropexy. J Urol 107:610, 1972.

Marshall VF, Segaul RM: Experience with suprapubic vesicourethral suspension after previous failures to correct stress incontinence in women. J Urol 100:647, 1968.

Noll LE, Hutch JA: The SCIPP line: An aid in interpreting the voiding lateral cystourethrogram. Obst Gynec 33:680, 1969.

Steinhausen TB & others: Chain urethrocystography before and after urethrovesical suspension for stress incontinence. Obst Gynec 35:405, 1970.

Susset JG & others: Stress incontinence and urethral obstruction in women: Value of uroflowmetry and voiding urethrography. J Urol 111:504, 1974.

Tanagho EA: Simplified cystography in stress urinary incontinence. Brit J Urol 46:295, 1974.

Tanagho EA, Miller ER: Functional considerations of urethral sphincter dynamics. J Urol 109:273, 1973.

Urinary Incontinence

Berry JL, Dahlen CP: Evaluation of a procedure for correction of urinary incontinence in men. J Urol 105:105, 1971.

Flocks RH, Boldus R: The surgical treatment and prevention of urinary incontinence associated with disturbance of the internal urethral sphincteric mechanism. J Urol 109:279, 1973.

Furlow WL: Evaluation of the Kaufman anti-incontinence procedure: Experience with 14 patients. J Urol 108:770, 1972.

Gleason DM, Bottaccini MR, Reilly RJ: Active and passive incontinence: Differential diagnosis. Urology 4:693, 1974.

Hinman FJ, Schmaelzle JF, Cass AS: Autogenous perineal bone graft for post-prostatectomy incontinence. 2. Technique and results of prosthetic fixation of urogenital diaphragm in man. J Urol 104:888, 1970.

Kaufman JJ: Treatment of post-prostatectomy urinary incontinence using a Silicone gel prosthesis. Brit J Urol 45:646, 1973.

Kaufman JJ: Urethral compression operations for the treatment of post-prostatectomy incontinence. J Urol 110:93, 1973.

Politano VA & others: Periurethral Teflon injection for urinary incontinence. J Urol 111:180, 1974.

Raney AM: Reconstruction of bladder neck and prostatic urethra: Clinical experience with bladder-flap. Urology 3:324, 1974.

Salcedo H: Surgical correction of post-prostatectomy urinary incontinence using Marlex mesh: Preliminary report. J Urol 107:441, 1972.

Scott FB, Bradley WE, Timm GW: Treatment of urinary incontinence by implantable prosthetic urinary sphincter. J Urol 112:75, 1974.

Symmonds RE: Loss of the urethral floor with total urinary incontinence: A technique for urethral reconstruction. Am J Obst Gynec 103:665, 1969.

Tanagho EA, Smith DR: Clinical evaluation of a surgical technique for the correction of complete urinary incontinence. J Urol 107:402, 1972.

Foreign Bodies Introduced into the Bladder & Urethra

Najafi E, Maynard JF: Foreign body in lower urinary

tract. Urology 5:117, 1975.

Prasad S & others: Foreign bodies in urinary bladder. Urology 2:258, 1973.

Vesical Manifestations of Allergy

Pastinszky I: The allergic diseases of the male genitourinary tract with special reference to allergic urethritis and cystitis. Urol Internat 9:288, 1960.

Rubin L, Pincus MB: Eosinophilic cystitis: The relationship of allergy in the urinary tract to eosinophilic cystitis and the pathophysiology of eosinophilia. J Urol 112:457, 1974.

Diverticulum

Bauer SB, Retik AB: Bladder diverticula in infants and children. Urology 3:712, 1974.

Goldman HJ: A rapid safe technique for removal of a large vesical diverticulum. J Urol 106:379, 1971.

Ostroff EB, Alperstein JB, Young JD Jr: Neoplasm in vesical diverticula: Report of 4 patients, including a 21-year-old. J Urol 110:65, 1973.

Peterson LJ, Paulson DF, Glenn JF: The histopathology of vesical diverticula. J Urol 110:62, 1973.

Reece RW & others: Evaluation of bladder diverticulum using fiberoptic bronchoscope. Urology 3:790, 1974.

Vesical Fistulas

Baumrucker GO: Ball repair of vesicovaginal fistula. Urology 3:333, 1974.

Boronow RC: Management of radiation-induced vaginal fistulas. Am J Obst Gynec 110:1, 1971.

Farringer JL Jr & others: Vesicolic fistula. South MJ 67:1043, 1974.

Glenn JF, Stevens PS: Simplified vesicovaginal fistulectomy. J Urol 110:521, 1973.

Gross M, Peng B: Appendico-vesical fistula. J Urol 102:697, 1969.

Hutch JA, Noll LE: Prevention of vesicovaginal fistulas. Obst Gynec 35:924, 1970.

Lawson J: Vesical fistulae into the vaginal vault. Brit J Urol 44:623, 1972.

Moir JC: Vesico-vaginal fistulae as seen in Britain. J Obstet Gynaec Brit Common 80:598, 1973.

Morse FP III, Dretler SP: Diagnosis and treatment of colovesical fistula. J Urol 111:22, 1974.

O'Conor VJ Jr & others: Suprapubic closure of vesicovaginal fistula. J Urol 109:51, 1973.

Raghavaiah NV: Double-dye test to diagnose various types of vaginal fistulas. J Urol 112:811, 1974.

Slade N, Gaches C: Vesico-intestinal fistulae. Brit J Surg 59:593, 1972.

Vargas AD, Quattlebaum RB Jr, Scardino PL: Vesicoenteric fistula. Urology 3:200, 1974.

Wolfson JS: Vaginography for demonstration of ureterovaginal, vesicovaginal and rectovaginal fistulas, with case reports. Radiology 83:438, 1964.

Perivesical Lipomatosis

Barry JM, Bilbao MK, Hodges CV: Pelvic lipomatosis: A rare cause of suprapubic mass. J Urol 109:592, 1973.

Blau JS, Janson KL: Pelvic lipomatosis. Arch Surg 105:498, 1972.

Carpenter AA: Pelvic lipomatosis: Successful surgical treatment. J Urol 110:397, 1973.

Long WW Jr & others: Perivesical lipomatosis. J Urol 109:238, 1973.

Lucey DT, Smith MJV: Pelvic lipomatosis. J Urol 105:341, 1971.

Morettin LB, Wilson M: Pelvic lipomatosis. Am J Roentgenol 113:181, 1971.

Schechter LS: Venous obstruction in pelvic lipomatosis. J Urol 111:757, 1974.

Radiation Cystitis

Mallik MKB: Study of radiation necrosis of the urinary bladder following treatment of carcinoma of the cervix. Am J Obst Gynec 83:393, 1962.

Noninfectious Hemorrhagic Cystitis

Bennett AH: Cyclophosphamide and hemorrhagic cystitis. J Urol 111:603, 1974.

Holstein P & others: Intravesical hydrostatic pressure treatment: New method for control of bleeding from bladder mucosa. J Urol 109:234, 1973.

McGuire EJ & others: Hemorrhagic radiation cystitis: Treatment. Urology 3:204, 1974.

Scott MP Jr, Marshall S, Lyon RP: Bladder rupture following formalin therapy for hemorrhage secondary to cyclophosphamide therapy. Urology 3:364, 1974.

Spiro LH & others: Formalin treatment for massive bladder hemorrhage. Urology 2:669, 1973.

Yalla SV & others: Cystitis glandularis with perivesical lipomatosis: Frequent association of two unusual proliferative conditions. Urology 5:383, 1975.

Empyema of the Bladder

Dretler SP: The occurrence of empyema cystitis: Management of the bladder to be defunctionalized. J Urol 108:82, 1972.

Spence HM, Allen TD: Vaginal vesicostomy for empyema of the defunctionalized bladder. J Urol 106:862, 1971.

Congenital Anomalies of the Prostate & Seminal Vesicles

Donohue RE, Greenslade NF: Seminal vesical cyst and ipsilateral renal agenesis. Urology 2:66, 1973.

Feldman RA, Weiss RM: Urinary retention secondary to Müllerian duct cyst in a child. J Urol 108:647, 1972.

Rieser C, Griffin TL: Cysts of the prostate. J Urol 91:282, 1964.

Warren MM, Greene LF: Calculus in the prostatic utricle. J Urol 107:82, 1972.

Bloody Ejaculation

Ross JC: Haemospermia. Practitioner 203:59, 1969.

27 . . .
Disorders of the
Penis & Male Urethra

CONGENITAL ANOMALIES OF THE PENIS & MALE URETHRA

Congenital absence of the penis is exceedingly rare. A few cases of duplication have been reported, occasionally with 2 complete urethral channels. Megalopenis (hyperplasia) may be seen in boys suffering from interstitial cell tumor or hyperplasia or tumor of the adrenal cortex. Micropenis (hypoplasia) is often seen in male intersexes who have other feminizing traits (eg, hypospadias). Some are observed in otherwise normal-appearing boys, though many have congenital anomalies elsewhere. Some growth may be observed following local application of 0.2% testosterone propionate in water-miscible ointment base twice daily. Guthrie & others (1973) recommend the IM injection of 25 mg of testosterone cypionate every 3 weeks for 3 months. Hinman (1972) finds that surgical release of the corpora affords a significant gain in length.

STENOSIS OF THE EXTERNAL URINARY MEATUS

Stenosis of the external meatus is common and should be sought in all newborn males. It may be congenital or can be acquired after circumcision, or from trauma to the meatus by rough diapers. If it is severe, dilatation of the entire urinary tract, up to and including the renal pelvis (hydronephrosis), may develop, and death from uremia may occur. The usual symptom is bloody spotting and crusting of the meatus, which is caused by infection and ulceration just within the orifice. Meatotomy is indicated, following which the parents must dilate the urethra once every day for 2 weeks and at lengthening intervals for 2 more weeks. The small end of an oral thermometer is an excellent and readily available instrument for this purpose.

URETHRAL STRICTURE

Congenital urethral stricture occasionally occurs in male infants. The 2 most common sites are in the region of the corona (fossa navicularis) and in the membranous urethra. Severe strictures cause back pressure (from obstruction), which is followed by dilatation of the urethra, hypertrophy of the vesical musculature, and functional ureterovesical obstruction or reflux, both leading to hydronephrosis. Symptoms may be those of obstruction (eg, urinary stream of small caliber, hyperdistended bladder) or secondary infection (eg, fever, dysuria).

Excretory urograms may show the changes caused by obstruction (vesical trabeculation, hydronephrosis). The postvoiding film may reveal residual urine. A urethrogram (Figs 6–9 and 27–1) will delineate the degree and length of the stricture.

Every child with the symptoms mentioned above should be examined cystoscopically. The passage of the instrument will be arrested by the stricture. Urethral dilatations with sounds or filiforms and followers will keep the stricture open, but the prognosis depends upon the degree of damage suffered by the upper urinary tract. Surgical repair of the stricture is usually necessary. Congenital diaphragmatic strictures respond to overdilatation or internal urethrotomy (Fig 27–1).

POSTERIOR OR PROSTATIC URETHRAL VALVES

Posterior (prostatic) urethral valves or diaphragms are folds of mucous membrane on the floor of the prostatic urethra (Fig 27–2). They are one of the most common causes of congenital urethral obstruction in boys. Since they are obstructive, they cause dilatation of the prostatic urethra, hypertrophy of the detrusor (trabeculation), vesical diverticula, and hypertrophy of the trigonal muscles. The latter development tends to cause a functional obstruction of the intravesical ureter; hydroureteronephrosis is therefore the rule. In the advanced stage, vesicoureteral reflux may occur, but less than half of these boys exhibit reflux. Infec-

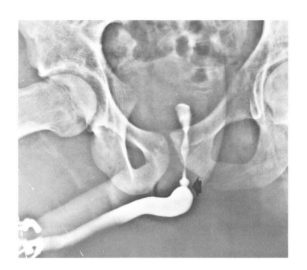

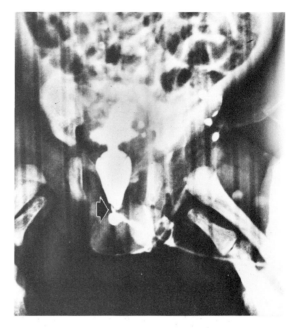

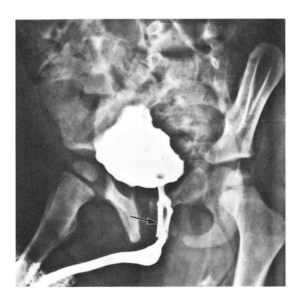

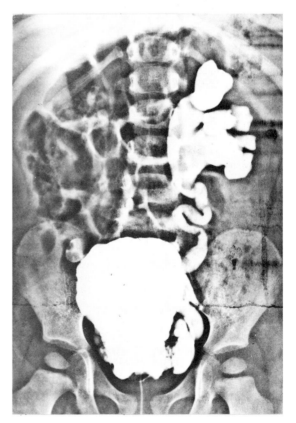

Figure 27–1. *Above left:* Retrograde urethrogram showing congenital diaphragmatic stricture. *Above right:* Posterior urethral valves revealed on voiding cystourethrography. Arrow points to area of severe stenosis at distal end of prostatic urethra. *Below left:* Posterior urethral valves. Patient would not void with cystography. Retrograde urethrogram showing valves (see arrow). *Below right:* Cystogram, same patient. Free vesicoureteral reflux and vesical trabeculation with diverticula.

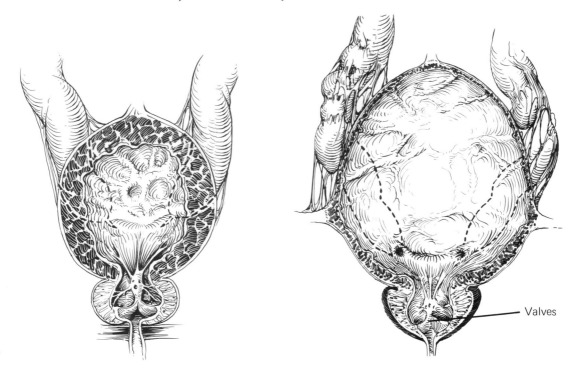

Figure 27–2. Posterior urethral valves. *Left:* Dilatation of the prostatic urethra, hypertrophy of vesical wall and trigone in stage of compensation; bilateral hydroureters secondary to trigonal hypertrophy. *Right:* Attenuation of bladder musculature in stage of decompensation; advanced ureteral dilatation and tortuosity, usually secondary to vesicoureteral reflux.

tion under these circumstances is almost inevitable, but it is apt to occur late because of the normally sterile proximal urethra. A number of cases of intraperitoneal rupture of the kidney with urinary ascites have been reported in such newborns. In a few, ascites is so severe as to cause respiratory difficulty. Paracentesis may be necessary to save life (Kellett, Turner & Levkoff, 1973). In milder cases, relief of the prostatic obstruction will cause the urinary extravasation to subside.

Clinical Findings

A. Symptoms: Difficulty in initiating urination and a very weak urinary stream are the principal symptoms. A distended bladder may be noted by the parents. Infection causes frequency, enuresis, and burning on urination. High fever suggests renal infection, but infection can be present without febrile response or vesical symptoms.

In the later stages, after renal insufficiency has developed, the child may suffer from anorexia, loss of weight, and anemia and fails to thrive.

B. Signs: A distended bladder may be seen, felt, or percussed. More commonly, however, a hard mass is felt deep in the pelvis. This represents the severely hypertrophied bladder. A poor urinary stream may be observed. Often, however, examination may reveal nothing more than evidence of chronic illness.

C. Laboratory Findings: Anemia due to chronic infection or uremia may be noted. The urine is often infected. Impairment of renal function may be discov-

ered by noting loss of concentrating power of the kidneys or elevation of the blood urea nitrogen and serum creatinine.

A diaper PSP test (see Chapter 5) should be performed on all infants suspected of having urinary tract obstruction. Excretion of less than 30% of the dye in 3 hours requires explanation. Little dye will be recovered when valves are present because of the combination of impaired renal function and transport of urine.

D. X-Ray Findings: Excretory urograms may demonstrate hydroureters and hydronephroses as well as irregularity in the outline of the bladder (trabeculation) or diverticula. The postvoiding film will reveal considerable retention of urine. Voiding cystourethrograms may reveal wide dilatation of the prostatic urethra and the negative shadows representing the valves (Fig 27–1). This procedure is the definitive diagnostic step. The cystograms may demonstrate reflux of the radiopaque material into the ureters and kidneys. The urograms which result usually preclude the need for ureteral catheterization and retrograde urograms. If the child cannot be induced to void, retrograde urethrography may show the valves (Fig 27–1).

E. Instrumental Examination: A catheter can usually be passed without difficulty, thereby ruling out stricture. These valves are only obstructive from within outward. Cystoscopy and panendoscopy show trabeculation of the bladder wall, occasionally diverticula, and hypertrophy of the trigone. The mucosal diaphragms may be visualized on the floor of the prostatic urethra, although they may be torn during instrumentation and therefore may be missed.

Treatment

Treatment consists of destruction of the valves. The simplest method is to pass very large sounds (up to 30F) through a perineal urethrotomy. Transurethral resection has its advocates. If the changes proximal to the valves are not severe, destruction of the valves is all that is necessary. Johnston & Kulatilake (1971) found that the majority of their cases fell into this category. Almost half of the boys will show vesicoureteral reflux, but in one-third reflux will cease after relief of the primary obstruction. Because of hypertrophy of the trigone, functional obstruction of the uretero-vesical junctions may develop. After treatment of the valves, the hypertrophy of the trigone subsides with lessening of the abnormal pull on the intramural ureters; secondary hydroureteronephrosis may subside.

In the most severe cases of hydronephrosis, removal of the primary obstruction may not be sufficient because of ureteral atony or obstruction, in which case loop cutaneous ureterostomies may have to be done to preserve renal function. This will lead to resolution of ureteral dilatation and hydronephrosis. When optimum repair is obtained, reconstruction of the urinary tract can be accomplished in most cases. In a few, this may not occur, and permanent drainage (eg, cutaneous ureterostomy) may be all that can be accomplished.

The period of urinary diversion should be as short as possible. Tanagho (1974) has observed that, after prolonged proximal diversion, permanent vesical contracture occurs in some patients.

Following destruction of the posterior urethral valves, about one-third will have normal urinary control, another third will suffer stress incontinence, and the remainder will have poor control (Whitaker, Keeton, & Williams, 1972). Johnston & Kulatilake (1971) have observed that control is apt to improve appreciably at puberty.

Complicating urosepsis should be treated by whatever drug is indicated by culture and sensitivity tests. In many cases infection cannot be eradicated even after definitive surgical repair; suppressive therapy should then be applied.

Prognosis

The prognosis depends upon the degree of destruction of the upper urinary tract. The diagnosis is too often not made until renal damage has become severe. Some of these children continue to lose function from incurable renal infection even after the obstruction has been relieved.

Early diagnosis requires that a competent nurse in the newborn nursery—or the pediatrician—make it a point to observe the size and force of the urinary stream in all male infants before they leave the hospital.

ANTERIOR URETHRAL VALVES

A few instances of anterior urethral valves in boys have been reported. They may suffer from enuresis or leakage of urine and an impaired urinary stream. A retrograde urethrogram will reveal the valve. The passage of a catheter to afford cystourethrography may rupture the valve. Panendoscopy will visualize the lesion, which can be destroyed by fulguration or fragmentation by the passage of sounds.

URETHRORECTAL & VESICORECTAL FISTULAS

Urethrorectal and, more rarely, vesicorectal fistulas are sometimes seen. They are almost always associated with imperforate anus occurring when the urorectal fold which divides the rectum from the urogenital sinus fails to develop completely. This permits a communication between the rectum and the urethra (in the region of the verumontanum) or bladder. (See Chapter 2.)

An infant with such a fistula passes fecal material and gas through the urethra. The anus may develop normally (open externally), in which case urine may be passed through the rectum.

Cystoscopy and panendoscopy usually visualize the fistulous opening. Barium given by mouth will reach the blind rectal pouch, and appropriate radiograms will measure the distance between the end of the rectum and the perineum. The imperforate anus must be opened immediately and the fistula closed, or, if the rectum lies quite high, temporary sigmoid colostomy must be performed. Definitive surgery, with repair of the urethral fistula, can be undertaken later.

HYPOSPADIAS

Hypospadias in the male is evidence of feminization. The hypospadiac penis presents ventral curvature (chordee) distal to the urethral meatus. The meatus opens on the ventral side of the penis proximal to the tip of the glans penis; it may present as far back as the perineum. When the orifice is in the scrotal or perineal area, the scrotum is bifid, thereby assuming the appearance of labia majora. The foreskin is deficient on the ventrum (Fig 27–3). In extreme degrees of hypospadias, the penis may be unusually small, simulating a hypertrophied clitoris.

The penoscrotal and perineal types (Fig 27–3) are usually associated with enlargement of the prostatic utricle, which represents a remnant of the fused ends of the Müllerian ducts. At times a rudimentary or even complete vaginal tract and uterus are present. For

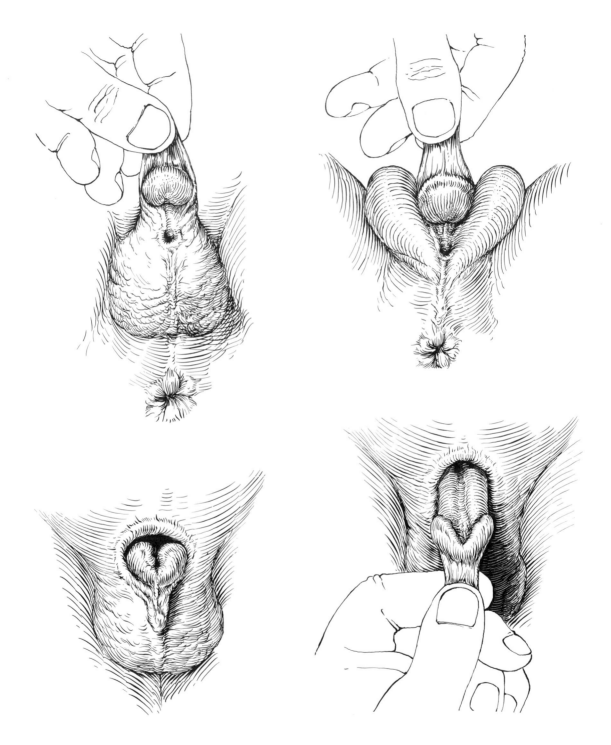

Figure 27–3. Hypospadias and epispadias. ***Above left:*** Hypospadias, penoscrotal type. Redundant dorsal foreskin which is deficient ventrally; ventral chordee. ***Above right:*** Hypospadias, midscrotal type. Chordee more marked. Penis often small. ***Below left:*** Epispadias. Redundant ventral foreskin which is absent dorsally; severe dorsal chordee. ***Below right:*** Traction on foreskin reveals dorsal defect.

this reason, chromatin (genetic) sex should be established by a buccal smear. The incidence of cryptorchism is high. Dwoskin & Kuhn (1974) have found that half of these patients have a hernia and, of these, 50% are bilateral. They demonstrated this by instilling radiopaque fluid into the peritoneal cavity. The patient was then placed in the prone position and 3–4 x-rays were taken during the next 45 minutes. There is no deficiency of the sphincters, so incontinence does not occur.

Adequate surgical correction demands, above all, straightening of the shaft so that normal intercourse is possible. This must be followed by formation of a urethra which extends to or near the tip of the glans so that semen can be deposited deep in the vagina. For psychologic reasons, it is best that this corrective surgery be completed before school age.

CHORDEE WITHOUT HYPOSPADIAS

Congenital ventral chordee without hypospadias is occasionally seen. It appears to be caused by a short urethra that acts as a bow-string, particularly with erection. Such a lesion interferes with intercourse. If the penis has adequate length, the dorsal surface can be shortened by excising elliptical portions of the tunica albuginea. Closing the defects will straighten the penis.

Devine & Horton (1973) find that in most cases fibrous tissue will be found in association with the urethra and corpus spongiosum. Resection of this tissue leads to a straight penis.

EPISPADIAS

Epispadias is considerably less common than hypospadias, but it is more disabling. It is quite rare in females. The urethra opens on the dorsum of the penis at some point proximal to the glans. The most common site is at the abdominopenile junction. Dorsal curvature (chordee) is also present (Fig 27–3). More serious, however, is the fact that this dorsal defect usually extends proximally, so that a defect of the urinary sphincters is present. This causes urinary incontinence. The pubic bones are separated as seen with exstrophy of the bladder. It should be noted that epispadias is but a relatively mild degree of exstrophy.

Treatment requires correction of urinary incontinence and of the inability to copulate. Repair of the urinary sphincters has not been too successful, but Tanagho & Smith (1972) have obtained complete continence by interposing a tubed flap of anterior bladder wall between the bladder and prostatic urethra. Plastic repair of the penis requires reduction of the chordee followed by urethroplasty, which advances the urinary orifice to the distal end of the shaft. If

urinary continence cannot be achieved, some type of urinary diversion may have to be provided (eg, ureteroileal conduit).

ACQUIRED DISEASES OF THE PENIS & MALE URETHRA

PRIAPISM

Priapism is a rather rare affliction. It consists of a prolonged erection, unassociated with sexual stimulation, which is usually painful. The blood in the cavernous spaces becomes sludgelike rather than clotted. It may last for many days. About 25% of the cases are associated with leukemia, metastatic carcinoma, or sickle cell disease, but as a rule the mechanism is not clear. Priapism is occasionally seen following injuries to the spinal cord.

Fitzpatrick (1973) has shown obstruction of the deep dorsal vein on cavernosograms as the basic cause for the erection.

If spontaneous subsidence of priapism does not occur within a few hours, the following regimen should be instituted: Ice water enemas should first be ordered; temporary (even permanent) subsidence of the erection may occur. Evacuation of the sludged blood of the corpora by needle and syringe should next be tried. The corpora should then be thoroughly irrigated with an anticoagulant followed by bandage compression. Unless the erection subsides promptly, either spontaneously or in response to treatment, the septa of the corpora cavernosa undergo fibrosis. This results in impotence—inability to gain an erection.

Evans & Young (1973) demonstrated occlusion of the internal pudendal arteries at the level of the urogenital diaphragm by arteriography. This appears to be an obvious cause of impotence.

In patients with sickle cell anemia, Seeler (1973) suggests the intensive transfusion of packed red cells to double the hematocrit. Cessation of pain and subsidence of the erection occurs in 24 hours. Shreibman, Gee, & Grabstald (1974) lowered the peripheral blood count in patients with chronic granulocytic leukemia by administering either cytarabine or hydroxyurea with good results.

If conservative treatment fails, prompt operation is mandatory. Either saphenous vein-corpus cavernosum or bilateral corpora cavernosa-spongiosum shunt should be done. Once the erection subsides, normal blood flow may return, in which case the shunts close spontaneously.

PLASTIC INDURATION OF THE PENIS
(Peyronie's Disease)

Fibrosis of the covering sheaths of the corpora cavernosa occurs without known cause, usually in men over 45 years of age. This fibrotic area will not permit lengthening of the involved surface (dorsum) with erection so that the penis bends toward the involved area (chordee). In the early stages, erection is accompanied by pain. The degree of curvature may finally preclude coitus. Apparently the process begins as vasculitis in the connective tissue beneath the tunica albuginea of the penis and then extends to adjacent structures. This leads to fibrosis and at times calcification or even ossification.

Palpation of the shaft reveals a well-demarcated, raised plaque of fibrosis which is usually in the midline of the dorsum near the base of the organ, although it may be placed more laterally or distally. X-ray may reveal areas of calcification within the indurated area.

Treatment is unsatisfactory. Low-dosage x-ray therapy has some value. Potassium para-aminobenzoate (Potaba), 12 g/day in divided doses, may decrease the chordee by softening the fibrous plaque. It should be continued for 6 months to 2 years. Recently there has been some enthusiasm for operation. Poutasse (1972) exposes the center of the plaque and chips away the scar tissue for a distance of 2–3 cm down to cavernous tissue. This maneuver allows separation of the remaining plaque. Devine & Horton (1974) excise the plaque and replace it with a dermal graft taken from the abdomen. Byström (1973) inserts a dermo-fat graft, the dermis being excised. Good results are claimed. Such procedures should be considered if intercourse is difficult or impossible.

PHIMOSIS

Phimosis is a disease in which it is impossible to retract the foreskin over the glans. It is usually secondary to infection beneath a redundant foreskin. Poor hygiene frequently contributes to the infection. Such a reaction causes tissue injury, and healing is by fibrosis. The preputial opening thereby becomes contracted, so that the foreskin cannot be retracted. This further facilitates the infectious process, usually by mixed organisms, including anaerobes, vibrios, and spirochetes. Such chronic irritation of many years' standing may be the cause of squamous epithelioma. Stones may form in the preputial sac.

The patient may merely complain of inability to retract the foreskin, but more commonly he is disturbed by symptoms and signs of infection (eg, redness and swelling of the foreskin, purulent discharge, and local pain).

Treatment consists of measures to control the infection (hot soaks, antibiotics). A dorsal slit of the foreskin is necessary if infection is marked. Circumcision should be performed when the inflammatory reaction has subsided.

PARAPHIMOSIS

Paraphimosis is a condition in which the foreskin, once retracted behind the glans, cannot be replaced in its normal position. This is due to chronic inflammation under the redundant foreskin, which leads to contracture of the preputial skin ring.

This tight ring of skin, caught behind the glans, causes venous occlusion which leads to edema of the glans and further disproportion between the size of the glans and the caliber of the preputial opening. If neglected, arterial occlusion may supervene and gangrene of the glans may develop.

Paraphimosis can usually be treated by squeezing the glans firmly for at least 5 minutes, thus reducing its size. The glans is then pushed proximally as the prepuce is moved distally. If manual reduction fails, incision of the constricting tissue is indicated. Once the inflammation and edema have subsided, circumcision should be performed.

CIRCUMCISION

In most countries, routine circumcision is practiced at birth. Unfortunately, in unskilled hands, the use of various mechanical devices has at times caused removal of too much penile skin or even resection of a portion or all of the glans. It seems that the most common cause of urethral meatal stenosis is excoriation of the denuded meatus following circumcision.

Circumcision does prevent phimosis, paraphimosis, and balanoposthitis in adolescence and adult life. The diabetic suffers a high incidence of the latter. Circumcision is indicated in this instance. It is rare for the male, circumcised at birth, to develop penile cancer, which carries a mortality rate of 33%. For these reasons, routine neonatal circumcision seems indicated.

URETHRAL STRICTURE

Acquired urethral stricture today is a rare complication of severe gonococcal urethritis but a common sequel of urethral injury. In either case the urethra heals by the proliferation of fibroblasts, producing contraction.

Pathogenesis & Pathology

A severe degree of stenosis causes changes typical of obstruction. These include (1) dilatation of the urethra proximal to the stricture, (2) compensatory changes in the bladder musculature, and (3) hydroureteronephrosis secondary to hypertrophy of the ureterotrigonal complex or vesicoureteral reflux. Because of stasis, infection occurs which may cause periurethral abscess, prostatitis, cystitis, and pyelonephritis. If the organisms split urea, vesical or renal calculi may form. Urethral stricture, then, may cause severe damage to the urinary tract.

Clinical Findings

A. Symptoms: The most common symptom is gradual diminution of the force and caliber of the urinary stream. Sudden urinary retention may occur if an infection at the site of stricture is exacerbated. A history of urethral injury or severe untreated gonorrhea can usually be obtained. Symptoms of cystitis may be noted. There may be fever secondary to prostatitis or pyelonephritis.

B. Signs: Periurethral induration may be found at the site of the stricture. A tender mass may be present if periurethral abscess has developed. Perineal urinary fistulas may be noted. A visible or palpable bladder may be found if urinary retention has supervened. Prostatic massage and culture of the secretions may reveal evidence of prostatitis.

C. Laboratory Findings: If infection is present, the white blood count may be elevated and pus and bacteria will be found in the urine. PSP excretion may be diminished if there is renal damage or residual urine.

D. X-Ray Findings: A urethrogram and voiding cystourethrogram will reveal the site and degree of the stricture. Fistulas may be demonstrated (Fig 27–4). After urethral dilatation, a cystogram may show a thickened, trabeculated bladder and, possibly, ureteral reflux. Excretory urograms may reveal urinary calculi or changes compatible with chronic pyelonephritis.

E. Instrumental Examination: A catheter or sound of average size (22F) will be arrested at the site of stricture. Panendoscopy may visualize it. Cystoscopy (done after urethral dilatation) will show hypertrophy of the vesical muscle and, often, inflammation.

Differential Diagnosis

Prostatic or bladder neck obstruction may cause similar symptoms, but in this instance a catheter passes through the urethra with ease. An enlarged (or cancerous) gland is usually found on rectal examination.

Carcinoma of the urethra can mimic urethral stricture, but panendoscopy and biopsy of the visualized tumor will establish the proper diagnosis.

Complications

Prostatis, cystisis, and pyelonephritis are common complications. Periurethral abscess may develop at the stricture site; it may resolve or rupture through the skin, causing a urethrocutaneous fistula. Urinary stones may form secondary to stasis and infection.

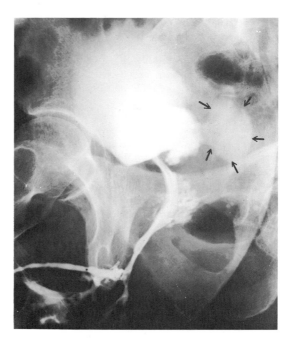

Figure 27–4. Urethral stricture with multiple perineal fistulas. Voiding cystourethrogram showing stricture of perineal urethra, multiple fistulas, dilated prostatic ducts, and vesical diverticulum outlined by arrows.

Treatment

A. Specific Measures:

1. Dilatation—After local urethral or general anesthesia has been obtained and the urethra distended with water-soluble lubricant, a 22F sound should be gently passed (Fig 9–4). If this is arrested, a 20F sound should be tried. Smaller sounds should not be used, for their tips may perforate the friable urethra at the site of the stricture.

Next, passage of a filiform should be attempted (Figs 9–5 and 9–6). If one passes to the bladder, an appropriate follower can be screwed onto its end. If the smallest follower will not penetrate the stricture, the filiform should be taped in place; the patient will be able to void around it. This maneuver will allow subsidence of the inflammatory reaction, so that after a day or so dilation will be possible. If a filiform cannot be passed and the patient is in urinary retention, suprapubic cystostomy must be done.

Once an instrument has been passed through the stricture, 2 methods for urethral dilatation are available:

a. The stricture should be dilated to 18–20F. A 14–16F catheter should then be passed into the bladder and left indwelling. After 48 hours, the next size can usually be easily passed; this procedure can be repeated every 2 days until a 24–26F catheter has been placed. This method is relatively painless.

b. Sounds of increasing sizes should be passed to the point of urethral tolerance. This procedure can then be repeated, using larger sounds at weekly intervals until a 24–26F sound can be passed. This method achieves results more quickly but is more painful.

Dilatation of a urethral stricture is a palliative treatment; it is not curative. Sounds should be passed at increasing intervals (eg, 2 weeks, 1 month, 3 months, 6 months). Periodic sounding must be done indefinitely.

2. Surgery—If the stricture contracts rapidly so that the use of sounds is not feasible, internal urethrotomy should be done; an indwelling 24F Silastic catheter should be left in place for 30 days. In most of these cases, periodic dilatations will still be required. Should this fail, urethroplasty should be performed. Complications are uncommon.

B. General Measures: Hot sitz baths may help combat local infection and decrease pain after instrumentation.

C. Treatment of Complications: Infection of the kidneys or bladder requires antimicrobial therapy, particularly at the time of urethral dilatation (which may exacerbate preexisting infection). Periurethral abscess may resolve with medical treatment. If it does not, surgical drainage will be necessary. Urethrocutaneous fistulas may close spontaneously once the stricture is dilated. If they do not, surgical correction must be done.

Prognosis

Most urethral strictures can be kept open by periodic dilatations; a few will require surgical treatment. Their deleterious effects on renal function must always be kept in mind.

URETHRAL WARTS
(Condylomata Acuminata)

In some men who have cutaneous condylomata (see Chapter 30), bloody spotting from the urethra may be noted; the patient may see a wart just inside the urethral meatus. Panendoscopy will reveal these lesions. A urethrogram may show their presence also. If they are few in number, transurethral fulguration should be done. When many lesions are present, extensive electrocoagulation could lead to stricture formation.

Rosenberg & Al-Askari (1973) recommend intraurethral instillation of thiotepa once a week for 7–10 weeks. Sixty milligrams of the drug are disolved in 5 ml of water and mixed with 10 ml of a mixture of water and water-soluble lubricant. The drug should be retained for 30 minutes by clamping the glans. Before each instillation, a white blood cell and platelet count must be done to be sure absorption has not caused an adverse hematopoietic effect.

Bissada, Redman, & Sulieman (1974) had similar success with the use of fluorouracil. They instilled 5 ml of a 5% solution for 20 minutes twice a week for 5 weeks. The drug was retained for 20 minutes. If a few lesions still persist, they recommend its use once a week for another 6–8 weeks.

Gigax & Robison (1971) have recommended the instillation of 0.5% colchicine. It was successful in eradicating the warts in 4 cases. The author, however, knows of 2 cases wherein urethral absorption of the drug was so severe that life was endangered.

FISTULA

Fistulas between the urethra and penile skin usually follow an exacerbation of infection just proximal to a stricture. A fistula may develop secondary to a carcinoma of the urethra or to a foreign body which has been inserted into the channel (eg, bobby pin). Periurethritis and abscess formation may then develop. Spontaneous drainage may occur. Urethroscopy (panendoscopy) and urethrography will reveal the site and cause of the fistulous opening. Biopsy may be indicated. When all evidence of inflammation has disappeared, surgical closure can be performed.

THROMBOPHLEBITIS OF
THE SUPERFICIAL PENILE VEINS

Not infrequently, thrombophlebitis of the circumferential veins just proximal to the corona develops. The patient notes a firm ridge of tender tissue and redness of the overlying skin. Examination reveals thrombosis of the vein; this may also involve the longitudinal superficial dorsal vein. No treatment is required. Recanalization takes place in a few months.

•   •   •

References

General

Wisdom A: *Color Atlas of Venereology.* Year Book, 1973.

CONGENITAL ANOMALIES

Penis and Male Urethra

Cullen TH: Duplication of the male urethra. Brit J Surg 60:751, 1973.

Farah R, Reno G: Congenital absence of the penis. J Urol 107:154, 1972.

Guthrie RD, Smith DW, Graham CB: Testosterone treatment for micropenis during early childhood. J Pediat 83:247, 1973.

Harada N, Sawada A: Surgical treatment for microphallus. J Urol 108:594, 1972.

Hinman F Jr: Microphallus: Characteristics and choice of treatment from a study of 20 cases. J Urol 107:499, 1972.

Johnson CF, Carlton CE Jr, Powell NB: Duplication of penis. Urology 4:722, 1974.

Kessler WO, McLaughlin AP: Agenesis of the penis: Embryology and management. Urology 1:226, 1973.

Sotiropoulos A, Uson A, Lattimer JK: Duplication of external genitalia in men. Urology 4:688, 1974.

Susan LP, Roth RB, Kaminsky ——: Complete duplication of urethra. Urology 5:390, 1975.

Stenosis of the External Urinary Meatus

Allen JS, Summers JL: Meatal stenosis in children. J Urol 112:526, 1974.

Allen JS, Summers JL, Wilkerson JE: Meatal calibration of newborn boys. J Urol 107:498, 1972.

Mowad JJ, Michaels MM: Meatal stenosis associated with vesicoureteral reflux in boys: Management of 25 cases. J Urol 111:100, 1974.

Urethral Stricture

Cobb BG, Wolf JA Jr, Ansell JS: Congenital stricture of the proximal urethral bulb. J Urol 99:629, 1968.

Leadbetter GW Jr: The etiology, symptoms, and treatment of urethral strictures in male children. Pediatrics 31:80, 1963.

Posterior or Prostatic Urethral Valves

Agusta VE, Howards SS: Posterior urethral valves. J Urol 112:280, 1974.

Arnold SJ, Ginsburg A: Radiographic and photoendoscopic studies in posterior urethral valves in enuretic boys. Urology 4:145, 1974.

Bueschen AJ, Garrett RA, Newman DM: Posterior urethral valves: Management. J Urol 110:682, 1973.

Cass AS, Stephens FD: Posterior urethral valves: Diagnosis and treatment. J Urol 112:519, 1974.

Johnston JH, Kulatilake AE: The sequelae of posterior urethral valves. Brit J Urol 43:743, 1971.

Kellett JW, Turner WR Jr, Levkoff AH: Paracentesis in the management of neonatal ascites. Urology 2:672, 1973.

Kendall AR, Karafin L: Obstructive posterior urethral valves: The light at the end of the tunnel. J Urol 113:266, 1975.

Milliken LD Jr, Hodgson NB: Renal dysplasia and urethral valves. J Urol 108:960, 1972.

Ramsey EW, Jarzylo SV, Bruce AW: Spontaneous extravasation of urine from the renal pelvis and ureter. J Urol 110:507, 1973.

Tanagho EA: Congenitally obstructed bladder: Fate after prolonged defunctionalization. J Urol 111:102, 1974.

Weller MH, Miller K: Unusual aspects of urine ascites. Radiology 109:665, 1973.

Whitaker RH: The ureter in posterior urethral valves. Brit J Urol 45:395, 1973.

Whitaker RH, Keeton JE, Williams DI: Posterior urethral valves: A study of urinary control after operation. J Urol 108:167, 1972.

Williams DI & others: Urethral valves. Brit J Urol 45:200, 1973.

Anterior Urethral Valves

Firlit CF, King LR: Anterior urethral valves in children. J Urol 108:972, 1972.

Malhoski WE, Frank IN: Anterior urethral valves. Urology 2:382, 1973.

Urethrorectal & Vesicorectal Fistulas

Wesolowski S, Bulinski W: Vesico-intestinal fistulae and recto-urethral fistulae. Brit J Urol 45:34, 1973.

Hypospadias

Aarskog D: Clinical and cytogenetic studies in hypospadias. Acta paediat scandinav, Suppl 203, 1970.

Allen TD, Spence HM: The surgical treatment of coronal hypospadias and related problems. J Urol 100:504, 1968.

Dwoskin JY, Kuhn JP: Herniograms and hypospadias. Urology 3:458, 1974.

Engel RME, Scott WW: Hypospadias: Results with the Hodgson urethroplasty. J Urol 109:115, 1973.

Fuqua F: Renaissance of urethroplasty: The Belt technique of hypospadias repair. J Urol 106:782, 1971.

Genetics of hypospadias. Brit MJ 4:189, 1972.

Hoffman WW, Hall WV: A modification of Spence's hood for one-stage surgical correction of distal shaft penile hypospadias. J Urol 109:1017, 1973.

Horton CE, Devine CJ Jr: One-stage repair for hypospadias cripples. Plast Reconstr Surg 45:425, 1970.

Lattimer JK, Vakili B, Smith AM: The dorsal tilt: An embellishment to any operation for hypospadias. J Urol 109:1035, 1973.

Nosti JC, Davis JW: Treatment of hypospadias by the Byars technique. Plast Reconstr Surg 52:128, 1973.

Sadlowski RW, Belman AB, King LR: Further experience with one-stage hypospadias repair. J Urol 112:677, 1974.

Smith DR: Repair of hypospadias in the preschool child: A report of 150 cases. J Urol 97:723, 1967.

Sykes PH, Ho LCY: Hypospadias: A report on 193 treated cases. Plast Reconstr Surg 50:452, 1972.

Wettlaufer JN: Cutaneous chordee: Fact or fancy? Urology 4:293, 1974.

Chordee Without Hypospadias

Devine CJ Jr, Horton CE: Chordee without hypospadias. J Urol 110:264, 1973.

Devine CJ Jr, Horton CE: Use of dermal graft to correct chordee. J Urol 113:56, 1975.

Pond HS, Brannan W: Correction of congenital curvature of the penis: Experiences with the Nesbit operation at Ochsner Clinic. J Urol 112:491, 1974.

Saalfeld J & others: Congenital curvature of the penis: Successful results with variations in corporoplasty. J Urol 109:64, 1973.

Epispadias

Bredin HC, Muecke EC: Surgical correction of male epispadias with total incontinence. J Urol 109:904, 1973.

Culp OS: Treatment of epispadias with and without urinary incontinence: Experience with 46 patients. J Urol 109:120, 1973.

Dey DL, Cohen D: The surgery of female epispadias. Surgery 69:542, 1971.

Klauber GT, Williams DI: Epispadias with incontinence. J Urol 111:110, 1974.

Tanagho EA, Smith DR: Clinical evaluation of a surgical technique for the correction of complete urinary incontinence. J Urol 107:402, 1972.

ACQUIRED DISEASES

Priapism

Cosgrove MD, LaRocque MA: Shunt surgery for priapism: Review of results. Urology 4:1, 1974.

Dahl DS, Middleton RG: Comparison between caverno-saphenous and cavernospongiosum shunting in the treatment of idiopathic priapism: A report of 5 operations. J Urol 112:614, 1974.

Darwish ME, Atassi B, Clark SS: Priapism: Evaluation of treatment regimens. J Urol 112:92, 1974.

Evans IL, Young AF: Internal pudendal arteriography after priapism. Brit J Surg 60:329, 1973.

Fitzpatrick TJ: Spongiograms and cavernosograms: A study of their value in priapism. J Urol 109:843, 1973.

Karayalcin G, Imran M, Rosner F: Priapism in sickle cell disease: Report of five cases. Am J Med Sc 264:289, 1972.

LaRocque MA, Cosgrove MD: Priapism: A review of 46 cases. J Urol 112:770, 1974.

Resnick MI & others: Priapism in boys: Management with cavernosaphenous shunt. Urology 5:492, 1975.

Rubin SO: Priapism as a probable sequel to medication. Scandinav J Urol Nephrol 2:81, 1968.

Sacher EC & others: Cavernospongiosum shunt in the treatment of priapism. J Urol 108:97, 1972.

Schreibman SM, Gee TS, Grabstald H: Management of priapism in patients with chronic granulocytic leukemia. J Urol 111:786, 1974.

Seeler RA: Intensive transfusion therapy for priapism in boys with sickle cell anemia. J Urol 110:360, 1973.

Stein JJ, Martin DC: Priapism. Urology 3:8, 1974.

Plastic Induration of the Penis

Byström J & others: Induratio penis plastica (Peyronie's disease). Scandinav J Plast Reconstr Surg 7:137, 1973.

Devine CJ Jr, Horton CE: Surgical treatment of Peyronie's disease with a dermal graft. J Urol 111:44, 1974.

Helvie WW, Ochsner SF: Radiation therapy in Peyronie's disease. South MJ 65:1192, 1972.

Poutasse EF: Peyronie's disease. J Urol 107:419, 1972.

Smith BH: Subclinical Peyronie's disease. Am J Clin Path 52:385, 1969.

Zarafonetis CJD: Antifibrotic therapy with Potaba. Am J Med Sc 248:550, 1964.

Paraphimosis

Øster J: Further fate of the foreskin: Incidence of preputial adhesions, phimosis, and smegma among Danish boys. Arch Dis Childhood 43:200, 1968.

Skoglund RW Jr, Chapman WH: Reduction of paraphimosis. J Urol 104:137, 1970.

Circumcision

Dagher R, Selzer ML, Lapides J: Carcinoma of the penis and the anti-circumcision parade. J Urol 110:79, 1973.

Murdock MI, Selikowitz SM: Diabetes-related need for circumcision. Urology 4:60, 1974.

Trier WC, Drach GW: Concealed penis: Another complication of circumcision. Am J Dis Child 125:276, 1973.

Urethral Stricture

Abrahams JI & others: Treatment of urethral stricture by free full-thickness skin graft (Devine) urethroplasty. Urology 1:93, 1973.

Anastasi GW, Olsson CA: Pedicle patch urethroplasty for cure of urethral stricture. Plast Reconstr Surg 51:1, 1973.

Ashken MH: A personal experience with 37 Turner-Warwick scrotal inlay urethroplasties. Brit J Urol 46:313, 1974.

Bissada NK & others: Urethrography in the investigation of proximal urethral strictures. J Urol 110:299, 1973.

Brannan W, Ochsner MG, Fuselier HA Jr: Anterior urethral strictures: Experience with free graft urethroplasty. J Urol 109:265, 1973.

Carlton FE, Scardino PL, Quattlebaum RB: Treatment of ureteral strictures with internal urethrotomy and 6 weeks of silastic catheter drainage. J Urol 111:191, 1974.

deLacey GJ & others: Urethral stricture and urethral rupture. Am J Roentgenol 119:822, 1973.

Devereux MH, Burfield GD: Prolonged follow-up of urethral strictures treated by intermittent dilatation. Brit J Urol 42:321, 1970.

Devereux MH, Williams DI: The treatment of urethral stricture in boys. J Urol 108:489, 1972.

Helmstein K: Internal urethrotomy: Modifications in the operative technique. Acta chir scandinav, Suppl 340, 1965.

Jessen C: Resection of urethral stricture and end-to-end anastomosis. Scandinav J Urol Nephrol 4:87, 1970.

Madduri S, Kamat MH, Seebode J: Urethral stricture treated with soft catheter dilatation: Reappraisal of an old technique. Urology 4:504, 1974.

McGuire EJ, Weiss RM: Scrotal flap urethroplasty for strictures of the deep urethra in infants and children. J Urol 110:599, 1973.

McKinney DE, Chenault OW Jr: Experiences with Devine inlay graft urethroplasty. Urology 5:487, 1975.

Pierce JM Jr: Urethroplasty for anterior urethral stricture. J Urol 109:422, 1973.

Torres SA: Urethral stricture: Treatment with internal urethrotomy and silastic catheter intubation. Urology 3:456, 1974.

Whitehead ED, Morales PA: Complications of urethroplasty for stricture. J Urol 107:412, 1972.

Wise HA II & others: Treatment of urethral strictures. J Urol 107:269, 1972.

Zinman L, Libertino JA: Surgical management of urethral strictures. S Clin North America 53:465, 1973.

Urethral Warts

Bissada NK, Cole AT, Fried FA: Extensive condylomas acuminata of the entire male urethra and the bladder. J Urol 112:201, 1974.

Bissada NK, Redman JF, Sulieman JS: Condyloma acuminatum of the male urethra: Successful management with 5-fluorouracil. Urology 3:499, 1974.

Dretler SP, Klein LA: The eradication of intraurethral condyloma acuminata with 5 percent 5-fluorouracil cream. J Urol 113:195, 1975.

Gigax JH, Robison JR: The successful treatment of intraurethral condyloma acuminata with colchicine. J Urol 105:809, 1971.

Rosenberg JW, Al-Askari S: Management of intraurethral condyloma acuminata. J Urol 110:686, 1973.

Fistula

Blandy JP, Singh M: Fistulae involving the adult male urethra. Brit J Urol 44:632, 1972.

Thrombophlebitis of the Superficial Penile Veins

Harrow BR, Sloane JA: Thrombophlebitis of superficial penile and scrotal veins. J Urol 89:841, 1963.

28 . . .

Disorders of the
Female Urethra

CONGENITAL ANOMALIES
OF THE FEMALE URETHRA

DISTAL URETHRAL STENOSIS
IN INFANCY & CHILDHOOD
(Spasm of the External Urinary Sphincter)

There has been considerable confusion about the site of lower tract obstruction in small girls who suffer from enuresis, a slow and interrupted urinary stream, recurrent cystitis, and pyelonephritis and who, on thorough examination, often exhibit vesicoureteral reflux. Treatment has largely been directed to the bladder neck on rather empirical grounds. Most of these children, however, have congenital distal urethral stenosis with secondary spasm of the striated external sphincter rather than bladder neck contracture.

At birth, calibration of the urethra with bougies á boule reveals no evidence of a distal ring of urethral stenosis (Fisher & others, 1969). Within a few months, however, such a ring develops as a normal anatomic structure. After puberty, the ring disappears. The inference is that the absence of estrogens leads to the development of this lesion. Lyon & Tanagho (1965) found that the ring calibrates at 14F at age 2 and at 16F between the ages of 4 and 10. They recognized, however, that from the hydrodynamic standpoint such a stenotic area should not be obstructive. Nonetheless, almost all observers recognize that destruction of the ring is successful in relieving symptoms and persistent infection or vesical dysfunction in 80% of these children. Lyon & Tanagho (1965) postulated that the basic cause of these urinary difficulties could be reflex spasm of the periurethral striated sphincter and noted that voiding cystourethrograms suggest this possibility (Fig 28–1).

Tanagho & others (1971), measuring pressures in the bladder and in the proximal and mid urethra simultaneously in symptomatic girls, found resting pressures in the midurethral segment as high as 200 cm of water. Normal is 100 cm of water. Attempts at voiding caused intravesical pressures as high as 225 cm of water (normal, 30–40) to develop. Under curare, the urethral closing pressures dropped to normal (40–50 cm of water), proving that these obstructing pressures were caused by spasm of the striated sphincter muscle. If the distal urethral ring was treated and symptoms abated, repeat pressure studies showed normal midurethral and intravesical voiding pressures. If, on the other hand, symptoms persisted, pressures were found to remain at their extremely high levels.

It seems clear, therefore, that the major cause of urinary problems in little girls is spasm of the external sphincter and not vesical neck stenosis (Smith, 1969).

In addition to recurrent urinary tract infection, these patients have hesitancy in initiating micturition and a slow, hesitant, or interrupted urinary stream. Enuresis and involuntary loss of urine during the day are common complaints. Abdominal straining may be required. Small amounts of residual urine are found, thus impairing the vesical defense mechanism (Hinman, 1966). A voiding cystourethrogram may reveal an open bladder neck and ballooning of the mid urethra secondary to the spastic external sphincter (Fig 28–1).

While the voiding cystourethrogram may reveal evidence of the distal ring, the typical findings are not always seen, particularly if the flow rate is slow. The definitive diagnosis is made by bougienage (see Chapter 10).

The simplest and least harmful treatment is overdilatation with sounds up to 32–36F or with the Kollmann dilator (Lyon & Tanagho, 1965, 1971; Hendry, Stanton, & Williams, 1973). In either instance, the ring "cracks" anteriorly, with some bleeding. Recurrence of the lesion is rare. Internal urethrotomy has its proponents (Immergut & Gilbert, 1973; Hradec & others, 1973), but Kaplan, Sammons, & King (1973) prefer dilatation; their poorest results were obtained from urethrotomy. Incising the entire length of the urethra cannot cut the external sphincter, whose abnormal tone is the cause of the obstruction. "Cracking" the ring by overdilatation accomplishes the same purpose. Walker & Richard (1973) were unimpressed by this syndrome; their bibliography, however, failed to cite the work of those who have found its treatment to be effective. In 80% of these children, a successful outcome is achieved: cessation of enuresis, normal free voiding pattern, cure of recurrent cystitis or persistent bacteriuria, and, at times, disappearance of vesicoureteral reflux (Lyon & Marshall, 1971). The latter is only to be expected of the "borderline" valve embar-

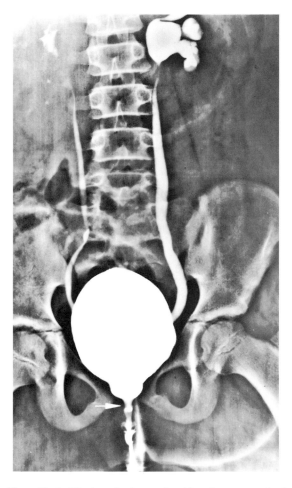 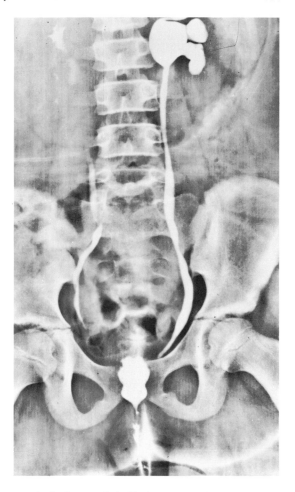

Figure 28—1. Distal urethral stenosis with reflux spasm of voluntary urethral sphincter. *Left:* Voiding cystourethrogram showing bilateral vesicoureteral reflux, a wide-open vesical neck, and severe spasm of the striated urethral sphincter in the midportion of the urethra (see arrow) secondary to distal urethral stenosis. *Right:* Postvoiding film. Bladder empty, vesical neck open, but dilated urethra contains radiopaque fluid proximal to the stenotic zone. Urethral bacteria thus can flow back into the bladder. (Courtesy of AD Amar.)

rassed by increased intravesical voiding pressure and infection. Since the ring disappears at puberty, it is probably this improvement in hydrodynamics that has caused spontaneous improvement in these girls. Even if this is true, however, the distal ring should be treated when found.

LABIAL FUSION
(Synechia Vulvae)

Some children with recurring urinary infection are found to have fusion of the labia minora, which is apt to cause obstruction to the flow of urine so that it tends to pool in the vagina. The local application of estrogen cream twice daily for 2—4 weeks usually causes spontaneous separation (Caparo & Greenberg,

1972). Forceful separation or dissection has its advocates (Podolsky, 1973; Christensen & Øster, 1971).

ACQUIRED DISEASES
OF THE FEMALE URETHRA

ACUTE URETHRITIS

Acute urethritis frequently occurs with gonorrheal infection in women. Urinary symptoms are often present at the onset of the disease. Cultures and smears establish the diagnosis. Cure is quickly effected by antibiotics. The detergents in bubble bath or certain spermatocidal jellies may lead to vaginitis and urethritis. Symptoms of vesical irritability may occur.

CHRONIC URETHRITIS

Because the distal portion of the channel normally harbors bacteria, chronic urethritis is one of the most common urologic difficulties affecting women. Chronic urethral inflammation may occur (1) because of increase in the urethral flora from contaminated diapers; (2) from the trauma of coitus or childbirth, particularly if urethral stenosis, either congenital or following childbirth, is present; (3) because of the need for an indwelling urethral catheter following surgical or cystoscopic operations; (4) from neighborhood cervicitis or vaginitis; or (5) following intercourse with an infected partner.

Clinical Findings

The urethral mucosa is reddened and quite sensitive. Granular areas are often seen, and polypoid masses may be noted just distal to the bladder neck. The urethra is often found to be stenotic.

A. Symptoms: The symptoms resemble those of cystitis, although the urine may be clear. Complaints include burning on urination, frequency, and nocturia. Discomfort in the urethra may be felt, particularly when walking.

B. Signs: Examination may disclose redness of the meatus, hypersensitivity of the meatus and of the urethra on vaginal palpation, and evidence of cervicitis or vaginitis. There is no urethral discharge.

C. Laboratory Findings: Collection of the initial and midstream urine in separate containers reveals pus in the first glass and none in the second (Marshall, Lyon, & Schieble, 1970). T-strain mycoplasmas are often identifiable in the first glass. These findings are similar to those observed in nonspecific urethritis in the male. Clinically, the presence of white blood cells in the absence of bacteria on a routine stain or culture suggests this cause.

In other instances, various bacteria may be found on culture (eg, *Streptococcus faecalis, Escherichia coli*) in both the urethral washings and in a specimen taken from the introitus. Bruce & others (1973) recommend the regular local application of an antiseptic (eg, hexachlorophene, chlorhexidine cream) to the introitus in order to prevent bacteria from the perineum-vagina -vulva from reinfecting the urethra.

D. Instrumental Examination: A catheter, bougie à boule, or sound may meet resistance because of urethral stenosis. Panendoscopy reveals redness and a granular appearance of the mucosa. Inflammatory polyps may be seen in the proximal portion of the urethra. Cystoscopy may show increased injection of the trigone (trigonitis), which often accompanies urethritis.

Differential Diagnosis

Differentiation from cystitis depends upon bacteriologic study of the urine; panendoscopy demonstrates the urethral lesion. Both diseases may be present.

Psychologic disorders may cause symptoms which are identical with those associated with chronic urethritis. A history of short bouts of frequency without nocturia is suggestive of functional illness. The neurotic makeup of the patient usually becomes obvious (Zufall, 1963).

Treatment & Prognosis

Successful treatment requires removal of the cause of the urethritis. Gradual urethral dilatations (up to 36F in the adult) should be given if there is urethral stenosis; this allows for some inevitable contracture. Immergut & Gilbert (1973) prefer internal urethrotomy. T-strain mycoplasmas are fairly sensitive to both tetracycline and erythromycin. Nonspecific bacteria usually respond to appropriate antibiotics.

SENILE URETHRITIS

After physiologic (or surgical) menopause, hypoestrogenism occurs and retrogressive (senile) changes take place in the vaginal epithelium; it becomes rather dry and pale. Since the urethra arises from the same embryologic tissues as the female generative organs, similar degenerative changes develop in the lower urinary tract. Some eversion of the mucosa about the urethral orifice, from foreshortening of the vaginal canal, is usually seen. This is commonly misdiagnosed as caruncle.

Clinical Findings

A. Symptoms: Many postmenopausal women have symptoms of vesical irritability (burning, frequency, urgency) and stress incontinence. They may complain of vaginal and vulval itching and some discharge.

B. Signs: The vaginal epithelium is dry and pale. The mucosa at the urethral orifice is often reddened and hypersensitive; eversion of its posterior lip due to foreshortening of the urethrovaginal wall is commonly seen.

C. Laboratory Findings: The urine is usually free of organisms. The diagnosis can be made by the following procedure: A dry smear of vaginal epithelial cells is stained with Lugol's solution. The slide is then washed with water and immediately examined microscopically while wet. In hypoestrogenism, the cells take up the iodine poorly and are therefore yellow. When the mucosa is normal, these cells stain deep brown because of their glycogen content. The diagnosis may also be confirmed by the Papanicolaou technic.

D. Instrumental Examination: Panendoscopy usually demonstrates a reddened and granular urethral mucosa. Some urethral stenosis may be noted.

Differential Diagnosis

Senile urethritis is often mistaken for urethral caruncle. Although there is eversion of the posterior lip of the urinary meatus in senile urethritis, a hypersensitive vascular tumor is lacking.

Before operations to relieve stress incontinence are performed, estrogenic (or androgenic) vaginal therapy should be given. It may preclude the need for surgery.

Treatment

Senile urethritis responds well to diethylstilbestrol vaginal suppositories, 0.1 mg nightly for 3 weeks. Estrogen creams applied locally are also effective. Estrogen urethral suppositories have been recommended, but they offer no advantages and patients have difficulty inserting them. After 3 weeks of treatment, the drug is withheld for 1 week and then the course is repeated. More than 2 courses are occasionally indicated, depending upon the symptoms and the appearance of the vaginal smear stained as outlined above.

Estrogen suppositories may cause considerable vaginal irritation or vaginal bleeding after withdrawal of the drug. If so, methyltestosterone linguets (5 mg) can be used as vaginal suppositories with equally good results. They should be inserted daily for 5–8 weeks. Diethylstilbestrol, 0.1 mg/day by mouth, is also effective.

Prognosis

Senile urethritis usually responds promptly to estrogen or androgen therapy.

CARUNCLE

Urethral caruncle is a benign, red, raspberrylike, friable vascular tumor involving the posterior lip of the external urinary meatus. It is rare before the menopause. Microscopically it consists of connective tissue containing many inflammatory cells and blood vessels, and is covered by an epithelial layer.

Clinical Findings

Symptoms include pain on urination, pain with intercourse, bloody spotting even from mild trauma, and the presence of a mass at the meatal orifice. A sessile or pedunculated red, friable, tender mass is seen at the posterior lip of the meatus.

Differential Diagnosis

Carcinoma of the urethra may involve the urethral meatus. Palpation reveals definite induration. Biopsy will establish the true diagnosis.

Senile urethritis is often associated with a polypoid reaction of the urinary meatus. In fact, it is the most common cause of masses in this region. The differentiation can be made by establishing the presence of hypoestrogenism and its response to replacement therapy. Biopsy should be done if doubt exists.

Thrombosis of the urethral vein presents as a bluish, swollen, tender lesion involving the posterior lip of the urinary meatus. It has the appearance of a thrombosed hemorrhoid. It subsides without treatment.

Treatment

Only if the lesion produces troublesome symptoms should local excision be done.

Prognosis

True caruncle is usually cured by excision, but in a few instances it does recur.

THROMBOSIS OF THE URETHRAL VEIN

Spontaneous thrombosis of the urethral vein which occupies the floor of the distal urethra occurs in older women. The patient is conscious of sudden local pain and, shortly thereafter, a mass at the urethral orifice. Examination reveals a purple mass protruding from the posterior lip of the urethra; at the onset it is quite tender. Its abrupt onset tends to rule out caruncle or malignancy. If there is doubt about its true nature, biopsy should be done.

No treatment is required in most instances; gradual resolution occurs. Evacuation of the clot has been recommended.

PROLAPSE

Prolapse of the urethra in the female is not common. It usually occurs only in children or in paraplegics suffering from a lower motor neuron lesion. The protruding urethral mucosa presents as an angry red mass which, if not reduced promptly, may become gangrenous. Such a protruding mass in a little girl must be differentiated from prolapse of a ureterocele.

After reduction, cystoscopy should be done to rule out ureterocele. Recurrences are rare once reduction has been accomplished; the accompanying inflammation probably "fixes" the tissue in place as healing progresses. If the prolapsed urethra cannot be reduced, or if it recurs, an indwelling catheter should be inserted, traction placed upon it, and a heavy piece of suture material tightly tied over the tissue and catheter just proximal to the mass. The tissue later sloughs off. Using this same technic, the tissue can be resected, preferably with an electrosurgical unit.

URETHROVAGINAL FISTULA

Urethrovaginal fistulas may follow local injury secondary to fracture of the pelvis or obstetric or surgical injury (see Chapter 16). A common cause is accidental trauma to the urethra or its blood supply in the course of surgical repair of a cystocele. Vaginal urethroplasty is indicated.

DIVERTICULUM

Diverticulation of the urethral wall is not common. Diverticula are at times multiple. Most cases are probably secondary to obstetric urethral trauma or severe urethral infection. A few cases of carcinoma in such diverticula have been reported. This disease is usually associated with recurrent attacks of cystitis. Purulent urethral discharge is sometimes noted as the infected diverticulum empties. Dyspareunia sometimes results. On occasion the diverticulum may be large enough to be discovered by the patient.

The diagnosis is usually made on feeling a rounded cystic mass in the anterior wall of the vagina which, upon pressure, leaks pus from the urethral orifice. Endoscopy may reveal its urethral opening. The postvoiding film of an excretory urographic series may reveal the lesion (Hauser & von Eschenbach, 1974). It may be possible to introduce a small catheter through which radiopaque fluid can be instilled. Appropriate x-ray films are then exposed (Fig 28–2). The plain film may show the presence of a stone in the diverticulum. Should these methods fail, the following procedures can be used:

(1) Empty the diverticulum manually. Catheterize, and instill 5 ml of indigo carmine and 60 ml of contrast medium into the bladder. Remove the catheter and have the patient begin to void. Occlude the meatus with a finger. This maneuver usually causes filling of the diverticulum with the test solution. Take appropriate x-rays and do panendoscopy, seeking leakage of blue dye from the mouth of the diverticulum (Borski & Stutzman, 1965).

(2) Insert a Davis-TeLinde catheter. This looks like a Foley catheter, but it is surrounded by a second movable balloon. Pass the catheter to the bladder and inflate the proximal balloon. With tension on the catheter, slide the second balloon against the urinary meatus and inflate it. In the catheter, between the balloons, is a hole through which injected radiopaque fluid will escape, thus filling the urethra and diverticulum. X-rays are then exposed.

Treatment consists of removal of the sac through an incision in the anterior vaginal wall. The defect in the urethra must be repaired. Ellik (1957) recommends opening the diverticulum and stuffing it with Oxycel, then closing the diverticulum. The inflammatory reaction that results destroys the cyst. An indwelling urethral catheter should be left in place for 10 days following treatment.

The outcome is usually good unless the diverticulum is so situated that its excision injures the external urinary sphincter mechanism. The risk of such a complication is lessened if Ellik's technic is used. In a few cases, urethrovaginal fistula may develop. If the fistula does not close with prolonged catheter drainage, surgical repair will be necessary.

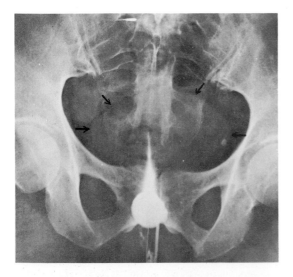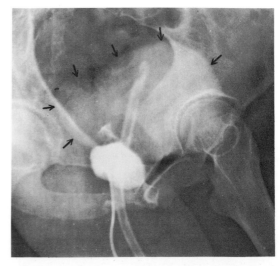

Figure 28–2. Urethral diverticulum containing stone. *Left:* Plain film showing stone. Arrows outline bladder. *Right:* Diverticulum filled with radiopaque fluid instilled through ureteral catheter. Bladder outlined by arrows.

STRICTURE

Stricture of the adult female urethra is quite common and is often found to be the primary cause of nonspecific urethritis or cystitis. It may be congenital or acquired. The trauma of intercourse and especially that associated with childbirth may lead to periurethral fibrosis with contracture, or the stricture may be caused by the surgeon during vaginal repair. It may develop secondary to acute or chronic urethritis.

Persistent hesitancy in initiating urination and a slow urinary stream are the principal symptoms of stricture. Burning, frequency, nocturia, and urethral pain may occur from secondary urethritis or cystitis. If secondary infection of the bladder is present, pus and bacteria will be found in the urine. A fairly large catheter (22F) may pass to the bladder only with difficulty. Panendoscopy may visualize the point of narrowness and disclose evidence of urethritis. Cystoscopy often reveals trabeculation (hypertrophy) of the bladder wall.

Chronic cystitis may cause similar symptoms, but urinalysis will reveal evidence of infection. Cancer of the urethra causes progressive narrowing of the urethra, but induration and infiltration of the urethra will be found on vaginal examination. Panendoscopy with biopsy establishes the diagnosis. Vesical tumor involving the bladder neck will cause hesitancy and impairment of the urinary stream. Cystoscopy is definitive. Chronic urethritis commonly accompanies urethral stenosis; either may be primary. Recurrent or chronic cystitis is often secondary to stenosis.

Treatment consists of gradual urethral dilatation (up to 36F) at weekly intervals. Slight overstretching is necessary since some contracture will occur after therapy is discontinued. Measures to combat urethritis and cystitis must also be employed. Internal urethrotomy also has its proponents.

With proper overdilatation of the urethra and specific therapy of the urethritis which is usually present, the prognosis is good.

• • •

References

Distal Urethral Stenosis in Infancy & Childhood

Fisher RE & others: Urethral calibration in newborn girls. J Urol 102:67, 1969.

Hendry WF, Stanton SL, Williams DI: Recurrent urinary infections in girls: Effects of urethral dilatation. Brit J Urol 45:72, 1973

Hinman F Jr: Mechanisms for the entry of bacteria and the establishment of urinary infection in female children. J Urol 96:546, 1966.

Hradec E & others: Significance of urethral obstruction in girls. Urol Internat 28:440, 1973.

Immergut MA, Gilbert EC: Internal urethrotomy in recurring urinary infections in girls. J Urol 109:126, 1973.

Kaplan GW, Sammons TA, King LR: A blind comparison of dilatation, urethrotomy and medication alone in the treatment of urinary tract infection in girls. J Urol 109:917, 1973.

Kedar SS: The urethra in the female child. Brit J Urol 40:441, 1968.

Lyon RP, Marshall S: Urinary tract infections and difficult urination in girls: Long-term followup. J Urol 105:314, 1971.

Lyon RP, Tanagho EA: Distal urethral stenosis in little girls. J Urol 93:379, 1965.

Smith DR: Critique on the concept of vesical obstruction in children. JAMA 207:1686, 1969.

Tanagho EA, Lyon RP: Urethral dilatation versus internal urethrotomy. J Urol 105:242, 1971.

Tanagho EA, Meyers FH, Smith DR: Urethral resistance: Its components and implications. I. Smooth muscle component. II. Striated muscle component. Invest Urol 7:136, 195, 1969.

Tanagho EA & others: Spastic external sphincter and urinary tract infection in girls. Brit J Urol 43:69, 1971.

Vermillion CD, Halverstadt DB, Leadbetter GW Jr: Internal urethrotomy and recurrent urinary tract infection in female children. 2. Long-term results in the management of infection. J Urol 106:154, 1971.

Walker D, Richard GA: A critical evaluation of urethral obstruction in female children. Pediatrics 51:272, 1973.

Labial Fusion

Capraro VJ, Greenberg H: Adhesions of the labia minora: A study of 50 patients. Obst Gynec 39:65, 1972.

Christensen EH, Øster J: Adhesions of labia minora (synechia vulvae) in childhood. Acta paediat scandinav 60:709, 1971.

Podolsky ML: Labial fusion: A cause of recurrent urinary tract infections. Clin Pediat 12:345, 1973.

Acute Urethritis

Bass HN: "Bubble bath" as an irritant to the urinary tract of children. Clin Pediat 7:174, 1968.

Marshall S: The effect of bubble bath on the urinary tract. J Urol 93:112, 1965.

Chronic Urethritis

Bruce AW & others: Recurrent urethritis in women. Canad MAJ 108:973, 1973.

Essenhigh DM, Ardran GM, Cope V: A study of the bladder outlet in lower urinary tract infections in women. Brit J Urol 40:268, 1968.

Immergut MA, Gilbert EC: The clinical response of women to internal urethrotomy. J Urol 109:90, 1973.

Marshall S, Lyon RP, Schieble J: Nonspecific urethritis in females. California Med 112:9, June 1970.

Moore T, Hira NR, Stirland RM: Differential urethrovesical urinary cell-count. Lancet 1:626, 1965.

Zimskind PD, Mannes HA: Approach to bladder neck and urethral obstruction in women. S Clin North America 53:571, 1973.

Zufall R: Treatment of the urethral syndrome in women. JAMA 184:894, 1963.

Senile Urethritis

Quinlivan LG: The treatment of senile vaginitis with low doses of synthetic estrogens. Am J Obst Gynec 92:172, 1965.

Smith P: Age changes in the female urethra. Brit J Urol 44:667, 1972.

Caruncle

Marshall FC, Uson AC, Melicow MM: Neoplasms and caruncles of the female urethra. Surg Gynec Obst 110:723, 1960.

Thrombosis of the Urethral Veins

Falk HC: Treatment of urethral vein thrombosis. Obst Gynec 23:85, 1964.

Harrow BR: The thrombosed urethral hemorrhoid: 3 case reports. J Urol 98:482, 1967.

Prolapse

Capraro VJ, Bayonet-Rivera NP, Magoss I: Vulvar tumor in children due to prolapse of urethral mucosa. Am J Obst Gynec 108:572, 1970.

Klaus H, Stein RT: Urethral prolapse in young girls. Pediatrics 52:645, 1973.

Potter BM: Urethral prolapse in girls. Radiology 98:287, 1971.

Turner RW: Urethral prolapse in female children. Urology 2:530, 1973.

Urethrovaginal Fistula

Gray L: Urethrovaginal fistulas. Am J Obst Gynec 101:28, 1968.

Diverticulum

Benjamin J & others: Urethral diverticulum in adult female: Clinical aspects, operative procedure, and pathology. Urology 3.1, 1974.

Borski AA, Stutzman RE: Diverticulum of female urethra: A simplified diagnostic aid. J Urol 93:60, 1965.

Dretler SP, Vermillion CD, McCullough DL: The roentgenographic diagnosis of female urethral diverticula. J Urol 107:72, 1972.

Ellik M: Diverticulum of the female urethra: A new method of ablation. J Urol 77:243, 1957.

Glassman TA, Weinerth JL, Glenn JF: Neonatal female urethral diverticulum. Urology 5:249, 1975.

Golimbu M, Al-Askari S: High pressure voiding urethrography. Urology 3:717, 1974.

Houser LM II, von Eschenbach AC: Diverticula of female urethra: Diagnostic importance of postvoiding film. Urology 3:453, 1974.

Presman D, Rolnick D, Zumerchek J: Calculus formation within a diverticulum of the female urethra. J Urol 91:376, 1964.

Sholem SL, Wechsler M, Roberts M: Management of the urethral diverticulum in women: A modified operative approach. J Urol 112:485, 1974.

Spence HM, Duckett JW Jr: Diverticulum of the female urethra: Clinical aspects and presentation of a simple operative technique for cure. J Urol 104:432, 1970.

Torres SA, Quattlebaum RB: Carcinoma in a urethral diverticulum. South MJ 65:1374, 1972.

Stricture

Essenhigh DM, Ardran GM, Cope V: A study of the bladder outlet in lower urinary tract infections in women. Brit J Urol 40:268, 1968.

Immergut MA, Gilbert EC: The clinical response of women to internal urethrotomy. J Urol 109:90, 1973.

29...
Disorders of the Testis, Scrotum, & Spermatic Cord

DISORDERS OF THE SCROTUM

Hypoplasia of the scrotum accompanies cryptorchism. Bifid scrotum is present with midscrotal or perineal hypospadias and in certain cases of intersexuality. In both instances the 2 scrotal sacs simulate labia majora.

Idiopathic edema of the scrotum is occasionally seen in children. It may be unilateral or may involve both sacs. The edema may involve the penis or may spread into the perineum or the inguinal region. The exact cause is not known; it may represent an allergic response. Antihistamines may be of value in treatment, though the process does resolve spontaneously.

Conn (1971) has observed scrotal edema following paracentesis for cirrhosis of the liver caused by development of a fistula between the peritoneum and the subcutaneous tissue. In women, the edema involves the labia. The possibility of torsion of the spermatic cord must, however, be kept in mind for it may affect the scrotal skin in a similar fashion.

In association with healed meconium peritonitis, masses may develop in the scrotum (or in the inguinal area). At birth, examination may lead to the diagnosis of hydrocele, but 1 month later the scrotal masses have become firm. A plain film of the abdomen will reveal calcification in the masses as well as in the abdomen. This will differentiate the masses from teratoma.

CONGENITAL ANOMALIES OF THE TESTIS

ANOMALIES OF NUMBER

Absence of one or both testes is very rare and can only be proved at autopsy. Polyorchism is very rare. A spermatocele or tumor of the spermatic cord is often mistaken for a third gonad.

HYPOGONADISM

Males suffering from either congenital or prepuberal primary testicular eunuchoidism or pituitary hypogonadism (congenital or secondary to a brain lesion) are tall and have disproportionately long extremities because of delay in fusion of the epiphyses. The testes are small. There is lack of development of secondary sexual characteristics associated with some deficiency in libido and potency. These men are sterile. A somewhat feminine fat distribution may be noted, and there are wrinkles about the eyes. The primary gonadal defect is often associated with color blindness and mental retardation.

X-ray studies of the bones reveal delay in closure of the epiphyses. The differential diagnosis of these 2 disorders often depends upon determination of FSH and 17-ketosteroid (or serum testosterone) excretion in the urine. The pituitary type will excrete no FSH; the androgen level is very low. The gonadal eunuch excretes high levels of FSH (above 80 mouse units/24 hours) but only moderately decreased amounts of 17-ketosteroids or serum testosterone. The pituitary eunuchoid male may have an enlarged sella turcica or visual field defects secondary to tumor.

Both types are treated with testosterone. Give long-acting esters of testosterone, 200 mg/month IM, or a comparable preparation by mouth daily.

For a discussion of Klinefelter's syndrome, see Chapter 31.

ECTOPY & CRYPTORCHISM

In ectopy the testicle has strayed from the path of normal descent; in cryptorchism it is arrested in the normal path of descent. Ectopy may be due to an abnormal connection of the distal end of the gubernaculum testis which leads the gonad to an abnormal position. The ectopic sites are as follows (Fig 29–1):

(1) **Superficial inguinal (most common site):** After passing through the external inguinal ring, the testis proceeds superolaterally to a position superficial

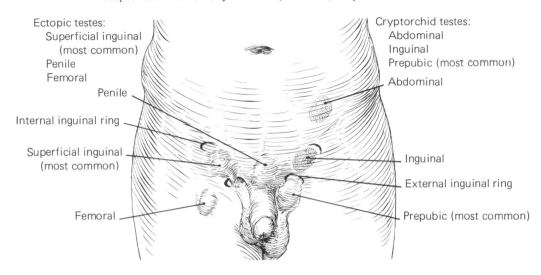

Figure 29–1. Undescended testes. Position of testes in various types of ectopy and cryptorchism.

to the aponeurosis of the external oblique muscle.

(2) Perineal (rare): The testis is found just in front of the anus and to one side of the midline.

(3) Femoral or crural (rare): The testis is found in Scarpa's triangle superficial to the femoral vessels. The cord passes under the inguinal ligament.

(4) Penile (rare): The testis is placed under the skin at the root of the dorsum of the penis.

(5) Transverse or paradoxical descent (rare): Both testes descend the same inguinal canal. This condition is accompanied by findings compatible with pseudo-hermaphroditism.

(6) Pelvic (rare): The testis is found in the true pelvis (discovered only by surgical exploration).

Cryptorchism is a condition in which a testicle is arrested at some point in its normal descent. Thus, it may be found anywhere between the renal and scrotal areas. At the time of birth (9-month gestation), the incidence of maldescent is 3.4%. Half of these descend in the first month of life. The incidence in the adult is 0.7–0.8%. In the premature, it is 30%. (Klauber, 1973; Levin & Sherman, 1973.) A few of the cryptorchid testes may descend at puberty.

Etiology

The cause of maldescent is not clear. The following possibilities must be considered.

A. Abnormality of the Gubernaculum Testis: The gubernaculum is a cordlike structure which extends from the lower pole of the testis to the scrotum. In the embryo, of course, it is exceedingly short; differential growth of the body of the embryo appears to cause "descent" of the gonad from its lumbar origin. Absence or abnormality of the gubernaculum testis could lead to maldescent.

B. Intrinsic Testicular Defect: It may be that maldescent is due to a congenital gonadal (dysgenetic)

defect which causes the testicle to be insensitive to gonadotropins. This theory best accounts for unilateral cryptorchism. It also would explain why many patients with bilateral cryptorchism, given definitive therapy at the optimum age, are sterile.

C. Deficient Gonadotropic Hormonal Stimulation: Lack of adequate maternal gonadotropins could account for incomplete descent. This seems to be the obvious explanation for bilateral cryptorchism in the premature infant, since the elaboration of maternal gonadotropins remains at a low level until the last 2 weeks of gestation. It is difficult, however, to apply this theory to unilateral cryptorchism, which is more common than bilateral arrest.

Pathogenesis & Pathology

The efficacy of the scrotum as a temperature regulator for the testes is well recognized. They are kept about 1 °C (1.5 °F) cooler than body temperature. The spermatogenic cells are quite sensitive to the latter. Most investigators recognize histologic changes in the retained testis by the age of 5 years or even earlier. Diminution in the size of spermatogenic tubules and in the number of spermatogonia is noted.

Moore has clearly shown the efficacy of the scrotum as a temperature regulator for the testes. The spermatogenic cells are quite sensitive to body temperature. Cooper has demonstrated microscopic changes in the retained organ in boys at the age of 2. Robinson and Engle and others have reported definite diminution in the size of spermatogenic tubules and the number of spermatogonia in undescended testes in boys as young as 6 years of age.

After 6 years of age, the changes become more obvious. The diameter of the tubules is smaller than normal. The number of spermatogonia decreases, and fibrosis between the tubules becomes marked. The cryptorchid testis after puberty may be fairly normal in size, but it is markedly deficient in spermatogenic components; infertility is the rule.

It must be borne in mind, however, that about 10% of these testes are congenitally defective (primary hypogonadism, hypogonadism secondary to hypopituitarism). These gonads will show subnormal spermatogenic activity in spite of proper treatment.

Fortunately, the Leydig cells are resistant to body temperature; they are therefore usually found in normal numbers in the cryptorchid organ. Impotence on an endocrinologic basis is therefore rare in this group.

Mininberg & Bingol (1973) have noted a high incidence of chromosome abnormalities in the undescended organ, but the blood chromosomes are normal. They postulate that this may be the cause of the maldescent and suggest that this defect might be the cause of later carcinomatous degeneration.

Clinical Findings

A. Symptoms: The cardinal symptom of ectopy or cryptorchism is absence of one or both testes from the scrotum. The patient may complain of pain in the testis due to trauma to the organ, which may be situated in a vulnerable position (eg, over the pubic bone). The adult patient with bilateral cryptorchism may present with a complaint of infertility.

B. Signs: In true maldescent, the scrotum on the affected side is atrophic. The testis is either not palpable (lying within or even proximal to the inguinal canal) or can be felt external to the inguinal ring. It cannot be manipulated into the scrotum. A common position for such a testis is in the region of the inguinal canal. If one is felt in this area, it must be a superficial inguinal ectopic testis (lying subcutaneously) for it would be impossible to feel a small testis through the heavy external oblique aponeurosis. Inguinal hernia may be demonstrated on the affected side.

C. Laboratory Findings: Studies of the urinary 17-ketosteroids, gonadotropins, and serum testosterone may help in tracing the cause of cryptorchism. In primary hypogonadism, the urinary gonadotropins (FSH) are markedly elevated, whereas the androgens are moderately reduced. In primary hypopituitarism, the androgens and pituitary gonadotropins are definitely depressed. In "primary" cryptorchism, the androgens and pituitary gonadotropins are often moderately diminished.

Differential Diagnosis

Physiologic cryptorchism (retractile or migratory testis) is a common phenomenon which requires no treatment. Because of the small mass of the prepuberal testis and the strength of the cremaster muscle, which inserts upon the spermatic cord, the testes are apt to be involuntarily retracted out of the scrotum in cold weather or with excitement or physical activity. The diagnosis is made by noting that the scrotum on the suspected side is normally developed and that the "inguinal" testis can be pushed into and to the bottom of the scrotum. It may be necessary to place the child in a warm tub to afford maximum muscular relaxation, in which case the testis is found in the normal position. Such a testis descends at puberty and has been found to be normal.

Complications

Associated inguinal hernia is found in 25% of patients with maldescent. At the time of surgery, 95% prove to have a patent processus vaginalis. Dwoskin & Kuhn (1973) recommend that radiopaque fluid be injected intraperitoneally. With the patient in the prone position, a hernia sac will fill and be shown on serial films.

Torsion of the spermatic cord is occasionally seen as a complication of cryptorchism. Phillips & Holmes (1972) believe it is most commonly seen in spastic neurologic disease. This must also be differentiated from strangulated hernia, appendicitis, and diverticulitis (Riegler, 1972).

Most authorities agree that the danger of malignancy in a misplaced testis is significantly higher than in the organ which is normally descended. This further substantiates the theory that many of these testes are dysgenetic.

Treatment

Since definite histologic change can be demonstrated in the cryptorchid testis by the age of 6 years, placement of the testis in the scrotum should be accomplished by the age of 5. Scorer (1967) feels that surgical correction should be accomplished at about the age of 1 year. He found that 83% had an associated inguinal hernia. However, a successful operation will not ensure fertility if the testis is congenitally defective.

A. Hormone Therapy: Chorionic gonadotropin should be administered in doses of 5000 IU intramuscularly daily for 3–5 days, depending upon the size of the child. Methyltestosterone, 5 mg/day, may be given by mouth for 1 month if the child refuses to accept the injections.

If physiologic cryptorchism has been carefully ruled out, hormone therapy will cause descent in a month or so in not more than 10–20% of cases. It is more successful in bilateral than in unilateral cryptorchism. Some of these may, in truth, have been physiologic retractile testes whose diagnosis has been missed despite frequent examination. Such descent will at least save the child an operation and the surgeon embarrassment. It is probably safe to say that if this treatment is successful the testis would have descended spontaneously at puberty.

B. Surgical Treatment: If hormone therapy fails, or if inguinal hernia can be demonstrated, orchiopexy (and hernioplasty) should be done immediately. The testis must be placed at the bottom of the scrotum without tension; the blood supply to the organ must be meticulously preserved. Should the testis not be discovered, or noted to be very atrophic and therefore removed, a prosthesis can be placed in the scrotum.

Prognosis

Success of treatment is measured by fertility. The man with one untreated cryptorchid testis produces fewer sperms than the man with normally descended testes. Untreated, bilateral cryptorchism almost always causes infertility. If treated at the optimal age, 60% of these males will be fertile.

CONGENITAL ANOMALIES OF THE EPIDIDYMIS

Congenital absence of the epididymis is rare. At times the epididymis may be anterior rather than posterior to the testis. Lack of fusion of the epididymis and testis has been reported.

DISORDERS OF THE SPERMATIC CORD*

SPERMATOCELE

A spermatocele is a painless cystic mass containing sperm. It lies just above and posterior to the testis but is separate from it (Fig 29—2). Most spermatoceles are less than 1 cm in diameter, although they are occasionally quite large and may be mistaken for hydro-

*The only congenital anomaly that affects the spermatic cord is absence of the vas deferens. If it is bilateral, infertility is the result.

celes. They may be firm, simulating solid tumor. The cause is not entirely clear, although they probably arise from the tubules that connect the rete testis to the head of the epididymides (vasa efferentia) or from cystic structures on the upper pole of the testis or epididymis.

Since they are relatively small, spermatoceles are usually discovered by the physician during routine examination of the genitalia; at times they may be large enough to come to the attention of the patient. Examination reveals a freely movable transilluminating cystic mass lying above the testicle. Microscopic examination of aspirated contents reveals sperms, usually dead. Grossly, the fluid is thin, white, and cloudy.

Spermatocele is differentiated from hydrocele of the tunica vaginalis in that the latter covers the entire anterior surface of the testicle. Aspiration of hydrocele recovers yellow but clear fluid. A tumor of the coverings of the spermatic cord (eg, mesothelioma, fibroma) may feel like a tense spermatocele. It does not, however, contain fluid, and will not transilluminate.

Spermatocele requires no therapy unless it is large enough to annoy the patient, in which case it should be excised.

VARICOCELE*

Varicocele is common in young men and consists of dilatation of the pampiniform plexus above the testis. The left side is most commonly affected. These veins drain into the internal spermatic vein in the region of the internal inguinal ring. This vein passes lateral to the vas deferens at the internal inguinal ring and, on the left side, drains into the renal vein. On the right it empties into the vena cava.

The left internal spermatic vein is particularly

See also p 456.

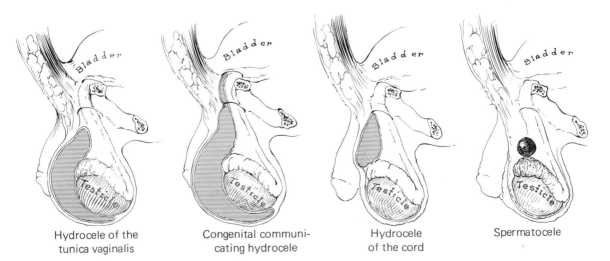

| Hydrocele of the tunica vaginalis | Congenital communicating hydrocele | Hydrocele of the cord | Spermatocele |

Figure 29—2. Hydrocele of the tunica vaginalis and cord; spermatocele.

liable to have incompetent valves. This fact, plus gravity, may lead to poor drainage of the pampiniform plexus, the veins of which gradually undergo dilatation and elongation. At times they are painful, particularly in sexually continent men. Sexual activity (including masturbation) in this instance may relieve symptoms.

The sudden development of a varicocele in an older man is sometimes seen as a late sign of renal tumor when tumor cells have invaded the renal vein, thereby occluding the spermatic vein.

Examination of a man with varicocele reveals a mass of dilated, tortuous veins lying posterior to and above the testis. It may extend up to the external inguinal ring and is often tender. The degree of dilatation can be increased by the Valsalva maneuver. Testicular atrophy from impaired circulation may be present.

No treatment is required unless the varicocele is thought to contribute to infertility or is painful or so large as to disturb the patient. A scrotal support will often relieve discomfort; otherwise, ligation of the internal spermatic vein at the internal inguinal ring is indicated. The results from this operation are uniformly excellent, particularly in the treatment of infertility.

HYDROCELE

A hydrocele consists of a collection of fluid within the tunica or processus vaginalis. Although it may occur within the spermatic cord, it is most often seen surrounding the testicle. A number of cases of hydrocele of the canal of Nuck have been reported. A hydrocele may develop rapidly secondary to local injury, acute nonspecific or tuberculous epididymitis, or orchitis. It may complicate testicular neoplasm. Chronic hydrocele is more common. Its cause is usually unknown, and it usually afflicts men past the age of 40 years. Fluid collects about the testis, and the mass grows gradually (Fig 29−2). It may be soft and cystic or quite tense. The fluid is clear and yellow.

Hydrocele of the tunica vaginalis is common in the newborn, probably as a result of late closure of the processus vaginalis, which is continuous with the peritoneum. Most of these fluid collections subside spontaneously during the first few weeks of life.

Clinical Findings

Young boys with hydrocele commonly have a history of a cystic mass which is small and soft in the morning but larger and more tense at night. One can only conclude, in these instances, that a small communication exists in the processus vaginalis between the peritoneal cavity and the tunica vaginalis (Fig 29−2). Hernia or communicating hydrocele is therefore the proper diagnosis. Hydrocele is painless unless it is accompanied by acute epididymal infection. The patient may, however, complain of its bulk or weight.

The diagnosis is made by finding a rounded cystic intrascrotal mass which is not tender unless underlying inflammatory disease is present. The mass transilluminates. If the hydrocele is enclosed within the spermatic cord, a cystic fusiform swelling is noted in the groin or in the upper scrotum.

A tense hydrocele must be differentiated from tumor of the testis, which does not transilluminate. However, if hydrocele develops in a young man without apparent cause, it should be aspirated so that careful palpation of the testicle and epididymis can be done in order to rule out cancer or tuberculosis.

Complications include compression of the blood supply of the testicle, which leads to atrophy; hemorrhage into the hydrocele sac following trauma or aspiration (hematocele); or, rarely, infection complicating aspiration.

Treatment

Unless complications are present, active therapy is not required. The indications for treatment are a very tense hydrocele which might embarrass circulation to the testicle or a large, bulky mass which is cosmetically unsightly and perhaps uncomfortable for the patient.

One aspiration of a hydrocele which is present during the first few months of life is often curative. Periodic aspiration is usually the treatment of choice in chronic hydrocele. Most chronic hydroceles refill slowly over a period of 6−20 weeks, at which time aspiration can be repeated. If the sac refills rapidly or if the patient requests definitive therapy, the parietal tunica vaginalis should be resected. Lord (1972) has described a simple operation for its repair wherein the hydrocele sac, after being opened, is merely stitched together to collapse the wall. The results of both procedures are good, though in a few cases the hydrocele recurs. Secondary infection may require incision and drainage. Hematocele should be treated by resection of the hydrocele sac.

TORSION OF THE SPERMATIC CORD

Torsion of the spermatic cord (torsion of the testicle) is an uncommon affliction which is almost completely limited to prepuberal males between the ages of 8 and 20 years. It has been observed in the newborn (Schneider, Laycob, & Griffin, 1973). It causes strangulation of the blood supply of the testis. Unless treatment is prompt (within 3 or 4 hours), testicular atrophy may occur.

The cryptorchid testis is prone to undergo torsion. In about half of patients, it occurs during sleep (Sparks, 1972). In most instances, congenital abnormality of the tunica vaginalis or spermatic cord is present. Torsion seems to be most often due to a voluminous tunica vaginalis which inserts well up on the cord. This allows the testis to rotate within the tunica. The initiating factor seems to be spasm of the cremaster muscle, which inserts obliquely on the cord. Its contraction causes the patient's left testis to rotate counterclockwise and his right testis clockwise (as the physician observes the patient from the foot of the bed) (Burton, 1972). With vascular occlusion there is edema of the testis and the cord up to the point of occlusion. This leads to gangrene of the testis and epididymis.

Clinical Findings

The diagnosis should suggest itself when a young boy suddenly develops severe pain in one testicle, followed by swelling of the organ, reddening of the scrotal skin, lower abdominal pain, and nausea and vomiting. However, as Lyon (1961) has pointed out, torsion of the cord may be accompanied only by moderate scrotal swelling and little or no pain.

Examination usually reveals a swollen, tender organ which is retracted upward as a result of shortening of the cord by volvulus. Pain may be increased by lifting the testicle up over the symphysis. (The pain from epididymitis, rare in children, is usually alleviated by this maneuver.) Within a few hours after onset, moderate fever and leukocytosis may develop.

The diagnosis may be made in the early stages if the epididymis can be felt in an abnormal position (eg, anterior). After a few hours, however, the entire gonad becomes so swollen that the epididymis cannot be distinguished from the testis by palpation. Hahn & others (1975) recommend the use of radioisotopes in the differential diagnosis of torsion and epididymitis. Since there is hypervascularity with epididymitis and testicular ischemia with torsion, a rectilinear scan following the intravenous injection of ^{99m}Tc will reveal this difference. A simpler and quicker method of diagnosis utilizes the Doppler stethoscope used in conjunction with ultrasound. There is no sound echoing from an ischemic testis; sound is increased with the hypervascularity of epididymitis (Levy, 1975).

Differential Diagnosis

The differential diagnosis includes acute epididymitis, acute mumps orchitis, and trauma. Epididymitis is rare before puberty. It is often accompanied by pyuria. Mumps orchitis is usually accompanied by parotitis; it is rare before puberty. Without a history or findings of injury, traumatic orchitis may be misdiagnosed as torsion of the cord.

Epididymitis is unusual before age 25. Differential diagnosis may be difficult if epididymitis is not complicated by pyuria, for fever is associated with both. In case of doubt, expose the testis (Del Villar, Ireland, & Cass, 1972).

Treatment

If the patient is seen within a few hours of onset, manual detorsion may be attempted (King & others, 1974). Knowing that torsion causes the left testis to rotate counterclockwise and the right clockwise, one may twist a testis in the opposite direction. The right testis should be "unscrewed" and the left one "screwed up" (Editorial BMI, 1972). This maneuver is facilitated by infiltration of the spermatic cord, near the external inguinal ring, with 10–20 ml of 1% procaine hydrochloride. If this fails, immediate surgical detorsion must be performed, although after 4–6 hours infarction usually will have occurred in those testes subjected to a 720-degree twist of the cord. Whether the testis appears to be viable or not, it should be sutured down to preclude subsequent torsion. Even though the seminiferous tubules may become necrotic, the more hardy interstitial cells may remain viable. Excision of the parietal tunica vaginalis will cause agglutination of the testicle to the scrotal wall. Since the opposite testicle usually is affected by the same abnormal attachments, prophylactic fixation of that organ is imperative.

Prognosis

Unfortunately, the diagnosis is usually made and treatment instituted too late, and atrophy is to be expected in most instances.

·   ·   ·

TORSION OF THE APPENDICES OF THE TESTIS AND EPIDIDYMIS

On the upper poles of both the testis and epididymis there are small vestigial appendages which may be sessile or pedunculated (Fig 1–8). The latter type may spontaneously undergo torsion, which leads to an inflammatory reaction followed by ischemic necrosis and absorption.

This phenomenon usually affects prepuberal boys up to the age of 16 years. Sudden onset of testicular pain is noted. Should the physician have the opportunity to examine the boy shortly after onset, a small tender lump may be felt at the upper pole of the testis or epididymis; this sign is pathognomonic, particularly if, with the skin held tight over the mass, it appears to be blue (Dresner, 1973).

If the patient is seen later, the entire testicle is swollen and tender. The differential diagnosis is then between torsion of these appendages and of the spermatic cord. Immediate surgical exploration is indicated, for time is a critical factor in the treatment of torsion of the cord. If an appendix is twisted, it should be excised.

●   ●   ●

References

SCROTUM

Berdon WE & others: Scrotal masses in healed meconium peritonitis. New England J Med 277:585, 1967.

Conn HO: Sudden scrotal edema in cirrhosis: A postparacentesis syndrome. Ann Int Med 74:943, 1971.

Nicholas JL, Morgan A, Zachary RB: Idiopathic edema of scrotum in young boys. Surgery 67:847, 1970.

Thompson RB, Rosen DI, Gross DM: Healed meconium peritonitis presenting as inguinal mass. J Urol 110:364, 1973.

TESTIS

Anomalies of Number

Goldberg LM, Skaist LB, Morrow JW: Congenital absence of the testes: Anorchism and monorchism. J Urol 111:840, 1974.

Lazarus BA, Tessler AN: Polyorchidism with normal spermatogenesis. Urology 3:615, 1974.

Hypogonadism

Bryson MF, Reichlin S: Neuroendocrine regulation of sexual function and growth. P Clin North America 13:423, 1966.

Federman DD: The assessment of organ function—the testis. New England J Med 285:901, 1971.

Longson D: Androgen therapy. Practitioner 208:338, 1972.

Wilson JD: Recent studies on the mechanism of action of testosterone. New England J Med 287:1284, 1972.

Ectopy & Cryptorchism

Altman BL, Malament M: Carcinoma of the testis following orchiopexy. J Urol 97:498, 1967.

Dajani AM: Transverse ectopia of the testes. Brit J Urol 41:80, 1969.

Dwoskin JY, Kuhn JP: Herniagrams in undescended testes and hydroceles. J Urol 109:520, 1973.

Ehrlich RM & others: Effect of gonadotropin in cryptorchism. J Urol 102:793, 1969.

Firor HV: Two-stage orchiopexy. Arch Surg 102:598, 1971.

Flinn RA, King LR: Experiences with the midline transabdominal approach in orchiopexy. Surg Gynec Obst 133:285, 1971.

Hortling H & others: An endocrinologic follow-up study of operated cases of cryptorchism. J Clin Endocrinol 27:120, 1967.

Kiesewetter WB, Shull WR, Fetterman GH: Histologic changes in the testes following anatomically successful orchidopexy. J Pediat Surg 4:59, 1969.

Klauber GT: Management of the undescended testis. Canad MAJ 108:1129, 1973.

Lattimer JK & others: A natural-feeling testicular prosthesis. J Urol 110:81, 1973.

Lattimer JK & others: The optimum time to operate for cryptorchidism. Pediatrics 53:96, 1974.

Levin A, Sherman JO: The undescended testis. Surg Gynec Obst 136:473, 1973.

Miller HC: Transseptal orchiopexy for cryptorchism. J Urol 98:503, 1967.

Mininberg DT, Bingol N: Chromosomal abnormality in undescended testes. Urology 1:98, 1973.

Persky L, Albert DJ: Staged orchiopexy. Surg Gynec Obst 132:43, 1971.

Phillips NB, Holmes TW Jr: Torsion infarction in ectopic cryptorchidism: A rare entity occurring most commonly with spastic neuromuscular disease. Surgery 71:335, 1972.

Pryn WJ: The maintenance of maldescended testicles within the scrotum using a dartos pouch. Brit J Surg 59:175, 1972.

Riegler HC: Torsion of intra-abdominal testis: An unusual problem in diagnosis of the acute surgical abdomen. S Clin North America 52:371, 1972.

Scorer CG: Early operation for the undescended testis. Brit J Surg 54:694, 1967.

SPERMATIC CORD

Spermatocele

Clarke BG, Bamford SB, Gherardi GJ: Spermatocele: Pathologic and surgical anatomy. Arch Surg 86:351, 1963.

Lord PH: A Bloodless operation for spermatocele or cyst of the epididymis. Brit J Surg 57:641, 1970.

Schoenberg HW, Murphy JJ: The differential diagnosis of intrascrotal masses. GP 25:82, March 1962.

Varicocele

Ahlberg NE & others: Phlebography in varicocele scroti. Acta radiol diag 4:517, 1966.

Clarke BG: Incidence of varicocele in normal men and among men of different age groups. JAMA 198:1121, 1966.

Kiska EF, Cowart GT: Treatment of varicocele by high ligation. J Urol 83:713, 1960.

Shafik A, Khalil AM, Saleh M: The fasciomuscular tube of the spermatic cord: A study of its surgical anatomy and relation to varicocele: A new concept for the pathogenesis of varicocele. Brit J Urol 44:147, 1972.

Hydrocele

Ahmed S: Abdominoscrotal hydrocele in an infant. Surgery 70:316, 1971.

Ariyan S: Hydrocele of the canal of Nuck. J Urol 110:172, 1973.

Dahl DS & others: Lord's operation for hydrocele compared with conventional techniques. Arch Surg 104:40, 1972.

Lord PH: Bloodless surgical procedures for the cure of idiopathic hydrocoele and epididymal cyst (spermatocoele). Progr Surg 10:94, 1972.

Ross JG: Treatment of primary hydroceles in infancy and childhood. Brit J Surg 49:415, 1962.

Wallace AF: Aetiology of the idiopathic hydrocele. Brit J Urol 32:79, 1960.

Wilkinson JL: An operation for large scrotal hydrocele. Brit J Surg 60:450, 1973.

Torsion of the Spermatic Cord

Burton JA: Atrophy following testicular torsion. Brit J Surg 59:422, 1972.

Corriere JN Jr: Horizontal lie of the testicle: A diagnostic sign of torsion of the testicle. J Urol 107:616, 1972.

Del Villar RG, Ireland GW, Cass AS: Early exploration in acute testicular conditions. J Urol 108:887, 1972.

Hahn LC & others: Testicular scanning: A new modality for the preoperative diagnosis of testicular torsion. J Urol 113:60, 1975.

Kaplan GW, King LR: Acute scrotal swelling in children. J Urol 104:219, 1970.

King LM & others: Untwisting in delayed treatment of torsion of the spermatic cord. J Urol 122:217, 1974.

Korbel EI: Torsion of the testis. J Urol 111:521, 1974.

Krarup T: Torsion of the testis. Scandinav J Urol Nephrol (Suppl 15):165, 1972.

Lattimer JK, Smith AM: Scrotal pouch technique: Adjunct to orchiopexy. Urology 5:137, 1975.

Levy BJ: The diagnosis of torsion of the testicle using the Doppler ultrasonic stethoscope. J Urol 113:63, 1975.

Lyon RP: Torsion of the testicle in childhood: A painless emergency requiring contralateral orchiopexy. JAMA 178:702, 1961.

Morgenlander HL, Wise GJ: Scrotal aspiration: Aid in early differentiation between torsion of spermatic cord and acute epididymo-orchitis. Urology 4:686, 1974.

Parker RM, Robison JR: Anatomy and diagnosis of torsion of the testicle. J Urol 106:243, 1971.

Pederson JF, Holm HH, Hald T: Torsion of the testis diagnosed by ultrasound. J Urol 113:66, 1975.

Schneider RE, Laycob LM, Griffin WT: Testicular torsion in utero. Am J Obst Gynec 117:1126, 1973.

Sparks JP: Torsion of the testis in adolescents and young adults. Clin Pediat 11:484, 1972.

Torsion of the testicle again. (Editorial.) Brit MJ 4:505, 1972.

Appendices of the Testis & Epididymis

Dresner ML: Torsed appendage diagnosis and management: Blue dot sign. Urology 1:63, 1973.

Rose MB, Pambakian H: Bilateral torsion of the appendix testis. J Urol 110:408, 1973.

Skoglund RW, McRoberts JW, Ragde H: Torsion of the testicular appendages: Presentation of 43 new cases are a collective review. J Urol 104:598, 1970.

30 . . .
Skin Diseases of the External Genitalia*

Rees B. Rees, Jr., MD*

Almost any skin condition, including psoriasis, seborrheic dermatitis, lichen planus, eczema, etc, can affect the region of the external genitalia and perineum. The patient should be questioned and examined for other possible areas of involvement. In any case of itching or infected dermatitis in this area, it is important to rule out diabetes and pediculosis or scabies.

Associated vaginal and other urologic conditions should be corrected. Self-treatment and overtreatment may alter and complicate genital lesions. Emotional factors associated with repeated scratching and rubbing tend to prolong and complicate genital conditions.

Many individuals with involvement in this area have a fear of venereal disease; if there is no question of this, the fear should be dispelled.

ECZEMATOID DERMATITIS

Eczematoid dermatitis is a broad descriptive term which denotes changes such as redness, vesiculation, scaling, weeping, lichenification (accentuation and thickening of skin markings), and excoriation. This type of eruption may become secondarily infected through scratching. Included in this group are such conditions as contact dermatitis, localized neurodermatitis, pruritus vulvae and scroti, atopic dermatitis, and intertriginous dermatitis. These conditions usually overlap in producing an eczematoid dermatitis, and treatment must take this into consideration.

Contact Dermatitis

Contact dermatitis includes changes produced both by primary irritants and true allergic sensitizers. Possible causes are cosmetics, feminine deodorant sprays, douches, contraceptives, soaps, local medications ("overtreatment dermatitis"), wearing apparel, plants (poison oak and ivy), etc.

*Venereal disease is discussed in Chapter 14; tumors in Chapter 18.

Rees B. Rees is Clinical Professor of Dermatology & Radiology, University of California School of Medicine, San Francisco.

Treatment must include removal of the suspected agent, if possible. Cool wet dressings constitute excellent treatment, and corticosteroid creams may be used topically if infection is not present. The fluorinated corticosteroid creams such as fluocinolone, triamcinolone, betamethasone, and fluocinonide are more likely to produce atrophic striae in the groin than is 0.25–1% hydrocortisone.

Circumscribed Neurodermatitis (Lichen Simplex Chronicus)

These thickened lesions are of great importance in the persistence of any vulval or scrotal skin condition regardless of the original cause. Rubbing and scratching can prolong any eruption indefinitely, and it is usually this problem that causes the patient to seek medical care. This may be done almost subconsciously. A continuing itch-scratch cycle is established which must be broken before healing can occur.

Treatment is as for contact dermatitis (above) plus counseling about the dangers of persistent trauma.

Itching of Vulva & Scrotum

These are merely nonspecific terms used to classify some cases of marked pruritus of these areas with little or no skin changes. Treatment is as for contact dermatitis (above).

Atopic Dermatitis

This lesion presents as dry lichenified dermatitis on the penis, scrotum, in the groins, and on the vulva. Similar changes are usually present also on the face and neck and in the antecubital and popliteal spaces. Generalized dryness is present. There is usually a personal or family history of asthma or hay fever.

A potent corticosteroid cream (0.2% fluocinolone or 0.5% triamcinolone) rubbed in thinly 4 or 5 times daily is effective, although striae may supervene. Hydrocortisone cream, 0.5–1%, should be tried first.

Intertrigo

Intertrigo (sodden, macerated dermatitis) is due to chafing and friction of contiguous surfaces. It occurs in the groins, inframammary areas, skin folds, etc, usually in obese individuals, and is more common during hot, humid weather. Treatment must be directed toward drying the area and reducing chafing.

Hydrocortisone, 1%, and iodochlorhydroxyquin, 0.5% in hydrophilic ointment base, may be rubbed into the areas twice daily, then dusted over with talc.

COMMON SUPERFICIAL INFECTIONS OF THE EXTERNAL GENITALIA

Pyodermas

Staphylococci are present in most of the infections discussed below, but streptococci may be found in as many as 40% of cases. A smear stained with Giemsa's stain will usually show many cocci within the polymorphonuclear leukocytes. Systemic antibiotic treatment is mandatory to prevent nephritis and other serious complications. Pediculosis and scabies should be ruled out.

Sodium cloxacillin is the drug of choice since it is not destroyed by penicillinase. If the patient is allergic to penicillin, the drug of second choice is erythromycin. A polymyxin-bacitracin ointment such as Polysporin may be used topically.

Pyodermas frequently complicate some other primary condition, such as pediculosis and scabies.

A. Folliculitis and Furunculosis: Infection of a hair follicle is usually acute but may be chronic and recurrent. Sharply pointed, extremely tender and hot swellings with central pustulation may be found.

B. Impetigo: Impetiginous involvement is more superficial and is characterized by "stuck-on crusts" and weeping. The mons pubis may be the sole site of involvement, but other areas are usually involved also.

C. Infectious Eczematoid Dermatitis: This is an acute reddened, weeping, spreading eruption. It is often associated with a draining process such as a furuncle or abscess or with vaginal discharge.

D. Hidradenitis Suppurativa: This is a deep chronic inflammatory infection of the apocrine sweat glands, characterized by cystic involvement and interconnecting sinus tracts. It usually involves the axillas and groins and may be an accompaniment of severe cystic acne. In addition to giving antibiotics, it may be necessary to unroof ("saucerize") or actually excise the lesions with or without grafting.

Fungal Infections

Heat, moisture, and darkness favor these infections. They are frequently aggravated by overtreatment.

A. Tinea Cruris: Tinea cruris is characterized by marginated, slightly elevated, scaling patches on the inner thighs and in the groins. There may be an active vesicular border. Pruritus may be intense. Direct microscopic examination of skin scrapings in 15% potassium or sodium hydroxide solution will reveal hyphae or spores. The differential diagnosis includes seborrheic dermatitis, psoriasis, intertrigo, and localized neurodermatitis. Tinea cruris usually responds to treatment with 3% precipitated sulfur and 1% salicylic acid in an emulsion base. Miconazole, 2% cream, is a good alternative. Griseofulvin (micronized), 500 mg orally, may be given daily after supper.

B. Anogenital Candidiasis: Infection with *Candida albicans* is characterized by erythematous, weeping, circumscribed lesions with peripheral epidermal undermining and satellite vesiculopustules. "Ping-pong" infections between sexual partners may occur. Pregnancy, diabetes, obesity, and hyperhidrosis are predisposing factors. Broad-spectrum antibiotic therapy or estrogen therapy may be followed by an overgrowth of candidal organisms. The skin involvement may be secondary to vaginal involvement. Lesions occur under the prepuce. High-power microscopic examination of skin scrapings in 15% potassium or sodium hydroxide solution shows clusters of tiny spores and fine mycelial filaments. Nystatin appears to be effective in most instances. It is available as dusting powder, cream, vaginal inserts, and oral tablets. Amphotericin B cream or lotion and miconazole cream (2%) are both good alternatives to nystatin.

Virus Infections

A. Warts: Warts are common in the vulval region, under the prepuce, and on the shaft of the penis. If present on the mucous or mucocutaneous surfaces, they are called condylomata acuminata. They are usually moist and macerated. They frequently respond to topical treatment with podophyllin, 25% in compound tincture of benzoin. If this fails, 25% in mineral oil should be tried. Severe discomfort may follow application of podophyllin. Fulguration may be necessary if podophyllin is not successful. Liquid nitrogen can be used either with a cotton-tipped applicator or a copper disk on a long steel wand. Each lesion may be frozen for 10–30 seconds.

B. Herpes Simplex (Cold Sore, Fever Blister): Genital herpes is usually due to recurrent herpesvirus type 2 and is characterized by grouped vesiculopustular lesions. There may be secondary adenopathy. This can be a painful recurrent condition and has been implicated in the genesis of cervical carcinoma. Rarely, a primary herpes simplex infection is seen, with severe vulvovaginitis and systemic manifestations. Uncomplicated herpes simplex may be treated with 0.1% proflavine dye solution topically after scarification. Any reading light may then be shined on the lesion for 15 minutes. For best results, the patient should reexpose the treated area to an incandescent light about 6–8 hours after office treatment, using the proflavine dye plus light. Fifteen minutes to one-half hour should be sufficient to inactivate all of the virus in the lesion.

This method of treatment is controversial because hamster cells in tissue culture infected with herpesvirus 2 have been shown to undergo malignant transformation. However, many defective virus particles occur in untreated herpes simplex lesions, and the risk is diminished, in all likelihood, by treating the lesions. Lupidon R, a herpesvirus 2 vaccine, is available in Germany. A simple dusting powder such as BFI (bismuth formic iodide) may be useful.

OTHER INFLAMMATORY DISORDERS

Drug Eruptions

Drug eruptions may involve the genitals. A fixed drug eruption, due usually to phenolphthalein, broad-spectrum antibiotics, or barbiturates may cause a perfectly round, bright-red to purplish macular lesion which comes and goes with each reexposure to the drug. Other drug eruptions usually have manifestations elsewhere as well as on the circumscribed area.

Urticaria & Angioneurotic Edema

These lesions ("hives" and "giant hives") may present on the vulva or male genitalia as a sole sign, at least initially. They may be confused with acute contact dermatitis, which can have an urticarial component. There may be a history of ingestion of an urticariogenic food such as shellfish, pork and pork products, strawberries, or yeast-containing foods. Penicillin is the most common drug cause. Treatment consists of removal of the cause plus cool wet dressings and antihistamines by mouth.

Erythema Multiforme

Erythema multiforme may present as an acute inflammatory erosive process on the genitalia, although signs are usually present elsewhere, eg, the lips, tongue, and mouth, possibly with conjunctivitis. Erythema multiforme and its more severe variant, Stevens-Johnson disease, may be idiopathic or may be caused by drug reaction, herpes simplex, or other infection. Finding a typical "target" herpes-iris or "bulls-eye" lesion may make the diagnosis. Severe forms must be managed symptomatically with supportive treatment and hospitalization. Systemic corticosteroids may be necessary (unless contraindicated), and broad-spectrum antibiotics may be helpful as well.

PAPULOSQUAMOUS ERUPTIONS

Psoriasis

Psoriasis may involve flexural surfaces (inverse psoriasis) such as the groin and the perianal, internatal cleft, and intermammary areas. It tends to be bright red and moist, and usually free of scales. Itching may be intense. Occasionally the only involvement may be in the anogenital area. A solitary plaque may present on the penis, leading to confusion with Bowen's disease or some other more serious disorder. The diagnosis usually can be made by inspection and by noting other areas of involvement such as in the scalp and on the elbows and knees. Pitting of the nails, when present, is almost pathognomonic of psoriasis. Treatment is with 0.1% anthralin ointment rubbed in sparingly morning and night for intertriginous lesions.

Seborrheic Dermatitis

Seborrheic dermatitis may appear as scurfy, scaly, erythematous patches and is easily confused with candidiasis, intertrigo, and psoriasis. Typical areas of involvement are usually present elsewhere, eg, the scalp, brows, creases of the cheeks and chin, in and around the ears, on the presternum, and in the axillas. Corticosteroid creams are very useful. Sulfur (3%) and salicylic acid (1%) in an emulsion base is also effective.

Lichen Planus

Lichen planus may appear on the glans penis or on the labia and introitus. The lesions are small polygonal violet-hued papules about 2–3 cm in diameter which have milky striations over their shiny surfaces. They may become clustered together to form plaques. Itching is usually a problem. There may be generalized involvement or typical lesions in the buccal mucosa which look like spilled milk.

Corticosteroid creams may be helpful in relieving the pruritus. The disease usually disappears after a course of several months.

LICHEN SCLEROSUS ET ATROPHICUS

This is a distinct entity characterized by flat-topped white papules which coalesce to form white patches without infiltration. The surface shows comedonelike plugs or dells. The end stages may resemble very thin parchment or tissue paper. It occurs most frequently in patches on the upper back, chest, and breasts, mostly in women. It almost inevitably involves the anogenital regions, where painful fissures may develop and severe itching may be a distressing symptom. On the penis this condition occurs as balanitis xerotica obliterans, which may lead to urethral stenosis and atrophy with telangiectasia about the meatus and on the glans, with some shrinkage of the prepuce. There is a direct relationship between these conditions and carcinoma. Anogenital lichen sclerosus et atrophicus may be misdiagnosed as kraurosis vulvae with or without leukoplakia. At present, kraurosis is regarded as a descriptive term for the manifestation in a number of diseases.

Lichen sclerosus et atrophicus may involute spontaneously, especially in young girls.

Vitamin A ointment may be tried. For severe itching, one may use intralesional corticosteroids such as triamcinolone (Kenalog) suspension injected into the skin with the Dermajet apparatus or by syringe. Topical corticosteroids may give relief.

Circumcision for balanitis xerotica obliterans which is lichen sclerosus is not particularly helpful.

• • •

References

General

Domonkos AN: *Andrews' Disease of the Skin: Clinical Dermatology,* 6th ed. Saunders, 1971.

Fitzpatrick TB & others: *Dermatology in General Medicine.* McGraw-Hill, 1971.

Rook A, Wilkinson DS, Ebling FJ: *Textbook of Dermatology.* Blackwell, 1973.

Contact Dermatitis

Fisher AA: *Contact Dermatitis.* Lea & Febiger, 1974.

Circumscribed Neurodermatitis

Marks R, Wells GC: Lichen simplex: Morphodynamic correlates. Brit J Dermat 88:249, 1973.

Atopic Dermatitis

Baer RL: *Atopic Dermatitis.* Lippincott, 1955.

Pyodermas

Maibach HI, Hildick-Smith G: *Skin Bacteria and Their Role in Infection.* McGraw-Hill, 1965.

Fungal Infections

Clayton YM: Therapy of fungal infections. Brit J Dermat 89:423, 1973.

Conant MF & others: *Manual of Clinical Mycology.* Saunders, 1971.

Virus Infections

Jarratt MT & others: Dye-photoinactivation and herpes simplex. Arch Dermat 109:570, 1974.

Drug Eruptions

Rees RB: Cutaneous drug reactions. Texas Med 66:92, 1970.

Urticaria

Warin RP, Champion RH: *Urticaria.* Saunders, 1974.

Erythema Multiforme

Yaffee HS: Erythema multiforme. In: *Newer Views of Skin Diseases.* Yaffee HS (editor). Little, Brown, 1966.

Psoriasis

Rees RB: Psoriasis. Mod Med 40:95, 1972.

Seborrheic Dermatitis

Rees RB: Dandruff and seborrhea. Cutis 9:669, 1972.

Lichen Planus

Irgang S: Lichen planus. Cutis 6:887, 1970.

Lichen Sclerosus et Atrophicus

Barker LP, Gross P: Lichen sclerosus et atrophicus of the female genitalia. Arch Dermat 85:362, 1962.

31...
Abnormalities of Sexual Differentiation

Felix A. Conte, MD, Edward O. Reiter, MD, & Melvin M. Grumbach, MD

Advances in cytogenetics, experimental embryology, steroid biochemistry, and methods of evaluation of the interaction between the hypothalamus, pituitary, and gonads have helped to clarify problems of sexual differentiation. Such anomalies may occur at any stage of intrauterine maturation and can lead to gross ambisexual development or to subtle abnormalities which do not become manifest until sexual maturity is achieved.

NORMAL SEXUAL DIFFERENTIATION

Chromosomal Sex

The normal human diploid cell contains 22 autosomal pairs of chromosomes and 2 sex chromosomes (2 X or one X and one Y). Arranged serially and numbered according to size and centromeric position, they are known as a karyotype. Recent advances in technics of staining chromosomes (Fig 31–1) permit positive identification of each chromosome by its unique "banding" pattern. Bands can be produced with a fluorescent dye, quinacrine (Q bands), at the centromeric position on the chromosome (C bands), and with Giemsa's stain (G bands). Fluorescent banding (Fig 31–2) is particularly useful because the Y chromosome stains so brightly that it can be identified easily in both interphase and metaphase cells. The standard nomenclature for describing the human karyotype is shown in Table 31–1.

Studies in patients with abnormalities of sexual differentiation indicate that the sex chromosomes, the X and Y chromosomes, carry genes that influence

Figs 31–1 to 31–10 and Tables 31–1, 31–2, and 31–4 are reproduced, with permission, from Grumbach MM, Van Wyk JJ: Disorders of sex differentiation. Chapter 8, pp 423–501, in: *Textbook of Endocrinology*, 5th ed. Williams RH (editor). Saunders, 1974.

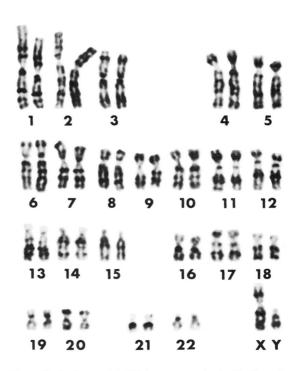

Figure 31–1. A normal 46,XY karyotype stained with Giemsa's stain to produce G bands. Note that each chromosome has a specific banding pattern.

Felix A. Conte is Assistant Professor of Pediatrics, University of California School of Medicine (San Francisco). Edward O. Reiter was a Fellow in Pediatric Endocrinology, University of California School of Medicine (San Francisco), and currently is Assistant Professor of Pediatrics, University of South Florida School of Medicine, and Co-Director of the Pediatric Endocrine Service, All Children's Hospital, St. Petersburg, Florida. Melvin M. Grumbach is Professor of Pediatrics and Chairman, Department of Pediatrics, University of California School of Medicine (San Francisco).

sexual differentiation by causing the bipotential gonad to develop either as a testis or an ovary. Genes on the short arm of the Y chromosome code specifically for a testis. Two normally functioning X chromosomes in the absence of a Y chromosome lead to the formation of an ovary.

Careful examination of the karyotype in humans reveals a marked discrepancy in size between the X and the Y chromosome. There is evidence that gene dosage

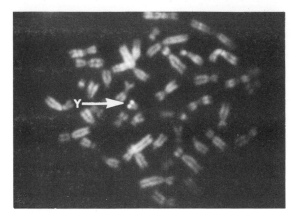
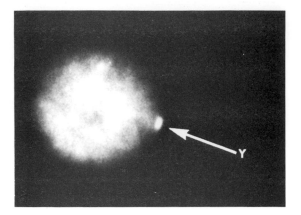

Figure 31—2. Metaphase chromosomes stained with quinacrine and examined through a fluorescent microscope. Note the bright fluorescence of the distal arms of the Y chromosome, which can also be seen in interphase cells ("Y body" at right).

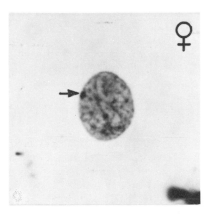
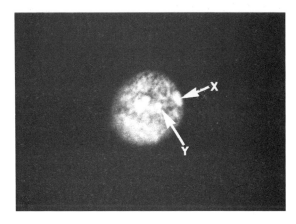

Figure 31—3. X chromatin body in the nucleus of a buccal mucosal cell from a normal female.

Figure 31—4. An interphase nucleus stained with quinacrine and examined by fluorescent microscopy. This cell reveals a "Y body" and an X chromatin body. The patient has a 47,XXY karyotype.

compensation is achieved in all persons with 2 or more X chromosomes in their genetic constitution by inactivation of all X chromosomes except one. This phenomenon, the so-called Lyon hypothesis, is thought to be a random process in each cell which occurs in the late blastocyst stage (days 12—18) of embryonic development. The result of this process is the formation of a sex chromatin body (Barr body) in the interphase cells of persons having 2 or more X chromosomes (Fig 31—3). In buccal mucosal smears of 46,XX females, a sex chromatin body is evident in 20—40% of the nuclei examined, whereas in normal 46,XY males a comparable sex chromatin body is absent. In patients with more that 2 X chromosomes, the maximum number of sex chromatin bodies in any diploid nucleus is one less than the total number of X chromosomes. By utilizing sex chromatin and Y fluorescent staining (Table 31—2), one can determine the sex chromosome complement of any individual from a buccal smear (Fig 31—4).

Testicular & Ovarian Differentiation (Fig 31—5)

Until the 12 mm stage (approximately 42 days of gestation), the embryonic gonads of males and females are indistinguishable. By 42 days, 300—1300 primordial germ cells have seeded the undifferentiated gonad. These large cells later become oogonia and spermatogonia, and lack of these cells is incompatible with further gonadal differentiation. Under the influence of a Y chromosome, the gonad will begin testicular differentiation by 43—50 days of gestation. Leydig cells are apparent by about 60 days, and differentiation of male external genitalia occurs by 65—77 days of gestation.

In the gonad destined to be an ovary, the lack of differentiation persists. At 77—84 days, long after differentiation of the testis in the male fetus, a significant number of germ cells enter meiotic prophase to characterize the transition of oogonia into oocytes which mark the onset of ovarian differentiation from the undifferentiated gonads.

Table 31—1. Nomenclature for describing the human karyotype pertinent to designating sex chromosome abnormalities.

Chicago and Paris Conferences	Description	Former Nomenclature
46,XX	Normal female karyotype	XX
46,XY	Normal male karyotype	XY
47,XXY	Karyotype with 47 chromosomes including an extra sex chromosome	XXY
45,X	One sex chromosome absent	XO
45,X/46,XY	Mosaic karyotype composed of 45,X and 46,XY cell lines	XO/XY
p	Short arm	S
q	Long arm	L
Xp—	Deletion of the short arm of the X	XDS
Xq—	Deletion of the long arm of the X	XDL
Xqi	Isochromosome of the long arm of X	XI
Xpi	Isochromosome of the short arm of X	
Xr	Ring X chromosome	XR
46,X,t (Xq—;9p+)	Translocation of the long arm of X onto the short arm of chromosome No. 9	X/9 translocation
Ydic	Dicentric Y chromosome	
Ypi	Isochromosome of the short arm of Y	
Yqi	Isochromosome of the long arm of Y	YI

Table 31-2. Sex chromosome complement correlated with X chromatin and Y bodies in somatic interphase nuclei.*

Sex Chromosomes	Maximum Number in Diploid Somatic Nuclei	
	X Bodies	Y Bodies
45,XO	0	0
46,XX	1	0
46,XY	0	1
47,XXX	2	0
47,XXY	1	1
47,XYY	0	2
48,XXXX	3	0
48,XXXY	2	1
48,XXYY	1	2
49,XXXXX	4	0
49,XXXXY	3	1
49,XXXYY	2	2

*The maximum number of X chromatin bodies in diploid somatic nuclei is one less than the number of Xs, whereas the maximum number of Y fluorescent bodies is equivalent to the number of Ys in the chromosome constitution.

Differentiation of Genital Ducts (Fig 31—6)

By the seventh week of intrauterine life, the fetus is equipped with the primordia of both male and female genital ducts. The Müllerian ducts, if allowed to persist, form the Fallopian tubes, the uterus, the cervix, and the upper third of the vagina. The Wolffian ducts, on the other hand, have the potentiality of differentiating into the epididymis, vas deferens, seminal vesicles, and ejaculatory ducts of the male. In the presence of a functional testis, the Müllerian ducts involute under the influence of the "Müllerian duct inhibitory factor," a nonsteroidal macromolecule secreted by Sertoli cells. This substance acts "locally" to cause Müllerian duct repression ipsilaterally. The differentiation of the Wolffian duct is stimulated by testosterone secretion from the testis. In the presence of an ovary or no gonad, Müllerian duct differentiation occurs and the Wolffian ducts involute.

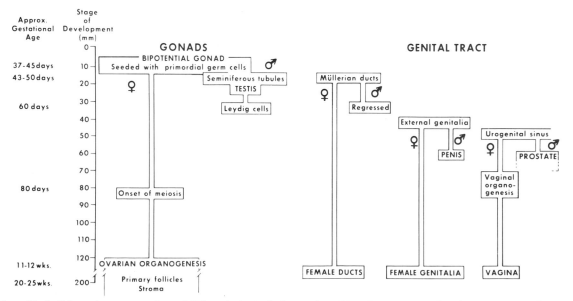

Figure 31—5. Schematic sequence of sexual differentiation in the human fetus. Note that testicular differentiation precedes all other forms of differentiation.

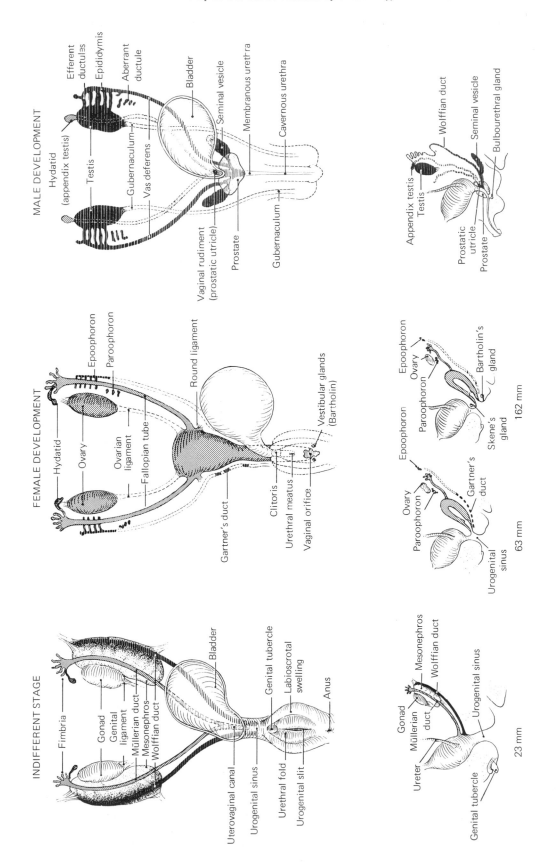

Figure 31—6. Embryonic differentiation of male and female genital ducts from Wolffian and Müllerian primordia. *A*: Indifferent stage showing large mesonephric body. *B*: Female ducts. Remnants of the mesonephros and Wolffian ducts are now termed the epoophoron, paroophoron, and Gartner's duct. *C*: Male ducts before descent into scrotum. The only Müllerian remnant is the testicular appendix. The prostatic utricle (vagina masculinus) is derived from the urogenital sinus. (Redrawn from Corning and Wilkins.)

Up to the eighth fetal week, the external genitalia of both sexes are identical and have the capacity to differentiate in either direction (Fig 31–7). There is an inherent tendency for the external genitalia to feminize, and this requires no hormonal stimulation. Differentiation along male lines is dependent upon stimulation by testosterone—specifically, its 5a reduced metabolite dihydrotestosterone. Under the influence of dihydrotestosterone, the following events take place: (1) the genital tubercle will enlarge to form a phallus; (2) fusion of the urogenital slit occurs to form a penile urethra; and (3) posterior descent of the labioscrotal swellings occurs to form the scrotum. Fig 31–8 is a diagrammatic summary of sex determination and differentiation.

PSYCHOSEXUAL DIFFERENTIATION

A person's legal and social designation of sex, as well as his psychosexual identification in relationship to his own and to the opposite sex, make up the gender role. Studies in man indicate that gender role is not coded by sex chromosomes, gonads, or sex steroids. Sexuality is apparently "imprinted" by words and attitudes of those around the child, by clothes, and by comparison of his own genitalia with those of others. In the absence of ambiguous attitudes on the part of the parents, sexual identity usually is well established by 18–30 months of age. Once gender identity is fixed, even the paradoxical development of secondary sexual characteristics of the opposite sex may not shake this conviction of sexual identity.

CLASSIFICATION OF ERRORS IN SEX DIFFERENTIATION

Disorders of sexual differentiation are the result of an abnormality in the complex process of differentiation which originates in genetic information on the X and Y chromosomes, as well as the autosomes, and results in the final product, the fertile adult male or female (Fig 31–8). A **true hermaphrodite** is defined as a person who possesses both ovarian and testicular tissue. A **male pseudohermaphrodite** is one whose gonads are exclusively testes but whose genital ducts or external genitalia, or both, exhibit incomplete masculinization in one or more respects (female phenotypic characteristics). A **female pseudohermaphrodite** is a person with exclusively ovarian gonadal tissue but whose genital development exhibits a masculine appearance.

CLASSIFICATION OF ANOMALOUS SEXUAL DEVELOPMENT
(Table 31–3)

1. SEMINIFEROUS TUBULE DYSGENESIS (STD): CHROMATIN-POSITIVE KLINEFELTER'S SYNDROME & ITS VARIANTS

STD or Klinefelter's syndrome is one of the most common forms (1:500 men) of primary hypogonadism and infertility in males. There is an increased incidence among mentally retarded males (1:100 in institutionalized patients). These patients usually have a 47,XXY karyotype and a chromatin-positive buccal smear, although patients with mosaicism have been reported.

The clinical features consist of a male phenotype: small, firm testes less than 3 cm in length, with extensive seminiferous tubule hyalinization and fibrosis, clumping of Leydig cells, and absent or severely deficient spermatogenesis, which results in sterility; a eunuchoid habitus with long legs, gynecomastia (in over half of patients); personality and behavior disorders, as well as a decrease in intellect (in one-fourth of patients); and a propensity for mild diabetes mellitus, varicose veins, and chronic pulmonary disease. Hypospadias and cryptorchism are rare. An increased frequency of carcinoma of the breast has been found in patients with Klinefelter's syndrome. Plasma and urinary concentrations of pituitary gonadotropins (especially FSH) are high, and plasma testosterone levels are frequently below the normal range, with poor testosterone responses to chorionic gonadotropin ("sick" Leydig cells).

Variants of Chromatin-Positive STD:

A. 48,XXYY: This variant comprises 3% of chromatin-positive males. They are usually mentally retarded, taller than XXY patients, and exhibit a prevalence for peripheral vascular disease. An increased incidence of delinquent behavior has been reported in this group.

B. 48,XXXY and 49,XXXYY: All of these patients are more severely mentally retarded than the XXY patients. Ten percent have minor skeletal anomalies, including radioulnar synostosis.

C. 49,XXXXY: Over 35 patients with this phenotype have been reported. They exhibit a variety of skeletal anomalies, especially radioulnar synostosis, mental retardation, and hypoplastic external genitalia. Testosterone deficiency is severe, but gynecomastia is absent. Congenital heart disease, cleft palate, strabismus, microcephaly, mandibular prognathism, and hypertelorism may be present.

D. 46,XX Males: The clinical features and hormonal values are similar to those of XXY patients, but in general these patients are shorter than XXY patients. Current evidence favors the hypothesis that

Table 31—3. Classification of anomalous sexual development.

Condition	Distinguishing Features
Disorders of gonadal differentiation Seminiferous tubule dysgenesis (Klinefelter's syndrome) Syndrome of gonadal dysgenesis and its variants (Turner's syndrome) Familial and sporadic XX and XY gonadal dysgenesis and their variants True hermaphroditism Other forms	Usually attributable to anomalous sex chromosomes: karyotype, X chromatin, and Y bodies variable. Differentiation of genital ducts, external genitalia, and hormonal sex concordant with gonadal histology. Frequently associated with mental retardation and somatic abnormalities.
Female pseudohermaphroditism Congenital virilizing adrenal hyperplasia Androgens and synthetic progestogens transferred from maternal circulation Malformations of intestine and urinary tract Other teratologic factors	X-chromatin-positive: XX karyotype. Ovaries and internal ducts normal female. External genitalia may range from mild clitoral hypertrophy to simulant cryptorchid male.

Male pseudohermaphroditism
Inborn errors of testosterone biosynthesis
  Errors affecting synthesis of both corticosteroids and testosterone (variants of congenital adrenal hyperplasia)
    Cholesterol 20a-hydroxylase deficiency (congenital lipoid adrenal hyperplasia)
    3β-Hydroxysteroid dehydrogenase deficiency
    17a-Hydroxylase deficiency
  Errors primarily affecting testosterone biosynthesis
    17,20-Desmolase (lyase) deficiency
    17β-Hydroxysteroid oxidoreductase deficiency (Reifenstein's syndrome?)
End organ insensitivity to androgenic hormones
  Complete syndrome of testicular feminization
  Incomplete syndrome of testicular feminization
Male pseudohermaphroditism with normal virilization at puberty (delay of onset of Leydig cell function, or transient fetal Leydig cell insufficiency)
  Familial perineal hypospadias with ambiguous development of urogenital sinus and male puberty (pseudovaginal perineoscrotal hypospadias; 5a-reductase deficiency)
Less severe forms of hypospadias
Ambiguous genitalia due to dysgenetic male pseudohermaphroditism
  X-chromatin-negative variants of the syndrome of gonadal dysgenesis (eg, XO, XY; XYp−)
  Incomplete form of XY gonadal dysgenesis
  Associated with degenerative renal disease
Female genital ducts in otherwise normal men (uteri herniae inguinale)
Maternal ingestion of estrogens or progestogens
Other forms
	X-chromatin-negative: XY karyotype. Testes only; some authors exclude dysgenetic testes due to chromosomal anomalies from this group, but for clinical consideration this category is regarded as belonging in the group of ambiguous genitalia due to dysgenetic male pseudohermaphroditism. The genital ducts are usually male. The external genitalia vary in appearance from mild hypospadias to structures simulating female genitalia, attributable to insufficient production of testosterone by fetal testes during period of sex differentiation and defects in response to target tissues to androgen.

Unclassified forms of abnormal sexual development
In males
  Cryptorchism
  Anorchia (the "vanishing testes" syndrome)
  Familial forms of primary hypogonadism and gynecomastia (Rosewater's syndrome)
In females
  Absence or anomalous development of uterus and Fallopian tubes
  Congenital absence of the vagina
  Rokitansky-Küstner syndrome
	A heterogeneous group of disorders of uncertain cause. Some may be variants of other forms of intersexuality. Sex chromosomes, however, are presumptively normal, and ambiguity of genitalia is not usually a prominent feature.

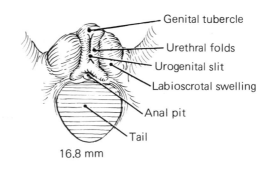

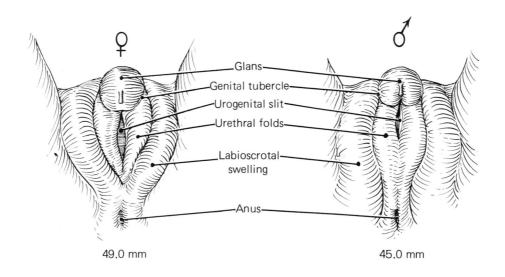

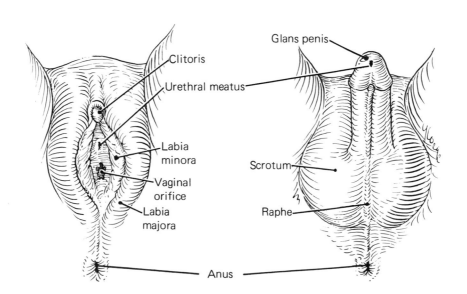

Figure 31—7. Differentiation of male and female external genitalia from bipotential primordia.

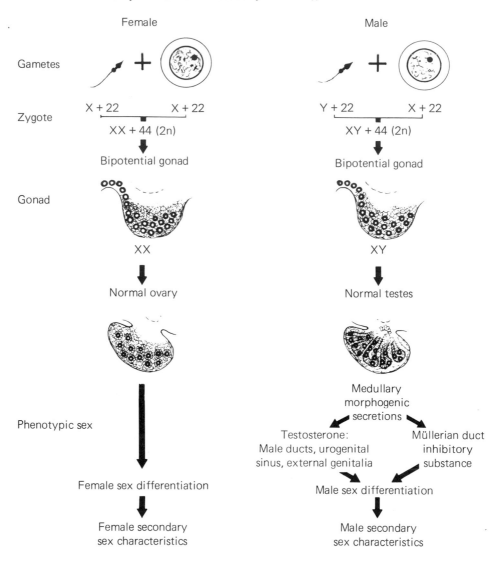

Figure 31—8. Diagrammatic summation of human sexual differentiation.

these patients have a mosaic karyotype with a cell line containing a Y chromosome which has been either lost or is undetected.

2. SYNDROME OF GONADAL DYSGENESIS: TURNER'S SYNDROME & ITS VARIANTS

Turner's Syndrome: 45,X Gonadal Dysgenesis

The 45,X karyotype may arise through a variety of chromosomal errors, either as a consequence of loss of an X or Y chromosome during meiosis in a parent cell or through mitotic errors after fertilization.

These patients are phenotypic sexually infantile females who have a constellation of somatic anomalies. They have a distinctive facies, with micrognathia,

epicanthal folds, low-set ears, and ptosis. The chest is shieldlike and the neck is short, broad, and webbed (40%). Other features include coarctation of the aorta (20%), unexplained hypertension (15%), structural abnormalities of the kidney (60%) such as horseshoe kidneys, double collection systems, retrocaval ureters, and other anomalies. A routine intravenous urogram is indicated in all patients with gonadal dysgenesis. Other features noted are lymphedema of the hands and feet, pigmented nevi, cubitus valgus, short fourth metacarpals (60%), and recurrent otitis media. The 2 least variable features are short stature (average height 55 inches with a range of 48—58 inches) and lack of gonadal function. The internal structures as well as the external genitalia are feminized but immature. The gonads are typically "streaklike" and contain only fibrous stroma arranged in whorls. Obesity, diabetes mellitus, thyroiditis, and osteoporosis are not infrequent. Plasma and urinary gonadotropins—particularly FSH—are elevated, especially in early infancy and after 10 years of age. Since ovarian function is absent, puberty does not ensue.

X-Chromatin-Positive Variants of Gonadal Dysgenesis

Patients with structural abnormalities of the X chromosome (deletions and additions) and mosaicism with XX cell lines may manifest the somatic as well as the gonadal features of the "syndrome of gonadal dysgenesis." Evidence suggests that genes on both the long and short arm of the X chromosome control gonadal differentiation, whereas genes on only the short arms of the X prevent the short stature and the somatic anomalies which are seen in 45,X patients. In general, mosaicism with a 46,XX cell line in association with a 45,X cell line will modify the phenotype toward normal. A few patients with 45,X/46,XX mosaicism have even had normal gonadal function.

X-Chromatin-Negative Variants of the
Syndrome of Gonadal Dysgenesis

These patients have mosaicism with a Y-bearing cell line: XO/XY, XO/XYY, XO/XY/XYY, or possibly a structurally abnormal Y chromosome. Phenotypically, these patients range from females with the features of Turner's syndrome through patients with ambiguous genitalia to (rarely) completely virilized males. Gonadal differentiation varies from bilateral streaks to bilateral dysgenetic testes, along with asymmetric development, ie, a streak on one side and a dysgenetic—or, rarely, a good testicle—on the other side. The development of the external genitalia as well as of the internal ducts usually correlates well with the degree of testicular differentiation and, presumably, the capacity of the fetal testes to secrete Müllerian duct inhibitory factor and testosterone. The propensity of these patients to develop gonadal tumors warrants prophylactic operative excision of the streaks or dysgenetic testicles. These patients invariably manifest some of the somatic stigmas of the syndrome of gonadal dysgenesis, especially short stature.

3. PURE GONADAL DYSGENESIS

These patients are phenotypic females with bilateral "streak" gonads and sexual infantilism. They have normal stature and lack the somatic stigmata of Turner's syndrome. The karyotype may be XX or XY, and familial cases have been reported.

4. TRUE HERMAPHRODITISM

By definition, these patients have both ovarian and testicular tissue present in either the same or opposite gonads. Clinically, the internal and external genitalia are usually ambiguous. Three-fourths of these patients have been reared as males, but they have variable degrees of hypospadias. Cryptorchism and inguinal hernia, which may contain a gonad or uterus, are present in 50% of cases. The differentiation of the internal ducts follows that of the ipsilateral gonad. Infertility is the invariable rule, and malignant degeneration of the gonads is common. Sixty percent of true hermaphrodites have a 46,XX karyotype, 20% have XY, and 10% have mosaicism or XX/XY chimerism.

Gonadal Neoplasms in Dysgenetic Gonads

The prevalence of gonadal neoplasms is greatly increased in patients with certain types of dysgenetic gonads. Dysgerminomas, seminomas, teratomas, and gonadoblastomas are found most frequently. Gonadal tumors are rare in patients with Klinefelter's syndrome and 45,X gonadal dysgenesis. The frequency is increased (1) in XO/XY mosaics and in other variants of the syndrome of gonadal dysgenesis in patients whose karyotypes contain a structurally normal or abnormal Y chromosome; and (2) in XY gonadal dysgenesis, either with a female phenotype or with ambiguous genitalia. Prophylactic castration is advised in these 2 categories as well as in individuals with gonadal dysgenesis who manifest signs of virilization, regardless of karyotype.

The gonad should be preserved in patients who are being raised as males only if it is a relatively normal testicle that can be relocated in the scrotum. The fact that a gonad is palpable in the scrotum does not preclude malignant degeneration and spread since seminomas tend to metastasize at an early stage before a local mass is obvious.

FEMALE PSEUDOHERMAPHRODITISM

These patients have normal ovaries and Müllerian derivatives associated with ambiguous external genitalia. In the absence of testes, a female fetus will masculinize if subjected to androgens from an extragonadal source. The degree of masculinization is dependent upon the stage of differentiation at the time of exposure. After 12 weeks of gestation, androgens will produce only clitoral hypertrophy. Rarely, ambiguous genitalia, which superficially resemble those produced by androgens, are the result of teratogenic malformations (Fig 31–9).

Congenital Adrenal Hyperplasia (Table 31–4)

There are 6 major types of adrenal hyperplasia, all inherited as an autosomal recessive gene. The common denominator of all 6 types is a defect in the synthesis of cortisol which results in an increase in ACTH and in adrenal hyperplasia. Both males and females can be affected, but males are rarely diagnosed at birth unless they are salt-losers and manifest adrenal crises. Types I–III are defects which are confined to the adrenal

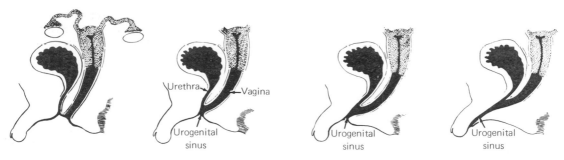

Figure 31–9. Female pseudohermaphroditism induced by prenatal exposure to androgens. Exposure after the 12th fetal week leads only to clitoral hypertrophy (diagram on left). Exposure at progressively earlier stages of differentiation (depicted from left to right in drawings) leads to retention of the urogenital sinus and labioscrotal fusion. If exposure occurs sufficiently early, the labia will fuse to form a penile urethra.

gland and produce virilization. Types IV–VI have in common blocks in cortisol and sex steroid synthesis, both in the adrenals and in the gonads. These latter types produce primarily incomplete masculinization in the male and little or no virilization in the female.

A. Type I–Partial C_{21} Hydroxylase Defect (Simple Virilization): This is the most common type of congenital adrenal hyperplasia. A partial defect in C_{21} hydroxylation leads to simple virilism. These patients conserve sodium normally since aldosterone secretion is normal or increased. The diagnosis can be confirmed by demonstrating elevated levels of 17-ketosteroids and pregnanetriol in the urine as well as elevated levels of plasma 17-hydroxyprogesterone.

B. Type II–Complete C_{21} Defect (Virilization With Salt-Losing Tendency): The salt-losing variant is a more severe defect in C_{21} hydroxylation and results in impairment of cortisol and aldosterone secretion. Patients with this defect manifest severe adrenal crises in the first few weeks of life, and, unless diagnosed and treated, they often die. The diagnosis is confirmed by finding elevated 17-ketosteroids in the urine and an elevated plasma 17-hydroxyprogesterone in a patient with a low serum sodium and elevated potassium.

C. Type III–C_{11} Hydroxylase Defect (Virilization With Hypertension): This is a rare form which results in virilization and hypertension due to the salt and water retaining effects of increased deoxycorticosterone secretion.

D. Type IV–3β-Hydroxysteroid Dehydrogenase Defect (Male or Female Pseudohermaphroditism and Adrenal Insufficiency): This is a rare form of adrenal hyperplasia which produces salt loss and a defect in cortisol and sex steroid secretion. Males are incompletely masculinized, and females are slightly virilized. The presence of high urinary 17-ketosteroids associated with urinary dehydroepiandrosterone and other 3β-hydroxysteroid elevations is diagnostic.

E. Type V–17α-Hydroxylase Defect (Male Pseudohermaphroditism, Sexual Infantilism, Hypertension, and Hypokalemic Alkalosis): These patients cannot make 17α-hydroxyprogesterone and its products—androgens, estrogens, and cortisol. Increased secretion of deoxycorticosterone leads to hypokalemic alkalosis. Affected males are incompletely masculinized and may appear to be phenotypic females, and affected females are sexually infantile.

F. Type VI–Cholesterol Desmolase Complex Defect (Male Pseudohermaphroditism, Sexual Infantilism, and Adrenal Insufficiency): This is a very early defect

Table 31–4. Clinical manifestations of various types of congenital adrenal hyperplasia.

Enzymatic Defect	Cholesterol Desmolase System (Cholesterol 20α-Hydroxylase)		3β-Hydroxysteroid Dehydrogenase		17α-Hydroxylase		11β-Hydroxylase	21α-Hydroxylase	
Type	VI		V		IV		III	II and I	
Chromosomal sex	XX	XY	XX	XY	XX	XY	XX	XY	XX	XY
External genitalia	Female	Female	Female (Clitoromegaly)	Ambiguous	Female	Female or ambiguous	Ambiguous	Male	Ambiguous	Male
Postnatal virilization	— (Sexual infantilism at puberty)		±	Mild to moderate	— (Sexual infantilism at puberty)		+	+		
Addisonian crises	+		+		—		—	+ in 40% (type II)		
Hypertension	—		—		+		+	—		

in the synthesis of all steroids which results in severe adrenal insufficiency and death in early infancy if untreated. Males exhibit pseudohermaphroditism, and those with a complete defect may appear to be phenotypic females.

Maternal Androgens & Synthetic Progestogens

Masculinization of the external genitalia of female infants can occur following ingestion by the mother of testosterone or synthetic progestational agents during the first trimester of pregnancy. Norethindrone, ethisterone, norethynodrel, and medroxyprogesterone acetate have been implicated. In rare instances, masculinization of a female fetus may be secondary to an ovarian or adrenal tumor in the mother.

Malformations of the Intestine & Urinary Tract

Anomalies such as imperforate anus, renal agenesis, and other malformations of the lower intestine and urinary tract are associated with genital abnormalities. The term nonspecific female pseudohermaphroditism has been suggested for this group of infants.

MALE PSEUDOHERMAPHRODITISM

Male pseudohermaphroditism is the condition in which the gonads are testes but the genital ducts or external genitalia are not completely virilized. Male pseudohermaphroditism can result from any of the following: (1) failure of testicular differentiation, (2) failure of secretion of testosterone and Müllerian duct

inhibiting substance, (3) failure of target tissues to respond to testosterone or dihydrotestosterone, and (4) failure of conversion of testosterone to dihydrotestosterone.

Inborn Errors of Testosterone Biosynthesis

Fig 31—10 demonstrates the major pathways in testosterone biosynthesis; each step is associated with an inherited (autosomal recessive) defect which results in incomplete masculinization. Steps 1, 2, and 3 are associated with errors in synthesis of both corticosteroid and testosterone synthesis:

(1) **20,22-Desmolase deficiency:** See Congenital Adrenal Hyperplasia.

(2) **3β-Hydroxysteroid deficiency:** See Congenital Adrenal Hyperplasia.

(3) **17α-Hydroxylase deficiency:** See Congenital Adrenal Hyperplasia.

The following errors affect only testosterone synthesis:

(4) **17,20-Desmolase deficiency:** These patients have ambiguous genitalia, inguinal or intra-abdominal testes, and an XY sex chromosome constitution. At puberty, incomplete virilization without gynecomastia may occur. If the diagnosis is made in infancy, these patients can be reared as males and treated with testosterone to induce male secondary sexual characteristics and phallic growth.

(5) **17β-Hydroxysteroid oxidoreductase deficiency:** These patients have female or ambiguous external genitalia, inguinal testes, male duct development, and progressive virilization with clitoral growth at puberty, often with concurrent breast development. Levels of plasma androstenedione and estrone are markedly ele-

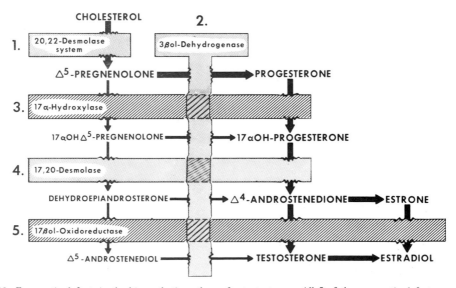

Figure 31—10. Enzymatic defects in the biosynthetic pathway for testosterone. All 5 of the enzymatic defects cause male pseudohermaphroditism in affected males. Even though all of the blocks affect both gonadal and adrenal cortical steroidogenesis, those at steps 1, 2, and 3 are associated with major abnormalities in the biosynthesis of glucocorticoids and mineralocorticoids.

vated because their conversion to testosterone and estradiol, respectively, is diminished. The usual androstenedione:testosterone ratio is reversed.

Previously, all familial cases of ambiguous external genitalia, male genital ducts, gynecomastia, and puberal virilization were grouped together as "incomplete feminizing testes syndrome." Some of these cases, as well as those of Reifenstein's syndrome (hypospadias, postpuberal testicular atrophy, azoospermia, androgen deficiency, and gynecomastia), may represent variable deficiencies of 17β-hydroxysteroid oxidoreductase.

End Organ Insensitivity to Androgenic Hormones (Complete Testicular Feminization)

The inability to utilize dihydrotestosterone as a result of a defect in cytoplasmic receptors for androgens results in a disorder in which XY males resemble females. In its complete form, these males have no sexual hair, have normal-appearing female external genitalia with a blind vaginal pouch, testes which are inguinal, intra-abdominal, or in the labioscrotal folds, and no Müllerian structure. At puberty, feminization occurs with normal breast development. These patients are usually diagnosed during evaluation for amenorrhea. The increased risk of malignant degeneration of the testes makes orchiectomy indicated.

Male Pseudohermaphroditism With Normal Virilization at Puberty

A. Familial Perineal Hypospadias With Ambiguous Development of the Urogenital Sinus and Male Puberty (Pseudovaginal Perineal Scrotal Hypospadias): These males are born with testicles and normal male internal genital ducts. The phallus is usually small and hypospadiac. There is persistence of the urogenital sinus with a blind vaginal pouch. In severe cases, a separate urethral and vaginal orifice is present. Recent studies indicate that these patients have a defect in 5a-reductase, so that they cannot convert testosterone to dihydrotestosterone (Fig 31–11). At puberty, they virilize and have phallic enlargement, male sexual hair, and a male sexual identity. No acne, facial hair, or temporal recession of the hairline occurs. Study of these patients demonstrates that virilization of the genital tubercle and urogenital sinus is under the control of dihydrotestosterone, while development of the

Wolffian structures is primarily testosterone dependent.

B. Hypospadias: Hypospadias occurs as an isolated finding in one in 700 newborn males. Although on embryologic grounds deficient virilization of the external genitalia implies subnormal Leydig cell function in utero or end organ resistance, in most patients there are few grounds for suspecting either mechanism. Thus, nonendocrine factors which affect differentiation of the primordia may be found in a variety of genetic syndromes. Aarskog studied 100 patients with hypospadias prospectively and found one patient to be a genetic female with congenital adrenal hyperplasia, 5 with sex chromosome abnormalities, and one with the incomplete form of XY gonadal dysgenesis. Nine patients were from pregnancies in which the mother had taken progestational compounds during the first trimester. Thus, a pathogenetic mechanism was found in 15% of these patients.

C. Ambiguous Genitalia Associated With Degenerative Renal Disease: Several cases are recorded of male pseudohermaphroditism associated with degenerative renal disease and hypertension. Defective masculinization has also been associated with Wilms's tumor. In this syndrome, both the kidneys and the testes are dysgenetic and, thus, a predisposition for renal neoplasms exists.

UNCLASSIFIED FORMS OF ABNORMAL SEXUAL DEVELOPMENT

Anorchia

Rarely, cryptorchid boys will have no gonadal tissue. The ducts are male but end blindly. The karyotype is XY, and the presence of normal male genitalia suggests that testes were present in fetal life to initiate male development; resorption must have occurred after that period. Administration of human chorionic gonadotropin, 500–2000 units IM daily for 5 days, is a useful test of Leydig cell function. In the presence of normal Leydig cell function, there will be a rise in plasma testosterone from concentrations less than 20 ng/100 ml to over 200 ng/100 ml. In infants under 4 years of age and children over 10, levels of plasma

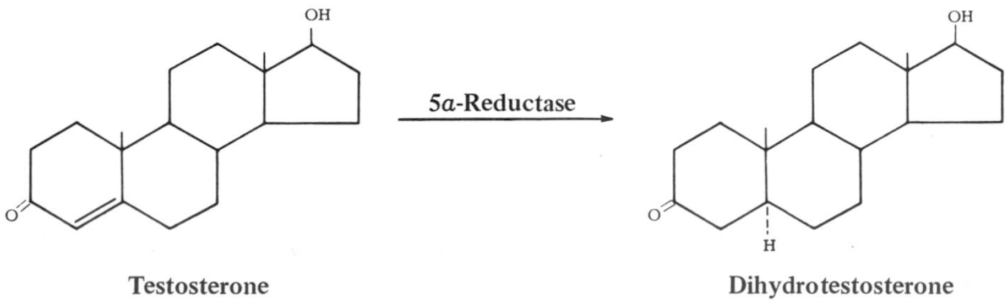

Figure 31–11. Metabolism of testosterone.

gonadotropin, particularly FSH, are a sensitive index of gonadal integrity. One can also utilize the LH and FSH response to the infusion of luteinizing hormone-releasing factor (LRF) to diagnose the absence of gonadal feedback on the hypothalamus and pituitary. In agonadal children, 100 μg of LRF infused as a bolus will elicit a marked rise in both LH and FSH which is greater than is achieved in both prepuberal and puberal children with normal gonadal function.

Micropenis

Males with congenital hypopituitarism can present with micropenis and hypoglycemia at birth. These infants will respond with phallic enlargement to either local testosterone ointment or 40 mg of testosterone enanthate IM monthly for 3 months.

MANAGEMENT OF PATIENTS WITH INTERSEX PROBLEMS

Choice of Sex

The goal of the physician who has a patient with ambiguous genitalia is to diagnose the problem and to assign a sex for rearing which is most compatible with a well-adjusted life and sexual adequacy. Once the sex for rearing is assigned, the gender role is reinforced by the appropriate employment of whatever surgical, hormonal, or psychologic measures are indicated. Except in female pseudohermaphrodites, ambiguities of the genitalia are caused by lesions that almost always make the patient infertile. In recommending male sex assignment, the adequacy of the size of the phallus should be the most important consideration. Except for those with hypopituitarism, boys with micropenis rarely develop a penis of adequate size. Therefore, unless one can expect the adult phallus to be of adequate size, it is much better to assign female sex to a child with

Table 31–5. Steps in the diagnosis of intersexuality in infancy and childhood.*

History: family history, pregnancy (hormones), "crises," virilization
Inspection
Palpation of inguinal region and labioscrotal folds and rectal examination
Oral mucosal smear—X chromatin pattern; karyotype—sex chromosome constitution
Excretion of 17-ketosteroids and pregnanetriol; serum 17-hydroxyprogesterone
Serum electrolytes and urea nitrogen
Provisional diagnosis

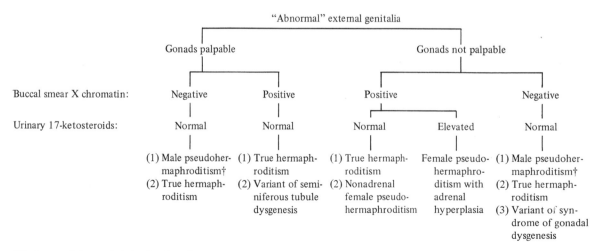

"Vaginogram" (urogenital sinus): selected cases
Endoscopy, laparotomy, gonadal biopsy: restricted to suspected male pseudohermaphrodites, true hermaphrodites, and selected instances of nonadrenal female pseudohermaphroditism

*From Grumbach MM: In: *Pediatrics,* 13th ed. Holt LE Jr, McIntosh R, Barnett HL (editors). Appleton-Century-Crofts, 1962.
†Excretion of 17-ketosteroids is increased in male pseudohermaphrodites who have congenital adrenal hyperplasia due to a defect in 3β-hydroxysteroid dehydrogenase.

ambiguous genitalia than to rear him as an inadequate male.

Differential Diagnosis

The steps in the diagnosis of intersexuality are delineated in Table 31–5.

Reassignment of Sex

Change of sex of assignment prior to 18 months of life is possible; after 2½ years of age, serious psychiatric consequences may result. Thus, a change of sex after 18 months of age should be undertaken only after much deliberation and with provision for long-term supervision and counseling.

Reconstructive Surgery

It is desirable to complete reconstructive surgery prior to 18 months of age. In children raised as females, the clitoris should be salvaged, if possible, by a clitoral recession procedure. Reconstruction of a vagina, if necessary, should be deferred until requested by the patient.

Removal of the gonads in children with the variant forms of gonadal dysgenesis should be performed at the time of initial repair of the external genitalia because gonadoblastomas, seminomas, and dysgerminomas have been reported to occur during the first decade.

In a patient with testicular feminization, the gonads should be left in situ if they are not situated in the labia majora to provide estrogen during early puberty. The patient may then undergo prophylactic castration, having had her female identity reinforced by normal feminization at puberty.

In patients reared as females with incomplete testicular feminization—or in those forms of errors of testosterone biosynthesis in which some degree of masculinization occurs at puberty (but in patients who will be reared as females)—gonadectomy should be performed prior to adolescence.

Hormonal Substitution Therapy

Cyclic estrogen and progestogen treatment is used in individuals reared as females with uterine tissue. Estrogen alone is utilized in a female without a uterus. In males, virilization is achieved by depot testosterone enanthate, 200 mg IM every 3–4 weeks.

Psychologic Management

The physician should recall that sex is not a single biologic entity but the summation of many morphogenetic, functional, and psychologic potentialities. There must never be any doubt in the mind of the parent or of the child as to his or her "true sex." Chromosomal and gonadal sex are secondary matters; the sex of rearing is paramount. With proper surgical reconstruction and hormone substitution, the individual whose psychosexual gender is discordant with chromosomal gender need not have any psychologic catastrophes as long as the sex of rearing is accepted with conviction by the family and others during the critical early years. Anatomic abnormalities, it must be stressed, do not predispose to homosexual tendencies. These individuals should reach adulthood as well-adjusted, virile men or feminine women capable of normal heterosexual interaction, albeit usually not of procreation.

●   ●   ●

References

Federman DD: *Abnormal Sexual Development.* Saunders, 1967.

Grumbach MM, Van Wyk JJ: Disorders of sex differentiation. Pages 423–501 in: *Textbook of Endocrinology,* 5th ed. Williams RH (editor). Saunders, 1974.

Hamerton JL: *Human Cytogenetics.* 2 vols. Academic Press, 1971.

Jones HW, Scott WW: *Hermaphroditism, Genital Anomalies, and Related Endocrine Disorders,* 2nd ed. Williams & Wilkins, 1971.

Levine H: *Clinical Cytogenetics.* Little, Brown, 1971.

Money J, Ehrhardt AA: *Man and Woman, Boy and Girl: The Differentiation and Dimorphism of Gender Identity From Conception to Maturity.* Johns Hopkins Univ Press, 1972.

Rimoin DL, Schimke RH: *Genetic Disorders of the Endocrine Glands.* Mosby, 1971.

32 ...
Renovascular Hypertension

Urologic renal disease is a not uncommon cause of hypertension. However, most cases of high blood pressure (ie, essential hypertension) are of unknown cause. Coarctation of the aorta, polycystic kidneys, glomerulonephritis, and polyarteritis nodosa are often accompanied by hypertension.

Etiology

Many years have passed since Goldblatt demonstrated in experimental animals that protracted renal ischemia could produce hypertension. In dogs, unilateral renal ischemia can cause transient hypertension, or it can cause no change at all if the other kidney is not removed or rendered ischemic. In man, however, there is unequivocal evidence that unilateral renal ischemia causes hypertension which can be cured by nephrectomy or reconstruction of the renal artery.

Pathogenesis

Why the ischemic kidney causes elevation of blood pressure is not known. The most attractive theory has been the following: Decreased blood flow through the afferent glomerular arteries leads to an increased number of secretory granules in the juxtaglomerular bodies, which are thought to elaborate renin. This enzyme reacts with an alpha$_2$ globulin to produce angiotensin I, a rather inert substance. When acted upon by a converting enzyme, it is changed to angiotensin II, a potent vasoconstrictor which also acts to increase aldosterone secretion by the adrenal cortex. Thus, hypertension is established.

It is true that, in severe hypertension caused by stenosis of the renal artery, renin has been recovered in increased amounts from the renal vein of the ischemic organ and evidence of hyperaldosteronism (hypokalemic alkalosis) has been observed. However, in milder hypertensives, such increased humoral activity may not be found.

Pathology

The common causes of stenosis of the renal artery are arteriosclerotic plaques, fibromuscular hyperplasia of the media (which usually affects relatively young females and children), neurofibromatosis (most often seen in children), and embolism or thrombosis. Stenosis in a renal artery may protect that kidney from the deleterious effects of hypertension while the other

kidney remains hypertensive. Thus, the ischemic kidney is ultimately the better of the two; it should be preserved unless considerable atrophy has occurred.

In autopsy material, poor correlation between the presence of hypertension and stenosis of the renal artery has been observed. A lesion producing at least a 50% (and probably even a 70%) reduction in luminal diameter appears to be necessary in order to reduce renal plasma flow to the point where clinically significant ischemia is produced. Thus, the significance of a stenosis shown on aortography can only be estimated by tests of differential renal function or estimation of renin levels of renal vein blood.

The changes observed in the pyelonephritic kidney have already been described (Chapter 12). From the standpoint of the genesis of hypertension, the most striking lesion is the marked thickening of the arteriolar walls. There is considerable variation in the arteriolar changes in the renal parenchyma involved by other renal lesions, such as tumor and hydronephrosis. Correlation of these changes with high blood pressure is poor, but postoperative return to normotension has been reported as a result of nephrectomy in many instances.

Other urologic renal lesions causing hypertension include ureteral and ureteropelvic junction obstruction with hydronephrosis, renal hypoplasia, ligation of a segmental branch of a renal artery, and tuberculosis. Preoperatively, elevated renin concentrations have been demonstrated in such cases. Hypertension is common with Wilms's tumor and is occasionally observed in patients with renal adenocarcinoma.

Clinical Findings

The clinical features of those renal diseases that may cause hypertension have already been discussed (see chronic pyelonephritis, thrombosis of the renal artery, aneurysm of the renal artery, hydronephrosis, renal tumors, and renal tuberculosis).

A. Symptoms: Hypertension caused by renal ischemia should be considered (1) if there is a recent onset of hypertension in the absence of a family history of hypertension, particularly if the patient is under 30 or over 50 years of age; (2) if the patient has had severe flank or abdominal pain or trauma (suggesting embolism or thrombosis of a renal artery), with or without hematuria; (3) if there is abrupt acceleration of a

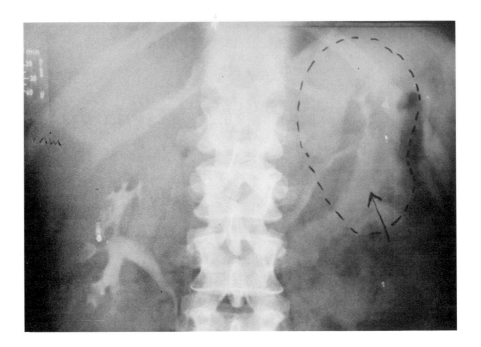

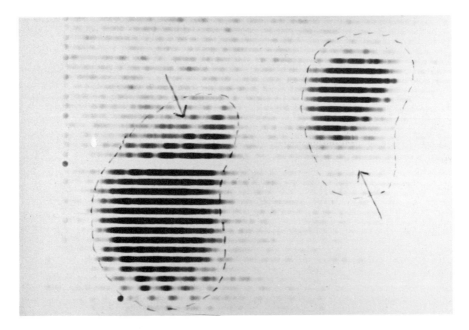

Figure 32—1. Renovascular hypertension. *Above:* Excretory urogram shows contraction of lower half of left kidney and failure of visualization of lower pole calyces. Right urogram normal. *Below:* Rectilinear scan, same patient, demonstrating ischemia of lower half of left kidney. Small area of upper pole of right kidney also ischemic. Renal angiogram showed stenosis of artery to lower pole of left kidney.

preexisting hypertension, especially in an older person; or (4) in the presence of severe hypertension at any age.

B. Signs: In addition to a relatively sustained diastolic hypertension, changes typical of malignant hypertension may be found in the retinas. A systolic bruit should be sought anteriorly and posteriorly over the renal areas. The presence of an aortic aneurysm or vascular insufficiency of the extremities is suggestive.

C. Laboratory Findings: Bacteria and pus cells in the urine may indicate chronic pyelonephritis. In the malignant phase of hypertension, proteinuria, casts, and red cells will be seen. Unless malignant hypertension, polycystic disease, bilateral atrophic pyelonephritis, or bilateral renal artery stenosis is present, total renal function (as measured by PSP test and creatinine clearance) is usually normal. Hypokalemic alkalosis suggestive of aldosteronism may be found. Lactic acid dehydrogenase may be elevated in the presence of bilateral chronic pyelonephritis or malignant hypertension.

D. X-Ray Findings: Excretory urography is the best generally available screening test for the presence of renal ischemia (Figs 32–1 and 32–2). It makes the presumptive diagnosis in 70–80% of cases. The bowel should be well prepared. Since delay in appearance of the radiopaque medium is an important sign, exposures should be made at 2, 3, and 5 minutes after rapid injection. The following findings are suggestive of renal ischemia: (1) a kidney at least 1 cm shorter than its mate (normally, the right kidney is 0.5 cm shorter than the left); (2) lack of function of one kidney (with normal pyelocalyceal architecture as shown by retrograde urography); (3) delayed appearance of visualization on the early films; (4) the occurrence, at times, of hyperconcentration of the radiopaque medium due to marked overreabsorption of water (a phenomenon which may be accentuated by making urograms with the patient hydrated); (5) narrow, delicate renal calyces, renal pelvis, and ureter because of diminution in the volume of urine excreted; (6) partial atrophy (contraction) of one pole; (7) normal, but small, calyceal pattern in a small kidney; and (8) scalloping or notching of the upper ureter caused by secondary arterial collaterals.

The urographic changes of chronic pyelonephritis, hydronephrosis, and polycystic kidneys should be obvious.

Although hyperconcentration of the radiopaque material typically occurs in the ischemic kidney because of overreabsorption of water, excretory urograms usually fail to reveal it. The urea washout test will more often reflect this phenomenon (Fournier & others, 1973). Osmotic diuresis is initiated with urea; the radiopaque material is "washed out" of the normal kidney on late films but will be visible in the ischemic organ because of the relative concentration of the iodide caused by over-reabsorption of water by the renal tubules.

Renal angiography (including selective angiography) will demonstrate stenosis of the renal artery caused by an atheromatous plaque (usually proximal), fibromuscular hyperplasia (usually distal), and neurofibromatosis (proximal) (Fig 32–3). When stenosis is severe, secondary periureteral collateral circulation may be seen (Fig 32–2).

E. Relative Renal Function Tests: If the history, physical examination, urinalysis, tests of total renal function, and excretory urograms suggest the possibility of renal hypertension, split function studies of the kidneys should be performed. In the presence of heart failure or shock (diminished renal blood flow), normal kidneys modify their function and respond in the following manner: Urine volume, urine sodium, chloride, and BUN concentrations, total PSP excretion (test of renal blood flow), and urinary pH are reduced; and responses to clearance tests, such as creatinine, iodopyracet (Diodrast), and PAH, are lowered. In addition, there is an increase in osmolality as well as increased concentration of creatinine, nitrogen, and potassium in the urine.

The ischemic kidney reacts in similar fashion. Its basic functional characteristic is marked reabsorption of water by the renal tubules; to an even greater extent, salt (both sodium and chloride) is absorbed. On the other hand, potassium and creatinine—though excreted in amounts smaller than those excreted by the normal kidney—are poorly reabsorbed, thus leading to an increase in their concentrations per unit volume.

In the presence of renal ischemia, urea—as opposed to creatinine—is significantly reabsorbed because of the slow flow of urine through the tubules. Thus, the urea nitrogen/creatinine ratio in the urine will be low. There is also a decrease in total PSP excretion but an increase in PSP concentration per milliliter of urine (because of overreabsorption of water) and an increase in osmolality of at least 15%.

1. Excretion of water, salt, and creatinine (Howard-Rapoport test)—

a. Technic—

(1) Normal salt diet for 3 days; no antihypertensive drugs for 5 days; good hydration. If performed under anesthesia, 1 liter of 10% glucose should be administered to ensure adequate urine flow.

(2) Ureteral catheters are properly placed in the renal pelves or ureters. Urine specimens are collected for bacteriologic study. Three specimens of urine are then collected from each kidney after urine flow has become stabilized. The volume of one of the specimens should be 40–60 ml. The volume of each is measured and sodium and creatinine concentrations determined.

b. Interpretation—The combinations of "positive" results shown in Table 32–1 suggest that nephrectomy or vascular reconstruction will tend to reduce hypertension.

Most cases of unilateral chronic pyelonephritis will yield a "negative" test (sodium concentration not decreased, or increased up to 40%; creatinine concentration decreased 33–66%). Nephrectomy, in this group, will not affect the hypertension. Bilateral renal lesions, particularly if they are of equal degree, may give a negative or equivocal test; such lesions are ob-

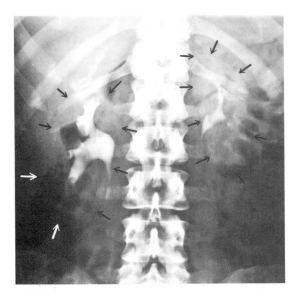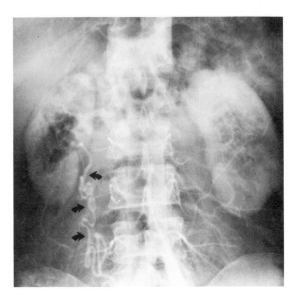

Figure 32—2. Hypertension caused by stenosis of left renal artery. ***Left:*** Ten-minute excretory urogram showing small left kidney with delayed and impaired excretion of radiopaque fluid. Because of diminution of urine volume, calyces and pelvis are smaller than in the contralateral kidney. ***Right:*** Angiogram in patient with complete occlusion of right main renal artery. Marked secondary periureteral collateral circulation allows persistence of some renal function.

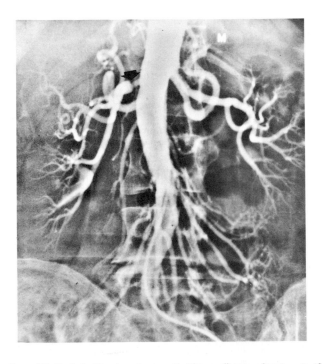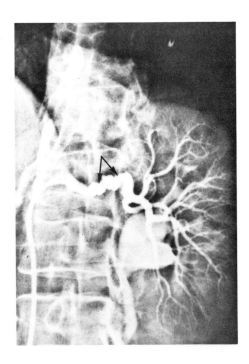

Figure 32—3. ***Left:*** Renal angiogram, "midstream" type, showing significant arteriosclerotic plaque at take-off of right renal artery (see arrow). ***Right:*** Selective angiogram of left kidney, right posterior oblique position. Fibromuscular hyperplasia of renal artery.

TABLE 32–1. Interpretation of Howard test.

Lesion	The ischemic kidney (in relation to the normal kidney) shows:		
	Urine Volume	Sodium Concentration	Creatinine Concentration
Stenosis of main renal artery	↓ 60% or more	↓ 15% or more	↑ 50–100%
Stenosis of branch of renal artery; chronic pyelonephritis with distal small artery disease	↓ 33–50%	↓ 0–20%	↑ 20–50%

TABLE 32–2. Interpretation of Stamey test.

Lesion	Urine Volume	PAH Concentration
Stenosis of main artery, unilateral	↓ 67% or more	↑ 100% or more
Stenosis of main artery, bilateral	↓ 40% or more	↑ 36% or more
Stenosis of segmental artery, unilateral. Also essential hypertension, glomerulonephritis, chronic pyelonephritis (rare).	↓ 50% or more	↑ 16% or more

viously more difficult to diagnose.

2. Sodium chloride-urea-ADH-PAH test (Stamey test)—This test is also based upon the demonstration of abnormal reabsorption of water by the ischemic kidney; it is designed to exaggerate the evidence of this phenomenon. A normal saline infusion containing 8% urea, vasopressin, and PAH is given after the placement of 8F plastic catheters in the midureters. (Stamey prefers to leave these catheters in place for 12–24 hours. This appears to lessen the incidence of postinstrumental ureteral obstruction.) Three collections of urine taken at 10-minute intervals from each kidney are analyzed for volume and PAH concentration. The latter is significantly increased by the kidney affected by renovascular disease. (The reader is referred to Stamey's monograph [1963] for a detailed description of the test technic.)

The ischemic kidney is revealed by its diminished urine volume and its increased concentration of PAH as compared to its mate (Table 32–2).

The combination of the Howard-Rapoport and Stamey tests increases the accuracy of diagnosis except when the arterial lesions are bilateral and equal. A "positive" test is an indication for renal aortography. Even when these tests are normal or equivocal, angiograms should still be made if the history, physical findings, and excretory urograms or isotope studies suggest the presence of renal ischemia.

3. Renal isotope studies—

a. The ^{131}I-hippurate isotope renogram—This has proved to be a good screening test for evidence of renovascular hypertension. Because of the overreabsorption of water by the tubules in the ischemic kidney, transport of the isotope to the pelvis is slow; its escape down the ureter is slowed. Furthermore, diminished renal blood flow decreases the amount of the iodide that reaches the kidney. Hence, the vascular spike from such a kidney is lower than that of its mate; its secretory phase is prolonged. Instead of the counts beginning to drop 3–5 minutes after injection, they tend to persist because of lack of "washout" (Fig 8–12).

b. The [203]Hg-chlormerodrin rectilinear scan—This measures renal tubular function and renal blood flow. It depicts the size and shape of the kidney. Thus, it

may reveal polar atrophy (Fig 32–1) but it does not differentiate chronic pyelonephritis or renal infarct from ischemia.

c. Anger camera scan—(Fig 8–5.) The ^{131}I-hippurate photos will show slow uptake of the isotope in the ischemic kidney. Because of the overreabsorption of water, there is slow transport of the iodide to the pelvis. Therefore, by 8–10 minutes there is apt to be hyperconcentration of the isotope in the parenchyma as compared to the normal kidney. At 15 minutes, the normal kidney may have cleared the isotope, yet it still lingers in the renal pelvis of the ischemic kidney. An isotope renogram can be constructed from the counts that are recorded.

The ^{99m}Tc scan will reflect diminution of blood supply to the ischemic kidney. These tests are of less help if the disease is bilateral.

F. Estimation of Renal Vein Renin Levels: Since the ischemic kidney elaborates increased amounts of renin, the precursor of angiotensin II, determination of the concentration of that substance recovered from each renal vein has proved to be of great value in establishing the diagnosis of renovascular hypertension. In order to accentuate the differences in these plasma concentrations, the patient should be on limited salt intake for a few days in order to decrease total blood volume. Kurtzman & others (1974) recommend that furosemide be given also.

If the plasma renin activity from the suspected side is 1½ or more times that recovered from the other vein, repair of that artery (or nephrectomy) has an excellent chance of relieving the hypertension. When the levels from both veins are about the same, only a few will respond to surgical treatment. Should the renal artery lesions be bilateral, this test may lose significance. It is of no value if there is only one kidney.

Summary of Plan of Study

Patients with clinical signs and symptoms of renovascular hypertension should be subjected to renal angiography. Those showing significantly stenotic lesions should have renal vein plasma renin determinations. If the involved kidney is found to elaborate at least 1½ times the renin activity of its mate, appropriate treatment is indicated. In equivocal cases, relative renal function studies should be done (Dean & Foster, 1973).

Differential Diagnosis

Essential hypertension usually develops between ages 30–50 in a person with a family history of hypertension. Intravenous urograms are normal. The tests for ischemia are negative.

Coarctation of the aorta is characterized by relatively low blood pressure in the legs, a bruit over the vascular lesion, and evidence of collateral circulation.

Pheochromocytoma may be considered, especially if hypertension occurs in paroxysms associated with sweating and palpitation. The glucagon test is usually positive (see Chapter 20). Urinary vanilmandelic acid or serum or urinary catecholamines are elevated during hypertensive seizures. Excretory urograms may reveal displacement of a kidney by the tumor. Angiography will reveal the tumor. Retroperitoneal gas insufflation will delineate a suprarenal mass.

Secondary aldosteronism may accompany renovascular hypertension. In both primary and secondary aldosteronism, hypokalemic alkalosis is present; it responds to the administration of spironolactone (Aldactone). Differentiation requires estimation of blood volume and serum sodium. In primary aldosteronism, both tend to be elevated. In secondary aldosteronism, they may be below normal.

Cushing's disease usually causes hypertension. Physical examination and hormonal assays establish the diagnosis.

The rare renal juxtaglomerular cell tumors elaborate increased amounts of renin. Findings consistent with hyperaldosteronism are found. Angiography reveals normal renal arteries but may show neovascularity in the tumor.

Treatment

Since there is some risk involved in reconstructive arterial repair, medical treatment for hypertension should be instituted. A good response is an indication for its continuance. If, however, significant hypertension persists, surgery should be done in order to protect renal function from the effects of high blood pressure. Nephrectomy is indicated for patients who have hypertension associated with serious unilateral renal lesions. The kidney should only be removed if its function is markedly deficient (eg, atrophic pyelonephritis, stenosis of the renal artery with marked atrophy, advanced hydronephrosis) or in order to save life (eg, cancer of the kidney). In the high-risk patient, nephrectomy should be considered, for it offers much lower mortality and morbidity rates than renal artery reconstruction.

Endarterectomy, homograft, sleeve resection of the involved arterial segment, or arterial shunt or graft is indicated in a case of unilateral renal artery stenosis when the involved kidney reveals fairly good function. This is potentially the best kidney since it has been protected from the adverse effects of hypertension. Postoperatively, a "reversal" of the Howard test occurs; the repaired kidney excretes more PSP, water, and salt than its mate.

Bilateral stenosis of the renal arteries, found in 50% of cases, should be treated in a similar manner, though Gittes & McLaughlin (1974) find that repair of the most serious lesion only affords control of hypertension in 85% of cases.

Since fibromuscular hyperplasia may involve intrarenal portions of the arteries, it may be necessary to remove the kidney and reconstruct them "on the bench." Autotransplantation is then accomplished.

Prognosis

If split function studies and plasma renin levels are positive and the pressure gradient between the aorta and a point distal to the renal artery lesion is at least 50 mm Hg, successful arterial repair or nephrectomy will cure the hypertension in about 40% of cases. In another 40% of cases, the hypertension will show significant improvement.

The best results are obtained in patients with fibromuscular hyperplasia (90%). Only 60% of those with atherosclerosis will respond. Nephrectomy, in unilateral lesions, offers the lowest mortality rate and the best response.

•   •   •

References

Amplatz K: Angiography in assessing renovascular hypertension: Past and present. Geriatrics 29:52, 1974.

Aurell M, Jonsson S, Vikgren P: Studies on arterial and renal venous plasma renin activity in hypertensive patients. Acta med scandinav 193:399, 1973.

Belzer FO & others: Surgical correction of advanced fibromuscular dysplasia of the renal arteries. Surgery 75:31, 1974.

Biglieri EG: Evaluation of renal vascular hypertension and primary hyperaldosteronism. California Med 115:40, Dec 1971.

Brolin I, Stener I: Collaterals in obstruction of the renal artery. Acta radiol diag 4:447, 1966.

Chassin MRG, Sullivan JM: Pharmacologic management of renovascular hypertension. JAMA 227:421, 1974.

Clayman AS, Bookstein JJ: The role of renal angiography in pediatric hypertension. Radiology 108:107, 1973.

Conn JW, Bookstein JJ, Cohen EL: Renin-secreting juxtaglomerular-cell adenoma: Preoperative clinical and angiographic diagnosis. Radiology 106:543, 1973.

Conn JW & others: The syndrome of hypertension, hyperreninemia, and secondary aldosteronism associated with renal juxtaglomerular cell tumor (primary reninism). J Urol 109:349, 1973.

Dean RH, Foster JH: Criteria for the diagnosis of renovascular hypertension. Surgery 74:926, 1973.

Fay R, Kaufman JJ: Renal hypertension in children. Urology 3:148, 1974.

Foster JH, Dean RH: Changing concepts in renovascular hypertension. S Clin North America 54:257, 1974.

Foster JH & others: Renovascular occlusive disease: Results of operative treatment. JAMA 231:1043, 1975.

Fournier A & others: Urography with urea wash-out in renovascular hypertension. Acta radiol diag 14:315, 1973.

Franklin SS & others: Operative morbidity and mortality in renovascular disease. JAMA 231:1148, 1975.

Gifford RW Jr & others: Controlling atherosclerotic renovascular hypertension. Geriatrics 28:124, 1973.

Gittes RF, McLaughlin AP III: Unilateral operation for bilateral renovascular disease. J Urol 111:292, 1974.

Grim CE & others: Unilateral "page kidney" hypertension in man. JAMA 231:42, 1975.

Howard JE, Connor TB: Use of differential renal function studies in the diagnosis of renovascular hypertension. Am J Surg 107:58, 1964.

Hunt JC & others: Renal and renovascular hypertension. Arch Int Med 133:988, 1974.

Jakobsen BE: Divided renal function studies in hypertension. Brit J Urol 46:149, 1974.

Juncos LI, Strong CG, Hunt JC: Prediction of results of surgery for renal and renovascular hypertension. Ann Int Med 134:655, 1974.

Kaufman JJ: Renal artery stenosis and azotemia. Surg Gynec Obst 137:949, 1973.

Klatte EC & others: The roentgenographic pre- and postoperative assessment of patients with renovascular disease. Am J Roentgenol 114:696 1972.

Knochel JP, White MG: The role of aldosterone in renal physiology. Arch Int Med 131:876, 1973.

Kurtzman NA & others: Renal vascular hypertension and low plasma renin activity: Interrelationship of volume and renin in the pathogenesis of hypertension. Arch Int Med 133:195, 1974.

Lawson RK, Hodges CV: Extracorporeal renal artery repair and autotransplantation. Urology 4:532, 1974.

Lecky JW, Craven JD: A refinement of the analysis of the rapid sequence excretory urogram in hypertensive patients—volume difference. J Urol 108:840, 1972.

Luke RG & others: Results of nephrectomy in hypertension associated with unilateral renal disease. Brit MJ 3:764, 1968.

Marks LS, Poutasse EF: Hypertension from renal tuberculosis: Operative cure predicted by renal vein renin. J Urol 109:149, 1973.

McCormach JL & others: Iatrogenic renal hypertension. Arch Surg 108:220, 1974.

Meares EM Jr, Gross DM: Hypertension owing to unilateral renal hypoplasia. J Urol 108:197, 1972.

Mena E & others: Neurofibromatosis and renovascular hypertension in children. Am J Roentgenol 118:39, 1973.

Michelakis AM: Effect of posture on renal vein renin in the diagnosis and followup of renovascular hypertension. J Urol 107:680, 1972.

Milsten R, Neifeld J, Koontz WW Jr: Extracorporeal renal surgery. J Urol 112:425, 1974.

Nemoy NJ, Fichman MP, Sellers A: Unilateral ureteral obstruction: A cause of reversible high renin content hypertension. JAMA 225:512, 1973.

Perry MO: Fibromuscular dysplasia. Surg Gynec Obst 139:97, 1974.

Rahill WJ & others: Hypertension and narrowing of the renal arteries in infancy. J Pediat 84:39, 1974.

Russell RP: Renal hypertension. S Clin North America 54:349, 1974.

Schaeffer AJ, Fair WR: Comparison of split function ratios with renal vein renin ratios in patients with curable hypertension caused by unilateral renal artery stenosis. J Urol 112:697, 1974.

Schambelan M & others: Role of renin and aldosterone in hypertension due to a renin-secreting tumor. Am J Med 55:86, 1973.

Schambelan M & others: Selective renal-vein renin sampling in hypertensive patients with segmental renal lesions. New England J Med 290:1153, 1974.

Schiff M Jr, McGuire EJ, Baskin AM: Hypertension and unilateral hydronephrosis. Urology 5:178, 1975.

Squitieri AP, Ceccarelli FC, Wurster JC: Hypertension with elevated renal vein renins secondary to ureteropelvic junction obstruction. J Urol 111:284, 1974.

Stamey TA: *Renovascular Hypertension*. Williams & Wilkins, 1963.

Stein JH, Ferris TF: The physiology of renin. Arch Int Med 131:860, 1973.

Symposium on renovascular hypertension. JAMA 200:1195, 1972.

Tilford DL, Kelsch RC: Renal artery stenosis in childhood neurofibromatosis. Am J Dis Child 126:665, 1973.

Vaughan TJ & others: Renal artery aneurysms and hypertension. Radiology 99:287, 1971.

33 . . .
Infertility, Vasectomy, & Impotence

INFERTILITY

A couple can be judged infertile if conception does not occur after 12 months of adequate cohabitation. About 10% of marriages are barren; spermatogenic deficiencies in the male are responsible in at least 30% of these. Joël (1966) observes that 6% of habitual abortions are noted in association with highly abnormal semen.

From the clinical standpoint, male fertility is judged through study of the sperms, including number, the percentage of motile sperms, and their viability and morphology. If sperms are absent from the ejaculate, testicular biopsy is indicated to differentiate between intrinsic deficiency of the germ cells (common) and obstruction of the conduction system (rare).

Pathogenesis

The common causes of male infertility are as follows:

A. Deficiencies in Maturation of Germ Cells: At least 85% of infertile men have intrinsic spermatogenic defects. The germ cells of the seminiferous tubules may be congenitally imperfect (aplastic), or incomplete maturation (spermatogenic arrest) may be observed secondary to hypogonadism or hypopituitarism.

Orchitis due to mumps or trauma and exposure to x-ray radiation frequently exert a deleterious effect upon spermatogenesis. In the cryptorchid testis, the temperature of the body causes injury to the germ cells.

B. Obstruction of the Conduction System: Bilateral epididymitis may cause occlusion of the ducts. Absence of connection between the vas deferens and the epididymis may be congenital or acquired (eg, vasoligation).

C. Hypothyroidism: Hypothyroidism is often associated with infertility and may have etiologic significance. A scientific explanation of this is lacking, but the administration of thyroid substance to hypothyroid infertile men with normal sperms may be followed by conception.

D. Hyperadrenalism: Hyperadrenalism causes an increase in volume of the ejaculate, diminished sperm count and motility, and an increased percentage of abnormal forms with evidence of desquamation. Plas-

ma testosterone is elevated. A similar picture is seen in association with varicocele.

E. Hypopituitarism: Hypopituitarism leads to lack of normal maturation of spermatogenic cells (germinal aplasia). Urine levels of FSH are low.

F. Hypogonadism: In testicular failure (eg, Klinefelter's syndrome), degeneration of the seminiferous tubules is seen. Urinary FSH is elevated. Serum testosterone or urinary 17-ketosteroid values are normal or only slightly subnormal since Leydig cells are numerous.

G. Sperm Antibodies: It would appear that 3 immune mechanisms are involved in some cases of infertility: (1) autoimmunization in men, (2) circulatory antibodies against sperms in women, and (3) tissue antibodies against semen in women.

In men, autoimmune antibodies cause sperm agglutination and may immobilize sperms. In women, penetrating sperms may be immobilized; their cervical mucus may become impenetrable. In the infertile couple, about 15% of each sex will be found to have such antibodies (Halim, 1974).

H. Tight Clothing: The use of shorts or supporters that hold the testes close to the body leads to increase in testicular temperature which is deleterious to spermatogenesis.

I. Varicocele: The presence of varicocele causes (1) an increase in the percentage of immature forms, (2) a decrease in sperm count, and (3) a decrease in the percentage of motile sperms. The cause is not known. It has been shown that it is not due to increased scrotal heat from the pooled blood. It has been postulated that adrenal corticosteroids might move in a retrograde manner down the spermatic vein to the testes. This theory has little support.

Testicular Histology & Pathology

A. Normal Development: Up to the age of 4 or 5 years, the testes are in a relatively quiescent state. The spermatogenic tubules are small. Adjacent to the basement membrane, a number of ovoid or round cells are seen. Few spermatogonia are present. The interstitial tissue contains a few clumps of Leydig cells.

Between the ages of 5 and 10 years, the germinal tubules become more tortuous and their lumens increase in diameter. More spermatogonia are present. The interstitial tissues show a decrease in the number of fibroblasts.

At puberty, probably stimulated by increasing amounts of pituitary gonadotropins (FSH, LH), active spermatogenesis begins and mature spermatozoa make their appearance. Hyperplasia of the interstitial (Leydig) cells develops (Fig 1–8).

B. Abnormal Development: The pathologic changes found in the infertile testis have been carefully studied by gonadal biopsy. Many degrees of damage may be noted.

1. Germinal aplasia—The seminiferous tubules show a complete or almost complete lack of germ cells. Normal numbers of Sertoli cells are present, however. The cause of this change may be either congenital or secondary to lack of follicle-stimulating hormone (FSH) from the pituitary gland. If pituitary function is normal, increased amounts of FSH may be found in the urine (Klinefelter's syndrome).

2. Spermatogenic arrest—The tubule and its cells are normal in appearance, but maturation fails to reach the adult stage.

3. Peritubular fibrosis—Normally, the basement membrane of the tubule is quite thin. For some unknown reason, progressive peritubular fibrosis may occur. In all probability, this impairs cellular nutrition and the sperm cells gradually disappear. At this stage, FSH excretion in the urine is increased.

4. Incomplete spermatogenesis—Some tubules may be quite normal, whereas others show lack of complete maturation. Both mature and immature sperms may be found in the tubular lumens. Men suffering from this defect have lowered sperm counts and an increase in the number of abnormal forms.

C. Spermatology: Clinically, there are 3 important criteria for normal semen.

1. Number—Most authorities state that "normal" semen contains at least 40 million sperms per milliliter in 2 ml of fluid. MacLeod (1969) found that 25% of fertile men have counts below 50 million/ml. He considers that true oligospermia consists of less than 20 million/ml, but he observes that, with excellent motility, conception may occur when the sperm count is as low as 10 million/ml.

2. Percentage of motile sperms and degree of motility—In most fertile men, at least 60% of the sperms are actively motile when the specimen is fresh. The fewer the motile forms, the greater the impairment of fertility. The degree of motility is also quite significant. The more sluggish the sperms, the greater the degree of infertility.

Generally speaking, the greater the percentage of motile forms, the more vigorous their motility.

3. Morphology—A differential count of normal and abnormal sperms affords considerable information. At least 60–70% of the sperms in most fertile men are normal (Fig 33–1).

Clinical Findings

A. History: The chief complaint of the patient is the inability to cause conception. Other information of importance includes childhood and adult illnesses (eg,

mumps orchitis, cryptorchism, tuberculosis); operations, especially those which might cause injury to the testes or their ducts (eg, repair of inguinal hernia, orchiopexy); trauma to the external genitalia; genital infections, particularly epididymitis; pregnancy in present or previous wife, frequency of intercourse, and exposure to toxins (eg, x-rays).

Evidence of retrograde ejaculation or lack of emission should be sought. This is common in diabetics, those undergoing repair of aortic aneurysms or radical retroperitoneal lymph node dissection (eg, testis tumor), and following any type of prostatectomy.

Certain drugs have a deleterious effect upon spermatogenesis. These include antitumor chemotherapeutic agents and nitrofurantoin. Vaginal lubricants are often spermatocidal.

The patient should be questioned about the use of shorts that support the scrotum, thus increasing testicular temperature.

B. Signs: A complete physical examination should never be neglected. Evidence of endocrinologic abnormality should be sought, including weight, height, body build, amount and distribution of hair, and gynecomastia. The degree of development of the penis should be noted and the scrotal contents carefully examined. (The testes of infertile men are usually normal in size and consistency.) Unilateral or bilateral changes may be noted. The small, flabby testes or the hard, pea-sized testes of Klinefelter's syndrome are usually azoospermic. Other testicular abnormalities may include cryptorchism and thickening of the epididymides (old epididymitis). The vas deferens should be carefully felt, for it may be absent or may fail to join the epididymis. Varicocele should be noted, for its presence offers the most hope when it comes to the point of treatment.

Rectal examination should include prostatic massage, although the significance of prostatitis in infertility is not clear. Fjällbrant (1970) believes that there is an increased incidence of sperm antibodies in some men who harbor this infection.

C. Laboratory Findings: Proteinuria or pyuria may be clues to chronic renal disease, which may depress spermatogenesis. Tests for nitrogen retention should be ordered.

1. Examination of the semen—This is the most important step in the investigation of suspected infertility.

a. Method of collection—The ejaculate should be obtained after at least 4 days of abstinence from intercourse. It is best produced by masturbation in the physician's office. This ensures that the entire specimen is collected in a clean, dry glass. Condoms must not be used, for the sperms are quickly killed on contact with them. The specimen must be examined within 2 hours of its collection. Normally, the semen is quite gelatinous and ropy. Within a few minutes, at room temperature, the fluid becomes thin and homogeneous. Failure to liquefy is abnormal.

b. Sperm count—The technic is simple, requiring

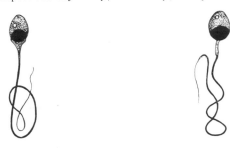

Oval or normal spermatozoa

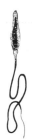 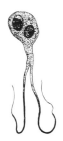 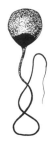 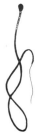 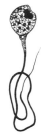

Abnormal spermatozoa

Figure 33–1. Normal and abnormal spermatozoa. (Redrawn and reproduced, with permission, from Hotchkiss: *Fertility in Men.* Lippincott, 1944.)

only a Neubauer blood cell counting chamber and a white cell pipet. Semen is drawn up to the 0.5 mark, and the rest of the chamber is filled with a saturated solution of sodium bicarbonate containing 1% phenol, which immobilizes the sperms. This mixture is then flooded over the counting chamber and covered with a coverslip. The number of sperms in the 5 blocks (80 small squares) is determined. To this number are added 6 zeros. This equals the number of sperms per milliliter.

Most fertile men have at least 40 million sperms per milliliter. The absence of sperms means a severe defect of the seminiferous tubules or obstruction of the conducting system. The finding of a few dead sperms rules out obstruction.

Oligospermia is almost always due to disease of the germ cells. The lower the count, the poorer the prognosis.

c. Percentage of motile sperms and degree of motility—Semen is placed on a slide and covered with a coverslip sealed with petroleum jelly. An estimate should be made of the percentage of motile forms, the degree of motility, and the duration of life of the sperms.

d. Morphology—(Fig 33–1.) Morphology may be judged by counting the normal and abnormal forms in a smear stained as follows:

(1) Dry a thin smear of semen in air.
(2) Flood with 10% formalin for 1 minute.
(3) Wash.
(4) Stain with Meyer's hematoxylin for 1½ minutes.

(5) Wash in lukewarm water.

2. Thyroid function test—Thyroid function should be evaluated by appropriate tests in all men presenting themselves as possibly infertile, whether the ejaculate is normal or not. The hypothyroid male with normal semen may become fertile only after thyroid has been administered.

3. Testicular biopsy—Biopsy is usually indicated only if azoospermia is present. Perhaps 40% of men showing defects on sperm examination will have serious irreversible lesions of the seminiferous tubules. Study of the seminiferous tubules will permit differentiation between severe intrinsic gonadal disease and blockage of the conducting system. In the latter case, spermatogenesis is normal. There is, however, evidence that sperm counts are apt to be temporarily depressed after biopsy.

4. Buccal smear—A buccal smear should receive nuclear chromatin analysis. If chromatin sex is positive (female), the diagnosis of Klinefelter's syndrome should be entertained. These patients are irreversibly sterile.

5. FSH test—Pituitary gonadotropins (FSH) in the urine should be measured. An increase means primary gonadal deficiency; if FSH is decreased, hypopituitarism is present.

6. Other tests—Estimation of plasma testosterone levels should be obtained. If this cannot be done, urinary 17-ketosteroids should be measured. These levels are depressed in chronic heavy marihuana users (Kolodney & others, 1974). They are elevated with hyperadrenocorticism.

D. X-Ray Findings: If blockage of the vasa is suspected, vasoseminal vesiculography may be indicated (Hébert, Bouchard, & Charron, 1971). A No. 23 needle is introduced into the lumen of the vas pointing to the epididymis. Two or 3 ml of radiopaque fluid are injected and films exposed. The needle is then pointed toward the prostate and the procedure is repeated.

E. Immunologic Survey: If both the man and the woman are found to have normal fertility or if the man's sperms show agglutination or are immobile, both should be tested for the presence of sperm antibodies.

Treatment

The results of treatment of infertility in the male are unsatisfactory except when a varicocele is found. Morphologic changes in the various components of the seminiferous tubules are largely irreversible.

A. Abnormalities Based on Spermatology:

1. Idiopathic oligospermia—Stewart & Montie (1973) suggest the use of 2.5 mg of cortisone acetate 4 times a day. Ansari, Wieland, & Klein (1972) have reported a good response from clomiphine citrate, 5 mg/day for 12 weeks. Schellen & Beek (1974) made similar observations. They recommend 50 mg/day for 60–90 days. Pregnancy occurred in 20%. Schachter, Goldman, & Zukerman (1973) find that 1 g of arginine per day improved the sperm count and motility in 65% of their patients. Hendry & others (1973) and Shellen & Beek (1972) recommend mesterolone, 75–100 mg/day for 1 year. They noted improvement in over half of their subjects.

2. Asthenospermia (low motility)—Stewart & Montie (1973) observed a good response from human chorionic gonadotropin (HCG), 10,000 units IM given twice a week for 3 months. Hendry & others (1973) had similar results using fluoxymesterone, 5 mg/day for 3–6 months.

3. Low volume of ejaculate (less than 1 ml)—Amelar & Dubin (1973) have observed improvement administering HCG, 2000–4000 units IM twice a week for 8 weeks. They suggest coitus interruptus in those with normal spermatology but with abnormally high volumes. The first portion of such ejaculate contains an increased concentration of sperms (Eliasson & Lindholmer, 1972).

B. Abnormal Endocrinologic Tests:

1. If hypothyroidism is found, appropriate replacement should be instituted.

2. If the plasma testosterone or urinary 17-ketosteroid levels are low, androgen therapy should be prescribed (Hendry & others, 1973). If the androgen levels are increased (hyperadrenalism), corticosteroid should be given to suppress adrenal activity.

3. If urinary FSH is low (hypopituitarism), give HCG, 2000–4000 units IM twice a week (Amelar & Dubin, 1973). An increased level of FSH reflects severe seminiferous tubular defects.

C. Retrograde Ejaculation or Lack of Emission: Immediately after ejaculation, the urine should be examined for the presence of sperms (retrograde ejaculation). Such urine should be centrifuged and the sperms instilled into the cervix. If the urine contains no sperms and an operation has been performed that might have damaged the thoracolumbar sympathetic nerves, prescribe ephedrine, 50–75 mg, one-half hour before coitus. This may cause ejaculation, which fluid may contain sperms. Stockamp, Schreiter, & Altwein (1974) noted some effect following the administration of 60 mg of phenylephrine IV.

D. General Measures: Sexual technic should be discussed with the couple. They should be apprised of the "fertile" period in the menstrual cycle. Intercourse should be avoided for 3 or 4 days before this time in order that the male can then deliver the best quantity and quality of semen. This is particularly important if the sperm count is deficient. Psychic factors should be sought.

If nonliquefaction of the semen is observed, Bunge (1968) has recommended that the woman insert a cocoa butter suppository containing 5 mg of alpha amylase powder into the vagina immediately after intercourse performed during the time of ovulation.

The general health of the patient should be improved by regulating his diet and eradicating infections, particularly of the prostate gland. A reducing diet should be utilized if the man is overweight. Alcoholic excesses should be curbed.

Vitamin B complex should be prescribed to ensure the normal inactivation of estrogens by the liver.

If the man wears a supporter or shorts that hold the scrotal contents close to the body, he should be instructed not to do so.

If treatment fails to improve the number, form, and motility of the sperms, and if conception does not occur, a cap containing the inadequate semen can be placed over the cervix. This may improve the chances for conception (Ulslein, 1973).

It has been recommended that large doses of testosterone (50 mg IM 3 times a week) should be administered for 3 months in men whose sperms are markedly inadequate in quality and quantity. This causes complete azoospermia, but after cessation of treatment a "rebound" phenomenon may occur and the semen may show improvement over its pretreatment level in 15% of patients. Ten percent may be made worse, however.

If the temperature of the testis is increased for a few months by hot soaks or by an insulated jockstrap, the sperm count is significantly decreased. Cessation of this treatment may result in a rebound of spermatogenic activity and a consequent increase in the sperm count that may culminate in pregnancy.

E. Surgical Measures: The surgical procedures available for the correction of specific abnormalities are as follows:

1. Vasovasostomy—If vasoligation has been performed, repair may be succcessful in almost 90% as judged by the recovery of normal numbers of sperms (Dorsey, 1973). Unfortunately, half of these men reveal autoimmunity to their own sperms, a complication of vasoligation (see below) (Howard & James,

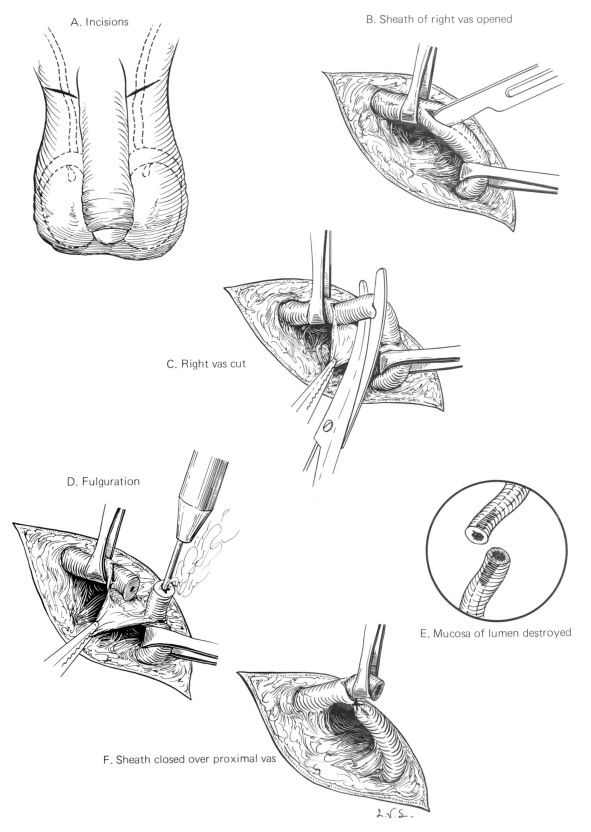

A. Incisions

B. Sheath of right vas opened

C. Right vas cut

D. Fulguration

E. Mucosa of lumen destroyed

F. Sheath closed over proximal vas

Figure 33–2. Steps in vasectomy. (Modified from a drawing by S Taft. Reproduced, with permission, from Schmidt S: Vasectomy should not fail. Contemporary Surgery 4:13, 1974.)

1973; Ansbacher, Keung-Yeung, & Wurster, 1972). Pregnancy may therefore result in only 25% of these couples.

2. Epididymovasostomy—If azoospermia is present but the testicular biopsy shows normal spermatogenesis and there is evidence of epididymal occlusion, epididymovasostomy should be considered. It may make conception possible in 10–20% of otherwise sterile matings.

3. Treatment of varicocele—Ligation of the spermatic vein at the internal inguinal ring as a cure for varicocele will usually improve the quality of the semen by improving motility of the sperms and their concentration. Pregnancy will occur in about half of this group.

4. Orchiopexy—Orchiopexy for undescended testes is of no value in the treatment of infertility after puberty.

F. Miscellaneous Factors in Therapy:

1. Noxious drugs should be stopped unless they appear to be lifesaving (Steward [1973], Timmermans [1974]).

2. Friberg & Gnarpe (1973) examined 54 infertile couples where the wives harbored T-mycoplasmas. They prescribed vibramycin, 100 mg/day from the 7th to the 16th day following the beginning of the last menstrual cycle, for 3 months. If the organism was still present, the dose of vibramycin was increased to 200 mg/day for 10 days. The partner was also treated for 10 days, and T-mycoplasmas were abolished in all. In 25%, pregnancy then occurred. De Louvois & others (1974) were, however, unable to corroborate these claims.

3. If the female is found to have sperm antibodies, her male partner should use a condom for 1 year. This allows subsidence of the antibody titer. Ansbacher, Keung-Yeung, & Behrman (1973) found that pregnancy then occurred in 50%.

Prognosis

The poorer the quality of the semen, the poorer the outlook for success in treatment. When the count is under 1 million/ml, there is little room for optimism. Azoospermia, unless caused by obstruction of the tubules of the epididymis, cannot be treated successfully.

VASECTOMY

During the past few years, there has been a striking increase in the utilization of vasectomy to prevent conception. Many women have had adverse reactions to the "pill"; others have suffered complications from the intrauterine device. Men are beginning to accept the fact that they must share the responsibility for population control. The usual indication for the operation, therefore, is the desire to be made sterile. The medical indications are (1) routine vasec-

tomy performed at the time of prostatectomy to prevent postoperative epididymitis, and (2) to prevent recurrent epididymitis.

Some men have deep-seated resistance to undergoing vasectomy. They may feel that the operation will cause them to become impotent out of some primitive feeling that if a man cannot cause conception he is not really a man. Thorough discussion of these matters before the operation is essential, for if a man expects to become impotent he will become so.

Preoperative Discussion With the Patient

The man must realize that 2 types of cells are harbored in the testes: seminiferous tubules and Leydig cells. Interrupting the vas stops sperm migration to the urethra. The Leydig cells are unaffected, for their androgens are picked up by blood vessels that continue to nourish them. Thus, androgen levels remain normal and the cells viable. Many men find intercourse even more satisfactory than before because the fear of conception has been removed (Nash & Rich, 1972).

The man must be told that he will suffer some discomfort during the operation from instillation of the local anesthetic. Minor discomfort for a few days postoperatively can be controlled with simple analgesics. Occasionally, an incision may open prematurely and drain for a few days. He must be warned that a small amount of bleeding may occur on the day of surgery. Some ecchymosis of the scrotal skin is to be expected. Significant bleeding (hematoscrotum) is rare but may require immediate operation.

The patient must realize that viable sperms are still harbored in the ampulla of the vas and that he cannot have intercourse for a time without continuing contraceptive practices. The ejaculate must be examined and shown to be free of sperms before the doctor can verify that he is infertile. This takes at least 12 ejaculations and often more (Marshall & Lyon, 1972).

In the discussion of vas repair it should be made clear that, although anatomically a high success rate can be expected, the formation of sperm antibodies as a complication of vasoligation will decrease the chance for conception to 25% or less (Dorsey, 1973; Howard & James, 1973).

Should the patient feel that he might desire a child later and if vasovasostomy is unacceptable, he may wish to deposit his semen in a frozen semen bank. There is a gradual loss of motility—approaching 50%—during the first 36 months; little change occurs thereafter (Smith & Steinberger, 1973). Friberg & Gemzell (1973) report 26 pregnancies out of 187 specimens after storing.

The patient must be told that recanalization as a complication of the formation of a sperm granuloma occurs in about 0.5% of cases (Esho, Ireland, & Cass, 1974), though Schmidt (1974) has not observed this in 1500 vasectomies accomplished by fulguration of the lumens of the cut vasa. For this reason, the ejaculate must be examined until no sperms, dead or alive, are found and a similar result is obtained 1 and 2 months later.

Technic of Vasectomy (Schmidt, 1974) (Fig 33—2)

The spermatic cord is isolated so that the skin over it is taut. The vas is manipulated so it is just under the skin, which is infiltrated with a local anesthetic. The needle is then advanced to infiltrate the perivasal tissues.

A 10 mm transverse incision should be made over the vas (Fig 33—2A). The tissues around the vas are separated and the vas is grasped with 2 Allis clamps (Fig 33—2B). The fascia covering the vas should be incised for a distance of 15 mm and the vas freed from it. The vas can then be divided (Fig 33—2C). Though occlusion by ligature is commonly practiced, there is a risk that the tissue distal to the tie may slough, allowing recanalization. Schmidt experienced no failures if he merely inserted the needle electrode of the electrosurgical machine into the lumen of each vasal end and delivered a mild coagulation current as he withdrew the electrode to destroy the mucous membrane (Fig 33—2D). (See also Esho, Ireland, & Cass, 1974.) Kraft & McQueen (1972) recommend the infusion of 20 ml of sterile water into the lumen of the proximal end of the vas. This hastened the day when motile sperms were found to be absent.

The proximal end of the vas is placed back in its fascial sheath, which is closed with plain catgut (Fig 33—2E). This burial technic further prevents recanalization. After hemostasis is achieved, the skin is closed with chromic catgut.

Hormonal Changes Following Vasectomy

Wieland & others (1972) and Rosenberg & others (1974) have found that the levels of serum testosterone and urinary FSH and LH were unchanged following the operation.

Complications of Vasectomy & Their Treatment

Sperm granuloma, due to extravasation of sperms, presents as a mass felt in the region of the vasectomy. The patient may complain of local pain, and the mass is found to be tender. At times, such a lesion is asymptomatic. The incidence has been estimated at 5—18% (Kwart & Coffey, 1973), most occurring when ligation of the vasa has been done. Electrocoagulation markedly reduces the incidence of this complication. Excision may be necessary to afford comfort.

Sperm granuloma may develop in the epididymis from rupture of the tubules due to high pressure distal to the vasectomy site. This will cause occlusion of the epididymal ducts, thus making later successful vasovasostomy impossible.

Congestive epididymitis is occasionally seen. The patient complains of testicular discomfort, and the organ is found to be enlarged and tender. It usually subsides with time.

Recanalization has an incidence of about 0.6% (Klapproth & Young, 1973). This can be reduced by using the surgical technic described above. Rarely, failure may be attributed to a mistake in properly identifying the vas (Leader & others, 1974); reoperation is indicated.

The development of both immobilizing and agglutinating sperm antibodies may occur as a result of extravasation of sperms. This reaction may also make later successful vasovasostomy impossible (Howard & James, 1973; Ansbacher, Keung-Yeung, & Wurster, 1972).

Profuse bleeding into the scrotum is rare. Because of the distensibility of the scrotal wall, it affords no hemostatic effect. Drainage is at times necessary.

Though the wound may open prematurely and drain for a few days, frank infection is rare. It may necessitate surgical drainage.

Prognosis

If the patient is well prepared psychologically by the physician and if the operation is properly performed, the success rate should approach 100%.

IMPOTENCE

Various degrees of impotence in men are common, and most cases are due to psychogenic causes. The complaints include inability to gain or maintain an erection, impaired erections, premature ejaculation, lack of emission with orgasm, loss of libido, or absence of normal sensation with ejaculation.

Most men are resistant to the suggestion that their troubles are on a psychologic basis. They are certain that the masturbation in which they indulged during adolescence or the gonorrhea they contracted later damaged their sexual organs. They have been taught that their symptoms are due to organic diseases, including prostatitis, verumontanitis, posterior urethritis, and decreased elaboration of androgens by the testes.

Physiology

The development of the male sexual attitude and power depends upon the presence of normal androgenic secretion at the time of puberty and the development of a male-oriented sexual attitude based on sociologic and psychogenic influences.

The ability to gain and maintain an erection that culminates in timed normal orgasm and ejaculation requires an intact nerve and blood supply to the lower genitourinary tract. The various aspects of potency are controlled by both autonomic and somatic nerves. Erection requires arteries of such caliber that an adequate flow of blood can be delivered to the penis.

A. Erection: This function is initiated by psychic or local influences. Sensory impulses reach the upper portion of the lumbar cord. Reflexes are set up through the sacral parasympathetic outflow (S2–4) which lead to relaxation of the arterioles to the corpora of the penis; the blood pressure within them approaches that of the carotid arteries. The cavernous bodies are thus engorged under pressure. Lack of psychic stimulus, atherosclerosis, or interruption of these nerves can impair the quality of erection.

Erection - parasympathetic S2-4
Emission - Thoracolumbar Sympathetic
Ejaculation Somatic S2-4 (motor & sensory)

B. Emission: Sensory nerve impulses from the glans penis reach the sacral cord and travel to the integrating center in the upper portion of the lumbar cord. These impulses set off a massive stimulus through the thoracolumbar sympathetic nerves which cause secretions from the prostate, seminal vesicles, and ejaculatory ducts to enter the prostatic urethra. Interruption of these nerves may preclude emission.

C. Ejaculation: Immediately after emission, spasmodic contractions of the muscles surrounding the urethra and those of the pelvic floor occur, thus forcing jets of semen down the urethra. The nerves involved are somatic S2–4. Accompanying the series of ejaculations is the rhythmic sensation of orgasm (S2–4). Hence, a lower motor neuron lesion in this zone could impair ejaculation and the sensation of orgasm.

D. Subsidence of Erection: The arterioles to the penis then contract and erection subsides.

Psychodynamics

With few exceptions, the causes of sexual difficulties in the male seen in office practice are psychic, ie, based on guilt, anxiety, jealousy, or frigidity on the part of the wife. Seldom is evidence of hypogonadism seen as an organic cause; androgen therapy as such is of little avail. Prostatitis may be an incidental finding; its treatment seldom improves sexual power unless the patient expects it to, in which case improvement is usually only temporary. After the age of 50 years, many men notice some diminution of desire and sexual power.

Organic Causes of Impotence

The patient with renal failure (eg, on dialysis) loses both desire and the power of gaining a normal erection.

Certain operations may damage the thoracolumbar sympathetic nerves, leading to lack of emission of ejaculate. These include (1) sympathectomy, (2) radical retroperitoneal lymph node dissection, and (3) surgical repair of aortic aneurysm. Complete impotence usually follows radical prostatectomy and prostatocystectomy. Even following simple perineal exposure and biopsy of the prostate, 37% notice some diminution of potency and 29% are truly impotent (Dahlen & Goodwin, 1957). Following abdominoperineal resection of the rectum, one-third of men will be impotent and another third will lose the power of emission.

Following any type of prostatectomy, the vesical neck remains open. Therefore, even though emission occurs, the ejaculate flows into the bladder (retrograde ejaculation).

Following radiotherapy for prostatic carcinoma, one-third of men will become impotent.

About 30–50% of men who sustain a fracture of the pelvis with damage to or avulsion of the membranous urethra will be impotent. Gibson (1970) believes that this disability is caused by thrombosis of the dorsal and deep arteries enclosed in the perineal pouch. A few will lose the power of emission.

Various neurologic lesions that affect the sexual integration center in the spinal cord (T12–L3), the thoracolumbar sympathetic nerves, the sacral parasympathetic outflow (S2–4), the cauda equina, or the pudendal nerves will have a deleterious effect upon sexual power.

Most patients with myelodysplasia and extensive spina bifida will be completely impotent. Acquired medical diseases of the cord or peripheral nerves may impair the power of erection or emission. They include tabes dorsalis, multiple sclerosis, and Parkinson's disease. Trauma to the spinal cord and peripheral nerves is one of the most common causes of organic impotence. In Comarr's (1971) series, 93% of patients with complete upper neuron lesions were able to achieve erection; of those with incomplete lesions, 98% were successful. In complete lower neuron lesions, only 26% achieved erection while in the incomplete group 83% had success. In both groups in whom erection was achieved, about 70–80% could have intercourse. The patients with complete upper neuron lesions lost the power of emission and orgasm, while those with lower neuron damage were more successful: 17% if the lesion was complete, 60% if incomplete.

Bilateral pudendal neurectomy leads to cessation of erections (Ross, 1956); unilateral resection usually has no such effect.

Subarachnoid alcohol block, cordotomy, or sacral neurectomy destroys the power of erection. Limited rhizotomy may preserve this power.

Certain drugs are apt to cause loss of erectile power. They include the ganglionic blocking agents used in the control of hypertension or certain bowel difficulties, methysergide, estrogens (in the treatment of prostatic cancer), antihistamines, tranquilizers, immunosuppressive agents, and heroin. Phenothiazine and phenoxybenzamine may interfere with emission.

Genital abnormalities that might preclude intercourse include exstrophy, epispadias, hypospadias, and congenital penile chordee. The dorsal tilt seen with Peyronie's disease may preclude intromission.

Endocrinologic abnormalities may reduce potency. This is seen in association with Cushing's and Addison's diseases, testicular failure, hypo- and hyperactivity of the pituitary (eg, acromegaly, pituitary ablation), and diabetes. In the latter, because of neuropathy, about half will develop an atonic neurogenic bladder. Damage to these parasympathetic nerves (S2–4) also prevents dilatation of the arteries to the corpora. In association with vesical atonicity, the bladder neck remains open; retrograde ejaculation then occurs.

Vascular lesions that will not allow a good influx of arterial blood into the corpora cavernosa will impair erections. In the Leriche syndrome, erections, if gained, cannot be retained. Generalized arteriolar sclerosis involving the vessels to the penis may preclude their dilatation.

Gaskell (1971), using a spectroscopic method, estimated the penile blood pressure in normal men and in men with erectile impotence. In the former group,

[handwritten notes at bottom of page:]
① renal failure   ④ Drugs   ⑦ Vascular inc p priapism
② Surgery   ⑤ genital anomalie ⑧ Radio k
③ Neurologic lesions ⑥ Endocrine   ⑨ Injuries

the penile blood pressure exceeded that in the brachial artery. In the latter, penile blood pressure was low.

Fitzpatrick (1974) studied the valves of the deep dorsal veins by cannulating them and injecting radiopaque fluid. In the normal men he found 1—3 competent valves. In those with poor or no erections, he found almost total absence of valves.

Malvar, Baron, & Clark (1974), using a Doppler flowmeter, found many impotent men to exhibit arterial insufficiency of the penile arteries.

Following an attack of priapism, inability to gain an erection is common. This is due to fibrosis of the septa in the cavernosa (Hinman, 1960).

Clinical Findings

A. Symptoms: Partial or complete impotence is the main complaint. The patient should be asked whether he has nocturnal erections, can masturbate with complete success, or whether he is potent with other than his usual sexual partner. Affirmative responses to these queries establish the cause as psychologic. Complaints referable to the vascular system should be explored with particular reference to intermittent claudication, which may reflect sclerosis of the arteries to the corpora cavernosa.

Symptoms suggesting vesical malfunction must be explored. Neurologic disease or diabetes may lead to an atonic bladder, in which case, because of damage to the sacral parasympathetic outflow, the arteries to the cavernosa cannot dilate.

A survey of drugs the patient might be taking may lead to the conclusion that stopping the drug will cure the impotence.

Past operations should be recorded, seeking one that might have damaged the thoracolumbar sympathetic nerves, the sacral parasympathetics, or the pudendal nerves.

A pelvic fracture sustained in the past is of importance, as is a history of radiation therapy for carcinoma of the prostate.

A history of penile abnormality, including priapism, may be obtained. Symptoms suggesting an endocrinologic abnormality may be discovered.

B. Signs: Changes compatible with endocrinologic disease should be sought: body build, gynecomastia, obesity, etc. The genitalia should be examined, noting any serious abnormality of the penis (eg, chordee, micropenis). The testes must be palpated for size and consistency though in most cases, psychogenic or organic, they are normal. Small size implies the possibility of hypoandrogenism or Klinefelter's syndrome. Evidence of bladder distention should be sought. Such a finding might suggest the presence of a neurogenic bladder. Prostatic secretion should be examined for the presence of infection.

A limited neurologic examination is indicated: anal sphincter tone, bulbocavernosus reflex, knee and ankle jerks, Babinski reflex, and perineal sensation. These steps will reveal any deficit of S2—4.

Peripheral circulation should be evaluated for evidence of aortic aneurysm, bruit over the femoral arteries, and peripheral pulses. Evidence of atherosclerosis may suggest similar changes in the arteries to the cavernosa.

C. Laboratory Findings: Urinalysis may reveal bacteriuria, suggesting vesical residual urine on a neurogenic basis. Glycosuria may be a clue to diabetic neuropathy. Proteinuria may suggest the possibility of renal insufficiency. A serum creatinine determination should be ordered, seeking serious renal disease.

The plasma testosterone level should be evaluated, though it is usually fairly normal even in older men. Other endocrinologic tests may be indicated.

D. X-Ray Findings: If there is a history of spinal injury, plain films may reveal evidence of an old fracture. Metastases to bone can cause pressure on the spinal cord or peripheral nerves. Calcification in an aortic aneurysm may be revealed.

E. Instrumental Findings: If the presence of neurogenic bladder is suspected, a PSP test should be done or a catheter should be passed to establish the fact. A cystometrogram will establish the diagnosis. It may show vesical hyperirritability if there is an upper neuron lesion and atonicity with a lower neuron lesion.

Differential Diagnosis

In office practice, a high percentage of normal examinations will be found. This psychogenic group comprises at least 90% of the patients examined.

In those who have suffered spinal cord trauma or undergone operations that affect the autonomic nervous system or the pudendal nerves, examination will reveal neurologic defects. Laboratory work will confirm endocrinopathy. If the proper equipment is at hand, impaired blood flow through the penile arteries can be documented.

Treatment

In patients without positive findings, drugs deleterious to sexual function should be discontinued unless they are considered lifesaving.

While psychiatric treatment may be needed for a few of these men, a counseling approach has been found to be increasingly successful. This consists of positive reassurance and reeducation concerning technics, attitudes, and psychology and the needs of the sexual partner, who should be included in these discussions. Though time-consuming, such therapy should be highly successful in the hands of most practitioners (Masters & Johnson, 1970).

Organic treatment is contraindicated in the psychogenic group. It only further assures the patient that masturbation or an attack of gonorrhea has caused damage to his sexual organs. Painful (and expensive) treatment (eg, prostatic massage, urethral dilatations, fulguration of the verumontanum) at times appears successful because guilt and anxiety are thus relieved.

Little can be done to improve function if organic disease is responsible, though treatment of aortic occlusion may restore normal blood flow to the penis (eg, Leriche syndrome). If absence of emission following damage to the sympathetic nerves occurs, epinephrine, 25–50 mg 30 minutes before intercourse, may cause the ejaculation of semen.

If the level of serum testosterone is low, replacement therapy should be applied. Give testosterone cypionate in oil, 200 mg IM every 3 weeks, or fluoxymesterone, 5 mg daily orally. If the impotence is secondary to diabetic neuropathy or renal insufficiency, such changes are irreversible.

In the organic group, the placement of a plastic

→ Halotestin (dose 2–10 mg/day).
not if ↑ Ca⁺⁺

prosthesis has afforded satisfaction in most patients. Such prostheses have also been used in the psychiatric group (Lash, 1968). At the very least, the prosthesis allows the sexual partner to gain sexual satisfaction.

Prognosis

Unless the patient's nonorganic difficulties are of short duration, he should be referred to a psychiatrist.

References

Infertility

Agger P: Scrotal and testicular temperature: Its relation to sperm count before and after operation for varicocele. Fertil Steril 22:286, 1971.

Albert PS, Mininberg DJ, Davis JE: Nitrofurans: sperm-immobilizing agents: Their tissue toxicity and clinical application. Urology 4:307, 1974.

Amelar RD, Dubin L: A coital technique for promotion of fertility. Urology 5:228, 1975.

Amelar RD, Dubin L: Male infertility: Current diagnosis and treatment. Urology 1:1, 1973.

Amelar RD, Dubin L, Schoenfeld C: Semen analysis: An office technique. Urology 2:605, 1973.

Andaloro VA Jr, Dube A: Treatment of retrograde ejaculation with brompheniramine. Urology 5:520, 1975.

Ansari AH, Wieland RG, Klein DE: Cisclomiphene citrate in the management of oligospermia. J Urol 108:131, 1972.

Ansbacher R, Keung-Yeung K, Behrman SJ: Clinical significance of sperm antibodies in infertile couples. Fertil Steril 24:305, 1973.

Bourne RB, Kretzschmar WA, Esser JH: Successful artificial insemination in a diabetic with retrograde ejaculation. Fertil Steril 22:275, 1971.

Brown JS & others: Venography in the subfertile man with varicocele. J Urol 89:388, 1967.

Bruce WR & others: Physical and chemical studies of sperm production. Canad MAJ 103:885, 1970.

Bunge RG: Alpha amylase suppositories and non-liquefaction of human semen. J Urol 99:350, 1968.

Cerruti RA & others: Vasovasostomy outpatient procedure for reversal of vasectomy. Urology 3:209, 1974.

Cochran JS: Immunobiology of reproductive processes in men. Urology 4:367, 1974.

DeKretser DM & others: Disordered spermatogenesis in patients with chronic renal failure undergoing maintenance haemodialysis. Australia New Zealand J Med 4:178, 1974.

DeLouvois J & others: Frequency of mycoplasma in fertile and infertile couples. Lancet 1:1073, 1974.

Dorsey JW: Surgical correction of post-vasectomy sterility. J Urol 110:554, 1973.

Eliasson R, Lindholmer C: Distribution and properties of spermatozoa in different fractions of split ejaculates. Fertil Steril 23:252, 1972.

Emery CB, Goldstein AMB, Morrow JW: Congenital absence of vas deferens with ipsilateral urinary anomalies. Urology 4:201, 1974.

Fjällbrant B: Localization of human male antibodies on spermatozoa. Am J Obst Gynec 108:550, 1970.

Frankel MS: Role of semen cryobanking in American medicine. Brit MJ 3:619, 1974.

Friberg J, Gnarpe H: Mycoplasma and human reproduction failure. Am J Obst Gynec 116:23, 1973.

Furuhjelm M, Carlström K, Johnson B: Endocrinological aspects of male infertility. Acta obst gynec scandinav 53:181, 1974.

Getzoff PL: Surgical management of male infertility: Results of a survey. Fertil Steril 24:553, 1973.

Hafez ESE: Transport of spermatozoa in the female reproductive tract. Am J Obst Gynec 115:703, 1973.

Hafez ESE, Thibault CG: International symposium on the biology of spermatozoa: Transport, survival, and fertilizing ability. Fertil Steril 25:825, 1974.

Halim A, Antoniou D: Autoantibodies to spermatozoa in relation to male infertility and vasectomy. Brit J Urol 45:559, 1973.

Halim A & others: Investigation and treatment of the infertile male. Proc Roy Soc Med 66:737, 1973.

Halim A & others: The significance of antibodies to sperm in infertile men and their wives. Brit J Urol 46:65, 1974.

Hansen KB: A comparative study of various methods for the detection of spermatozoal antibodies. Acta obst gynec scandinav 53:69, 1974.

Hébert G, Bouchard R, Charron J: Vasoseminal vesiculography. Am J Roengentol 113:735, 1971.

Hendry WF & others: Investigation and treatment of the subfertile male. Brit J Urol 45:684, 1973.

Hinkes E, Plotkin D: Reversible drug-induced sterility in a patient with acute leukemia. JAMA 223:1490, 1973.

Joël CA: Male factor in habitual abortion. Fertil Steril 17:374, 1966.

Klotz PG: Congenital absence of the vas deferens. J Urol 109:662, 1973.

Kolodny RC & others: Depression of plasma testosterone levels after chronic intensive marihuana use. New England J Med 290:872, 1974.

Kom C, Mulholland SG, Edson M: Etiology of infertility after retroperitoneal lymphadenectomy. J Urol 105:528, 1971.

Lehfeldt H, Guze H: Psychologic factors in contraceptive failure. Fertil Steril 17:110, 1966.

Li TS: Sperm immunology, infertility, and fertility control. Obst Gynec 44:607, 1974.

MacLeod J: Further observations on the role of varicocele in human male infertility. Fertil Steril 20:545, 1969.

Mann T: Advances in male reproduction physiology. Fertil Steril 23:699, 1972.

Meinhard E, McRae CU, Chisholm GD: Testicular biopsy in evaluation of male infertility. Brit MJ 3:577, 1973.

Nelson CMK, Bunge RG: Semen analysis: Evidence for changing parameters of male fertility potential. Fertil Steril 25:503, 1974.

Orecklin JR, Kaufman JJ, Thompson RW: Fertility in patients treated for malignant testicular tumors. J Urol 109:293, 1973.

Paulson DF, Lindsey CM, Anderson EE: Simplified technique for vasography. Fertil Steril 25:906, 1974.

Pardanani DS & others: Surgical restoration of vas continuity after vasectomy: Further clinical evaluation of a new operation technique. Fertil Steril 25:319, 1974.

Pedersen H: The human spermatozoon. Danish Med Bull 21 (Suppl 1):1, 1974.

Raboch J, Stárka L: Hormonal testicular activity in men with a varicocele. Fertil Steril 22:152, 1971.

Robinson D, Rock J: Intrascrotal hyperthermia induced by scrotal insulation: Effect of spermatogenesis. Obst Gynec 29:217, 1967.

Rowley MJ, O'Keefe KB, Heller CG: Decreases in sperm concentration due to testicular biopsy procedure in men. J Urol 101:347, 1969.

Sandeman TF: The effects of x irradiation on male human fertility. Brit J Radiol 39:901, 1966.

Santomauro AG, Sciarra JJ, Varma AO: A clinical investigation of the role of the semen analysis and postcoital test in the evaluation of male infertility. Fertil Steril 23:245, 1972.

Schachter A, Goldman JA, Zukerman Z: Treatment of oligospermia with the amino acid arginine. J Urol 110:311, 1973.

Schellen TM, Beek JM: The influence of high doses of mesterolone on the spermiogram. Steril Fertil 23:712, 1972.

Schellen TM, Beek JM: The use of clomiphene treatment for male sterility. Fertil Steril 25:407, 1974.

Sciarra JJ, Markland C, Speidel JJ: *Control of Male Fertility.* Harper & Row, 1975.

Scott LS: Mumps and male fertility. Brit J Urol 32:183, 1960.

Sohval AR: Sex chromatin, chromosomes, and male infertility. Fertil Steril 14:180, 1963.

Stewart BH: Drugs as cause and cure in male infertility. Drug Therap 3:34, 1973.

Stewart BH: Varicocele in infertility: Incidence and results of surgical therapy. J Urol 112:222, 1974.

Stewart BH, Montie JE: Male infertility: An optimistic report. J Urol 110:216, 1973.

Stockamp K, Schreiter F, Altwein JE: a-Adrenergic drugs in retrograde ejaculation. Fertil Steril 25:817, 1974.

Tagatz GE, Okagaki T, Sciarra JJ: The effect of vaginal lubricants on sperm motility and viability in vitro. Am J Obst Gynec 113:88, 1972.

Timmermans L: Influence of antibiotics on spermatogenesis. J Urol 112:348, 1974.

Ulstein M: Fertility of husbands at homologous insemination. Acta obst gynec scandinav 52:5, 1973.

VanderVliet WL: Survival and aging of spermatozoa: A review. Am J Obst Gynec 118:1006, 1974.

Wong TW, Straus FH, Warner NE: Testicular biopsy in the study of male infertility. 1. Testicular causes of infertility. Arch Path 95:151, 1973.

Vasectomy

Albert PS & others: The nitrofurans as sperm immobilizing agents. J Urol 113:69, 1975.

Ansbacher R, Keung-Yeung K, Wurster JC: Sperm antibodies in vasectomized men. Fertil Steril 23:640, 1972.

Craft I, McQueen J: Effect of irrigation of the vas on post-vasectomy semen-counts. Lancet 1:515, 1972.

Esho JO, Cass AS, Ireland GW: Morbidity associated with vasectomy. J Urol 110:413, 1974.

Esho JO, Ireland GW, Cass AS: Recanalization following vasectomy. Urology 3:211, 1974.

Esho JO, Ireland GW, Cass AS: Vasectomy: Comparison of ligation and fulgeration methods. Urology 3:337, 1974.

Friberg J, Gemzell C: Inseminations of human sperm after freezing in liquid nitrogen vapors with glycerol or glycerol-egg-yolk-citrate as protection media. Am J Obst Gynec 116:330, 1973.

Howard PJ Jr, James LP: Immunological implications of vasectomy. J Urol 109:76, 1973.

Hulka JF, Davis JE: Vasectomy and reversible vasocclusion. Fertil Steril 23:683, 1972.

Kaplan KA, Huether CA: A clinical study of vasectomy failure and recanalization. J Urol 113:71, 1975.

Kase S, Goldfarb M: Office vasectomy: Review of 500 cases. Urology 1:60, 1973.

Klapproth HJ, Young IS: Vasectomy, vas ligation and vas occlusion. Urology 1:292, 1973.

Kwart AM, Coffey DS: Sperm granulomas: An adverse effect of vasectomy. J Urol 110:416, 1973.

Leader AJ & others: Complications of 2711 vasectomies. J Urol 111:365, 1974.

Lear H: Psychosocial characteristics of patients requesting vasectomy. J Urol 108:767, 1972.

Marshall S, Lyon RP: Transient reappearance of sperm after vasectomy. JAMA 219:1753, 1972.

Marshall S, Lyon RP: Variability of sperm disappearance from the ejaculate after vasectomy. J Urol 107:815, 1972.

Nash JL, Rich JD: The sexual aftereffects of vasectomy. Fertil Steril 23:715, 1972.

Rosenberg E & others: Serum levels of follicle stimulating and luteinizing hormones before and after vasectomy in men. J Urol 111:626, 1974.

Schmidt SS: Vasectomy should not fail. Contemporary Surg 4:13, 1074.

Schmidt SS & others: Vas cautery: Battery powered instrument for vasectomy. Urology 3:604, 1974.

Sherman JK: Synopsis of the use of frozen human semen since 1964: State of the art of human semen banking. Fertil Steril 24:397, 1973.

Smith KD, Steinberger E: Survival of spermatozoa in a human sperm bank. JAMA 223:774, 1973.

Tyler ET: The clinical use of frozen semen banks. Fertil Steril 24:413, 1973.

Uehling DT, Wear JB: Patient attitudes towards vasectomy. Fertil Steril 23:838, 1972.

Wieland RG & others: Pituitary-gonadal function before and after vasectomy. Fertil Steril 23:779, 1972.

Impotence

Bancroft J: Sexual inadequacy in the male. Postgrad MJ 47:562, 1971.

Bias HI & others: Implantable penile prosthesis in impotent males. Urology 5:224, 1975.

Bors E, Comarr AE: *Neurological Urology: Physiology of Micturition, Its Neurological Disorders and Sequelae.* Univ Park Press, 1971.

Comarr AE: Sexual concepts in traumatic cord and cauda equina lesions. J Urol 106:375, 1971.

Cooper AJ & others: Androgen function in "psychogenic" and "constitutional" types of impotence. Brit MJ 3:17, 1970.

Cooper AJ: Diagnosis and management of "endocrine impotence." Brit MJ 2:34, 1972.

Dahlen CP, Goodwin WE: Sexual potency after perineal biopsy. J Urol 77:660, 1957.

Ellenberg M: Impotence in diabetes: The neurologic factor. Ann Int Med 75:213, 1971.

Fitzpatrick TJ: Venography of the deep dorsal venous and valvular systems. J Urol 111:518, 1974.

Gaskell P: The importance of penile blood pressure in cases of impotence. Canad MAJ 105:1047, 1971.

Gee WF & others: The impotent patient: Surgical treatment with penile prosthesis and psychiatric evaluation. J Urol 111:41, 1974.

Gibson GR: Impotence following fractured pelvis and ruptured urethra. Brit J Urol 42:86, 1970.

Hinman F Jr: Priapism: Reasons for failure of therapy. J Urol 83:420, 1960.

Lash H: Silicone implant for impotence. J Urol 100:709, 1968.

Lawrence DM, Swyer GIM: Plasma testosterone and testosterone binding affinities in men with impotence, oligospermia, azoospermia, and hypogonadism. Brit J Med 1:349, 1974.

Malvar T, Baron T, Clark SS: Assessment of potency with the Doppler flowmeter. Urology 2:396, 1973.

Manfredi RA, Leal JF: Selective sacral rhizotomy for the spastic bladder syndrome in patients with spinal cord injuries. J Urol 100:17, 1968.

Masters WH, Johnson VE: *Human Sexual Inadequacy.* Little, Brown, 1970.

Pearman RO: Insertion of a silastic penile prothesis for the treatment of organic sexual impotence. J Urol 107:802, 1972.

Ross JC: Treatment of the bladder in paraplegia. Brit J Urol 28:14, 1956.

Sabri S, Cotton LT: Sexual function following aortoiliac reconstruction. Lancet 2:1218, 1971.

Scott FB, Bradley WE, Timm GW: Management of erectile impotence: Use of implantable prosthesis. Urology 2:80, 1973.

Shader RI: Sexual dysfunction associated with thioridazine hydrochloride. JAMA 188:1007, 1964.

Small MP, Carrion HM, Gordon JA: Small-Carrion penile prosthesis: New implant for management of impotence. Urology 5:479, 1975.

Smith DR, Auerback A: Functional diseases. Pages 34—57 in: *Encyclopedia of Urology.* Vol 12. Springer-Verlag, 1960.

Stewart BL: Impotence in the male. J Lancet 83:2, 1963.

Stewart BH, Bergant JA: Correction of retrograde ejaculation by sympathomimetic medication: Preliminary report. Fertil Steril 25:1073, 1974.

Weiss HD: The physiology of human penile erection. Ann Int Med 76:793, 1972.

34...
Psychosomatic Urinary Frequency & Retention

Psychologic disturbances are not infrequently reflected in dysfunction of the bladder and kidneys. Little literature on this subject is available to the interested clinician despite the fact that such aberrations of function of the gastrointestinal tract, cardiovascular and respiratory systems, and skin are well documented. These organ systems are affected by various hormones as well as autonomic nerve impulses which affect the tone of smooth muscle. Since the bladder is also innervated by the parasympathetics and is composed of smooth muscle, one might expect the development of vesical spasm or atony under conditions of stress. Kidney function is influenced by changes in renal blood flow and by various hormones, including antidiuretic hormone (ADH), aldosterone, and epinephrine.

Both hormonal and autonomic influences on urinary tract function have been recorded in the literature. A summary of this literature is included in the discussions of specific entities that are the subject matter of this chapter.

EFFECTS OF THE PSYCHE
ON VESICAL FUNCTION

Mosso and Pellacani in 1881 were the first investigators to perform cystometry in both dogs and humans. They found that psychic stimuli had a profound effect on vesical tone and function. Such things as loud noises, the sound of running water, strong emotional reactions, or intense intellectual work caused vesical contractions.

Straub, Ripley, & Wolf (1949) studied, by cystometry, a group of neurotic patients who complained of vesical dysfunction. Small elevations of pressure occurred with cough or straining. When the patient was tranquil, the pressure remained low. If, however, the interviewer touched upon sensitive subjects (eg, relations with the husband, conditions of employment), intravesical pressure would immediately rise to 40–70 cm of water. When the conversation returned to more prosaic subjects, intravesical pressure returned to normal. Often, even though the patient complained of frequency, at the end of the interview the volume of fluid in the bladder, augmented by urine secretion, was apt to be 700 ml; yet the patient complained of no feeling of fullness.

In those patients who had gone into acute urinary retention without apparent previous urinary difficulty, cystometrograms showed vesical atony. After acute psychotherapy and resumption of voiding, the test reverted to normal.

The most common group were those complaining of frequency. They were found to be tense, anxious, and resentful. Those who suffered from urinary retention had feelings of hysteria and of being overwhelmed.

Many people develop acute vesical irritability under stress. A student may suffer from urinary frequency before final examinations. Even the female dog may wet the floor when the family returns from vacation.

EFFECTS OF THE PSYCHE
ON RENAL FUNCTION

Bloomstrand & Löfgren (1956) demonstrated the effects on renal blood flow associated with fear or rage. Catheters were passed to the level of the renal arteries of cats. In the controls, after the injection of India ink, diffuse staining of the renal cortex and, to a lesser extent, the medulla was found. Seventeen such cats were then subjected to the trauma of a barking dog. The India ink was then infused. The renal cortices were blanched. The authors believed that this phenomenon was caused by liberation of epinephrine. They noted that Homer Smith had recorded altered diuretic reactions which he thought were secondary to psychogenic renal vasoconstriction. They cited the work of Bycow and Alexjew-Berkman, who had dogs drink water while a bell rang. Once the conditioned reflex had been established, merely ringing the bell led to diuresis.

Levi (1956) studied the urinary excretions of epinephrine and norepinephrine in various psychologic states. Women were shown moving pictures that contained some exciting episodes. In the tranquil portions, catecholamine excretion was low. During the more exciting scenes or those leading to anxiety, the urinary catecholamines rose significantly.

DeMaria & others (1963) performed isotope renograms on a group of students. When feelings of fear or anxiety were induced, the renograms were compatible with an increased secretion of catecholamines.

Verney (1958) and Wakim (1967) showed that emotional tension causes increased secretion of ADH. Tranquility led to diuresis. Schottstaedt, Grace, & Wolff (1956) studied the excretion of water and electrolytes in a group of neurotic people. They found that when patients were subjected to stress, diuresis or antidiuresis occurred. When the patient was alert and tense (eg, occupied by intellectual work), urinary excretion fell 20%. Return to tranquility was followed by diuresis. If, however, the patient became angry, a 300% increase in urine excretion was immediately observed. If, on the other hand, the patient was listless and depressed, 30% less urine was passed. A return to normal feelings was accompanied by diuresis.

Barnes & Schottstaedt (1960) noted that patients with congestive heart failure retained even more water and salt if they suffered from excitement, anger, or apprehension.

Gerbner, Altman, & Mészáros (1959) hypnotized a group of patients and had them drink water. The point came when drinking from an empty glass resulted in diuresis.

The experimental work quoted above makes it clear that vesical function—both of the detrusor and of the sphincters—is influenced by psychic stimuli and that renal function is affected by changes in the secretion of catecholamines and ADH.

Jules Janet published a monograph on the effects of the psyche on vesical observations. Montassut, Chertok, & Aboulker (1951) and Chertok, Aboulker, & Cahen (1952) have written excellent studies.

PSYCHOGENIC SPASTIC BLADDER REACTION

Clinical Findings

The majority of these patients are women. A few cases occur in children. It would appear that during childhood each person develops pathways to an organ and that later, when under tension or anxiety, he expresses his tensions or anger through that organ. A history of prolonged enuresis is often obtained. Men are more apt to develop peptic ulcer.

A. Symptoms: An anxious patient complains of periodic frequency, mostly in the morning. It may be noticed for a few days and then subside spontaneously. Comparable nocturia is absent. With an attack, urgency to the point of incontinence may occur (Jeffcoate & Francis, 1966; Frewen, 1972). The patient may complain of "burning," but careful questioning reveals that

this sensation is not related to urination. It is probably secondary to spasm of the external urinary sphincter.

Frequency is initiated or increased following emotional upsets (eg, "scenes" with husband or children) and after sexual intercourse, which is, almost without exception, unsatisfactory. The common denominator seems to be unrelieved pelvic congestion precipitated by sexual frustration. A history of prolonged enuresis is often obtained.

Careful questioning reveals that the tense woman develops a small-capacity bladder so that she voids small amounts. Sleeping all night, however, she voids a normal volume on arising. It is this change in vesical capacity from hour to hour that affords an important clue to the psychosomatic spastic bladder.

Many of these women complain of obstructive voiding, but further questioning will reveal that, though some voidings are slow and hesitant, others are quite free. This rules out organic obstruction and can only be caused by periodic spasm of the striated external urinary sphincter as a result of tension.

Some patients may ask whether their "nerves" might cause these symptoms. Even if they do not, it is wise, when psychosomatic bladder reaction is suspected, to ask what they believe to be the cause. A surprising number will volunteer the information that they relate their attacks to acute emotional upsets.

B. Signs: The woman suffering from this syndrome tends to be aggressive, seemingly confident, yet tense and anxious. The men are usually meek and mild, with a poor sense of masculinity. The anal sphincter in women may be hypertonic. On vaginal examination, the urethra, the base of the bladder, and the cervix may be unduly sensitive but no lesion is found.

C. Laboratory Findings: Urinalysis is normal. Renal function is intact.

D. Instrumental Examination: Cystoscopy may be unduly painful (low pain threshold). The trigone and urethra may be hyperemic, often leading to the organic diagnosis of "urethrotrigonitis." These changes are secondary to pelvic congestion resulting from the incomplete sexual act. The bladder wall may be trabeculated. This change is secondary to spasm of the external urinary sphincter and must not be regarded as evidence of organic obstruction (eg, vesical neck stenosis). There is no residual urine. Cystometry may reveal a response compatible with uninhibited neurogenic bladder yet often, with reassurance, the capacity is found to be normal.

E. Recording of Intake and Output: Have the patient record, over a period of a few days, the time and volume of fluid intake and the time and volume of each voiding. During an attack, each urine volume in the morning may be 60–100 ml, whereas the rest of the day and at night the volumes are normal (350–400 ml). No organic disease will show this phenomenon.

Differential Diagnosis

Psychogenic diuresis (see below) also causes periodic morning frequency, but the volumes of each voiding are normal.

In true cystitis, both acute and chronic, the urine will contain bacteria. Frequency is consistent both day and night.

Nonspecific urethritis causes symptoms similar to those of bacterial cystitis. Symptoms are not periodic, nor do they occur only in the morning.

Senile urethritis may cause some vesical irritability or even stress incontinence, but symptoms are persistent. Senile vaginitis is observed, and the vaginal epithelium fails to stain with iodine.

Multiple sclerosis often causes aberrations in vesical function typified by urgency, frequency, and nocturia. These symptoms, however, are not periodic as are those caused by psychic stimuli.

Complications

Some cases of interstitial cystitis may actually be the end stage of the psychogenic bladder (Bowers, Schwartz, & Leon, 1958), though there is evidence that this disease may be due to an autoimmune collagen reaction.

Treatment

It is helpful to explain to these patients how "nerves" can play tricks on vesical function. They often fear that they have cancer or some other serious disease. Understanding the mechanism of the symptoms often allows them to accept such symptoms with equanimity. Since their troubles are secondary to significant psychosexual problems, they are best referred to a psychiatrist.

Anticholinergics taken during an attack may allay, in some degree, its severity.

Mistaken organic diagnoses are apt to lead to various empirical treatments, including urethral dilatations and even transurethral resection of the bladder neck. Such procedures are not only harmful but they further convince the patient that she has some serious disease.

Prognosis

This type of urinary frequency is difficult to relieve by medical means. Considerable relief is usually afforded by psychotherapy.

EFFECTS OF THE PSYCHE
ON VESICAL FUNCTION IN GIRLS

Little girls may suffer from the acute spastic bladder reaction, manifested by bouts of frequency and urgency. Enuresis is common in this group; even pantswetting may occur. Constipation is often noted. Voiding at times may seem obstructed yet at other times it is free (Malmquist, 1971; Galdston & Perlmutter, 1973). There are usually manifest behavioral problems which are further reflected in the parents' attitudes.

Urinalysis is usually negative, although, in the little girl who suffers from periodic spasm of the external sphincter, bacteria in the proximal urethra may be

washed back into the bladder by the resulting turbulent flow (see Distal Urethral Stenosis in Chapter 25). Excretory urograms are usually normal. The postvoiding film reveals no significant residual urine. If urethrocystoscopy is done, the findings are usually normal, though at times some vesical trabeculation secondary to sphincter spasm may be seen.

Bacterial cystitis is differentiated from this disorder because it usually is associated with urgency, frequency, nocturia, and burning on urination. Bacteriuria is found. There may be attacks of febrile pyelonephritis if vesicoureteral reflux is present.

No significant complications—except cystitis—are seen.

There is need for psychologic counseling of the parents. At times, the child may also require such guidance.

Most of these children respond to psychotherapy of their parents or themselves. Even without this, vesical irritability may subside by puberty. In adult life, however, under stressful situations, psychosomatic symptoms may recur.

EFFECTS OF THE PSYCHE
ON VESICAL FUNCTION IN BOYS

Two important papers dealing with this subject have been published recently (Hinman & Bauman, 1973; Bauman & Hinman, 1974). These authors recognize 2 groups of boys who have personality problems which lead to incoordination of the function of the vesical detrusor and its sphincters. All of these boys suffered from enuresis, pantswetting, urinary tract infection, and constipation with soiling. Secondary changes in the morphology of the urinary tract ranged from mild to severe.

Neurologic examination was normal in all patients. Thorough urologic survey failed to reveal any evidence of organic lower tract obstruction on endoscopy or voiding cystourography, though vesical trabeculation and residual urine were found. The majority (73 boys) had normal upper tracts without renal infection. Fourteen patients, however, had significant upper tract damage (hydroureteronephrosis) caused by ureterovesical obstruction, though a few did have vesicoureteral reflux (Fig 34–1 left).

These authors were impressed by the psychologic outlook of these patients. Their attitude was that of failure. They were shy, timid, depressed, and anxious. These observers concluded that the constipation, enuresis, residual urine, and urinary infection were secondary to spasm of the entire pelvic floor, including the external urinary sphincter which caused functional urethral obstruction.

In the more advanced cases, severe hypertrophy of the trigone led to functional ureteral obstruction caused by an increased pull on the ureterovesical junctions.

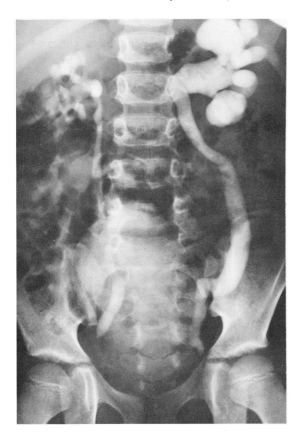 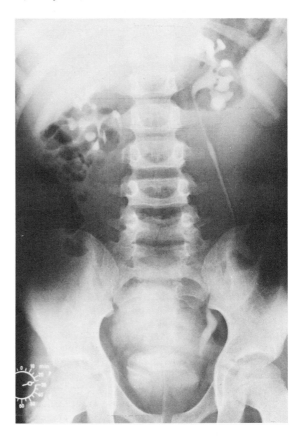

Figure 34—1. Pretreatment x-ray studies. *Left:* Excretory urogram showing dilated bladder reaching top of L5. Right ureter dilated throughout its length. Advanced hydroureteronephrosis, left. Voiding cystogram showed left vesicoureteral reflux. *Right:* Excretory urogram 1 year following institution of therapy. Right ureter now normal, left hydroureteronephrosis almost completely resolved. Cystogram negative. (Reproduced, with permission, from Hinman F, Baumann FW: Vesical and ureteral damage from voiding dysfunction in boys without neurologic or obstructive disease. J Urol 64:116, 1972.)

Treatment was given as follows: (1) Antibiotic therapy for the infection. (2) Anticholinergic medication. (Most efficacious was imipramine hydrochloride [Tofranil], 25 mg 4 times a day.) (3) Treatment of constipation with cleansing enemas followed by a stool softener at bedtime. (4) Instructing the parents to praise all successes but never to punish for wetting. They were taught to be positive in their approach, including giving rewards for dryness.

The physician must take a positive approach in his suggestions to the patient on how urinary function can be improved. The boy is encouraged to try hard to please himself (not the doctor or the parents). Positive suggestive therapy can be further enhanced by means of hypnosis.

In patients with lower tract findings only, 85% were relieved of all symptoms and infection. In the 14 boys with upper tract damage, all complaints were resolved, infection was eradicated, and moderate to marked improvement of the upper urinary tracts was demonstrated (Fig 34—1 right).

These authors warn against operation for this condition since the cause is functional and not organic.

ENURESIS

Enuresis originally meant "incontinence of urine," but usage has caused the term to be restricted to bedwetting after the age of 3 years. Most children have achieved normal bladder control by the age of 2½ years. Girls gain this control earlier than boys. At least 50% of cases are of psychic origin; 30% seem to be caused by delayed maturation of the nervous system or an intrinsic myoneurogenic bladder dysfunction; and perhaps 20% are secondary to more obvious organic disease. Most children with functional enuresis gain spontaneous nocturnal control by the age of 10 years.

Psychodynamics

Training in bladder control should begin after the age of 1½ years; attempts made before this are usually fruitless and may be harmful. If the parents fail in this teaching, the child may not develop cerebral inhibitory control over the infantile uninhibited bladder until much later in childhood. If the parents are emotionally unstable, their anxieties may be transmitted to the child, who may express his tensions through enuresis.

The birth of a sibling may cause a child to lose his paramount position in the family. He may then regress to an infancy pattern in order to recapture his parents' affection. An acute illness may be accompanied or followed by recurrence of incomplete nocturnal control. Physiologic or psychologic stress (fear and anxiety) may reestablish an uninhibited bladder.

Possibly 50% of enuretic children have electroencephalograms which are borderline or compatible with epilepsy. Many of these children have been shown to have bladders of small capacity.

Clinical Findings

A. Symptoms: The child may wet his bed occasionally or regularly. Careful questioning of the parents or observation by the physician reveals that the patient voids a free stream of normal caliber. This tends to rule out obstruction of the lower tract as a cause of the enuresis. Children with daytime incontinence usually have more than psychogenic enuresis.

There is no burning, although frequency and urgency are common. The urine is clear.

Careful observation of the parents usually reveals that they are anxious and tense; these traits are only increased by the child's bedwetting.

B. Signs: General physical and urologic examinations are normal.

C. Laboratory Findings: In the emotional group, all tests, including urinalysis, are normal. An electroencephalogram may be abnormal, however.

D. X-Ray Findings: Excretory urograms show no abnormality. The accompanying cystogram reveals no trabeculation; a film of the bladder taken immediately after voiding shows no residual urine.

E. Instrumental Examination: A catheter of suitable size passes readily to the bladder, thereby ruling out stricture. If passed after urination, no residual urine is found. Urethrocystoscopy is normal. Cystometric studies are usually normal, but a curve typical of the "uninhibited" (hyperirritable) neurogenic bladder (Fig 19–4) is often obtained.

Differential Diagnosis

A. Obstruction: Lower tract obstruction (eg, posterior urethral valves, meatal stenosis) causes a urinary stream of decreased caliber. Painful, frequent urination during the day and night, pyuria, and fever (eg, pyelonephritis) are often present, and the bladder may be distended. Urinalysis almost always reveals evidence of infection. Anemia and impairment of renal function may be demonstrated.

Excretory urograms may show dilatation of the bladder and the upper urinary tract. Incomplete vesical emptying may be seen on the postvoiding film. Cystography may demonstrate distal urethral stenosis or reflux. Urethrocystoscopy will reveal the organic cause.

Severe obstruction from severe spasm of the entire pelvic floor musculature on a psychosomatic basis can cause damage to the bladder and kidneys; infection is the rule.

B. Infection: Chronic urinary tract infection not due to obstruction usually produces frequency both day and night and pain on urination, although such infections may occur without symptoms of vesical irritability. Recurrent fever with exacerbations is common.

General examination may be normal. Anemia may be noted. Urinalysis will show pus cells or bacteria, or both. Renal function may be deficient. Excretory urograms may be essentially normal, although changes compatible with healed pyelonephritis are often seen. Cystoscopy will show the changes caused by infection. Urine specimens obtained by urethral catheter may reveal renal infection. Cystography may show vesicoureteral reflux.

C. Neurogenic Disease: Children suffering from sacral cord or root abnormality (eg, myelodysplasia) may have incomplete urinary control both day and night. Since they ordinarily have significant amounts of residual urine, infection is usually found on urinalysis. The passage of a catheter, or the postvoiding film taken in conjunction with excretory urograms, will demonstrate the presence of residual urine. A plain film of the abdomen may reveal spina bifida.

The cystometrogram is usually typical of a flaccid neurogenic bladder. Cystoscopy demonstrates an atonic bladder, with moderate trabeculation and evidence of infection.

D. Distal Urethral Stenosis: This congenital anomaly is the cause of enuresis in many young girls, even in the absence of cystitis. Urethral calibration will establish this diagnosis.

Complications

The complications of functional enuresis are psychic, not organic. These children are particularly disturbed when they begin to attend school. Even more pressure is brought to bear by their parents; the child finds it impossible to stay overnight at the homes of his playmates. Unhealthy introversion may be his lot. Enuresis may be prolonged because of undue emphasis on dryness or as a result of punitive or shaming measures.

Late Sequelae

Occasionally an adult is seen who, under stress, develops nocturnal frequency without comparable diurnal frequency. Thorough urologic investigation proves to be negative. Many of these people will give histories of enuresis of long duration in childhood. It is suggested that their cerebrovesical pathways again break down under undue emotional tension; nocturnal frequency may be the adult expression of enuresis.

Treatment

Treatment should be considered if enuresis persists after the age of 3 years.

A. General Measures: Fluids should be limited after supper. The child should empty his bladder at bedtime and be completely awakened a little before the usual time of bedwetting and allowed to void.

Drug therapy has its proponents.

1. Imipramine has been reported to cure 50–70% of patients and is probably the drug of choice. Start with 25 mg at bedtime. Increase the dose as needed to 50 mg. Twenty-five mg usually suffice.

2. Parasympatholytic drugs such as atropine or belladonna, by decreasing the tone of the detrusor, may at times be of value. Methantheline bromide, 25–75 mg at bedtime, is more potent.

3. Sympathomimetic drugs, eg, dextroamphetamine sulfate, 5–10 mg at bedtime, may cause enough wakefulness so that the child perceives the urge to void.

4. Diphenylhydantoin has been found to control some of those children whose electroencephalograms are abnormal.

5. The use of mechanical devices such as metal-covered pads which when wet cause an alarm to ring may be of benefit in cases of delayed maturation by setting up a conditioned reflex.

6. Urologic treatments (eg, urethral dilatation, urethral instillations of silver nitrate), though often recommended, should be condemned in the absence of demonstrable local disease. They are physically and psychically traumatic and can only cause further apprehension and fear in an already disturbed child.

B. Psychotherapy: Analytic evaluation and treatment may be indicated for the child and his parents. Responsibility for correction of the patient's feelings of insecurity rests with the parents, who must be cautioned not to punish the child nor in any way contribute further to his feelings of guilt and insecurity. The handling of the parents may prove difficult, in which case psychiatric referral may be necessary.

Prognosis

Retraining the enuretic child and, above all, reeducating the parents is difficult and time-consuming. Psychiatric referral for the parents and, at times, for the child may be necessary. Most patients conquer their enuresis by the age of 10 years. A few, however, do not, and may later develop vesical irritability of the psychogenic type in response to acute or chronic tension or anxiety.

PSYCHOGENIC URINARY RETENTION

This phenomenon is much less common than acute spastic bladder reaction. The majority of patients are women, though the author has observed psychogenic urinary retention in homosexuals following acute psychosexual stress. Women who suffer from sudden urinary retention express feelings of being overwhelmed (eg, the threat of rape) and exhibit severe depressive reactions.

Typically, the patient has been voiding in a perfectly normal manner when, suddenly, acute urinary retention occurs. It is difficult to think of any organic disease that would cause this symptom in an otherwise well person. The patient may give a history of periodic difficulty with urination, suggesting external sphincter spasm.

The patient appears depressed. Some acute psychologic trauma precipitated the attack. Abdominal examination will usually reveal a distended bladder. Neurologic examination is normal. Urinalysis and renal function tests are normal.

A catheter passes to the bladder with ease. A cystometrogram usually reveals changes compatible with an atonic bladder. Cystoscopy may reveal some trabeculation secondary to prolonged intermittent sphincter spasm. The urethra is normal.

An acute neurologic deficit (eg, stroke, trauma) may cause urinary retention, but neurologic signs are usually obvious. Postoperative urinary retention usually responds to one or more catheterizations.

Bacterial cystitis may occur as a complication resulting from periodic catheterization or the use of an indwelling catheter.

Intermittent catheterization is mandatory until normal vesical function returns. Prophylactic antimicrobial therapy should be considered.

Psychosomatic urinary retention usually responds well to acute psychotherapy, but further analysis is required to solve these patients' basic difficulties.

Cholinergic drugs (eg, bethanechol chloride) may be tried, but in the author's experience little is to be gained. Allen (1972), suspecting severe spasm of the external urinary sphincter in his 6 patients, observed spontaneous voiding after bilateral block of the pudendal nerves.

The diagnosis of some organic disease (eg, urethral or vesical neck stenosis) leads to useless empirical therapy that further convinces the patient that a serious local lesion exists. Such therapy should be condemned.

Prolonged psychotherapy may be required because of these patients' basic psychologic problems. In the author's experience, most patients respond.

PSYCHOSOMATIC ANTIDIURESIS–DIURESIS

Most patients suffering from periodic diuresis are women. They may be tense, anxious, and seemingly competent. On the other hand, some are subdued and repressed.

Clinical Findings

A. Symptoms: These patients complain of periodic frequency, mostly in the morning; there is usually no nocturia. A few, however, may note significant periodic nocturia without day frequency. Questioning reveals that, during the attacks of frequency, each voiding is of normal volume—in contrast to acute spastic bladder reaction. Such a history immediately suggests diuresis as the cause.

The patient should be asked about significant changes in body weight (most women have bathroom scales). There is usually a history of weight gain of 2–5 kg over a period of 2–4 days. After the inevitable diuresis, weight returns promptly to normal. As weight increases, signs of edema appear: rings tightening on the fingers, ankle swelling, and puffy facies. These changes subside following diuresis. This type of history is pathognomonic of the syndrome.

The attack usually follows an acute emotional experience (eg, an argument with husband, an incomplete sexual act, trouble with the children at school). It resolves when tension or anxiety subsides.

With anger or rage, immediate diuresis may occur without the usual antecedent antidiuresis.

B. Signs: Examination reveals little unless the patient is in an antidiuretic stage, in which case evidence of fluid retention may be noted.

C. Laboratory Findings: Noncontributory.

D. Instrumental Findings: Urethrocystoscopy hardly seems indicated, and in any case the findings are normal.

E. Recording of Intake and Output: Have the patient record the time and volume of fluid taken and voided as well as the body weight both morning and night for a few days. The typical response is a gradual increase in body weight and relative oliguria. When diuresis occurs, the patient will void frequent but normal volumes of urine over a period of 3–4 hours in the morning; weight is normal by evening.

Differential Diagnosis

Patients suffering from acute spastic bladder reaction have frequency in the morning but each voiding is of small volume.

Organic diseases of the bladder tend to cause frequency both day and night; their symptoms are not periodic. These include either a contracted bladder, significant residual urine, or bladder infection.

Complications

The only complications are those that may occur as a result of misdiagnosis and the employment of organic therapy (eg, transurethral resection of the bladder neck).

Treatment

Most patients are helped by an explanation of the cause of the diuresis. Some relief may be gained by limiting salt intake. When the patient notes the beginning of an increase in body weight, administration of a diuretic may abort the attack. Psychotherapy, however, should be encouraged, for these patients have significant psychosexual problems.

Prognosis

The treatment outlined above tends to ease or abolish the attacks. Even if attacks of frequency recur, these patients are better able to live with the problem if they understand the mechanism. Women often understand better than men the relationship between emotions and bodily functions.

COMPULSIVE POLYDIPSIA

Another cause of frequency of urination is drinking large volumes of fluid, which may not be consciously recognized by the patient. Some mothers teach their children that the kidneys are as dirty as the bowel and therefore must be flushed clean. Thus, polydipsia may begin in childhood. Some tense, nervous people develop a dry mouth which they confuse with thirst, and this may lead to excessive fluid intake.

The patient complains of frequency day and night. Questioning reveals that each voiding is of good volume. There is no burning or other symptom. The patient may deny polydipsia. Most revealing on urinalysis is a consistently low specific gravity, approaching 1.000. Infection is absent.

Excretory urograms are usually normal, though some hydroureteronephrosis may be noted (as in diabetes insipidus) because more urine is excreted than the ureterovesical junctions can pass.

Instruct the patient to record the time and volume of each fluid intake and the time and volume of each voiding. The typical patient will reveal an intake of 6–8 liters of fluid and frequent voidings of 350–450 ml. This establishes the diagnosis.

Despite the physiologic explanation given the patient, he may have difficulty in reducing his fluid intake to normal. Chapdelaine & Lanthier (1963) have described 2 such patients who finally lost their power to concentrate urine. Psychotherapy may be needed to bring about cure.

•   •   •

References

General

Smith DR, Auerback A: Functional diseases. Pages 1–57 in: *Encyclopedia of Urology.* Vol 12. Springer, 1960.

Turner RD, Bors E: Some interesting observations in neurological urology. Urol Internat 16:30, 1963.

Effects of Psyche on Vesical Function

Allen JD: Psychogenic urinary retention. South MJ 65:302, 1972.

Straub LR, Ripley HS, Wolf S: Disturbances of bladder function associated with emotional states. JAMA 141:1139, 1949.

Zufall R: Treatment of the urethral syndrome in women. JAMA 184:894, 1963.

Effects of Psyche on Renal Function

Barnes R, Schottstaedt WW: The relation of emotional state to renal excretion of water and electrolytes in patients with congestive heart failure. Am J Med 29:217, 1960.

Blomstrand R, Löfgren F: Influence of emotional stress on the renal circulation. Psychosom Med 18:420, 1956.

Chertok L, Aboulker P, Cahen M: Perspectives psychosomatiques en urologie. Evol Psychiatr 3:457, 1953.

DeMaria WJA & others: Renal conditioning. Psychosom Med 25:538, 1963.

Dykman RA & others: Inhibition of urine flow as a component of the conditioned defense reaction. Psychosom Med 24:177, 1962.

Gerbner M, Altman K, Mészáros I: The mechanism of the increase in diuresis induced by hypnotic suggestion. J Psychosom Res 3:282, 1959.

Janet J: Les troubles psychopathiques de la miction. Essai de psycho-physiologie normale et pathologique. Librairie Lefrançais (Paris), 1890.

Levi L: The urinary output of adrenalin and noradrenalin during pleasant and unpleasant emotional states. Psychosom Med 27:80, 1965.

Montassut ML, Chertok L, Aboulker P: De quelques investigations psychiatriques en urologie. Sem Hôp Paris 27:3002, 1951.

Schottstaedt WW, Grace WJ, Wolff HG: Life situations, behavior, attitudes, emotions and renal excretion of fluid and electrolytes. (5 parts.) J Psychosom Res 1:75, 147, 203, 287, 292, 1956.

Verney EB: Some aspects of water and electrolyte excretion. Surg Gynec Obst 106:441, 1958.

Wakim KG: Reassessment of the source, mode and locus of action of antidiuretic hormone. Am J Med 42:394, 1967.

Psychogenic Spastic Bladder Reaction

Bowers JE, Schwarz BE, Leon MJ: Masochism and interstitial cystitis: Report of case. Psychosom Med 20:296, 1958.

Frewen WK: Urgency incontinence: Review of 100 cases. J Obstet Gynaec Brit Common 79:77, 1972.

Jeffcoate TNA, Francis WJA: Urgency incontinence in the female. Am J Obst Gynec 94:604, 1966.

Effects of the Psyche on Vesical Function in Girls

Galdston R, Perlmutter AD: The urinary manifestations of anxiety in child. Pediatrics 52:818, 1973.

Malmquist CP: Hysteria in childhood. Postgrad Med 50:112, 1971.

Effects of the Psyche on Vesical Function in Boys

Baumann FW, Hinman F: Treatment of incontinent boys with non-obstructive disease. J Urol 111:114, 1974.

Hinman F: Urinary tract damage in children who wet. Pediatrics 54:143, 1974.

Hinman F, Baumann FW: Vesical and ureteral damage from voiding dysfunction in boys without neurologic or obstructive disease. J Urol 109:727, 1973.

Psychogenic Urinary Retention

Allen JD: Psychogenic urinary retention. South MJ 65:302, 1972.

Khan AU: Psychogenic urinary retention in a boy. J Urol 106:432, 1971.

Larson JW & others: Psychogenic urinary retention in women. JAMA 184:697, 1963.

Wahl CM, Golden JS: Psychogenic urinary retention. Psychosom Med 25:543, 1973.

Enuresis

Andersen OO, Petersen KE: Enuresis: An attempt at classification of genesis. Acta paediat scandinav 63:512, 1974.

Arnold ST, Ginsburg A: Enuresis: Incidence and pertinence of genitourinary disease in healthy enuretic children. Urology 2:437, 1973.

Butcher C, Donnai D: Vaginal reflux and enuresis. Brit J Radiol 45:501, 1972.

Campbell EW, Young JD Jr: Enuresis and its relationship to electroencephalographic disturbances. J Urol 96:947, 1966.

Forsythe WI, Redmond A: Enuresis and spontaneous cure rate: Study of 1129 enuretics. Arch Dis Childhood 49:259, 1974.

Fraser MS: Nocturnal enuresis. Practitioner 208:203, 1972.

Gibbon NO & others: Transection of the bladder for adult enuresis and allied conditions. Brit J Urol 45:306, 1973.

Linderholm BE: The cystometric findings in enuresis. J Urol 96:718, 1966.

Marshall S, Marshall HH, Lyon RP: Enuresis: An analysis of various therapeutic approaches. Pediatrics 52:813, 1973.

Martin GI: Imipramine pamoate in the treatment of childhood enuresis. Am J Dis Child 122:42, 1971.

Murphy S & others: Adolescent enuresis: A multiple contingency hypothesis. JAMA 218:1189, 1971.

Oppel WC, Harper PA, Rider RV: Social, psychological, and neurological factors associated with nocturnal enuresis. Pediatrics 42:627, 1968.

Compulsive Polydipsia

Chapdelaine A, Lanthier A: Compulsive polydipsia with defective renal concentrating powers. Canad MAJ 88:1184, 1963.

Linshaw MA, Hipp T, Gruskin A: Infantile psychogenic water drinking. J Pediat 85:520, 1974.

Stevko RM, Balsley M, Segar WE: Primary polydipsia: Compulsive water drinking. J Pediat 73:845, 1968.

Index